# Foundations of Maternal & Pediatric Nursing

## Third Edition

# DEDICATIONS

**Lois White:**
To my beloved husband, John, who is on his last great adventure and learning experience.

**Gena Duncan:**
To my husband, who gives me unconditional love and brings balance, calmness, and excitement to my life.
To Lois White, who modeled the role of an author and committed much of her life to this textbook.
To Wendy Baumle, for her hard work and dedication in developing this textbook. Thanks.
To future nurses who are caring and competent.

**Wendy Baumle:**
This book is dedicated to my beloved family—Patrick, Taylor, Madeline, Blair, Connor, Janet, and Robert—for their love and support, to Juliet Steiner for inspiring me and for making a difference in my life, to Gena Duncan for her guidance and friendship, and to my friends, colleagues, and students for their support and valuable insight into today's nursing education.

# Foundations of Maternal & Pediatric Nursing

## Third Edition

### Lois White, RN, PhD
Former Chairperson and Professor Department of Vocational Nurse Education, Del Mar College, Corpus Christi, Texas

### Gena Duncan, RN, MSEd, MSN
Former Associate Professor of Nursing, Ivy Tech Community College, Fort Wayne, Indiana

### Wendy Baumle, RN, MSN
James A. Rhodes State College, School of Nursing, Lima, Ohio

CENGAGE
Learning™

Australia • Brazil • Japan • Korea • Mexico • Singapore • Spain • United Kingdom • United States

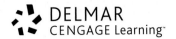
**DELMAR**
CENGAGE Learning

**Foundations of Maternal & Pediatric Nursing, Third Edition**
**Lois White, RN, PhD, Gena Duncan, RN, MSEd, MSN, and Wendy Baumle, RN, MSN**

Vice President, Career and Professional Editorial: Dave Garza

Director of Learning Solutions: Matt Kane

Executive Editor: Steven Helba

Managing Editor: Marah Bellegarde

Senior Product Manager: Juliet Steiner

Editorial Assistant: Meghan E. Orvis

Vice President, Career and Professional Marketing: Jennifer Ann Baker

Marketing Director: Wendy Mapstone

Senior Marketing Manager: Michele McTighe

Marketing Coordinator: Scott Chrysler

Production Director: Carolyn Miller

Production Manager: Andrew Crouth

Senior Content Project Manager: James Zayicek

Senior Art Director: Jack Pendleton

Technology Project Manager: Mary Colleen Liburdi

Production Technology Analyst: Patricia Allen

Production Technology Analyst: Ben Knapp

For product information and technology assistance, contact us at
**Cengage Learning Customer & Sales Support, 1-800-354-9706**
For permission to use material from this text or product,
submit all requests online at **www.cengage.com/permissions**.
Further permissions questions can be e-mailed to
**permissionrequest@cengage.com**

Library of Congress Control Number: 2010920488
ISBN-13: 978-1-428-31776-5
ISBN-10: 1-428-31776-7

**Delmar**
5 Maxwell Drive
Clifton Park, NY 12065-2919
USA

Cengage Learning is a leading provider of customized learning solutions with office locations around the globe, including Singapore, the United Kingdom, Australia, Mexico, Brazil, and Japan. Locate your local office at: **international.cengage.com/region**

Cengage Learning products are represented in Canada by Nelson Education, Ltd.

To learn more about Delmar, visit **www.cengage.com/delmar**

Purchase any of our products at your local college store or at our preferred online store **www.CengageBrain.com**

**Notice to the Reader**

Publisher does not warrant or guarantee any of the products described herein or perform any independent analysis in connection with any of the product information contained herein. Publisher does not assume, and expressly disclaims, any obligation to obtain and include information other than that provided to it by the manufacturer. The reader is expressly warned to consider and adopt all safety precautions that might be indicated by the activities described herein and to avoid all potential hazards. By following the instructions contained herein, the reader willingly assumes all risks in connection with such instructions. The publisher makes no representations or warranties of any kind, including but not limited to, the warranties of fitness for particular purpose or merchantability, nor are any such representations implied with respect to the material set forth herein, and the publisher takes no responsibility with respect to such material. The publisher shall not be liable for any special, consequential, or exemplary damages resulting, in whole or part, from the readers' use of, or reliance upon, this material.

Printed in the United States of America
1 2 3 4 5 6 7 12 11 10

# CONTENTS

## UNIT 1

## Nursing Care of the Client: Childbearing / 1

### CHAPTER 1: PRENATAL CARE / 2

## CHAPTER 3:  THE BIRTH
PROCESS / 70

# UNIT 2

# Nursing Care of the Client: Childrearing / 169

## CHAPTER 6: BASICS OF PEDIATRIC CARE / 170

## CHAPTER 7: INFANTS WITH SPECIAL NEEDS: BIRTH TO 12 MONTHS / 189

# CHAPTER 8: COMMON PROBLEMS:1 TO 18 YEARS / 232

# CONTRIBUTORS

**Jennifer Einhorn, MS, RN**
Nursing Instructor
Chamberlain College of Nursing
Addison, IL
  *Chapter 4, Postpartum Care*
  *Chapter 5, Newborn Care*

**Mary Jane Hamilton, RN, C, PhD**
Professor of Nursing
Texas A&M University-Corpus Christi
Corpus Christi, TX
  *Chapter 6, Basics of Pediatric Care*

**Carla McCuan MS, RN**
Sanford Brown College
St. Peters, MO
  *Chapter 1, Prenatal Care*

**Patricia Sunderhaus, MSN, RN**
Senior Instructor, Nursing
Brown Mackie College
Cincinnati, OH
  *Chapter 6, Basics of Pediatric Care*
  *Chapter 8, Common Problems: 1 to 18 Years*

**Donna Wofford, RN, PhD**
Professor
Department of RN Education
Del Mar College
Corpus Christi, TX
  *Chapter 7, Infants with Special Needs: Birth to 12 Months*
  *Chapter 8, Common Problems: 1 to 18 Years*

**Zayda Yeoh, RN, MSN**
Practical Nursing Department Chair
Brown Mackie College
Fort Wayne, IN
  *Chapter 7, Infants with Special Needs: Birth to 12 Months*

# REVIEWERS

**Charlene Bell, RN, MSN, NCSN**
Instructor
Associate Degree Nursing Program
Southwest Texas Junior College
Uvalde, TX

**Donna Burleson, RN, MS**
Chair of Nursing Department
Cisco Junior College
Abilene, TX

**Dotty Cales, RN**
Instructor
North Coast Medical Training Academy
Kent, OH

**Carolyn Du, BSN, MSN, NP, CDe**
Director of Education
Pacific College
Costa Mesa, CA

**Jennifer Einhorn, RN, MS**
Nursing Instructor
Chamberlain College of Nursing
Addison, IL

**Patricia Fennessy, RN, MSN**
Education Consultant
Connecticut Technical High School
  System
Middletown, CT

**Helena L. Jermalovic, RN, MSN**
Assistant Professor
University of Alaska
Anchorage, AK

**Sharon Knarr, RN**
Clinical Instructor
LPN Program
Northcoast Medical Training
  Academy
Kent, OH

**Christine Levandowski,
  RN, BSN, MSN**
Director of Nursing
Baker College
Auburn Hills, MI

**Wendy Maleki, RN, MS**
Director
Vocational Nursing Program
American Career College
Ontario, CA

**Katherine C. Pellerin, RN,
  BS, MS**
Department Head LPN Program
Norwich Technical High School
Norwich, CT

**Jennifer Ponto, RN, BSN**
Faculty
Vocational Nursing Program
South Plains College
Levelland, TX

**Cheryl Pratt, RN, MA,
  CNAA**
Regional Dean of Nursing
Rasmussen College
Mankato, MN

**Cherie R. Rebar, RN, MSN,
  MBA, FNP**
Chair, Associate Professor, Nursing
  Program
Kettering College of Medical Arts
Kettering, OH

**Patricia Schrull, RN, MSN, MBA,
  MEd, CNE**
Director, Practical Nursing Program
Lorain County Community College
Elyria, OH

**Laura Spinelli**
Keiser Career College
Miami Lakes, FL

**Frances S. Stoner, RN, BSN, PHN**
Instructor, NCLEX® Coordintor
American Career College
Anaheim, CA

**Tina Terpening**
Associate Nursing Faculty
University of Phoenix, Southern
  California Campus

**Lori Theodore, RN, BSN**
Orlando Tech
Orlando, FL

**Kimberly Valich, RN, MSN**
Nursing Faculty, Department
  Chairperson
South Suburban College
South Holland, IL

Sarah Elizabeth Youth
Whitaker, DNS, RN
Nursing Program Director
Computer Career Center
El Paso, TX

Shawn White, RN, BSN
Clinical Coordinator, Nursing
Instructor
Griffin Technical College
Griffin, GA

Christina R. Wilson, RN, BAN,
PHN
Faculty, Practical Nursing Program
Anoka Technical College
Anoka, MN

## MARKET REVIEWERS AND CLASS TEST PARTICIPANTS

Deborah Ain
Nursing Professor
College of Southern Nevada
Las Vegas, NV

Mary Ann Ambrose, MSN, FNP
Program Director
Cuesta Community College Vocational
Nursing Program
Paso Robles, CA

Jennie Applegate, RN, BSN
Practical Nursing Instructor
Keiser Career College
Greenacres, FL

Charlotte A. Armstrong, RN, BSN
Instructor
Northcoast Medical Training Academy
Kent, OH

Camille Baldwin
High Tech Central
Fort Myers, FL

Priscilla Burks, RN, BSN
Practical Nursing Instructor
Hinds Community College
Pearl, MS

Virginia Chacon
Colorado Technical University
Pueblo, CO

Sherri Comfort, RN
Practical Nursing Instructor
Department Chair
Holmes Community College
Goodman, MS

Brandy Coward, BNS, MA
Director of Nursing
Angeles Institute
Lakewood, CA

Scott Coward, RN
Campus Director
Angeles Institute
Lakewood, CA

Jennifer Decker
Clinical Instructor
College of Eastern Utah
Price, UT

C. Kay Devereux
Professor
Department Chair, Vocational
Nurse Education
Tyler Junior College
Tyler, TX

Carolyn Du, BSN, MSN, NP, CDe
Director of Education
Pacific College
Costa Mesa, CA

Laura R. Durbin, RN, BSN, CHPN
Instructor
West Kentucky Community and
Technical College
Paducah, KY

Robin Ellis, BSN, MS
Nursing Faculty
Provo College
Provo, UT

Suzanne D. Fox, RN
Practical Nursing Instructor
Arkansas State University Technical
Center
Marked Tree, AR

Judie Fritz, RN, MSN
Instructor
Keiser Career College
Miami Lakes, FL

Edith Gerdes, RN, MSN, BHCA
Associate Professor of Nursing
Ivy Tech Community College
South Bend, IN

Juanita Hamilton-Gonzalez
Professor
Coordinator—Practical Nursing Program
City University of New York–Medgar Evers
Brooklyn, NY

Jane Harper
Assistant Professor
Southeast Kentucky Community &
Technical College
Pineville, KY

Angie Headley
Nursing Instructor
Swainsboro Technical College
Swainsboro, GA

Lillie Hill
Clinical Coordinator/Instructor
Practical Nursing
Durham Technical Community
College
Durham, NC

Michelle Hopper
Sanford-Brown College
St. Peters, MO

Karla Huntsman, RN, MSN
Instructor
Nursing Program
AmeriTech College
Draper, UT

Connie M. Hyde, RN, BSN
Practical Nursing Instructor
Louisiana Technical College
Lafayette, LA

Kimball Johnson, RN, MS
Nursing Professor
College of Eastern Utah
Price, UT

Sandy Kamhoot, BSN
Faculty
Santa Fe College
Gainesville, FL

Juanita Kaness, MSN, RN, CRNP
Nursing Program Coordinator
Lehigh Carbon Community
College
Schnecksville, PA

**Mary E. Kilbourn-Huey, MSN**
Assistant Professor
Maysville Community and Technical
    College
Maysville, KY

**Gloria D. Kline, RN**
Practical Nursing Instructor
Hinds Community College
Vicksburg, MS

**Christine Levandowski, RN, BSN,
    MSN**
Director of Nursing
Baker College
Auburn Hills, MI

**Mary Luckett, RN, MS**
Professor Vocational Nursing
Level 1 Coordinator
Houston Community College
Coleman College for Health Sciences
Houston, TX

**Wendy Maleki, RN, MS**
Director
Vocational Nursing Program
American Career College
Ontario, CA

**Luzviminda A. Malihan**
Assistant Professor
Hostos Community College
Bronx, NY

**Vanessa Norwood McGregor,
    RN, BSN, MBA**
Practical Nursing Instructor
West Kentucky Community and
    Technical College
Paducah, KY

**Kristie Oles, RN, MSN**
Practical Nursing Chair
Brown Mackie College
North Canton, OH

**Beverly Pacas**
Department Head/Instructor
Practical Nursing
Louisiana Technical College
Baton Rouge, LA

**Debra Perry, RN, MSN**
Instructor
Lorain County Community College
Elyria, OH

**Cheryl Pratt, RN, MA, CNAA**
Regional Dean of Nursing
Rasmussen College
Mankato, MN

**Charlotte Prewitt, RN, BSN**
Practical Nursing Instructor
Meridian Technology Center
Stillwater, OK

**Stephanie Price**
Faculty, Practical Nursing
Holmes Community College
Goodman, MS

**Patricia Schrull, RN, MSN, MBA,
    MEd, CNE**
Director, Practical Nursing Program
Lorain County Community College
Elyria, OH

**Margi J. Schutlz, RN, MSN,
    Ph.D.**
Director, Nursing Division
GateWay Community College
Phoenix, AZ

**Sherie A. Shupe, RN, MSN**
Director of Nursing
Computer Career Center
Las Cruces, NM

**Sherri Smith, RN**
Chairwoman
Arkansas State University Technical
    Center
Jonesboro, AR

**Cheryl Smith, RN, BSN**
Practical Nursing Instructor
Colorado Technical University
North Kansas City, MO

**Laura Spinelli**
Keiser Career College
Miami Lakes, FL

**Jennifer Teerlink, RN, MSN**
Nursing Faculty
Provo College
Provo, UT

**Dana L. Trowell, RN, BSN**
LPN Program Director
Dalton State College
Dalton, GA

**Racheal Vargas, LVN**
Clinical Liaison
Medical Assisting/Vocational Nursing
Lake College
Reading, CA

**Sarah Elizabeth Youth Whitaker,
    DNS, RN**
Nursing Program Director
Computer Career Center
El Paso, TX

**Shawn White, RN, BSN**
Clinical Coordinator, Nursing Instructor
Griffin Technical College
Griffin, GA

**Sharon Wilson**
Program Director/Instructor, Practical
    Nursing
Durham Technical Community College
Durham, NC

**Vladmir Yarosh, LVN, BS**
Program Coordinator—Vocational Nurse
    Program
Gurnick Academy of Medical Arts
San Mateo, CA

**DiAnn Zimmerman**
Director, Instructor
Dakota County Technical College
Rosemount, MN

# PREFACE

*Foundations of Maternal & Pediatric Nursing*, third edition, concisely and comprehensively presents prenatal care, complications of pregnancy, birth, postpartum care, and newborn care. There is a strong emphasis on life span development and includes childrearing from birth through 18 years of age.

Although a systems approach is presented, the concept of holistic care is fundamental to this text. Throughout the book, boxes highlight special topics regarding critical thinking questions, memory tricks, life span development, client teaching, cultural considerations, professional tips, community/home health care, safety, and infection control. Pharmacology basics, medication administration, and diagnostic testing are presented. Chapter presentation is based on the nursing process that incorporates the 2009–2011 NANDA-I diagnoses and NIC/NOC references. The student is provided with opportunities to demonstrate knowledge and develop critical thinking skills by completing Case Studies included in many of the chapters. Concept Maps and Concept Care Maps challenge the student to incorporate the interrelatedness of nursing concepts in preparation for clinical practice. The student has the opportunity to assess knowledge and critical thinking of essential nursing concepts by answering NCLEX®-style review questions at the end of each chapter.

Health care settings are changing, multifaceted, challenging, and rewarding. Critical thinking and sound nursing judgments are essential in the present health care environment. Practical/Vocational nursing students confront and adapt to changes in technology, information, and resources by building a solid foundation of accurate, essential information. A firm knowledge base also allows nurses to meet the changing needs of clients. This text was written to equip the LPN/VN with current knowledge, basic problem-solving and critical thinking skills to successfully pass the NCLEX®-PN exam and meet the demanding challenges of today's health care.

## ORGANIZATION

*Foundations of Maternal & Pediatric Nursing*, third edition, consists of 2 units divided into 8 chapters. The units concisely and thoroughly discuss nursing care of the client in childbearing and childrearing.

- **Unit 1:** NURSING CARE OF THE CLIENT: CHILD-BEARING—covers preconception education, prenatal care, fetal development, complications of pregnancy, the birth process, postpartum care, and care of the newborn.
- **Unit 2:** NURSING CARE OF THE CLIENT: CHILD-REARING—presents the basics of pediatric care. The two chapters in this unit, Infants with Special Needs: Birth to 12 Months and Common Problems: 1 to 18 years, address the major situations of pediatric care.

## FEATURES

Each chapter includes a variety of learning aids designed to help the reader further a basic understanding of key concepts. Each chapter opens with a **Making the Connection** box that guides the reader to other key chapters related to the current chapter. This highlights the integration of the text material. **Learning Objectives** are presented at the beginning of each chapter as well. These help students focus their study and use their time efficiently. A listing of **Key Terms** is provided to identify the terms the student should know or learn for a better understanding of the subject matter. These are bolded and defined at first use in the chapter.

The content of each chapter is presented in nursing process format. Where appropriate, a **Sample Nursing Care Plan** is provided in the chapter. These serve as models for students to refer to as they create their own care plans based on case studies. **Case Studies** are presented at the conclusion of most chapters. These call for students to draw upon their knowledge base and synthesize information to develop their own solutions to realistic cases. **Nursing Diagnoses, Planning/Outcomes, and Interventions** are presented in a convenient table format for quick reference. **Concept Maps** and **Concept Care Maps** are visual pictures of interrelated concepts as they relate to nursing.

A bulleted **Summary** list and multiple-choice **NCLEX®-style Review Questions** at the end of each chapter assist the student in remembering and using the material presented. **References/Suggested Readings** allow the student to find the source of the material presented and also to find additional information concerning topics covered. **Resources** are also listed and provide names and internet addresses of organizations specializing in a specific area of health care.

Boxes used throughout the text emphasize key points and provide specific types of information. The boxes are:

- **Critical Thinking**: encourages the student to use the knowledge gained to think critically about a situation.
- **Memory Trick**: provides an easy-to-remember saying or mnemonic to assist the student in remembering important information presented.
- **Life Span Considerations**: provides information related to the care of specific age groups during the life span.
- **Client Teaching**: identifies specific items that the client should know related to the various disorders.
- **Cultural Considerations**: shares beliefs, manners, and ways of providing care, communication, and relationships of various cultural and ethnic groups as a way to provide holistic care.
- **Professional Tip**: offers tips and technical hints for the nurse to ensure quality care.
- **Safety:** emphasizes the importance of and ways to maintain safe care.
- **Community/Home Health Care**: describes factors to consider when providing care in the community or in a client's home, and adaptation in care that may be necessary.
- **Drug Icon**: highlights pharmacological treatments and interventions that may be appropriate for certain conditions and disorders.
- **Collaborative Care**: mentions members of the care team and their roles in providing comprehensive care to clients.
- **Infection Control**: indicates reminders of methods to prevent the spread of infections.

The back matter includes a **Glossary of Terms**. The appendices include **NANDA-I Nursing Diagnoses**; **Recommended Childhood, Adolescent, and Adult Immunization Schedules**; **Abbreviations**, **Acronyms** and **Symbols**; and **English/ Spanish Words and Phrases**. **Standard Precautions** are found on the inside back cover.

## NEW TO THIS EDITION

### Updated content within chapters:

- Included 3 categories of fetal heart rate patterns to guide obstetrical health care providers.
- HELLP syndrome is related to the complication of preeclampsia/eclampsia and explained at an appropriate level for the LP/VN student.
- Included current maternity and pediatric terminology and nursing trends.
- Discussed current medications for maternal and pediatric care.

### Other additions

- Added case studies to all chapters as appropriate; case studies have a mixture of critical thinking and nursing process questions.

- Added concept care maps to chapters as appropriate for visual picture of the nursing process.
- Increased number of challenging and applicable critical thinking questions.
- Cultural considerations updated and cultural content included throughout the text.
- Added Adult Immunization Schedule along with Childhood and Adolescent Immunization Schedules.
- Cited research articles in understandable manner for easy application of evidence-based practice.
- Added current NANDA diagnoses according to *NANDA-International Nursing Diagnoses, 2009-11 Edition: Definitions and Classification (NANDA Nursing Diagnosis)*.
- Added new NCLEX®-style review questions at the end of chapters to help students challenge their understanding of content while gaining practice with this important question style.
- Added memory tricks for ease of student recall of pertinent information.
- Numerous new photos and illustrations for improved presentation of concepts.
- New, free, StudyWARE™ CD-ROM provides interactive games, animations, videos, heart and lung sounds, and much more to augment the learning experience and support mastery of concepts.

## EXTENSIVE TEACHING/ LEARNING PACKAGE

The complete supplements package for *Foundations of Maternal & Pediatric Nursing*, third edition, was developed to achieve two goals:

1. To assist students in learning the information and procedures presented in the text.
2. To assist instructors in planning and implementing their programs for the most efficient use of time and other resources.

## INSTRUCTOR RESOURCES

### Foundations of Nursing Instructor's Resource, third edition

ISBN-10: 1-428-31780-5
ISBN-13: 978-1-428-31780-2

The Instructor's Resource has four components to assist the instructor and enhance classroom activities and discussion.

### Instructor's Guide

- **Instructional Approaches**: Ideas and concepts to help educators manage different presentation methods. Suggestions for approaching topics with rich discussion topics and lecture ideas are provided.
- **Student Learning Activities:** Ideas for activities such as classroom discussions, role play, and individual assignments designed to encourage student critical thinking as they engage with the concepts presented in the text.

- **Resources:** Additional books, videos, and resources for use in developing and implementing your curriculum.
- **Web Activities:** Suggestions for student learning experiences online, including specific websites and accompanying activities.
- **Suggested Responses to the Case Study:** Case studies located throughout the core book challenge student critical thinking with questions about nursing care. Suggested responses are included.
- **Answers to Review Questions:** Answers and rationales for all end-of-chapter NCLEX®-style questions are provided.

## Computerized Testbank

- Includes a rich bank of questions that test students on retention and application of material in the text.
- Many questions are now presented in NCLEX® style, with each question providing the answer and rationale, as well as cognitive levels.
- Allows the instructor to mix questions from each of the didactic chapters to customize tests.

## Instructor Slides Created in PowerPoint

- A robust offering of instructor slides created in PowerPoint outlines the concepts from text in order to assist the instructor with lectures.
- Ideas presented stimulate discussion and critical thinking.

## Image Library

A searchable Image Library of more than 800 illustrations and photographs that can be incorporated into lectures, class materials, or electronic presentations.

# STUDENT RESOURCES

## Foundations of Maternal & Pediatric Nursing Study Guide, third edition

ISBN-10: 1-428-31786-4
ISBN-13: 978-1-4283-1786-4

A valuable companion to the core book, this student resource provides additional review on all 8 chapters of *Foundations of Maternal & Pediatric Health Nursing* with Key Term matching review questions, Abbreviation Review Exercises, Self-Assessment Questions, and other Review Exercises and Activities. Answers to questions are provided at the back of the book, making this an excellent resource for self-study and review.

## Foundations of Nursing Online Companion

ISBN-10: 1-428-31779-1
ISBN-13: 978-1-428-31779-6

The Online Companion gives you online access to all the components in the Instructor's Resource as well as additional tools to reinforce the content in each chapter and enhance classroom teaching. Multimedia animations, additional chapters, and resources related to workplace transition are just some of the many resources found on this robust site.

## CL eBook to Accompany Foundations of Maternal & Pediatric Nursing, third edition

printed access code ISBN-10: 1-435-48786-9
printed access code ISBN-13: 978-1-4354-8786-4
instant access code ISBN-10: 1-435-48785-0
instant access code ISBN-13: 978-1-4354-8785-7

## Foundations of Nursing WebTutor Advantage on Blackboard

ISBN-10: 1-428-31781-3
ISBN-13: 978-1-428-31781-9

## Foundations of Nursing WebTutor Advantage on WebCT

ISBN-10: 1-428-31782-1
ISBN-13: 978-1-428-31782-6

- A complete online environment that supplements the course provided in both Blackboard and WebCT format.
- Includes chapter overviews, chapter outlines, and competencies.
- Useful classroom management tools include chats and calendars, as well as instructor resources such as the instructor slides created in PowerPoint.
- Multimedia offering includes video clips and 3D animations.

# ABOUT THE AUTHORS

Lois Elain Wacker White earned a diploma in nursing from Memorial Hospital School of Nursing, Springfield, Illinois; an Associate degree in Science from Del Mar College, Corpus Christi, Texas; a Bachelor of Science in Nursing from Texas A & I University—Corpus Christi, Corpus Christi, Texas; a Master of Science in Education from Corpus Christi State University, Corpus Christi, Texas; and a Doctor of Philosophy degree in education administration—community college from the University of Texas, Austin, Texas.

She has taught at Del Mar College, Corpus Christi, Texas, in both the Associate Degree Nursing program and the Vocational Nursing program. For 14 years, she was also chairperson of the Department of Vocational Nurse Education. Dr. White has taught fundamentals of nursing, mental health/mental illness, medical-surgical nursing, and maternal/pediatric nursing. Her professional career has also included 15 years of clinical practice.

Dr. White has served on the Nursing Education Advisory Committee of the Board of Nurse Examiners for the State of Texas and the Board of Vocational Nurse Examiners, which developed competencies expected of graduates for each level of nursing.

Gena Duncan has worked as an RN for 36 years in the clinical, community health, and educational arenas. This has equipped Mrs. Duncan with a wide range of nursing experiences and varied skills to meet the educational needs of today's students. She has a MSEd and MSN.

During her professional career, Mrs. Duncan served as a staff nurse, an assistant head nurse of a medical-surgical unit, a continuing education instructor, an associate professor in an LPN program, and director of an Associate degree nursing program. She has taught LPN, ADN, BSN, and MSN nursing students. As a faculty member she taught many nursing courses and served on a statewide curriculum committee for a state college. As director of an Associate degree nursing program, she was instrumental in starting and obtaining state board approval of an LPN-RN nursing program.

Her master's research thesis was entitled, An Investigation of Learning Styles of Practical and Baccalaureate Students. The results of the study are published in the *Journal of Nursing Education*. She has coauthored two textbooks, a medical-surgical textbook, and a transitions text for LPN to RN students. She has been an active member of Sigma Theta Tau.

Wendy Baumle is currently a nursing instructor at James A. Rhodes State College in Ohio. She has spent 19 years as a clinician, educator, school district health coordinator, and academician. Mrs. Baumle has taught fundamentals of nursing, medical-surgical nursing, pediatrics, obstetrics, pharmacology, anatomy and physiology, and ethics in health care in practical nursing and associate nursing degree programs. She has previously taught at Lutheran College, Fort Wayne, Indiana, at Northwest State Community College, Archbold, Ohio, and at James. A. Rhodes State College in Lima, Ohio. Mrs. Baumle earned her Bachelor of Science degree in Nursing from The University of Toledo, Toledo, Ohio and her Master's degree in Nursing from The Medical College of Ohio, Toledo, Ohio. Mrs. Baumle is a member of a number of professional nursing organizations, including Sigma Theta Tau, the American Nurses Association, the National League for Nursing, and the Ohio Nurses Association.

# ACKNOWLEDGMENTS

Many people must work together to produce any textbook, but a comprehensive book such as this requires even more people with various areas of expertise. We would like to thank the contributors for their time and effort to share their knowledge gained through years of experience in both the clinical and academic settings.

To the reviewers, we thank you for your time spent critically reading the manuscript, expertise, and valuable suggestions that have added to this text.

We would like to acknowledge and sincerely thank the entire team at Delmar Cengage Learning who has worked to make this textbook a reality. Juliet Steiner, senior product manager, receives a special thank you. She has kept us on track and provided guidance with humor, enthusiasm, sensitivity, and expertise. We extend a special thank you to Steve Helba, executive editor, for his vision for this text, calm demeanor, and patience. Other members on the team—Marah Bellegarde, managing editor, James Zayicek, senior content product manager, Jack Pendleton, senior art director, and Meghan Orvis, editorial assistant, have all worked diligently for the completion of this textbook. Thank you to all.

# HOW TO USE THIS TEXT

This text is designed with you, the reader, in mind. Special elements and feature boxes appear throughout the text to guide you in reading and to assist you in learning the material. Following are suggestions for how you can use these features to increase your understanding and mastery of the content.

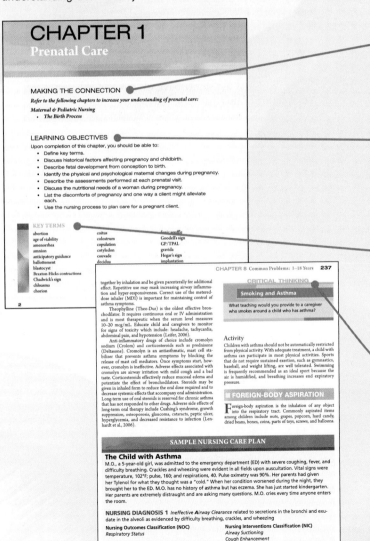

## MAKING THE CONNECTION

Read these boxes before beginning a chapter to link material across the holistic care continuum and to tie new content to the material you have already encountered.

## LEARNING OBJECTIVES

Read the chapter objectives before reading the chapter to set the stage for learning. Revisit the objectives when preparing for an exam to see which entries you can respond to with "yes, I can do that."

## KEY TERMS

Review this list before reading the chapter to familiarize yourself with the new terms and to revisit those terms you already know to link them to the content in the new chapter.

## CRITICAL THINKING

Visit these boxes after reading the entire chapter to check your understanding of the concepts presented.

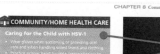

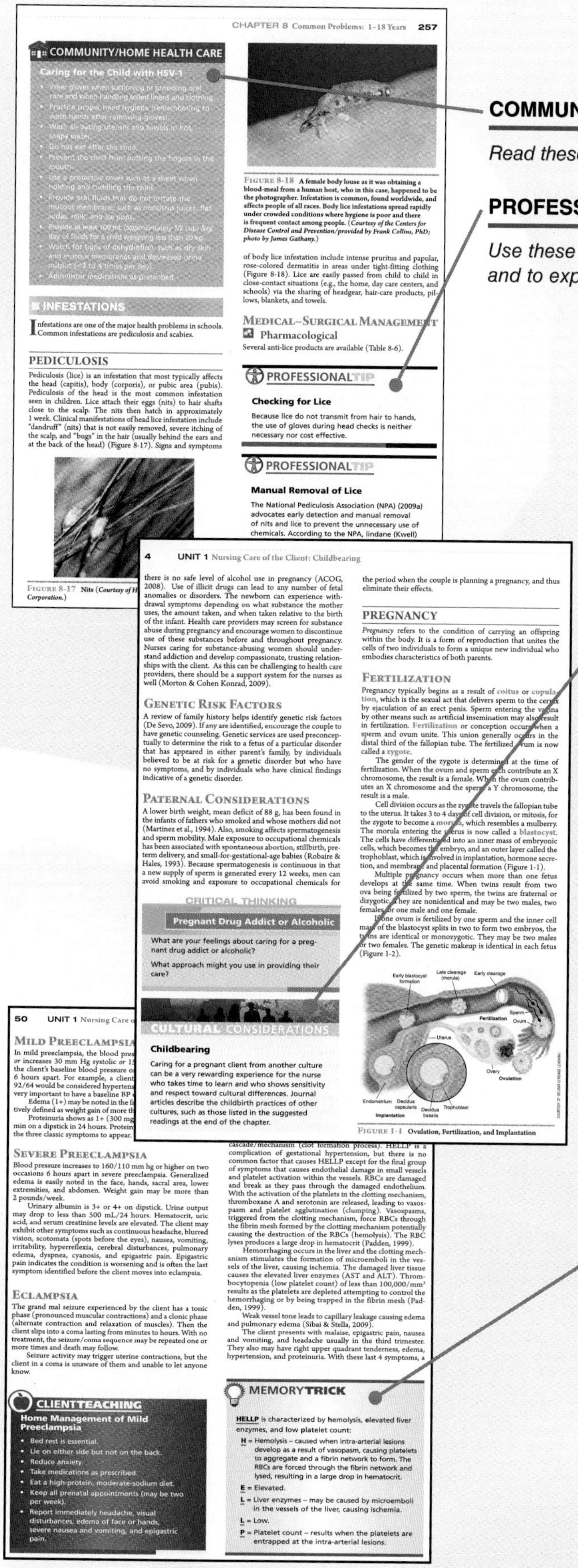

### COMMUNITY/HOME HEALTH CARE

**Caring for the Child with HSV-1**

- Wear gloves when suctioning or providing oral care and when handling soiled linens and clothing.
- Practice proper hand hygiene (remembering to wash hands after removing gloves).
- Wash all eating utensils and towels in hot, soapy water.
- Do not wear after the child.
- Prevent the child from putting the fingers in the mouth.
- Use a protective cover such as a sheet when bathing and cuddling the child.
- Provide oral fluids that do not irritate the mucous membrane, such as noncitrus juices, flat sodas, milk, and ice pops.
- Provide at least 100 mL (approximately 1/2 cup) /kg/ day of fluids for a child weighing less than 20 kg.
- Watch for signs of dehydration such as dry skin and mucous membranes and decreased urine output (<3 to 4 times per day).
- Administer medications as prescribed.

### INFESTATIONS

Infestations are one of the major health problems in schools. Common infestations are pediculosis and scabies.

#### PEDICULOSIS

Pediculosis (lice) is an infestation that most typically affects the head (capitis), body (corporis), or pubic area (pubis). Pediculosis of the head is the most common infestation seen in children. Lice attach their eggs (nits) to hair shafts close to the scalp. The nits then hatch in approximately 1 week. Clinical manifestations of head lice infestation include "dandruff" (nits) that is not easily removed, severe itching of the scalp, and "bugs" in the hair (usually behind the ears and at the back of the head) (Figure 8-17). Signs and symptoms

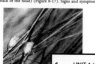

FIGURE 8-17 Nits (Courtesy of Hogil Corporation.)

FIGURE 8-18 A female body louse as it was obtaining a blood-meal from a human host, who in this case, happened to be the photographer. Infestation is common, found worldwide, and affects people of all races. Body lice infestations spread rapidly under crowded conditions where hygiene is poor and there is frequent contact among people. (Courtesy of the Centers for Disease Control and Prevention/provided by Frank Collins, PhD; photo by James Gathany.)

of body lice infestation include intense pruritus and papular, rose-colored dermatitis in areas under tight-fitting clothing (Figure 8-18). Lice are easily passed from child to child in close-contact situations (e.g., the home, day care centers, and schools) via the sharing of headgear, hair-care products, pillows, blankets, and towels.

#### MEDICAL–SURGICAL MANAGEMENT

**Pharmacological**

Several anti-lice products are available (Table 8-6).

#### PROFESSIONAL TIP

**Checking for Lice**

Because lice do not transmit from hair to hands, the use of gloves during head checks is neither necessary nor cost effective.

#### PROFESSIONAL TIP

**Manual Removal of Lice**

The National Pediculosis Association (NPA) (2009a) advocates early detection and manual removal of nits and lice to prevent the unnecessary use of chemicals. According to the NPA, lindane (Kwell)

---

there is no safe level of alcohol use in pregnancy (ACOG, 2008). Use of illicit drugs can lead to any number of fetal anomalies or disorders. The newborn can experience withdrawal symptoms depending on what substance the mother uses, the amount taken, and when taken relative to the birth of the infant. Health care providers may screen for substance abuse during pregnancy and encourage women to discontinue use of these substances before and throughout pregnancy. Nurses caring for substance-abusing women should understand addiction and develop compassionate, trusting relationships with the client. As this can be challenging to health care providers, there should be a support system for the nurses as well (Morton & Cohen Konrad, 2009).

#### GENETIC RISK FACTORS

A review of family history helps identify genetic risk factors (De Sevo, 2009). If any are identified, encourage the couple to have genetic counseling. Genetic services are used preconceptually to determine the risk to a fetus of a particular disorder that has appeared in either parent's family, by individuals believed to be at risk for a genetic disorder but who have no symptoms, and by individuals who have clinical findings indicative of a genetic disorder.

#### PATERNAL CONSIDERATIONS

A lower birth weight, mean deficit of 88 g, has been found in the infants of fathers who smoked and whose mothers did not (Martinez et al., 1994). Also, smoking affects spermatogenesis and sperm mobility. Male exposure to occupational chemicals has been associated with spontaneous abortion, stillbirth, preterm delivery, and small-for-gestational-age babies (Robaire & Hales, 1993). Because spermatogenesis is continuous in that a new supply of sperm is generated every 12 months, men can avoid smoking and exposure to occupational chemicals for

#### CRITICAL THINKING

**Pregnant Drug Addict or Alcoholic**

What are your feelings about caring for a pregnant drug addict or alcoholic?

What approach might you use in providing their care?

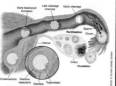

#### CULTURAL CONSIDERATIONS

**Childbearing**

Caring for a pregnant client from another culture can be a very rewarding experience for the nurse who takes time to learn and who shows sensitivity and respect toward cultural differences. Journal articles describe the childbirth practices of other cultures, such as those listed in the suggested readings at the end of the chapter.

the period when the couple is planning a pregnancy, and thus eliminate their effects.

#### PREGNANCY

*Pregnancy* refers to the condition of carrying an offspring within the body. It is a form of reproduction that unites the cells of two individuals to form a unique new individual who embodies characteristics of both parents.

#### FERTILIZATION

Pregnancy typically begins as a result of *coitus* or *copulation*, which is the sexual act that delivers sperm to the cervix by ejaculation of an erect penis. Sperm entering the vagina by other means such as artificial insemination may also result in fertilization. *Fertilization* or conception occurs when a sperm and ovum unite. This union generally occurs in the distal third of the fallopian tube. The fertilized ovum is now called a *zygote*.

The gender of the zygote is determined at the time of fertilization. When the ovum and sperm each contribute an X chromosome, the result is a female. When the ovum contributes an X chromosome and the sperm a Y chromosome, the result is a male.

Cell division occurs as the zygote travels the fallopian tube to the uterus. It takes 3 to 4 days of cell division, or mitosis, for the zygote to become a *morula*, which resembles a mulberry. The morula entering the uterus is now called a *blastocyst*. The cells have differentiated into an inner mass of embryonic cells, which becomes the embryo, and an outer layer called the trophoblast, which is involved in implantation, hormone secretion, and membrane and placental formation (Figure 1-1).

Multiple pregnancy occurs when more than one fetus develops at the same time. When twins result from two ova being fertilized by two sperm, the twins are fraternal or dizygotic; they are nonidentical and may be two males, two females or one male and one female.

If one ovum is fertilized by one sperm and the inner cell mass of the blastocyst splits in two to form two embryos, the twins are identical or monozygotic. They may be two males or two females. The genetic makeup is identical in each fetus (Figure 1-2).

FIGURE 1-1 Ovulation, Fertilization, and Implantation

---

#### MILD PREECLAMPSIA

In mild preeclampsia, the blood pressure either increases or increases 30 mm Hg systolic or 15 mm Hg diastolic above the client's baseline blood pressure on two occasions at least 6 hours apart. For example, a client with a baseline BP of 92/64 would be considered hypertensive. It is therefore very important to have a baseline BP reading.

Edema (1+) may be noted in the face, hands, or abdomen tively defined as weight gain of more than 2 pounds/week.

Proteinuria shows as 1+ (300 mg/L or 30 mg/dL) protein min on a dipstick in 24 hours. Proteinuria is defined as one of the three classic symptoms to appear.

#### SEVERE PREECLAMPSIA

Blood pressure increases to 160/110 mm Hg or higher on two occasions 6 hours apart in severe preeclampsia. Generalized edema is easily noted in the face, hands, sacral area, lower extremities, and abdomen. Weight gain may be more than 2 pounds/week.

Urinary albumin is 3+ or 4+ on dipstick. Urine output may drop to less than 500 mL/24 hours. Hematocrit, uric acid, and serum creatinine levels are elevated. The client may exhibit other symptoms such as continuous headache, blurred vision, scotomata (spots before the eyes), nausea, vomiting, irritability, hyperreflexia, cerebral disturbances, pulmonary edema, dyspnea, cyanosis, and epigastric pain. Epigastric pain indicates the condition is worsening and is often the last symptom identified before the client moves into eclampsia.

#### ECLAMPSIA

The grand mal seizure experienced by the client has a tonic phase (pronounced muscular contractions) and a clonic phase (alternate contraction and relaxation of muscles). Then the client slips into a coma lasting from minutes to hours. With no treatment, the seizure/coma sequence may be repeated one or more times and death may follow.

Seizure activity may trigger uterine contractions, but the client in a coma is unaware of them and unable to let know.

#### CLIENT TEACHING

**Home Management of Mild Preeclampsia**

- Bed rest is essential.
- Lie on either side but not on the back.
- Reduce anxiety.
- Take medications as prescribed.
- Eat a high-protein, moderate-sodium diet.
- Keep all prenatal appointments (may be two per week).
- Report immediately headache, visual disturbances, edema of face or hands, severe nausea and vomiting, and epigastric pain.

cascade/mechanism (clot formation process). HELLP is a complication of gestational hypertension, but there is no common factor that causes HELLP except for the final group of symptoms that causes endothelial damage in small vessels and platelet activation within the vessels. RBCs are damaged and break as they pass through the damaged endothelium. With the activation of the platelets in the clotting mechanism, thromboxane A and serotonin are released, leading to vasospasm and platelet agglutination (clumping). Vasospasms, triggered from the clotting mechanism, force RBCs through the fibrin mesh formed by the clotting mechanism potentially causing the destruction of the RBCs (hemolysis). The RBC lyses produces a large drop in hematocrit (Padden, 1999).

Hemorrhaging occurs in the liver and the clotting mechanism stimulates the formation of microemboli in the vessels of the liver, causing ischemia. The damaged liver tissue causes the elevated liver enzymes (AST and ALT). Thrombocytopenia (low platelet count) of less than 100,000/mm³ results as the platelets are depleted attempting to control the hemorrhaging or by being trapped in the fibrin mesh (Padden, 1999).

Weak vessel tone leads to capillary leakage causing edema and pulmonary edema (Sibai & Stella, 2009).

The client presents with malaise, epigastric pain, nausea and vomiting, and headache usually in the third trimester. They also may have right upper quadrant tenderness, edema, hypertension, and proteinuria. With these last 4 symptoms, a

#### MEMORY TRICK

**HELLP** is characterized by hemolysis, elevated liver enzymes, and low platelet count:

**H** = Hemolysis – caused when intra-arterial lesions develop as a result of vasospasm, causing platelets to aggregate and a fibrin network to form. The RBCs are forced through the fibrin network and lysed, resulting in a large drop in hematocrit.

**E** = Elevated.

**L** = Liver enzymes – may be caused by microemboli in the vessels of the liver, causing ischemia.

**L** = Low.

**P** = Platelet count – results when the platelets are entrapped at the intra-arterial lesions.

---

## COMMUNITY/HOME HEALTH CARE

*Read these boxes before making a home visit to a client with a given disorder.*

## PROFESSIONAL TIP

*Use these boxes to increase your professional competence and confidence, and to expand your knowledge base.*

## CULTURAL CONSIDERATIONS

*Test your sensitivity to cultural and ethnic diversity by scanning these boxes and using the guidelines and suggestions in your practice. You may also want to ask yourself what biases or preconceptions you have about different cultural practices before reading a chapter and then read these boxes for information that may help you be more sensitive in your nursing care and approach to clients.*

## MEMORY TRICK

*Use the mnemonic devices provided in the new Memory Trick feature to help you remember the correct steps or proper order of information when working with clients.*

# HOW TO USE THIS TEXT (Continued)

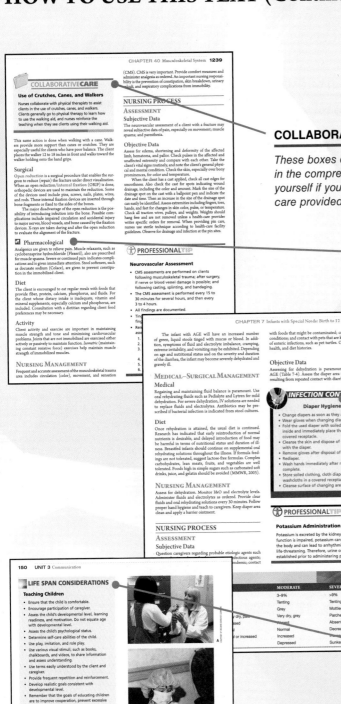

## COLLABORATIVE CARE

These boxes explain which other health care professionals may be involved in the comprehensive care offered to clients. Review these boxes and ask yourself if you understand how your role as a nurse will complement the care provided by others on the health care team.

## DRUG ICONS

These symbols draw attention to information relating to the pharmacological management available for certain disorders. Review these sections to understand the pharmacological treatments appropriate for your clients' conditions.

## INFECTION CONTROL

When reading a chapter, stop and pay attention to these features and ask yourself, "Had I thought of that? Do I practice these precautions?"

## LIFE SPAN CONSIDERATIONS

Use these boxes to increase your awareness of variations in care based on client age; this will help you deliver more effective and appropriate care.

## CLIENT TEACHING

Read these boxes to gain insight into client learning needs related to the specific disorder or condition. You may want to make your own index cards or electronic notes listing these teaching guidelines to use when you are working with clients.

# HOW TO USE THIS TEXT (Continued)

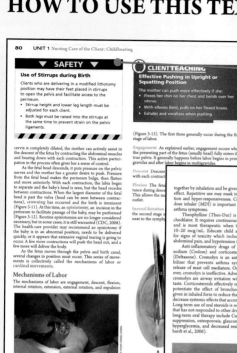

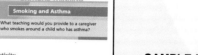

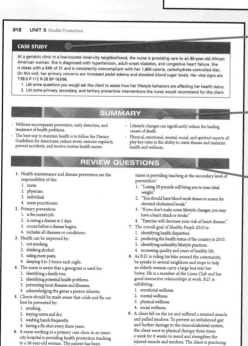

## SAFETY

*Pause while reading to consider these elements and quiz yourself: "Do I take steps such as these to ensure my own and the client's safety? Do I follow these guidelines in every practice encounter?"*

## SAMPLE NURSING CARE PLAN

*Use this feature to test your understanding and application of the content presented. Ask yourself "Would I have come up with the same nursing diagnoses? Are these the interventions that I would have proposed? What other interventions would be appropriate?"*

## CONCEPT CARE MAPS

*Review these graphical tools to help incorporate the interrelatedness of nursing concepts in preparation for clinical practice.*

## CASE STUDY

*Read over these boxes within the text. Draw on the knowledge you have gained and synthesize information to develop your own educated responses to the case study challenges.*

## SUMMARY

*Carefully read the bulleted list to review key concepts discussed. This is an excellent resource when studying or preparing for exams.*

## REVIEW QUESTIONS

*Test your knowledge and understanding by answering the NCLEX®-style review questions with each chapter. These are an excellent way to test your mastery of the concepts covered in the chapter, and a good opportunity to become familiar with answering NCLEX®-style review questions.*

# HOW TO USE STUDYWARE™ TO ACCOMPANY FOUNDATIONS OF MATERNAL & PEDIATRIC NURSING, THIRD EDITION

## MINIMUM SYSTEM REQUIREMENTS

- Operating systems: Microsoft Windows XP w/SP 2, Windows Vista w/ SP 1, Windows 7
- Processor: Minimum required by Operating System
- Memory: Minimum required by Operating System
- Hard Drive Space: 500 MB
- Screen resolution: 1024 x 768 pixels
- CD-ROM drive
- Sound card & listening device required for audio features
- Flash Player 10. The Adobe Flash Player is free, and can be downloaded from http://www.adobe.com/products/flashplayer/

## Setup Instructions

1. Insert disc into CD-ROM drive. The StudyWare™ installation program should start automatically. If it does not, go to step 2.
2. From My Computer, double-click the icon for the CD drive.
3. Double-click the *setup.exe* file to start the program.

## Technical Support

Telephone: 1-800-648-7450
8:30 A.M.-6:30 P.M. Eastern Time
E-mail: delmar.help@cengage.com

StudyWARE™ is a trademark used herein under license.

Microsoft® and Windows® are registered trademarks of the Microsoft Corporation.

Pentium® is a registered trademark of the Intel Corporation.

## GETTING STARTED

The StudyWARE™ software helps you learn terms and concepts in *Foundations of Maternal & Pediatric Nursing*, third edition. As you study each chapter in the text, be sure to explore the activities in the corresponding chapter in the software. Use StudyWARE™ as your own private tutor to help you learn the material in your *Foundations of Maternal & Pediatric Nursing*, third edition textbook.

Getting started is easy! Install the software by following the installation instructions provided above. When you open the software, enter your first and last name so the software can store your quiz results. Then choose a chapter or section from the menu to take a quiz or explore media and activities.

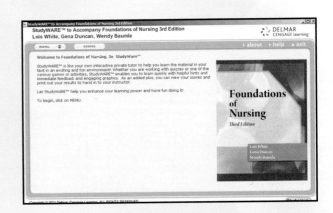

# HOW TO USE STUDYWARE™ (Continued)

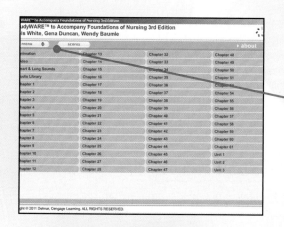

## MENU

*You can access the menu from wherever you are in the program. The Menu includes Animations, Video, Heart & Lung Sounds, Chapter activities for all didactic chapters, and NCLEX®-Style Quizzes for each major unit. You can also access your scores from the button to the right of the main menu button.*

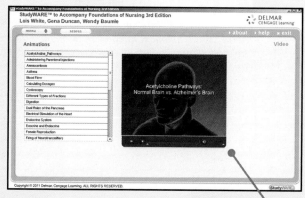

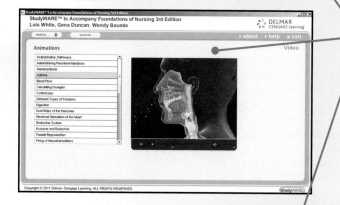

## ANIMATION

*This section on your StudyWARE™ CD-ROM provides 35 multimedia animations of biological, anatomical, and pharmacological processes. These animations visually explain some of the more difficult concepts and are an engaging resource to support your understanding.*

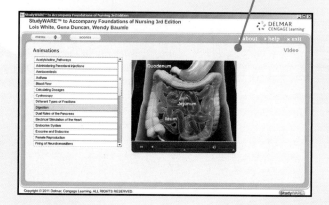

# HOW TO USE STUDYWARE™ (Continued)

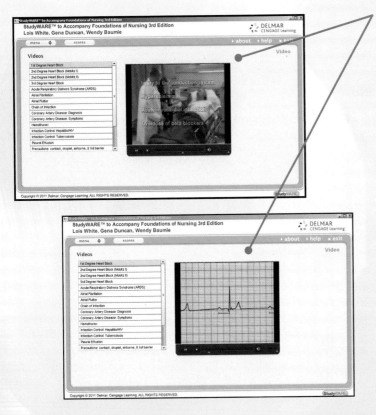

## VIDEO

A selection of 20 high quality video clips on topics ranging from infection control to the cardiovascular and respiratory systems has been provided. Click on the clip you would like to view, then click on the play button on the media viewer in the center of the screen. These video clips, many of which were developed by Concept Media, are a wonderful resource to help visualize difficult processes and skills.

## HEART & LUNG SOUNDS

This searchable multimedia program provides a comprehensive library of audio files for different heart and lung sounds that will be encountered by nurses. Sounds can be viewed according to category or specific sounds can be found by using the alphabetical term search function. In addition to hearing the sounds, related information about etiology and auscultation is provided.

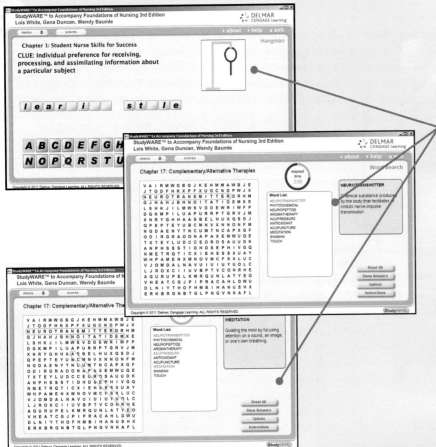

## CHAPTER ACTIVITIES

For each chapter from Foundations of Maternal & Pediatric Nursing, *third edition*, that contains glossary terms, games and activities are provided to help you master the terminology in a fun and interesting way. Concentration is a memory game that asks you to flip cards to match definitions with their terms. Flash Cards allow you to test your knowledge of a term by reading the term, thinking about the definition, then checking the actual definition. Hangman follows the traditional hangman game format and can be played by one or two players, challenging you to fill in the blanks for a term before the puzzle is completed. Crossword Puzzles provide definitions of key terms as clues so you can fill in the appropriate term and clear the board.

# HOW TO USE STUDYWARE™ (Continued)

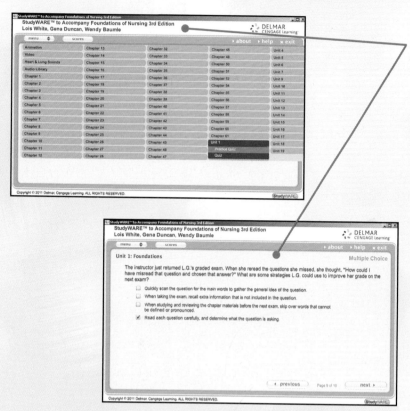

## QUIZZES

For each unit in Foundations of Maternal & Pediatric Nursing, *third edition, both practice and live quizzes are provided to test your understanding of critical concepts. The quiz program keeps track of your answers and a report can be generated at the end of the quiz outlining the questions, your answer, and the correct answer. Once the quiz has been completed, click on the Scores button for these details. Use the questions you missed as topic areas for additional study.*

# UNIT 1

# Nursing Care of the Client: Childbearing

# CHAPTER 1
## Prenatal Care

## MAKING THE CONNECTION

*Refer to the following chapters to increase your understanding of prenatal care:*

**Maternal & Pediatric Nursing**
- ◆ **The Birth Process**

## LEARNING OBJECTIVES

Upon completion of this chapter, you should be able to:

- Define key terms.
- Discuss historical factors affecting pregnancy and childbirth.
- Describe fetal development from conception to birth.
- Identify the physical and psychological maternal changes during pregnancy.
- Describe the assessments performed at each prenatal visit.
- Discuss the nutritional needs of a woman during pregnancy.
- List the discomforts of pregnancy and one way a client might alleviate each.
- Use the nursing process to plan care for a pregnant client.

## KEY TERMS

| | | |
|---|---|---|
| abortion | coitus | funic souffle |
| age of viability | colostrum | Goodell's sign |
| amenorrhea | copulation | GP/TPAL |
| amnion | cotyledon | gravida |
| anticipatory guidance | couvade | Hegar's sign |
| ballottement | decidua | implantation |
| blastocyst | ductus arteriosus | lanugo |
| Braxton-Hicks contractions | ductus venosus | Leopold's maneuvers |
| Chadwick's sign | fertilization | linea nigra |
| chloasma | foramen ovale | meconium |
| chorion | fundus | morula |

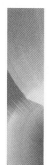

| | | |
|---|---|---|
| multigravida | polyhydramnios | striae gravidarum |
| multipara | postterm | supine hypotensive syndrome |
| nesting | prenatal care | teratogen |
| nulligravida | preterm | term |
| nullipara | primigravida | umbilical cord |
| para | primipara | uterine souffle |
| physiologic anemia of pregnancy | pseudocyesis | vernix caseosa |
| pica | psychoprophylaxis | Wharton's jelly |
| placenta | quickening | zygote |

# INTRODUCTION

For centuries, birth was part of family life and took place at home. Women learned about pregnancy and childbirth by asking female family members or friends and by being present when other women gave birth. In the United States in 1900, more than 90% of births were in the home.

In 1908, the American Red Cross and the Maternity Center Association offered the first formal programs for prenatal education. These early classes taught women about pregnancy, nutrition, and health care during pregnancy. By the 1950s, the classes included preparation for birth. In 1960, the American Society for Psychoprophylaxis in Obstetrics (ASPO/Lamaze) and the International Childbirth Education Association (ICEA) were founded. They both promote the idea that birth is a healthy process and that parents should have choices about the process.

In 1969, the Nurses Association of the American College of Obstetricians and Gynecologists (NAACOG) was formed with a goal of improving the health of women and newborn infants. The organization was renamed the Association of Women's Health, Obstetric and Neonatal Nurses (AWHONN) in 1993. The National Certification Corporation (NCC) is a not-for-profit organization that has provided a nationally accredited certification program for nurses and other health care professionals in obstetric, gynecologic and neonatal specialties since 1975.

Today, many couples postpone pregnancy to obtain advanced education or establish careers; they may expect to participate in every aspect of the pregnancy, including decision making, and are much more informed than in the past of the educational offerings available. Today's nurse must have a firm understanding of the physical and psychological changes brought about by pregnancy, as well as the application of the nursing process in meeting the needs of the childbearing family.

# PRECONCEPTION EDUCATION AND CARE

It has long been known that prenatal education and care identifies and reduces some problems in pregnancy and improves many outcomes. Yet, in 2004, the United States ranked 29th in the world in infant mortality, tied with Poland and Slovakia (CDC, 2008). More perinatal health experts are recognizing that a healthy pregnancy begins before conception.

Preconception education and care are focused on helping a couple prepare to conceive and identifying their reproductive risks before conception. The main goal is to protect the fetus during embryogenesis. Unhealthy habits can harm the fetus before the mother knows she is pregnant. Adopting a healthy lifestyle before pregnancy means eating a low-fat, high-fiber diet rich in vegetables and fruits; exercising at least 3 times a week; and getting to within 15 pounds of one's ideal weight. To prevent neural tube defects, all women who could possibly become pregnant should have an intake of 400 mcg of folic acid from a vitamin supplement and/or fortified foods and eat a healthful diet (Hasenau & Covington, 2002). Another goal is to help the couple identify genetic factors that may affect a pregnancy.

## IMMUNIZATIONS AND DISEASE STATUS

Immunization status is confirmed, and needed immunizations, especially rubella and hepatitis B, are administered before pregnancy. Tests are completed for infectious diseases such as syphilis, hepatitis B, HIV, Chlamydia, gonorrhea, human papilloma virus and herpes simplex. Some states also test for group B streptococcus. These diseases are treated to minimize adverse effects on the mother and fetus. Chronic diseases such as hypertension, cardiac disease, diabetes, epilepsy, thyroid dysfunction, asthma, renal disease, and phenylketonuria should be under control for the best outcome of pregnancy.

## MEDICATIONS

Known teratogens to avoid are warfarin (Coumadin), gold salts, isotretinoin (Accutane), valproic acid (Depakene), lithium (Eskalith), diazepam (Valium), phenytoin (Dilantin), tetracycline, diethylstilbestrol, DES (stilphostrol), live-virus vaccines, and folic acid antagonists. Taking any medication, either over-the-counter (OTC) or prescription, should first be discussed with the health care provider. It is best to have the system cleared of medications before conception, if possible.

## SMOKING, ALCOHOL, AND ILLICIT DRUGS

Smoking, alcohol, and illicit drugs all have negative effects on pregnancy. Smoking is associated with major complications for pregnancy and low-birth-weight infants. Nearly 12% of pregnant women report drinking while pregnant, although there is no safe level of alcohol use in pregnancy (ACOG, 2008). Use of illicit drugs can lead to any number of fetal anomalies or disorders. The newborn can experience withdrawal symptoms depending on what substance the mother uses, the amount taken, and when taken relative to the birth of the infant. Health care providers may screen for substance abuse during pregnancy and encourage women to discontinue use of these substances before and throughout pregnancy. Nurses caring for substance-abusing women should understand addiction and develop compassionate, trusting relationships with the client. As this can be challenging to health care providers, there should be a support system for the nurses as well (Morton & Cohen Konrad, 2009).

## GENETIC RISK FACTORS

A review of family history helps identify genetic risk factors (De Sevo, 2009). If any are identified, encourage the couple to have genetic counseling. Genetic services are used preconceptually to determine the risk to a fetus of a particular disorder that has appeared in either parent's family, by individuals believed to be at risk for a genetic disorder but who have no symptoms, and by individuals who have clinical findings indicative of a genetic disorder.

## PATERNAL CONSIDERATIONS

A lower birth weight, mean deficit of 88 g, has been found in the infants of fathers who smoked and whose mothers did not (Martinez et al., 1994). Also, smoking affects spermatogenesis and sperm mobility. Male exposure to occupational chemicals has been associated with spontaneous abortion, stillbirth, preterm delivery, and small-for-gestational-age babies (Robaire & Hales, 1993). Because spermatogenesis is continuous in that a new supply of sperm is generated every 12 weeks, men can avoid smoking and exposure to occupational chemicals for

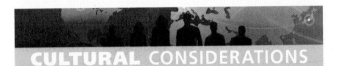

### CRITICAL THINKING

#### Pregnant Drug Addict or Alcoholic

What are your feelings about caring for a pregnant drug addict or alcoholic?

What approach might you use in providing their care?

### CULTURAL CONSIDERATIONS

#### Childbearing

Caring for a pregnant client from another culture can be a very rewarding experience for the nurse who takes time to learn and who shows sensitivity and respect toward cultural differences. Journal articles describe the childbirth practices of other cultures, such as those listed in the suggested readings at the end of the chapter.

the period when the couple is planning a pregnancy, and thus eliminate their effects.

## PREGNANCY

*Pregnancy* refers to the condition of carrying an offspring within the body. It is a form of reproduction that unites the cells of two individuals to form a unique new individual who embodies characteristics of both parents.

### FERTILIZATION

Pregnancy typically begins as a result of **coitus** or **copulation**, which is the sexual act that delivers sperm to the cervix by ejaculation of an erect penis. Sperm entering the vagina by other means such as artificial insemination may also result in fertilization. **Fertilization** or conception occurs when a sperm and ovum unite. This union generally occurs in the distal third of the fallopian tube. The fertilized ovum is now called a **zygote**.

The gender of the zygote is determined at the time of fertilization. When the ovum and sperm each contribute an X chromosome, the result is a female. When the ovum contributes an X chromosome and the sperm a Y chromosome, the result is a male.

Cell division occurs as the zygote travels the fallopian tube to the uterus. It takes 3 to 4 days of cell division, or mitosis, for the zygote to become a **morula**, which resembles a mulberry. The morula entering the uterus is now called a **blastocyst**. The cells have differentiated into an inner mass of embryonic cells, which becomes the embryo, and an outer layer called the trophoblast, which is involved in implantation, hormone secretion, and membrane and placental formation (Figure 1-1).

Multiple pregnancy occurs when more than one fetus develops at the same time. When twins result from two ova being fertilized by two sperm, the twins are fraternal or dizygotic. They are nonidentical and may be two males, two females, or one male and one female.

If one ovum is fertilized by one sperm and the inner cell mass of the blastocyst splits in two to form two embryos, the twins are identical or monozygotic. They may be two males or two females. The genetic makeup is identical in each fetus (Figure 1-2).

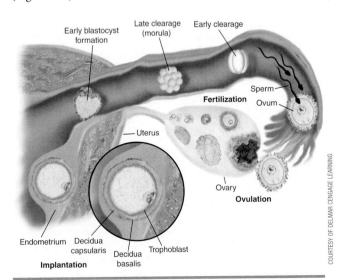

**FIGURE 1-1** Ovulation, Fertilization, and Implantation

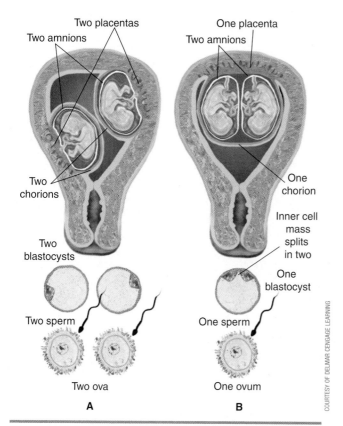

**FIGURE 1-2**  Formation of Twins; *A*, Fraternal (nonidentical); *B*, Identical

## IMPLANTATION

About 7 days after ovulation or 5 days after fertilization, the trophoblast burrows into the endometrium, usually in the upper part of the uterus. This process is called **implantation**, or embedding of the fertilized egg into the uterine lining. The endometrium is now called the **decidua**. The trophoblast puts out villi, fingerlike projections, to anchor the blastocyst.

The outer fetal membrane is the **chorion**, formed from the trophoblast. The chorionic villi degenerate, except for those attached to the uterine wall, which become the maternal side of the placenta. The inner membrane (fetal side), the **amnion**, originates in the blastocyst during the early stages of development. The amnion expands as the fetus grows until it slightly adheres to the chorion. These two fetal membranes form the amniotic sac or bag of water (BOW).

## AMNIOTIC FLUID

The amniotic fluid is formed by the secretions from the amniotic cells, lungs and skin of the fetus, and fetal urine. It is 98% water, but also contains  glucose, protein, sodium, urea, creatinine, **lanugo** (fine hair covering body of fetus), and **vernix caseosa** (white, creamy covering on the fetus's body). Amniotic fluid is slightly alkaline. Approximately every 3 hours, the fluid is replaced. The amnionic cells and the fetus urinating and swallowing regulate the secretion and reabsorption of the fluid.

The amniotic fluid has several important functions in that it:

- Equalizes the pressure around the fetus
- Cushions the fetus from external compression
- Provides a constant temperature and fluid for the fetus to swallow

- Allows freedom of movement for the fetus
- Lubricates the membranes and the fetus

The yolk sac develops as a second cavity in the blastocyst. It forms primitive red blood cells until the liver is able to take over the process in about 6 weeks. Gradually, the yolk sac is incorporated into the umbilical cord.

## PLACENTA AND UMBILICAL CORD

The chorionic villi at the base of the implanted fertilized ovum and the decidua basalis, the endometrium at the site of implantation, form the placenta. The **placenta** is a membranous vascular organ connecting the fetus to the mother, which produces hormones to sustain a pregnancy, supplies the fetus with oxygen and food, and transports waste products out of the fetal system. The development of the placenta, stimulated by progesterone secreted by the corpus luteum, begins about the third week following fertilization. The placenta is fully functional by the 12th week.

There is a maternal side to the placenta and a fetal side. The maternal side is irregular and is divided into subdivisions called **cotyledons**. It resembles liver both in color and texture. The fetal side is covered by the amnion, so it is smooth and shiny.

The chorionic villi contain blood vessels that join to form larger and larger vessels, eventually becoming the umbilical cord. The **umbilical cord**, a structure that connects the fetus to the placenta, has two arteries and one vein. It is surrounded and protected by a thick substance called **Wharton's jelly** and covered by the amnion. The two umbilical arteries carry deoxygenated blood from the fetus to the placenta, where carbon dioxide and other waste products are eliminated. The one umbilical vein carries oxygenated blood to the fetus along with nutrients, hormones, antibodies, and whatever drugs or toxic substances the mother may have in her body. This is one instance in which arteries carry deoxygenated blood and a vein transports oxygenated blood. Generally, the cord is attached to the center of the placenta, but it can be attached any place on the placenta.

The circulatory systems of the mother and fetus are separate. Maternal blood enters the intervillous spaces of the placenta. Fetal blood is in the vessels of the chorionic villi. Thus the cells of the fetal blood vessels and the chorion keep maternal blood and fetal blood separate (Figure 1-3).

### Functions of the Placenta

The placenta has three major functions: transport, endocrine, and metabolic. All are necessary to maintain the pregnancy and promote normal fetal growth and development. The placenta provides the respiratory and excretory functions for the fetus as well as providing nutrition to the fetus.

**Transport**  There are several mechanisms by which the placenta transports substances.

- Some substances move by diffusion from an area of higher concentration to an area of lower concentration. Those substances transported by this mechanism are oxygen, carbon dioxide, carbon monoxide, water, electrolytes, fat-soluble vitamins, anesthetic gases, and drugs.
- Facilitated diffusion uses a carrier system to move molecules more rapidly than simple diffusion. Some glucose and oxygen are transported by this method.

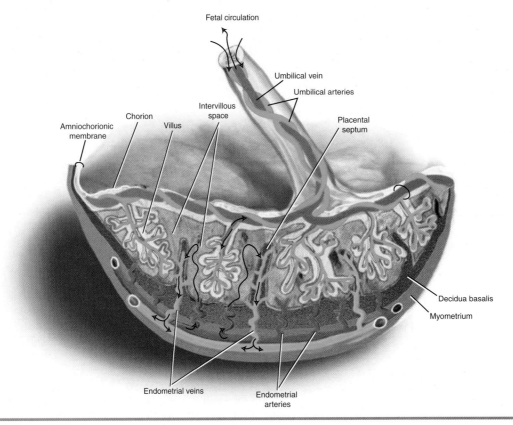

COURTESY OF DELMAR CENGAGE LEARNING

**FIGURE 1-3** **Placental Circulation**

- Active transport allows molecules to move from an area of lower concentration to an area of higher concentration. Substances moved across the placenta by active transport are amino acids, glucose, iron, calcium, iodine, and water-soluble vitamins.
- Pinocytosis transfers larger molecules such as albumin, globulins, antibodies, and viruses through cell membranes.
- Osmotic pressure and hydrostatic pressure move most of the water.

Very large molecules such as insulin, heparin, IgM, and blood cells do not move across the placenta unless there is a tear in the placenta.

**Endocrine** The placenta secretes five hormones that are essential to pregnancy: human chorionic gonadotropin (hCG), which is the basis for pregnancy tests; human placental lactogen (hPL); estrogen; progesterone; and relaxin.

The trophoblast secretes hCG during early pregnancy. The hCG prevents involution of the corpus luteum and stimulates it to continue producing progesterone and estrogen for 11 to 12 weeks. Eight to ten days after fertilization, hCG is present in maternal blood serum; a few days after the missed menstrual period, hCG is found in maternal urine. After 11 weeks, the placenta is producing enough estrogen and progesterone to maintain the pregnancy.

Human placental lactogen makes a sufficient supply of protein, glucose, and minerals available to the fetus by stimulating changes in maternal metabolism. Human placental lactogen is an insulin antagonist, thus decreasing maternal metabolism of glucose. It also ensures that the mother's body is prepared for lactation.

The placenta secretes primarily the estrogen estriol. Estrogen stimulates development of uterine and breast tissues in the mother. It also increases vascularity and vasodilation in the villous capillaries.

After 11 weeks of pregnancy, the placenta takes over the production of progesterone from the corpus luteum. Progesterone, a smooth muscle relaxant, prevents uterine contractions by decreasing its contractility. It also maintains the endometrium.

Relaxin causes changes in collagen. The connective tissue of the symphysis pubis and sacroiliac joints are softened and become slightly flexible.

**Metabolic** The placenta produces fatty acids, glycogen, and cholesterol for fetal use and hormone production. The enzymes required for fetoplacental transfer are also produced by the placenta. It breaks down epinephrine and histamine and stores glycogen and iron.

# FETAL DEVELOPMENT

Fetal development is divided into three stages. The pre-embryonic or germinal stage is the first 14 days after fertilization. The second stage, the embryonic stage, is from the beginning of the third week (day 15) through week eight. The fetal stage is from week 9 until 38 to 40 weeks or full term.

Development occurs in a systematic manner from head to toe (cephalo-caudal), from proximal to distal (close to body–farthest from body), and from general to specific. This means that the head develops before the arms and the arms develop before the legs; the arms and legs develop before the fingers and toes; and the fetus moves its arms before grasping with the hands.

Fetal development is sometimes described in general terms of trimester. The first trimester is the first 12 weeks, second trimester weeks 13 through 27, and third trimester weeks 28 to 40.

Pregnancy generally lasts 10 lunar (28-day) months, 40 weeks, or 280 days. It is calculated from the first day of the mother's last menstrual period (LMP). Table 1-1 identifies

**TABLE 1-1  Stages of Fetal Development**

| STAGE | FETAL DEVELOPMENT | STAGE | FETAL DEVELOPMENT |
|---|---|---|---|
| **Preembryonic or Germinal Stage** | | Week 10 | Head growth slows. |
| Weeks 1 and 2 | Rapid cell division and differentiation. | Wt 14 g (1/2 oz) | Islets of Langerhans differentiated. |
| | Germinal layers form. | L 5–6 cm (2 in) | Bone marrow forms, RBCs produced. |
| **Embryonic Stage** | | crown-heel (C–H) | Bladder sac forms |
| Week 3 | Primitive nervous system, eyes, ears, red blood cells present. | | Kidneys make urine. |
| | Heart begins to beat day 21. | Week 11 | Tooth buds appear. |
| Week 4 | Half the size of a pea. | | Liver secretes bile. |
| Wt 0.4 g | Brain differentiates. | | Urinary system functions. |
| L 4–6 mm | GI tract begins to form. | | Insulin forms in pancreas. |
| (crown–rump, C–R) | Limb buds appear. | Week 12 | Lungs take shape. |
| Week 5 | Cranial nerves present. | Wt 45 g (1.5 oz) | Palate fuses. |
| L6–8 mm (C–R) | Muscles have innervation. | L 9 cm (3.5 in) (C–R) | Heart beat heard with Doppler. |
| Week 6 | Fetal circulation established. | 11.5 cm (4.5 in) (C–H) | Ossification established. |
| L 10–14 mm (C–R) | Liver produces red blood cells. | | Swallowing reflex present. |
| | Central autonomic nervous system forms. | | External genitalia, male or female distinguished. |
| | Primitive kidneys form. | **Second Trimester** | |
| | Lung buds present. | Week 16 | Meconium forms in bowels. |
| | Cartilage forms. | Wt 200 g (7 oz) | Scalp hair appears. |
| | Primitive skeleton forms. | L 13.5 cm (5.5 in) (C–R) | Frequent fetal movement. |
| | Muscles differentiate. | 15 cm (6 in) (C–H) | Skin thin, pink. |
| Week 7 | Eyelids form. | | Sensitive to light. |
| L 22–28 mm (C–R) | Palate and tongue form. | | 200 mL amniotic fluid. (Amniocentesis possible.) |
| | Stomach formed. | Week 20 | Myelination of spinal cord begins. |
| | Diaphragm formed. | Wt 435 g (15 oz) | Peristalsis begins. |
| | Arms, legs move. | L 19 cm (7.5 in) (C–R) | Lanugo covers body. |
| Week 8 | Resembles human being. | 25 cm (10 in) (C–H) | Vernix caseosa covers body. |
| Wt 2 g | Eyes moved to face front. | | Brown fat deposits begun. |
| L 3 cm (1.5 in) (C–R) | Heart development complete. | | Sucks and swallows amniotic fluid. |
| | Hands and feet well formed. | | Heart beat heard with fetoscope. |
| | Bone cells begin replacing cartilage. | | Hands can grasp. |
| | All body organs have begun forming. | | Regular schedule of sucking, kicking, and sleeping. |
| **Fetal Stage** | | Week 24 | Alveoli present in lungs, begin producing surfactant. |
| Week 9 | Finger and toe nails form. | Wt 780 g | Eyes completely formed. |
| | Eyelids fuse shut. | (1 lb, 12 oz) | Eyelashes and eyebrows appear. |
| | | L 23 cm (9 in) (C–R) | Many reflexes appear. |
| | | 28 cm (11 in) (C–H) | Chance of survival if born. |

*(Continues)*

**TABLE 1-1  Stages of Fetal Development (Continued)**

| STAGE | FETAL DEVELOPMENT | STAGE | FETAL DEVELOPMENT |
|---|---|---|---|
| **Third Trimester** | | Week 36 | A few creases on soles of feet. |
| Week 28 | Subcutaneous fat deposits begun. | Wt 2,500–2,750 g | Skin less wrinkled. |
| Wt 1200 g | Lanugo begins to disappear. | (5 lb, 8 oz) | Fingernails reach fingertips. |
| (2 lb, 10 oz) | Nails appear. | L 35 cm (14 in) (C–R) | Sleep-wake cycle fairly definite. |
| L 28 cm (11 in) (C–R) | Eyelids open and close. | 48 cm (19 in) (C–H) | Transfer of maternal antibodies. |
| 35 cm (14 in) (C–H) | Testes begin to descend. | Week 38 | L/S ratio 2:1 |
| Week 32 | More reflexes present. | Week 40 | Lanugo only on shoulders and upper back. |
| Wt 2,000 g | CNS directs rhythmic breathing movements. | Wt 3,000–3,600 g | Creases cover sole. |
| (4 lb, 6.5 oz) | CNS partially controls body temperature. | (6 lb, 10 oz-7 lb, 15 oz) | Vernix mainly in folds of skin. |
| L 31 cm (12 in) (C–R) | Begins storing iron, calcium, phosphorus. | L 50 cm (20 in) (C–H) | Ear cartilage firm. |
| 41 cm (16 in) (C–H) | Ratio of the lung surfactants lecithin and sphingomyelin (L/S) is 1.2:2. | | Less active, limited space. |
| | | | Ready to be born. |

COURTESY OF DELMAR CENGAGE LEARNING

stages of fetal development and gives the weight and length (crown-rump length, or C-R) or crown-heel (C-H) beginning in week 4.

## SYSTEM DEVELOPMENT

All systems in the fetus have begun forming by the eighth week. They grow, develop, and mature at different rates, and some do not mature until years after birth.

## Cardiovascular System

With the primitive heart beginning to beat on the 21st day after conception, the cardiovascular system is the first to function in the embryo. Most congenital malformations of the heart and great vessels develop during the sixth to eighth weeks.

**Fetal Circulation** Fetal circulation has several unique features. Oxygenated blood comes from the placenta and enters the fetus, at the umbilicus, through the umbilical vein. It divides at the liver with a small branch going to the liver and the other branch, the **ductus venosus**, entering the inferior vena cava. The blood is now partially deoxygenated by the blood coming from the lower part of the fetus's body.

This blood enters the right atrium and moves through the **foramen ovale** (a flap opening in the atrial septum that allows only right-to-left movement of blood) to the left atrium and then to the left ventricle. A small portion of this blood passes into the right ventricle. The left ventricle pumps the blood out through the aorta.

Blood entering the right atrium from the superior vena cava flows to the right ventricle. It is pumped out through the pulmonary arteries. Most of this blood goes into the aorta through the **ductus arteriosus**, a fetal vessel connecting the pulmonary trunk to the aorta. Normally this closes at birth.

A small amount of blood goes to the lungs to nourish the lung tissue.

The aorta and its branches supply blood to the rest of the body. The two umbilical arteries branch from the internal iliac arteries and return blood to the placenta to be oxygenated. Figure 1-4 shows fetal circulation.

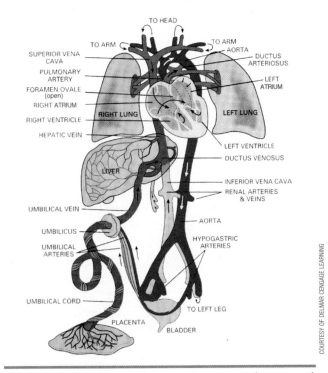

**FIGURE 1-4  Fetal Circulation. Red is arterial (oxygenated) blood, light purple is venous (unoxygenated) blood, and dark purple is mixed arterial-venous blood.**

COURTESY OF DELMAR CENGAGE LEARNING

**Hematologic Development** The formation of blood goes along with cardiovascular development. About day 14, primitive blood cells are formed in the yolk sac. It is the fifth week of gestation before the fetal liver begins hematopoiesis.

Fetal hemoglobin (Hgb F), found only during gestation and the early neonatal period, has a great attraction for oxygen. This ensures an adequate oxygen supply. Blood type is genetically determined at conception.

## Gastrointestinal System

During the fourth week of gestation, the gastrointestinal tract begins forming. The fetus begins swallowing amniotic fluid by the 20th week, but there is no coordination of the swallow and suck reflexes until 34 weeks or later.

Meconium (fecal material stored in the fetal intestines) begins to form about week 16; however, there should not be passage of meconium in utero. If the fetus encounters hypoxic stress, the anal sphincter may relax and meconium may be passed, causing meconium staining of the amniotic fluid.

## Musculoskeletal System

Limb buds appear late in the fourth week and development is complete by the eighth week. Growth of the skeleton is determined by genetics and maternal supply of calcium and phosphorus. Cartilage is noted about 5 weeks and ossification begins about 12 weeks but is not completed until after puberty.

By the end of the 12th week, skeletal muscles begin involuntary movements. Skeletal muscle development depends on an adequate volume of amniotic fluid to allow plenty of fetal movement.

## Genitourinary System

Kidneys begin forming at about 3 weeks and pass through several changes. Around 12 weeks, they begin to produce a hypotonic urine. The placenta and the maternal kidneys are still responsible for fetal waste removal. All the nephrons are in the kidneys at birth.

The reproductive system develops at the same time as the urinary system. Testes can be seen in the abdomen by 7 weeks and begin descending to the scrotum about 30 weeks. The ovaries develop in the abdomen and stay in the pelvic cavity. All of the ova a female will ever have are in the ovaries at birth. Visual determination of fetal gender can be made through ultrasound by the end of week 12.

## Integumentary System

The skin protects the underlying tissues. Vernix caseosa protects the skin, with the amount present decreasing as the pregnancy progresses. Creases form on the palms, fingers, and soles during week 11, with permanent designs formed by week 17. Skin color is genetically determined.

Lanugo appears during week 20 and slowly disappears; most is gone by birth. Tooth buds for the deciduous (baby) teeth appear during week 6 while tooth buds for permanent teeth do not appear until week 10. Second and third permanent molar tooth buds do not appear until after birth. Mammary glands develop during the 6th week.

## Respiratory System

Lung buds begin forming during week 6, with bronchi forming by week 16. Primitive lungs are formed by 23 weeks, but there are not enough alveoli for sufficient gas exchange. Surfactant production begins between weeks 20 and 24. Surfactant reduces the surface tension of the fluid lining the alveoli in the lungs, thus facilitating breathing by keeping the alveoli from collapsing with expiration. Surfactant production matures between weeks 35 and 37. The age of viability, or gestational age at which a fetus could live outside the uterus, is considered to be 20 weeks. Adequate lung functioning also depends on surfactant production and neurologic maturation.

## Immunologic System

Between the 12th and 15th weeks, immune capability begins developing. It functions very minimally because the fetus lives in a sterile environment. The fetus produces small amounts of the immunoglobins IgG, IgA, and IgE before 20 weeks. IgG provides the most immunity. Maternal IgG is actively transported across the placenta to provide passive immunity against many infectious diseases. Blood group antibodies are a type of IgG. They can move across the placenta by active transport and cause hemolytic disease of the newborn.

## FACTORS AFFECTING FETAL DEVELOPMENT

Many factors influence fetal development, especially during the first trimester. Even before the mother knows she is pregnant, factors are affecting embryonic development. One of the very first is the quality of the sperm and the ovum and the genetic code. Teratogens (any agent, such as radiation, drugs, viruses, or other microorganisms, capable of causing abnormal fetal development) exert the greatest influence on cells undergoing the most rapid growth. Each organ has a period when teratogenic agents or other insults can cause physical and functional defects.

A well-provided maternal environment is also important. Maternal malnutrition, acute and chronic diseases, drugs, alcohol, and smoking all can exert potentially harmful effects on the fetus before birth.

# MATERNAL PHYSIOLOGICAL CHANGES OF PREGNANCY

Many physiological changes take place when a woman is pregnant. Every system of the mother's body undergoes some change during pregnancy.

## REPRODUCTIVE SYSTEM

The most obvious physiological changes occur in the reproductive system.

## Uterus

The most dramatic change occurs in the size of the uterus. Before pregnancy, it is a small, pear-shaped, thick-walled, muscular organ weighing 60 g (2 oz). At the end of pregnancy, it is a large, thin-walled organ weighing 1,000 g (2 lb). Its capacity has increased from 10 mL to 5 L. The uterus enlarges mainly by hypertrophy of the muscle cells stimulated by estrogen and the growing fetus. There are three layers of smooth (involuntary)

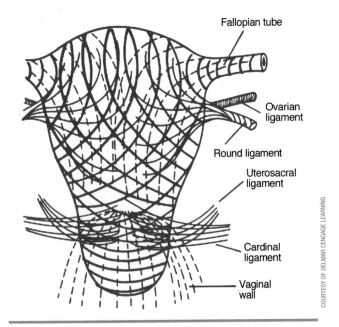

**FIGURE 1-5** **Muscle Layers of the Uterus**

muscles in the uterus (Figure 1-5). The outer layer is made of longitudinal muscles. The muscle fibers of the middle layer are interlaced in a figure eight pattern. Circular fibers that form sphincters at the openings of the fallopian tubes and at the internal os of the cervix make up the inner layer of uterine muscle. This configuration of muscle layers allows the uterus to expand evenly in all directions during pregnancy. One-sixth of the mother's blood volume is in the vascular system of the uterus by the end of pregnancy.

Irregular uterine contractions occur throughout pregnancy. About 16 weeks or later, the mother may become aware of these **Braxton-Hicks contractions**. These generally painless contractions assist in uterine and placental circulation. Pain is an individual perceptual experience. A softening of the uterine isthmus about the sixth week of pregnancy, noted during a pelvic exam, is called **Hegar's sign**.

## Cervix

The cervix increases in cell number by the influence of estrogen. It secretes a thick, sticky mucus that forms a plug in the cervix. This plug prevents microorganisms from entering through the vagina. During labor, as the cervix dilates, this mucus plug is expelled. **Goodell's sign** (softening of the cervix) and **Chadwick's sign** (a purplish-blue color of the cervix and vagina caused by the increased vascularity) are both noted at about 8 weeks.

## Ovaries

Follicles do not mature and ovulation does not occur during pregnancy. The corpus luteum produces progesterone and estrogen for about 12 weeks, at which time the placenta takes over the production.

## Vagina

Estrogen causes a loosening of connective tissue and an increase in vaginal secretions. The acidic secretions prevent bacterial infections. The increased level of glycogen in cells may enhance growth of organisms such as *Trichomonas vaginalis* or *Candida albicans*.

## Breasts

In addition to breast enlargement from hormonal influence, the nipples become more erect, the areolas darken, and Montgomery's tubercles enlarge. **Colostrum**, an antibody-rich yellow fluid, is secreted by the breasts during the last trimester and first 2–3 days after birth, and gradually changes to milk a few days after delivery.

## CARDIOVASCULAR SYSTEM

Blood flow increases to the uterus and kidneys, where the workload is increased. The pulse increases by 10 to 15 beats/minute by the end of pregnancy. Cardiac output increases 30% to 50% early in pregnancy. Blood pressure decreases, is lowest during the second trimester, and increases gradually to near the prepregnant level during the third trimester. This occurs because of the progesterone's relaxing effect on the smooth muscles.

Stasis of blood in the lower extremities, caused by the enlarged uterus interfering with return blood flow, may lead to dependent edema and varicose veins of the legs, vulva, or rectum.

**Supine hypotensive syndrome**, also known as vena caval syndrome, occurs when the mother lies supine. The enlarged, heavy uterus presses on the inferior vena cava, causing a reduced blood flow back to the right atrium (Figure 1-6). The mother experiences dizziness, clammy-pale skin, nausea, and a lowering of her blood pressure. This decreases placental perfusion, which can affect fetal reserve. The situation is relieved when the mother lies on her side.

Maternal blood volume increases 30% to 50%, reaching its peak at about 30 weeks. There is some increase in red blood cells, but most of the increase is plasma. This hemodilution is manifested by a lower hematocrit (34% to 40%) and is termed **physiologic anemia of pregnancy**.

The white blood cell count begins to increase by about 8 weeks and may reach 18,000/mm³ by the time of delivery. Platelets, fibrin, fibrinogen, and coagulation factors VII, IX, and X increase. This increase with possible venous stasis in late pregnancy increases the risk of venous thrombosis.

## RESPIRATORY SYSTEM

Progesterone decreases airway resistance, allowing an increase in oxygen consumption. The depth of respirations increases,

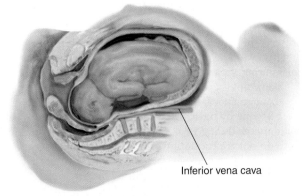

Inferior vena cava

**FIGURE 1-6** **Supine Hypotensive Syndrome. Enlarged uterus presses on vena cava when mother is supine. Side-lying position relieves pressure.**

causing a mild respiratory alkalosis, which is compensated by increased renal secretion of bicarbonate (Littleton & Engebretson, 2002). The enlarging uterus presses upward on the diaphragm. The rib cage flares and the chest circumference expands to keep the intrathoracic volume the same as when not pregnant. Estrogen causes edema and vascular congestion of the nasal mucosa.

## MUSCULOSKELETAL SYSTEM

The relaxation of the pelvic joints in preparation for delivery is caused by relaxin. As pregnancy progresses, the mother's center of gravity gradually changes because of the increased size and weight of the uterus anteriorly. To compensate, the mother increases the curve of the lumbosacral spine (lordosis), which frequently results in a low backache, and may cause the woman to have a waddling gait. Figure 1-7 illustrates this change throughout pregnancy.

## GASTROINTESTINAL SYSTEM

Nausea and/or vomiting, known as "morning sickness," are common in early pregnancy but usually disappear by 12 weeks. The smooth muscle relaxation effect of progesterone results in delayed gastric emptying and decreased peristalsis. The enlarging uterus displaces the stomach and intestines. All of these changes contribute to constipation. Relaxation of the cardiac sphincter allows reflux of acidic gastric contents into the esophagus, giving the mother heartburn.

## URINARY SYSTEM

Urinary frequency occurs in the first trimester as the enlarging uterus presses on the bladder and in the third trimester as the fetus settles into the pelvis and presses on the bladder. Progesterone causes the ureters to relax and dilate. Glomerular filtration rate (GFR) begins rising in the second trimester. Tubular reabsorption also increases.

Glycosuria (excretion of glucose in the urine) develops if the kidneys are unable to reabsorb all of the glucose filtered by the glomeruli. Any amount more than a trace of glucose in the urine is investigated.

## INTEGUMENTARY SYSTEM

Several skin pigment changes generally occur during pregnancy. The nipples, areola, vulva, and perineal area darken. **Linea nigra** is a pigmented line on the abdomen from umbilicus to symphysis pubis. **Chloasma**, also called "mask of pregnancy," is a darkening of the skin of the forehead and around the eyes. It is generally more pronounced in

dark-haired women. **Striae gravidarum**, or "stretch marks," are reddish streaks frequently found on the abdomen, thighs, buttocks, and breasts. They are the result of separation of the underlying connective tissue of the skin (Figure 1-8). As the skin stretches, the client may experience itching.

## ENDOCRINE SYSTEM

The anterior pituitary hormone prolactin is responsible for initial milk production. The posterior pituitary hormone oxytocin causes uterine contractions and the ejection of milk from the breasts (let-down reflex) after delivery.

The placental hormones, especially hPL, are insulin antagonists, so a greater insulin production is required. This puts an increased stress on the islets of Langerhans in the pancreas to put out more insulin. A woman with a marginally functioning pancreas may show signs of gestational diabetes in the latter half of pregnancy.

A slight increase in the size of the thyroid often occurs, as well as an increase in its capacity to bind thyroxine. Maternal thyroxine is important for fetal neural development throughout pregnancy, especially during the first trimester. This results in a higher level of serum protein-bound iodine (PBI).

## METABOLISM

The metabolic rate of the mother increases during pregnancy as the demands of the growing fetus increase. The mother must meet her own and the fetus's nutritional needs.

# SIGNS OF PREGNANCY

The many physiological changes that a woman experiences during pregnancy are categorized as presumptive, probable, or positive signs of pregnancy.

## PRESUMPTIVE SIGNS

Changes that the woman experiences and reports are termed presumptive or subjective signs. They may be caused by other conditions, so are not diagnostic of pregnancy. Presumptive signs include:

- **Amenorrhea** (absence of menses), usually the first sign that a woman notices causing her to think she is pregnant.
- Nausea and vomiting, often referred to as "morning sickness," but can occur any time of the day. This sign usually disappears by 12 weeks of pregnancy.

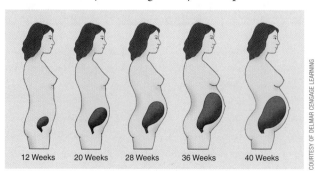

FIGURE 1-7    **Lordosis increases throughout pregnancy.**

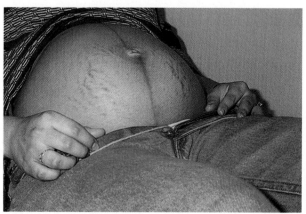

FIGURE 1-8    **Linea Nigra and Striae Gravidarum**

- Breast changes, tenderness, or tingling.
- Urinary frequency, as the growing uterus presses against the bladder, giving the woman the sensation of needing to urinate.
- Excessive fatigue, often noted after the first missed menstrual period. It may last for several months.
- Abdominal enlargement usually noticed by the woman, generally after 12 weeks.
- **Quickening**, perception of fetal movement by the mother, usually between 16 and 20 weeks. It begins as a fluttering sensation and gradually gets stronger and more frequent.

A positive diagnosis of pregnancy is usually made before these last two signs are noted by the woman; however, there is a condition called **pseudocyesis** or false pregnancy, in which the woman believes so strongly that she is pregnant that she appears to have all the early presumptive signs of pregnancy.

## PROBABLE SIGNS

The examiner can identify these objective changes, but since they can be caused by conditions other than pregnancy, they are not diagnostic of pregnancy.

### Pelvic Signs

Goodell's sign (softening of the cervix), Hegar's sign (softening of the uterine isthmus), and Chadwick's sign (purplish discoloration of the vagina, cervix, and vulva) can be identified by the examiner during the first 12 weeks of pregnancy.

Uterine enlargement is identified after the eighth week of pregnancy. The fundus is palpable just above the symphysis at 12 weeks and at the umbilicus at 20 weeks (Figure 1-9). If these uterine enlargement milestones are reached earlier, multiple pregnancy, or **polyhydramnios**, excessive amniotic fluid, is suspected.

### Braxton-Hicks Contractions

After the 28th week, these contractions can be felt by the examiner and also by the client.

### Increased Pigmentation

The nipples and areola darken. Linea nigra may appear on the abdomen, chloasma may mark the face, and striae gravidarum may be noticed on the breasts and abdomen.

### Ballottement

During the fourth or fifth month, if the fetus is pushed upward through the vagina or abdomen, the floating fetus rebounds against the examiner's fingers; this is known as **ballottement** (Figure 1-10).

### Pregnancy Test

The basis for a pregnancy test is the presence of hCG in either the urine or blood of the woman. A test of the blood is positive 8 days after conception, and a test of the urine is positive 10 to 14 days after conception.

## POSITIVE SIGNS

A positive sign of pregnancy proves conclusively that the woman is pregnant. No other condition can cause these signs to appear. There are only three positive signs of pregnancy: hearing the fetal heartbeat, visualization of the fetus, and the examiner feeling fetal movement.

### Hearing the Fetal Heartbeat

The fetal heartbeat can be detected at 10 to 12 weeks using the Doppler ultrasound method (Figure 1-11).

When auscultating the abdomen over the uterus, a soft, blowing sound may be heard. The sound occurring at the same rate as the mother's pulse is called the **uterine souffle**, caused by the blood pulsating through the uterus and placenta. The sound occurring at the same rate as the fetal heart rate is called the **funic souffle**, caused by blood pulsating through the umbilical cord.

### Visualization of the Fetus

An abdominal ultrasound examination can detect a pregnancy by the sixth week after the last menstrual period (LMP). An endovaginal ultrasound examination, using a vaginal probe, can detect a gestational sac 10 days after implantation.

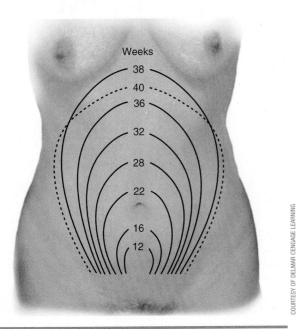

**FIGURE 1-9** Fundal Height Milestones

COURTESY OF DELMAR CENGAGE LEARNING

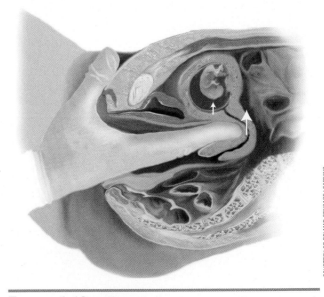

**FIGURE 1-10** Ballottement

COURTESY OF DELMAR CENGAGE LEARNING

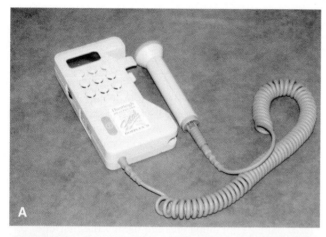

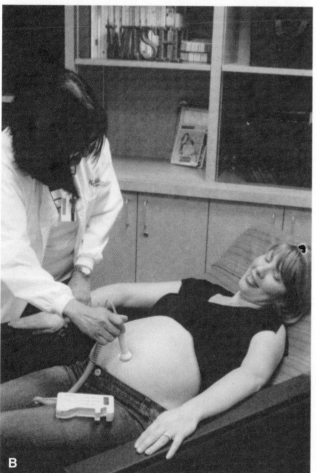

PHOTOS COURTESY OF DELMAR CENGAGE LEARNING

FIGURE 1-11  *A,* Fetal Doppler; *B,* Fetal Doppler in Use

## Examiner Feeling Fetal Movement

Fetal movement felt by the examiner, not the mother, is a positive sign of pregnancy.

## PSYCHOLOGICAL ADAPTATION TO PREGNANCY

Pregnancy is often viewed as a developmental stage having its own developmental tasks. Both the expectant mother and father deal with significant changes and major psychosocial adjustment.

## DEVELOPMENTAL TASKS

Four major developmental tasks are identified for pregnancy. They are pregnancy validation, fetal embodiment, fetal distinction, and role transition. These developmental tasks are met in this order. The rate at which they are met varies. According to Malnory (1996), completion of the developmental tasks is critical to positive parenting.

### Pregnancy Validation

During the first trimester, the pregnant woman's task is to validate and accept the pregnancy. Until the woman meets this task, she cannot meet the rest of the developmental tasks. Even when pregnancy is planned, there are normal feelings of ambivalence and disbelief about the pregnancy. Many women become introspective or have mood swings caused by hormone fluctuations.

### Fetal Embodiment

Fetal embodiment occurs as the mother incorporates the growing fetus into her body image. The physical changes she is experiencing, especially the growing uterus, help her meet this task. She feels that the fetus is a part of her. Self-involvement, depression, or regressive behavior are signs of difficulty in meeting this task.

### Fetal Distinction

When fetal movement is felt, it becomes easier for the mother to think of the fetus as a separate being. She may daydream about what the baby will be like and think about the kind of mother she wants to be.

### Role Transition

The last trimester is a time of preparation. Many expectant parents attend childbirth classes to learn about and prepare for labor, delivery, infant care, and self-care. Preparing a nursery, buying baby clothes, and selecting a day care are all ways of preparing for the infant's arrival. Role transition also includes parents exploring together the meaning of fathering and mothering, learning parenting skills, the amazing skills of a newborn for interactions, and the physical maturing and behavioral changes of the first 12 months of life. Another aspect is learning to enjoy watching the other parent interact with the newborn.

At the end of pregnancy, many mothers experience a surge of energy and see to it that the entire household is organized for the coming of the infant. This is called **nesting**. All of these preparations assist the pregnant woman in the transition to her new role of mother.

### Partners' Tasks

Fathers and other partners must meet the same developmental tasks as the expectant mother but in a more abstract way. Accepting the fact that they (as a couple) are pregnant and announcing it to family and friends meets the first task. The partner may also have ambivalent feelings about the pregnancy. By accepting the changes in the pregnant partner, both physical and psychological, the task of fetal embodiment is met. Fetal distinction is generally met when the partner hears the fetal heartbeat and feels the fetus moving. Role transition is met in virtually the same way as is done by the pregnant woman.

# FACTORS AFFECTING PSYCHOLOGICAL RESPONSE

Factors that contribute to a woman's psychological response to her pregnancy include body image, financial situation, cultural expectations, emotional security, and support from significant others.

## Body Image

The mother's body image, or perception of her own body, may change in several areas. The noticeable changes in body shape and the speed with which those changes occur may be very threatening to some women. Some women feel "fat" and "ugly" when they are pregnant, and others feel "so good" and "beautiful" when they are pregnant.

The physical discomforts of pregnancy may cause the mother to feel a lack of control over her own body. For example, urinary frequency or urinary incontinence may increase negative feelings about the pregnancy.

Pregnant women often feel restricted in their physical activities. As long as there is no problem with the pregnancy, encourage the mother to continue regular activities, keeping in mind that moderation is the key.

## Financial Situation

A poor financial situation may cause anxiety about paying bills, buying needed items for infant care, or having enough and proper foods for good nutrition. Financial consideration may also be a significant concern for the expectant mother's partner.

## Cultural Expectations

Cultural expectations of the family may cause conflicts for the pregnant woman and her partner if their ideas are different from their families' expectations. Conflicts occur if the cultural expectations of the mother are different from the cultural expectations of the father or partner.

## Emotional Security

A pregnant woman's satisfaction with herself and her life situation has an impact on how she responds to being pregnant. If the woman is secure in her feelings about herself and her perceived abilities as a mother, the pregnancy is more likely to be enjoyable. A pregnancy that was planned or long anticipated will likely be received with joy and excitement, whereas an unexpected or unwanted pregnancy may be met with fear, dread, or uncertainty.

## Support from Significant Others

It is important for the nurse and the expectant mother to take into consideration the psychological responses of significant others, namely, the father/partner, siblings, and grandparents.

Father/Partner  The expectant father or partner must shift thinking from being a person without children to a person with a child. He may feel left out, neglected, or resent the attention focused on the expectant mother.

Couvade is the development of physical symptoms by the expectant father such as fatigue, depression, headache, backache, and nausea. Longobucco and Freston (1989) found that men who show couvade have greater paternal role preparation.

Siblings  A new baby may be seen by siblings as a threat to their relationship with the parents. Siblings should be included in the pregnancy and preparations for the new baby on an age-appropriate basis. Feeling the fetus kick and hearing the heartbeat often are helpful activities for siblings. Parents must be sure to maintain some special time just for the siblings. Many areas have classes for siblings to help them understand what is happening in their lives.

Grandparents  Grandparents are usually the first ones told about the pregnancy. It is often difficult for grandparents to know how much to become involved in the process. Some grandparents feel they are not ready or are too young to become grandparents.

Practices of childbearing and childrearing often change greatly from one generation to another. Some areas have classes to provide information to grandparents about these changes.

# PRENATAL EDUCATION AND CARE

Prenatal care (care of a woman during pregnancy, before labor) is credited with the reduction of perinatal mortality over the last 50 years. The earlier prenatal care is begun, the better. This provides an opportunity for the health care provider to obtain baseline data on physical assessments and laboratory test results. Women who do not seek prenatal care in a timely fashion often have an underlying mental illness or substance abuse problem, or may be in denial of their pregnancy (Hatters Friedman, Heneghan, & Rosenthal, 2009). Cost may also be a major barrier to prenatal care.

Anticipatory guidance (providing information, teaching, or guidance to a client in anticipation of an expected event) is probably the most important aspect of prenatal care. It is based on the assessment of mother and fetus and knowledge of the normal process of pregnancy and possible complications.

## PRENATAL CARE

The goals of prenatal care are as follows:

- A healthy, prepared mother having minimal discomforts
- Identification of potential problems or complications as early as possible
- Safe delivery of a healthy infant
- A prepared father or partner who participates as much or as little as the couple desires
- Prepared siblings and grandparents

### Initial Visit

A comfortable environment, open communication, and the nurse's attitude will help put the woman at ease during the initial prenatal visit. The first visit is often quite lengthy. A complete history is recorded to identify factors that may

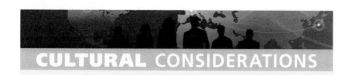

## CULTURAL CONSIDERATIONS

### Beliefs Influencing Pregnancy

Some cultural practices may not always be observed by a client, but some general practices that have cultural influences include the following:

- Muslim women are to keep hair, body, arms to the wrist, and legs to the ankles covered at all times. Also, a Muslim woman may not be alone in the presence of a man other than her husband or a male relative, including during a physical examination (Hutchinson & Baqi-Aziz, 1994).
- Korean women defer to elders, especially the mother-in-law, for care decisions (Schneiderman, 1996).
- Native American women should not look at a deformed, injured, or blind person, or the baby will have the same defect (Cesario, 2001).
- Orthodox Jewish women must keep their hair covered at all times except in the presence of their husbands. They may wear wigs or scarves. Men may not touch any woman except his wife, so he may not shake hands. The nurse may nod rather than offer to shake hands. A husband is not allowed to touch his wife when she is in *niddah*, whenever she is pregnant, menstruating, or nursing and there is blood from the vagina. Thus, he is unable to touch her or pass her anything when she is in labor (Zauderer C, 2009).
- Mexican women consider pregnancy a "hot" state and will avoid cold liquids, fearing they will cause an imbalance resulting in illness or miscarriage (Holtz C. 2008).
- Guatemalan women believe that a pregnant woman and her unborn child are physically and spiritually weak and may be vulnerable to illnesses and evil forces (Callister & Vega, 1998).
- In Malawi, Africa, the father determines family size and the timing of the pregnancies (Gennaro et al., 1998).

### TABLE 1-2  Terms Used in Describing a Pregnant Client

**Abortion** Loss of pregnancy before the age of viability (20 weeks gestation)

**GP/TPAL** Gravida, para/term, preterm, abortions, living

*Examples*: Mary Jo is G2 P1/T2 P0 A0 L2; second pregnancy, one delivery/two infants at term (twins), both living.

Susan is G4 P2/T1 P1 A1 L2; fourth pregnancy, two deliveries/one term infant, one preterm infant, one abortion, two living children.

**Gravida** Pregnancy, regardless of duration, includes present pregnancy

**Para** Delivery (birth) after 20 weeks' gestation, whether infant born alive or dead or number of infants born

**Preterm** Delivery after 20 weeks' gestation but before 38 weeks (full term)

**Term** A pregnancy between 38 and 42 weeks' gestation

**Nulligravida** Never been pregnant

**Primigravida** Pregnant for first time

**Multigravida** Pregnant two or more times

**Nullipara** Never having delivered an infant after 20 weeks' gestation

**Primipara** Has delivered once after 20 weeks' gestation

**Multipara** Has delivered twice or more after 20 weeks' gestation

**Postterm** Delivery after 42 weeks' gestation

COURTESY OF DELMAR CENGAGE LEARNING

negatively affect the pregnancy, and a physical examination is performed. If the woman did not seek preconception care, all of the topics covered in that section would then be discussed at the first prenatal visit. Important terms used in describing a pregnant client are provided in Table 1-2.

**Initial History** The history provides the health care provider with the client's past and present health. Figure 1-12 shows a sample health history summary.

**Estimating Duration of Pregnancy** Every family wants to know the "due date," the estimated date when the infant is to be born. The estimated date of birth (EDB) or estimated date of delivery (EDD) is 40 weeks from the first day of the

woman's LMP. Many women do not keep track of their menstrual periods, or have irregular periods; but an EDB can be identified based on other factors such as uterine size, date of quickening, date when the fetal heartbeat is heard, and ultrasound fetal measurements.

***Naegele's Rule*** Naegele's rule is the most common method of calculating the EDB. The rule is: Take the date of the first day of the last menstrual period, subtract 3 months, and add 7 days. For instance, if the LMP was June 28, the calculation would be as follows:

| Month | Day |
|---|---|
| 6  (June) | 28 |
| −3   months | +7  days |
| 3  (March) | 35 |

Because there are 31 days in March, the EDB moves forward to April 4.

***Gestation Calculator*** A gestation calculator, in the shape of either a chart or a wheel, allows a quick EDB calculation. The wheel generally provides other information also, such as fetal weight and body length for each week (Figure 1-13).

***Fundal Height*** Fundal height generally indicates gestational age through the second trimester (refer back to Figure 1-9).

Hollister™

**Health History Summary**
Hollister Maternal/Newborn Record System   Page 2 of 2
To order call: 1.800.323.4060   Re-order No. 5700

Patient's Name
ID. No.

Check and detail positive findings below. Use reference numbers.

**Cardiovascular**
37. Heart Disease
38. Rheumatic Fever
39. Mitral Valve Prolapse
40. Chronic Hypertension
41. Varicosities
42. Thrombophlebitis
  Previous Pulmonary Embolism
43. Blood Disorders
44. Anemia/Hemoglobinopathy
45. Blood Transfusions

**Pulmonary**
46. Asthma
47. Tuberculosis
48. Chronic Obstructive Pulmonary Disease

**Endocrine**
49. Diabetes
50. Thyroid Dysfunction
51. Maternal PKU
52. Endocrinopathy
53. Gastrointestinal
54. Liver Disease

**Genetic History**
73. Age ≥ 35 (♀) ≥ 50 (♂)
74. Cerebral Palsy
75. Cleft Lip/Palate
76. Congenital Anomalies
77. Congenital Heart Disease
78. Consanguinity
79. Cystic Fibrosis
80. Down's Syndrome
81. Hemophilia
82. Huntington's Chorea

Renal Disease
55. Cystitis
56. Pyelonephritis
57. Asymptomatic Bacteriuria
58. Chronic Renal Disease
59. Neurologic/Seizure Disorder
60. Autoimmune Disease
61. Cancer
62. Other

**Other**
63. Psychiatric Disease
64. Physical Abuse or Neglect
65. Emotional Abuse or Neglect
66. Addiction (Drug, Alcohol, Nicotine)
67. Major Accidents
68. Surgery
69. Anesthetic Complications
70. Non-Surgical Hospitalization
71. Other
72. No Known Disease/Problems

83. Mental Retardation
84. Muscular Dystrophy
85. Neural Tube Defect
86. Sickle Cell Disease or Trait
87. Tay-Sachs Disease
88. Test for Fragile X
89. Thalassemia A or B
90. Other
91. Other
92. Other

**Historical Risk Status** ☐ No Risk Factors Noted
☐ At Risk (Identify)

Signature

---

Hollister™

**Health History Summary**
Hollister Maternal/Newborn Record System   Page 1 of 2
To order call: 1.800.323.4060   Re-order No. 5700

Patient's Name
ID. No.

**Demographic Data**
Date of Birth
Age
Religion ☐ N/A
Marital Status S M SEP D W
Language ☐ English
Interpreter
☐ None
Race/Ethnicity

Father of Baby's Name
Patient / Father of Baby
Education   Occupation   Full Part Self Unemp   Work Tel No   Home Tel No

**Allergies/Sensitivities**
Medication ☐ None
Other ☐ None

Primary/Referring Physician

**Menstrual History**
Menarche   Interval   Length
yrs   days   days
Certain ☐ Yes ☐ No
Normal ☐ Yes ☐ No
LMP
Positive Pregnancy Test
Abnormalities ☐ None

**EDD**
By Dates
By Ultrasound
Date of Ultrasound

**Pregnancy History**

| No | Month/Year | Infant Sex | Weight at Birth | Wks Gest | Gravida | Full Term | Premature | Hours In Labor | Type of Delivery | Anesthesia | Spontaneous Ab | Induced Ab | Ectopic | Multiple Births | Live | Comments/Complications |
|----|-----------|-----------|-----------------|----------|---------|-----------|-----------|----------------|------------------|------------|----------------|------------|---------|-----------------|------|------------------------|
| 1 | | | | | | | | | | | | | | | | |
| 2 | | | | | | | | | | | | | | | | |
| 3 | | | | | | | | | | | | | | | | |
| 4 | | | | | | | | | | | | | | | | |
| 5 | | | | | | | | | | | | | | | | |
| 6 | | | | | | | | | | | | | | | | |
| 7 | | | | | | | | | | | | | | | | |

☐ Blood ☐ Urine

Check and detail positive findings below. Use reference numbers.

**Medical History**
**Obstetric**
1. Anemia
2. Fetal/Neonatal Death or Anomaly
3. Gestational Diabetes
4. Hemorrhage
5. Hyperemesis
6. Incompetent Cervix
7. Intrauterine Growth Retardation
8. Isoimmunization
9. Polyhydramnios
10. Postpartum Depression
11. Pregnancy Induced Hypertension
12. Preterm Labor or Birth
13. PROM-Chorioamnionitis
14. Rhogam Given
15. RH Neg

**Gynecologic**
16. Contraceptive Use
17. Abnormal PAP
18. Fibroids
19. GYN Surgery

**Gynecologic (Cont'd.)**
20. Infertility
21. In Utero Exposure to DES
22. Uterine/Cervical Anomaly

**Sexually Transmitted Diseases**
23. Chlamydia
24. Gonorrhea
25. Herpes (HSV)
26. Syphilis

**Vaginal/Genital Infections**
27. Trichomonas
28. Condylomata
29. Candidiasis

**Other Infections**
30. Toxoplasmosis
31. Group B Streptococcus
32. Rubella
33. Varicella
34. Cytomegalovirus (CMV)
35. AIDS (HIV)
36. Hepatitis (type ____)

FIGURE 1-12   *Representative Health History Forms (Permission to use this copyrighted material has been granted by the owner, Hollister Incorporated.)*

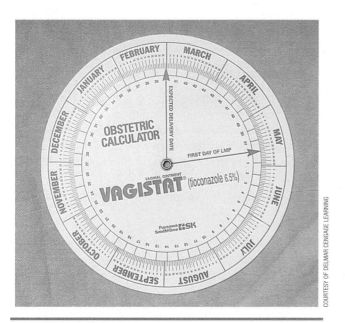

**FIGURE 1-13** Gestation Calculation Wheel. Place arrow labeled *first day of LMP* on that date. Read date at arrow labeled *expected delivery date.*

The **fundus** (top of the uterus) is measured in centimeters from the top of the pubic symphysis to the top of the uterine fundus (McDonald's method). This is fairly accurate between 18 and 30 weeks' gestation. The fundal height, for example, is generally 20 cm (at the umbilicus) at 20 weeks' gestation and 25 cm at 25 weeks' gestation in the average-height woman. Evaluating the visit-to-visit fundal height measurements provides a general pattern of fetal growth. A sudden increase may indicate twins or hydramnios (excessive amount of amniotic fluid), whereas a smaller increase may indicate growth restriction (Figure 1-14).

*Other Indicators* Additional assessments that indicate the gestational week of pregnancy include ultrasound, fetal heartbeat, and quickening.

- *Ultrasound:* Five to six weeks after the LMP, an ultrasound can detect a gestational sac. It shows fetal heartbeat activity at 9 to 10 weeks' gestation. By 12 to 13 weeks, the biparietal diameter (BPD), or distance between the parietal bones of the fetal skull, can be measured.

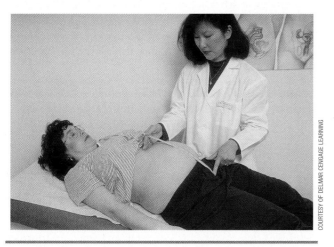

**FIGURE 1-14** Measuring Fundal Height

- *Fetal Heartbeat:* The fetal heartbeat is generally heard by 10 to 12 weeks with the fetal Doppler but may be heard as early as 8 weeks' gestation. It is usually 18 to 20 weeks before the fetal heartbeat can be heard with a fetoscope.
- *Quickening:* Fetal movement is usually felt by the mother at about 20 weeks' gestation. Women identify these movements as early as 16 weeks or as late as 22 weeks. Typically, the woman will detect this movement earlier with a second pregnancy than with a first.

**Physical Examination** The physical examination begins with measuring the client's height and weight and vital signs. A head-to-toe examination is performed by the health care provider. Special attention is given to the assessment of the heart, lungs, pelvis, breasts, and nipples. Figure 1-15 shows an initial pregnancy profile form, and Figure 1-16 shows a prenatal flow record.

The pelvic examination is performed last. The external genitalia are examined for scars, lesions, or infection. A Pap smear for cervical cancer and a specimen of cervical mucous for gonorrhea are usually obtained. A bimanual examination is performed to determine uterine changes (Figure 1-17) and pelvic size to estimate adequacy of the pelvic opening for delivery.

Pelvic size is estimated by the examiner during the manual examination. The diagonal conjugate (distance from the lower border of the pubic symphysis to the sacral promontory) is an estimate of the pelvic inlet. It is generally 11.5 cm. The antero-posterior diameter (9.5 to 11.5 cm), measured from the lower border of the pubic symphysis to the tip of the sacrum, is an estimate of the pelvic outlet.

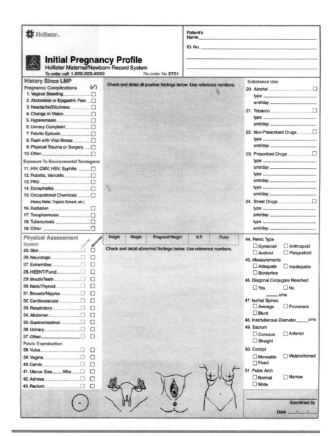

**FIGURE 1-15** Representative Initial Pregnancy Profile (*Permission to use this copyrighted material has been granted by the owner, Hollister Incorporated.*)

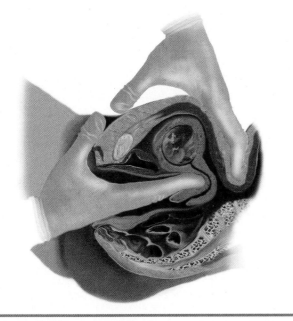

**FIGURE 1-16** **Representative Prenatal Flow Record** (*Permission to use this copyrighted material has been granted by the owner, Hollister Incorporated.*)

**FIGURE 1-17** **Bimanual Examination to Determine Uterine Changes**

## Screening Tests

During the first visit, screening tests are performed to determine the mother's health and to have baseline data with which to compare subsequent test results. Other screening tests are gestational age dependent and are ordered at a later time in pregnancy. Tests may vary for a specific client but generally include those listed in Table 1-3.

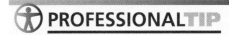

### Prenatal Diagnostic Tests

"AFP testing is accepted as the standard of care and must be offered to pregnant women between the 16th and 20th weeks of pregnancy. . . . [H]ealth care providers need to keep a record of patients' refusal of any diagnostic tests offered to them" (Rhodes, 1995).

## Return Visits

Return visits for an uncomplicated pregnancy generally are:

- Every 4 weeks for the first 28 weeks
- Every 2 weeks during weeks 29 to 36
- Every week, after 36 weeks, until birth of infant

**Subjective Data** The following subjective data should be collected at each return visit:

- How the client is feeling
- Any discomforts, concerns, or questions the client may have
- Any body changes noticed by the client
- How developmental tasks are being met

At an early return visit, the mother's expectations for childbirth should be discussed. Closer to the EDB, preparations for the baby should also be covered.

**Objective Data** On each return visit, the following objective data should be collected and compared with data collected on previous visits and to prepregnant data, if known.

**Blood Pressure** Any increase of 30 mm Hg systolic or 15 mm Hg diastolic from one visit to the next is reported to the health care provider. If there is no previous BP to compare to, a blood pressure of 140/90 or greater is reported.

**Weight** Total weight gain in a normal-weighted woman should be approximately 25 to 35 pounds, distributed as follows:

- Weeks 1 to 12:    2 to 4 pounds
- Weeks 13 to 40:    1 pound/week

The ACOG recommends that underweight women gain 28–40 pounds during pregnancy and that overweight women gain 15–25 pounds. Weight gain is more if the woman is carrying multiples.

**Uterine Size** The fundal height in centimeters indicates the weeks of gestation between 18 and 30 weeks.

**Edema** A small amount of dependent edema is often present in the last few weeks of pregnancy. Edema of the hands and face is reported to the health care provider. Sometimes it is difficult to detect small amounts of edema in the hands, so ask the client if her rings are tighter or if she has had to remove her rings.

**Fetal Position** Assessment of fetal position is performed using **Leopold's maneuvers**, a series of specific palpations

### TABLE 1-3  Screening Tests in Pregnancy

| TEST | RESULTS |
| --- | --- |
| **Initial visit** | |
| Complete Blood Count | |
| RBC | 3.75 million/mm³ due to hemodilution. |
| WBC | Rises to 18,000/mm³ by late pregnancy. Mostly an increase in neutrophils. |
| Hemoglobin (Hgb) | May decrease to 11.5g/dL later in pregnancy due to hemodilution. Repeat at 28 and 36 weeks. |
| Hematocrit (Hct) | 33% lowest acceptable, due to hemodilution. |
| Blood Type | A, B, AB, or O |
| Rh factor | Positive or negative. If negative, do indirect Coomb's test. Check father's Rh. |
| Coomb's Test | Should remain negative. Retest Rh negative women at 28 weeks. |
| Rubella Titer (HAI) | >1:10 indicates immunity. <1:10, immunize after birth of infant. |
| Blood Glucose | Should be 70–110 mg/dL. Retest at 24 and 32 weeks. |
| VDRL or RPR (Syphilis) | Should be negative. |
| Cervical/Vaginal Culture | Should be negative. |
| Gonorrhea | |
| Chlamydia | |
| Group B *Streptococcus* | |
| Hepatitis B Surface Antigen ($HB_sAg$) | Positive indicates either active hepatitis or carrier state. |
| Antibody Titer $HB_sAg$ | Positive indicates immunity to hepatitis. |
| HIV (many states mandate that it be offered) | Should be negative. |
| Tuberculosis | Should be negative. |
| Skin tests: Mantoux or Tine | If positive, do chest x-ray. |
| Urinalysis | |
| Color, specific Gravity, pH, ketones, albumin, glucose | Same as nonpregnant. Repeat at 28 weeks. Trace of glycosuria may occur in pregnancy. |
| **Subsequent visits** | |
| Alpha-fetoprotein (AFP) | Check with laboratory for normal range for each week of gestation. If elevated, may have neural tube defects. If decreased, may have Down syndrome. |
| Glucose tolerance test/glucose challenge test | Completed near 28 weeks' gestation to determine the client's ability to metabolize glucose. Normal values are less than 130 or 140, depending upon the reference used by the laboratory. |

of the pregnant uterus to determine fetal position and presentation. The client is placed in the supine position with knees bent, and the examiner stands at the client's right side facing her head.

- First, the examiner palpates to determine which fetal part is in the fundus. Generally, it is the breech (buttocks).
- Second, the examiner moves hands to the sides of the uterus and determines on which side of the mother the fetal back is located.
- Third, the examiner's right hand is placed above the symphysis pubis to note whether the head or breech is near the pubic symphysis (this should correlate with the first maneuver).
- Fourth, the examiner changes position to face the client's feet, and palpates the sides of the abdomen to determine on which side the cephalic prominence presents (Figure 1-18).

**Fetal Heartbeat**  After Leopold's maneuvers have determined fetal position, the fetal heartbeat is assessed over the location of the fetal back. The rate should be 110 to 160 beats/minute. The rate is recorded, indicating the abdominal quadrant in which the heartbeat was noted.

**Laboratory Tests**  At each visit, a urine sample is tested with a dipstick for protein, glucose, and ketones. If the results are positive for any of these three, the health care provider is notified.

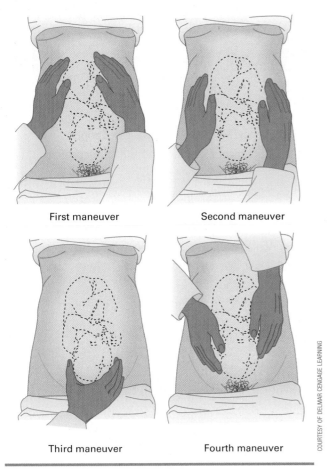

First maneuver          Second maneuver

Third maneuver          Fourth maneuver

COURTESY OF DELMAR CENGAGE LEARNING

**FIGURE 1-18** Leopold's Maneuvers

# ANTICIPATORY GUIDANCE

Many of the nursing interventions during pregnancy are anticipatory guidance (teaching). The order in which topics are covered and the time frame when topics are covered may vary from client to client, depending on when prenatal care was begun and if there are any complications.

## Environmental Hazards

Any chemicals, metals, anesthetic agents, antineoplastic and viral drugs, and x-ray examinations should be avoided. Excessive heat from saunas, hot tubs, or exercise in hot, humid weather should be avoided to prevent maternal hyperthermia (core temperature above 38.9°C/102°F). This has been associated with neural tube defects. Rogers and Davis (1995) report that the time needed to reach this core temperature is 15 minutes in a 39°C (102.2°F) tub and 10 minutes in a 41.1°C (106°F) tub.

## Discomforts of Pregnancy

The physiological changes in pregnancy often cause discomforts to the woman. Table 1-4 identifies the common discomforts of pregnancy, possible causes, and interventions the client can try to alleviate or reduce the discomfort.

## Warning Signs

The client is taught to immediately report to the health care provider the warning signs listed in Table 1-5. They may indicate complications of pregnancy. Generally, the sooner interventions are begun, the better the outcome.

| TABLE 1-4 Discomforts of Pregnancy | | |
|---|---|---|
| **DISCOMFORT** | **CAUSE** | **CLIENT INTERVENTIONS** |
| Nausea/vomiting | Elevated hCG level | Limit fluid intake at meals and upon waking. |
| | Decreased gastric emptying time due to progesterone | Eat crackers or toast upon waking. |
| | Ambivalence about pregnancy | Eat small amounts more frequently. |
| | Fatigue | Avoid fried, spicy, odorous, or gas-forming foods. |
| Heartburn (pyrosis) | Gastric reflux—cardiac sphincter relaxed due to progesterone | Avoid overeating. Eat small, frequent meals. |
| | | Avoid greasy foods. |
| | | Sit up for 1 hour after eating. |
| | | Take antacid only with health care provider's approval. |
| Urinary frequency | Pressure of uterus on bladder (early and late in pregnancy) | Empty bladder when urge is felt. |
| | | Do not restrict fluid intake. |
| | Urinary tract infection | Avoid fluids containing caffeine. |
| Breast tenderness | Effect of estrogen and progesterone | Wear well-fitting, supportive bra. |
| Flatulence | Relaxation of GI tract due to progesterone | Eat small meals. |
| | | Omit gas-forming foods from diet. |
| | | Have regular elimination. |

**TABLE 1-4  Discomforts of Pregnancy (Continued)**

| DISCOMFORT | CAUSE | CLIENT INTERVENTIONS |
|---|---|---|
| Constipation | Bowel sluggishness due to progesterone | Have regular schedule for bowel movement. |
| | Pressure of uterus on bowel | Increase activity and fluid intake. |
| | Decreased activity and fluid intake | Increase fiber in diet (raisins, prunes, fresh fruits and vegetables). |
| | Inadequate fiber in diet | |
| | Iron supplement | |
| Hemorrhoids | Constipation | Prevent constipation (see above). |
| | Straining to have bowel movement | Apply ice packs. |
| | Pressure of gravid (pregnant) uterus on veins | Use topical anesthetic ointments. |
| | Prolonged standing | Take sitz bath. |
| | | Gently push hemorrhoids back into rectum. |
| Ankle edema | Prolonged standing or sitting | Dorsiflex feet when prolonged standing or sitting necessary. |
| | Sodium and water retention from hormonal influence | Elevate legs when sitting or resting. |
| | Increased capillary permeability | Increase number of rest periods. |
| Varicose veins (legs) | Increased blood volume | Rest with feet and legs elevated. |
| | Congenital predisposition to weak vascular walls | Avoid crossing legs, standing still, garters and restrictive clothing. |
| | Relaxation of vessel walls due to progesterone | Wear support hose. |
| | Inactivity | |
| | Poor muscle tone | |
| | Prolonged standing | |
| | Obesity | |
| Backache | Relaxation of joints due to estrogen and relaxin | Get adequate rest. |
| | Exaggerated lordosis from change in center of gravity | Use proper posture. |
| | Wearing high-heeled shoes | Use proper body mechanics. |
| | Excessive weight | Wear low-heeled shoes. |
| | Fatigue | |
| | Poor body mechanics | |
| Dyspnea | Supine hypotensive syndrome | Lie on either side. |
| | Decreased lung capacity from pressure of uterus on diaphragm | Sleep in semi-Fowler's position. |
| | | Maintain proper posture. |
| Leg cramps | Calcium/phosphorus imbalance | Evaluate diet for adequate calcium and phosphorus intake. |
| | Pointing toes | |
| | Fatigue or muscle strain | Pull toes up toward knees. |
| | Pressure of gravid uterus impairs circulation to legs | Rest with legs elevated. |
| Dizziness and Fainting | Supine hypotensive syndrome | Lie on either side, not on back. |
| | Sudden change of position | Arise slowly. |
| | Standing for long period in warm area | Avoid standing in warm area. |
| | Hyperventilation | Practice slow, deep respirations. |
| | Hypoglycemia | Drink orange juice for fast-acting sugar. |
| | Anemia | |

*(Continues)*

**TABLE 1-4 Discomforts of Pregnancy (Continued)**

| DISCOMFORT | CAUSE | CLIENT INTERVENTIONS |
|---|---|---|
| Bleeding gums, nasal stuffiness, and epistaxis | Increased estrogen level<br>Increased blood volume<br>Lack of vitamin C | Avoid use of decongestants.<br>Use cool vaporizer or humidifier.<br>Use saline nasal spray several times a day.<br>Drink orange juice.<br>Have dental checkup. |
| Vaginal discharge | Increased estrogen causes more cervical Mucous | Bathe or shower daily. Avoid douching.<br>Wear absorbent cotton underwear. |
| Itchy skin | Tissue stretching<br>Soap use<br>Dehydration | Use lotion on skin.<br>Change soap, rinse well.<br>Drink more fluids. |
| Mood swings | Hormonal changes<br>Inadequate rest<br>Inadequate diet<br>Ambivalence about pregnancy | Get more rest.<br>Eat balanced diet.<br>Express fears, feelings, and concerns. |

COURTESY OF DELMAR CENGAGE LEARNING

**TABLE 1-5 Warning Signs during Pregnancy**

| WARNING SIGN | POSSIBLE CAUSE |
|---|---|
| Vaginal bleeding (any), "bloody show" | Abortion (miscarriage), placenta previa, placenta abruptio, lesions of cervix or vagina |
| Sudden gush of fluid from vagina | Rupture of membranes |
| Persistent vomiting | Hyperemesis gravidarum, infection |
| Severe, continuous headache | Hypertension, preeclampsia |
| Swelling of face, hands, legs, feet when arising in morning | Preeclampsia |
| Visual disturbances: blurring, double vision, flashes of light, spots before eyes | Hypertension, preeclampsia |
| Dizziness | Hypertension, preeclampsia |
| Fever over 100°F (37.8°C) and chills | Infection |
| Pain in abdomen or cramping | Ectopic pregnancy, abortion (miscarriage), placenta abruptio, labor |
| Epigastric pain | Preeclampsia |
| Irritating vaginal discharge | Vaginal infection |
| Dysuria | Urinary tract infection |
| Oliguria | Dehydration, renal impairment |
| Noticeable reduction or absence of fetal movement | Fetal distress, fetal death |

COURTESY OF DELMAR CENGAGE LEARNING

# Nutrition

There is very little change needed in the diet of a pregnant woman if she is already following the food guide pyramid. A woman eating a balanced, adequate diet needs to add only 300 kcalories a day to her diet when pregnant and 500 kcalories a day when breastfeeding. The addition of two milk servings and one meat serving will meet the 300 kcalorie increase as well as the increased need for calcium and protein.

Many health care providers have their pregnant clients take a multivitamin with calcium and iron to ensure an

## CLIENT**TEACHING**
### Pregnancy and Fluid Intake

A pregnant woman should drink at least 8 to 10 (8 oz) glasses of fluids each day. At least 4 to 6 of these should be water.

## CLIENT**TEACHING**
### Exercises for Pregnancy

Specific exercises are taught to clients to strengthen muscle tone in preparation for birth.

- The pelvic tilt reduces back strain and strengthens the abdominal muscles. Figure 1-19 illustrates how to perform the pelvic tilt in both a standing and kneeling position. Exhale, roll the hips and buttocks forward, hold for a count of five, then inhale and relax.
- Abdominal muscle tightening with every breath increases abdominal muscle tone. This can be done anywhere in any position. While slowly taking in a deep breath, expand the abdomen. Then exhale slowly while pulling the abdomen in until the muscles are completely contracted. Relax a few seconds and repeat the exercise.
- Kegel's exercises strengthen and tighten the perineal muscles. Tighten these muscles and pull them up toward the vagina as if trying to stop urination midstream. This exercise also can be done anytime, anyplace.
- The tailor sit (cross-legged sit) stretches the inner thigh muscles; adding arm reaches stretches the sides and upper body and helps relieve upper backache. Sit cross-legged and stretch one arm high over head, then release and exhale and repeat on the other side. Figure 1-20 illustrates the tailor sit and arm reaches.

adequate intake of these essential nutrients. Folic acid in the multivitamin prevents neural tube defects, calcium is needed for bone and teeth, and iron prevents anemia in mother and fetus. On the basis of a nutritional assessment, suggestions can be made to the client for a more adequate dietary intake, taking into account personal and cultural preferences.

Some pregnant women eat substances that are not considered edible and have no nutritive value. This is called **pica**. Eating ice, freezer frost, clay, soil or starch may interfere with the absorption of nutrients, cause constipation and most commonly cause iron deficiency anemia in the mother. Pica may be related to the mother's cultural beliefs. Kenyan woman believe eating soil increases fertility and reproductive success. Pica is underreported due to women's embarrassment in discussing the practice (Mills, 2007).

Factors that place a woman at risk for nutritional inadequacy during pregnancy include:

- Adolescence, due to demands for own growth and pregnancy; possible poor dietary habits; and possibility of trying to hide pregnancy
- Inadequate nutritional intake
- Pica
- Low income
- Smoking, alcohol, or drug use
- Short interval between pregnancies—no time to replenish nutrient stores
- Medical conditions such as diabetes or kidney problems
- Depression

## SELF-CARE

Physical care during pregnancy generally involves minor adjustments in or moderation of normal habits.

### Breast Care

Proper support of the breasts is important during pregnancy whether the woman is planning to breast-feed or bottle-feed her baby. A properly fitted maternity or nursing bra promotes comfort, retains breast shape, and prevents back strain if breasts are very large.

Cleanliness of the breasts is very important. Washing with water is sufficient because soap removes the natural lubricant provided by Montgomery's tubercles, causing drying and possible cracking of the nipples. If leakage is experienced, a nursing pad can be worn inside the bra, and the pregnant woman encouraged to rub the fluid into the nipple to lubricate the skin. Air-drying the nipples after leaking will also promote breast health.

### Personal Hygiene

Daily bathing is important because the pregnant woman generally has increased perspiration and vaginal mucous. Either a tub bath or shower may be taken, depending on the woman's preference and facilities available. Later in pregnancy, a tub bath may require that the mother have help in getting out of the tub. Douching should not be done because it changes the pH of the vagina and alters the normal flora.

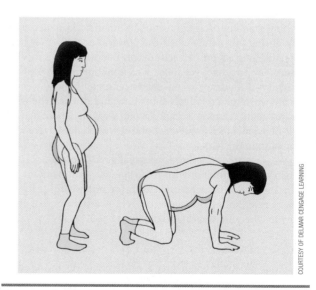

FIGURE 1-19  Pelvic Tilt

COURTESY OF DELMAR CENGAGE LEARNING

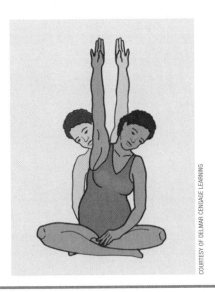

COURTESY OF DELMAR CENGAGE LEARNING

**FIGURE 1-20** **Tailor Sit and Arm Reaches**

## Activity/Rest

The pregnant woman should have some type of regular physical activity. Walking, swimming, and cycling are perhaps the best activities for most women. Women who routinely participate in exercise before pregnancy should continue and nonexercising women should begin exercising. Fatigue should be avoided. Exercise during pregnancy could reduce the risk of cesarean birth (Bungum, Peaslee, Jackson, & Perez, 2000). They should avoid hyperthermia and drink plenty of water before and after exercise to prevent dehydration. Exercise is contraindicated during pregnancy when the following are present: pregnancy-induced hypertension, preterm rupture of membranes, preterm labor during a prior or present pregnancy, incompetent cervix, persistent second or third trimester bleeding, or fetal growth restriction (Bungum et al., 2000).

Adequate rest is important for the pregnant woman. It is a challenge to find rest time during the day, especially for women who work outside the home or have small children. More sleep is needed, especially during the first and last trimester. Most women experience significant sleep problems throughout pregnancy (Mindell & Jacobson, 2000).

## Clothing

Clothing is an important aspect of a woman's self-image, especially during pregnancy when the physical changes may have a negative impact on her self-image. Encourage the mother to dress in attractive, yet loose and nonconstricting clothes. Maternity clothes are often shared among friends because they are worn for a relatively short time and can be expensive. The pregnant woman should avoid wearing knee-high or thigh-high stockings or garters because they can interfere with circulation in the legs.

Wearing low-heeled shoes is usually recommended. If the woman has no problem with backache *and* can maintain her balance, there is no medical reason for not wearing slightly higher-heeled shoes. Edema in the feet toward the end of pregnancy may require wearing a larger size shoe.

## Employment

How long to work when pregnant depends on the type of work done by the woman and how the pregnancy is progressing. The major factors to consider are whether there are teratogenic hazards in the work environment, if the woman is subject to physical strain or overfatigue, and if there are obstetrical or medical complications of the pregnancy. Rest periods should be available during the workday.

## Travel

Unless there are obstetrical or medical complications, travel is not restricted. When traveling by car, the pregnant client is encouraged to stop every 2 hours and walk around for 10 minutes or so. It is imperative always to wear the seat belt, both lap and shoulder, and to keep the lap belt snug below the abdomen. Possible bladder trauma, in case of an accident, is decreased by keeping the bladder empty. Travel by air is best for long trips. Many airlines and cruise ships will not accept passengers past a certain week of pregnancy.

## Dental Care

Regular oral hygiene should continue during pregnancy, and dental care can be performed. The woman should inform her dentist that she is pregnant. If possible, x-rays are delayed until after the infant is born. If x-rays must be done, a lead apron must be used.

## Sexual Activity

There is no reason to limit sexual activity in a healthy pregnancy. Only when the woman has a history of preterm labor, there is bleeding, or the membranes have ruptured is sexual intercourse contraindicated. As always, barrier protection should be used to prevent sexually transmitted diseases.

The expectant woman's sexual desire may decrease during the first trimester because of fatigue, nausea/vomiting, and breast tenderness. Often, during the second trimester, when the discomforts have lessened, she has greater sexual satisfaction than when not pregnant. By the third trimester, the discomforts of fatigue, dyspnea, urinary frequency, and painful pelvic ligaments may decrease her sexual desire.

After the fourth month, the woman should not lie flat on her back during intercourse because of supine hypotensive syndrome. A pillow can be placed under her right hip to displace the uterus or an alternate position used.

Men may find a change in their desire too. This may be related to their feelings about their partner's changing appearance, concern about hurting her or the fetus, and having sexual intercourse with a pregnant woman.

## CHILDBIRTH EDUCATION

Many health care providers recommend that their clients attend a prepared childbirth class. Several persons are recognized for developing childbirth education programs. The three most commonly known are Dick-Read, Bradley, and Lamaze.

In the 1930s, Dr Grantly Dick-Read believed women experience fear during childbirth because they do not understand what is happening in their bodies. This causes tension, which causes the woman to perceive pain more intensely. Later, Dr Robert Bradley stressed that labor is a normal process and felt that the partner support is most important. Dr Fernand Lamaze introduced the childbirth preparation method called **psychoprophylaxis**, teaching mental and physical preparation for childbirth. Further research is needed to conclude that other methods of relaxation and stress reduction, such as acupuncture, hypnotherapy and yoga produce positive outcomes (Beddoe & Lee, 2008).

Most childbirth education today combines these principles, teaching mothers and their support persons basic physiology of labor and how to relax to promote a safe and most comfortable delivery. Included is information regarding controlled breathing, contraction and relaxation of isolated muscles, guided imagery, counter pressure to the back for pain relief, positioning for comfort, use of massage and others. There are also classes teaching care of the newborn, infant massage, CPR, sibling rivalry and grandparenting.

Some women employ a doula to assist with birth or in the postpartum period. The term doula is a Greek term meaning "a woman who serves." Doulas are specially trained birth companions who provide information and emotional support during pregnancy, birth and in the postpartum period. Certification programs exist as well as professional organizations (DONA.org, 2009).

## NURSING PROCESS

The nurse's role centers on helping the client maintain a healthy pregnancy and preparing the client for childbirth and delivery.

### ASSESSMENT

The information presented in this chapter encompasses the possible subjective data and objective data that may be gathered about a specific client.

### NURSING DIAGNOSES

Nursing diagnoses applicable to a pregnant client may include:

- *Activity Intolerance*
- *Anxiety*
- *Disturbed **B**ody Image*
- *Ineffective **B**reathing Pattern*

- *Constipation*
- *Ineffective **C**oping*
- *Readiness for Enhanced Family **C**oping*
- *Fatigue*
- *Fear*
- *Deficient **F**luid Volume*
- *Excess **F**luid Volume*
- *Ineffective **H**ealth Maintenance*
- *Health Seeking Behaviors* (specify)
- *Risk for **I**njury*
- *Deficient **K**nowledge* (specify)
- *Impaired Physical **M**obility*
- *Noncompliance*
- *Imbalanced **N**utrition: Less Than Body Requirements*
- *Disturbed **S**leep Pattern*
- *Sexual Dysfunction*

### PLANNING/OUTCOME IDENTIFICATION

Set appropriate goals with the client and her family to meet needs as identified by the nursing diagnoses.

### NURSING INTERVENTIONS

Nursing interventions are individualized and specific for the client based on the assessment, nursing diagnoses, and goals. Nursing interventions for prenatal care are focused on teaching the client and providing anticipatory guidance.

### EVALUATION

Each goal is evaluated to determine how it has been met by the client.

## SAMPLE NURSING CARE PLAN

### Prenatal Care

P.S., age 23, first pregnancy, states she has been nauseated and has not eaten for about 3 weeks, feels very tired all the time, takes a nap after work, and then has trouble sleeping because she has to go to the bathroom frequently. Her LMP was 6 weeks ago, menstrual periods have always been regular every 28 days. She smokes 1 pack/day and drinks beer on the weekends. She does not like to cook, so most meals are eaten out. She has lost 3 pounds in the last month. She is unmarried, lives alone, and did not plan to get pregnant.

**NURSING DIAGNOSIS 1** *Knowledge Deficit (Self-Care in Pregnancy)* related to inexperience as evidenced by eating, drinking, and smoking habits

**Nursing Outcomes Classification (NOC)**
*Knowledge: Pregnancy*

**Nursing Interventions Classification (NIC)**
*Prenatal Care*

| PLANNING/OUTCOMES | NURSING INTERVENTIONS | RATIONALE |
|---|---|---|
| P.S. will competently care for herself during pregnancy. | Teach physiology of pregnancy, discomforts of pregnancy, things she can do to relieve the discomforts, self-care aspects, and fetal development. | Provides reasons for P.S. to take care of herself. |

*(Continues)*

## SAMPLE NURSING CARE PLAN (Continued)

| PLANNING/OUTCOMES | NURSING INTERVENTIONS | RATIONALE |
|---|---|---|
| | Gather more data about her work environment and psychosocial aspects of nutrition, smoking, and drinking. | Provides data for additional teaching regarding self-care. |

### EVALUATION
P.S. states that she now understands the changes pregnancy makes in her body.

### NURSING DIAGNOSIS 2 *Imbalanced Nutrition: Less than Body Requirements* related to inadequate food intake as evidenced by nausea and weight loss

**Nursing Outcomes Classification (NOC)**
*Nutritional Status: Energy*
*Nutritional Status: Nutrient Intake*

**Nursing Interventions Classification (NIC)**
*Nutrition Management*
*Teaching: Individual*

| PLANNING/OUTCOMES | NURSING INTERVENTIONS | RATIONALE |
|---|---|---|
| P.S. will have sufficient nutritional intake during pregnancy | Have P.S. keep a food diary for 3 days. | To determine current eating habits. |
| | Assess P.S.'s knowledge of healthy eating habits and her food and drink preferences. | To determine her knowledge base and to incorporate her preferences into her dietary plan. |
| | Teach basic nutrition, food guide pyramid, and nutritional needs during pregnancy. | May encourage changes in P.S.'s eating pattern. |

### EVALUATION
P.S. follows the food guide pyramid most of the time and is drinking 4 glasses of milk a day.

### NURSING DIAGNOSIS 3 *Risk for Injury* related to teratogenic substances as evidenced by smoking and alcohol consumption

**Nursing Outcomes Classification (NOC)**
*Risk Control: Tobacco Use*
*Risk Control: Alcohol*
*Risk Control: Unintended Pregnancy*

**Nursing Interventions Classification (NIC)**
*Teaching: Individual*
*Risk Identification: Childbearing Family*

| PLANNING/OUTCOMES | NURSING INTERVENTIONS | RATIONALE |
|---|---|---|
| P.S. will stop smoking and drinking alcohol. | Assess when P.S. is most likely to smoke cigarettes or drink alcohol. | May find behaviors/situations that P.S. can avoid to prevent craving cigarettes and alcohol. |
| | Refer to smoking-cessation programs. | To provide needed support while trying to quit. |
| | Teach effects of smoking and alcohol on fetal development. | May encourage P.S. to abstain from both. |

### EVALUATION
P.S. has cut her smoking in half and only drinks one beer on the weekend.

## CASE STUDY

B.W., age 30, and J.W., age 30, have been married 4 years. B.W.'s LMP was 12 weeks ago, but her menstrual periods have always been very irregular. She is tired all the time and nauseated every day, her clothes are very tight around her waist, and her abdomen is protruding.

The following questions will guide your development of a nursing care plan for the case study.

1. What other data would you collect about B.W.?
2. What diagnostic tests would you anticipate the health care provider performing or ordering?
3. What anticipatory guidance would be appropriate for B.W.?
4. When should B.W. return for a checkup?

## SUMMARY

- Ideally, planning for pregnancy begins before conception.
- Fetal development proceeds in an orderly and predictable manner.
- Prenatal care involves all aspects of the couple's life.
- A complete history for a pregnant client includes her own medical and obstetrical history, family history, and the fetus's father's history.
- Nutrition increase for pregnancy is 300 kcalories/day. Two extra glasses of milk and one extra serving of meat meets this need and supplies the extra calcium and protein needed.
- Anticipatory guidance comprises the majority of nursing interventions when caring for a pregnant client.

## REVIEW QUESTIONS

1. A woman arrives for her first prenatal visit. Her history reveals three pregnancies, including one spontaneous abortion. Her 2-year-old son was born at 36 weeks. The nurse accurately records which of the following into the medical record?
   1. G3 P2 T1 P1 A1 L1
   2. G3 P1 T0 P1 A1 L1
   3. G3 P1 T1 P0 A1 L1
   4. G2 P1 T0 P1 A1 L1

2. The pregnant client states her last menstrual period began on July 8th. Using Naegele's Rule, her due date would be identified as:
   1. April 15.
   2. October 15.
   3. October 1.
   4. April 1.

3. A client weighs 178 pounds at her 26 week prenatal visit. Her pre-pregnancy weight was162 pounds. Which is correct regarding her weight gain?
   1. She has gained too little weight.
   2. She has gained too much weight.
   3. She has gained the appropriate amount of weight.
   4. She is too early to determine appropriate weight gain.

4. A client in her first trimester complains of nausea and vomiting occurring nearly every morning. The nurse appropriately explains the reason for her symptoms when she says:
   1. "Estrogen increases vascularity, which causes pressure on the stomach from surrounding organs."
   2. "Progesterone promotes smooth muscle relaxation, causing food to stay in the stomach longer than when she is not pregnant."
   3. "Hormones cause changes in the gastric lining, resulting in increased acid production in the stomach."
   4. "The effects of estrogen cause the cardiac sphincter to relax, resulting in acid reflux, nausea and vomiting."

5. A nurse preceptor asks the novice nurse to tell her about the purpose of amniotic fluid. The preceptor knows the novice nurse needs further instruction when she says the amniotic fluid:
   1. provides a constant temperature for the fetus.
   2. allows the fetus to swallow and urinate.
   3. increases the pressure around the fetus.
   4. allows the fetus to move more freely.

6. Which statement indicates the nurse understands the treatment of supine hypotension?
   1. Have the client breathe into a paper bag slowly.
   2. Give the client a bolus of intravenous fluids over one hour.
   3. Check the client's blood pressure lying, sitting and standing.
   4. Have the client turn to either side to relieve symptoms.

7. A 34-week pregnant woman is at the mall, buying items for her nursery. She stops and smiles as she

watches a mother talking to her own baby. The client is most likely experiencing which developmental task of pregnancy?
1. Fetal embodiment.
2. Pregnancy validation.
3. Role transition.
4. Fetal distinction.

8. The client is fourteen weeks pregnant at her second prenatal visit. During her assessment, the health care provider measures her fundal height at 17cm. She suspects the client has:
1. a twin gestation.
2. gained more weight than expected.
3. a baby with congenital anomalies.
4. an ectopic pregnancy.

9. A Korean woman is admitted to the labor and delivery unit in active labor. During the admission assessment, she lets her mother answer all of the questions. The nurse understands that the client:
1. is mentally limited and doesn't understand the questions.
2. does not speak English as well as her mother.
3. does not feel comfortable in the hospital setting.
4. is following her own cultural standards.

10. A nurse is instructing a client in ways to minimize heartburn in pregnancy. She knows the client understands her teaching when she says: (Select all that apply.)
1. "I will eat small, frequent meals."
2. "I will lie down for one hour after meals."
3. "I should take a laxative each evening."
4. "I should avoid gassy foods."
5. "I should contact my physician before taking an antacid."
6. "I should avoid fatty foods."

# REFERENCES/SUGGESTED READINGS

American College of Obstetrics & Gynecology. (2005). ACOG Updates Definitive Guide to Pregnancy. Retrieved March 9, 2009, from ACOG News Release Web site, http://www.acog.org.

American College of Obstetrics & Gynecology. (2008). Alcohol and Pregnancy: Know the Facts. Retrieved March 9, 2009, from ACOG News Release Web site, http://www.acog.org.

American College of Obstetrics & Gynecology. (2008). All Patients Should be Asked About Alcohol and Drug Abuse. Retrieved March 9, 2009, from ACOG News Release Web site, http://www.acog.org.

American College of Obstetrics & Gynecology. (2008). Pregnant Women Reminded to Get Flu Vaccine. Retrieved March 9, 2009, from ACOG News Release Web site http://www.acog.org.

Allard-Hendren, R. (2000). Alcohol use and adolescent pregnancy. *MCN, 25*(3), 159–162.

Beckmann, C., Buford, T., & Witt, J. (2000). Perceived barriers to prenatal care services. *MCN, 25*(1), 43–46.

Beddoe, A., & Lee, K. (2008). Mind-body interventions during pregnancy. *Journal of Obstetric Gynecologic and Neonatal Nursing, 37*(2), 165–175.

Brucker, M., & Reedy, N. (2000). Nurse-midwifery: Yesterday, today, and tomorrow. *MCN, 25*(6), 322–326.

Bryan, A. (2000). Enhancing parent-child interaction with a prenatal couple intervention. *MCN, 25*(3), 139–144.

Bulechek, G., Butcher, H., McCloskey, J., & Dochterman, J., eds. (2008). *Nursing Interventions Classification (NIC)* (5th ed.). St. Louis, MO: Mosby/Elsevier.

Bungum, T., Peaslee, D., Jackson, A., & Perez, M. (2000). Exercise during pregnancy and type of delivery in nulliparae. *JOGNN, 29*(1), 258–264.

Callister, L., & Vega, R. (1998). Giving birth: Guatemalan women's voices. *JOGNN, 27*(3), 289–295.

Cesario, S. (2001). Care of the Native American woman: Strategies for practice, education, and research. *JOGNN, 30*(1), 13–19.

Cordero, S. (2003). Assessing fetal heart sounds. *Nursing2003, 33*(10), 54–55.

De Sevo, M. (2009). Unlocking the Clues of Family Health History, the Importance of Creating a Pedigree. *Nursing for Women's Health, 11*(3), 122–131.

Dick-Read, G. (1933). *Natural childbirth*. London: Heinemann.

Dick-Read, G. (1944). *Childbirth without fear*. New York: Harper & Row.

Dickason, E., Silverman, B., & Kaplan J. (1998). *Maternal-infant nursing care* (3rd ed.). St. Louis, MO: Mosby-Year Book.

Freda, M. (1998). Confronting the myths. *MCN, 23*(2), 107.

Gennaro, S., Kamwendo, L., Mbweza, E., & Kershbaumer, R. (1998). Childbearing in Malawi, Africa. *JOGNN, 27*(2), 191–196.

Giarelli, E. (2001). A legal look at genetic testing. *RN, 64*(10), 73–75.

Hall, S. (2002). Amniotomy: Necessary intervention or bad habit. *AWHONN Lifelines, 5*(6), 10–13.

Hasenau, S., & Covington, C. (2002). Neural tube defects: Prevention and folic acid. *MCN, 27*(2), 87–91.

Hatters Friedman, S., Heneghan, A., & Rosenthal, M. (2009). Characteristics of Women Who Do Not Seek Prenatal Care and Implications for Prevention. *Journal of Obstetric, Gynecologic & Neonatal Nursing, 38*(2), 174–181.

Holtz, C. (2008). *Global health care: issues and policies* (p. 459). Boston: Jones and Bartlett.

Howard, J., & Berbiglia, V. (1997). Caring for childbearing Korean women. *JOGNN, 26*(6), 665–671.

Hutchinson, M., & Baqi-Aziz, M. (1994). Nursing care of the childbearing Muslim family. *JOGNN, 23*(9), 767–771.

Jones, S. (1996). Genetics: Changing health care in the 21st century. *JOGNN, 25*(9), 777–783.

Ladewig, P., Moberly, S., Olds, S., & London, M. (2001). *Contemporary maternal-newborn nursing care* (5th ed.). Menlo Park, CA: Addison-Wesley Longman.

Lamaze, F. (1965). *Painless childbirth*. New York: Dimon & Schuster.

Littleton, L., & Engebretson, J. (2002). *Maternal, neonatal, and women's health nursing*. Clifton Park, NY: Delmar Cengage Learning.

Longobucco, D., & Freston, M. (1989). Relation of somatic symptoms to degree of paternal-role preparation of first-time expectant fathers. *JOGNN, 18*, 482.

Malnory, M. (1996). Developmental care of the pregnant couple. *JOGNN, 25*(6), 525–532.

Martinez, F., Wright, A., & Taussig, L. (1994, Sept.). The effect of paternal smoking on the birthweight of newborns whose mothers did not smoke. The Health Medical Associates. *Am J Public Health, 84*, 1489–1491.

Matthews, T. (1998). Smoking during pregnancy 1990-1996. *National Vital Statistics Reports, 47*(10), 1–12.

Mills, M. (2007). Craving more than food, the implications of pica. *Nursing for Women's Health*, 11(3), 266–273.

Mindell, J., & Jacobson, B. (2000). Sleep disturbances during pregnancy. *JOGNN*, 29(6), 590–597.

Moorhead, S., Johnson, M., & Maas, M. (2007). Nursing *Outcomes Classification (NOC)* (4th ed.). St. Louis, MO: Mosby.

Morton, J., and Choen Knorad, S. (2009). Introducing a caring/relational framework for building relationships with addicted mothers. *Journal of Obstetric, Gynecologic & Neonatal Nursing*, 38(2), 206–213.

Nasso, J. (1997). Planning for pregnancy—A preconception health program. *MCN*, 22(3), 142–146.

North American Nursing Diagnosis Association International. (2010). *NANDA-I nursing diagnoses: Definitions & classification 2009–2011*. Ames, IA: Wiley-Blackwell.

Pletsch, P., Morgan, S., & Pieper, A. (2003). Context & beliefs about smoking & smoking cessation. *MCN*, 28(5), 320–325.

Reifsnider, E., & Gill, S. (2000). Nutrition for childbearing years. *JOGNN*, 29(1), 43–55.

Remich, M. (1997). Promoting a healthy pregnancy. In E. Q. Younkin & M. S. Davis (Eds.), *Women's health: A primary care clinical guide* (2d ed.). Norwalk, CT: Appleton & Lange.

Rentschler, D. (2003). Pregnant adolescent's perspectives of pregnancy. *MCN*, 28(6), 377–383.

Rhodes, A. (1995). Liability for failure to offer prenatal AFP testing. *MCN*, 20(3), 169.

Robaire, B., & Hales, B. (1993, August). Paternal exposure to chemicals before conception. *BMI*, 307, 341–342.

Rogers, J., & Davis, B. (1995). How risky are hot tubs and saunas for pregnant women? *MCN*, 20(3), 137–140.

Rossner, S. (1998). Obesity and pregnancy. In G. Bray, C. Bouchard, & W. James (Eds.). *Handbook of obesity* (pp. 575–590). New York: Marcel Dekker.

Schneiderman, J. (1996). Postpartum nursing for Korean mothers. *MCN*, 21(3), 155–158.

Simpson, K., & Creehan, P. (2001). *AWHONN perinatal nursing* (2nd ed.). Philadelphia: Lippincott Williams & Wilkins.

Todd, S., LaSala, K., & Neil-Urban, S. (2001). An integrated approach to prenatal smoking cessation interventions. *MCN*, 26(4), 185–190.

Wisborg, K., Kesmodel, U., Bech B., et al. (2003). Maternal consumption of coffee during pregnancy and stillbirth and infant death in first year of life: Prospective study. *British Medical Journal*, 326(7386), 420.

Zauderer, C. (2009). Maternity Care for Orthodox Jewish Couples, Implications for Nurses in the Obstetric Setting. *Nursing for Women's Health*, 13(2), 112–120.

## RESOURCES

**American Dietetic Association,** http://www.eatright.org

**Association of Women's Health, Obstetric, and Neonatal Nurses (AWHONN),** http://www.awhonn.org

**Center for Disease Control and Prevention (CDC), National Center for Health Statistics,** http://www.cdc.gov/nchs

**DONA International,** http://www.dona.org

**Food and Nutrition Information Center,** http://www.nal.usda.gov

**International Childbirth Education Association (ICEA),** http://www.icea.org

**Lamaze International,** http://www.lamaze.org

**March of Dimes,** http://www.modimes.org

**National Certification Corporation (NCC),** http://www.nccwebsite.org

# CHAPTER 2
## Complications of Pregnancy

## MAKING THE CONNECTION

*Refer to the following chapters to increase your understanding of the complications of pregnancy:*

### Maternal & Pediatric Nursing

- **Prenatal Care**
- **The Birth Process**

## LEARNING OBJECTIVES

Upon completion of this chapter, you should be able to:

- Define key terms.
- Explain medical and nursing interventions for a client with hyperemesis gravidarum.
- Compare and contrast the etiology, medical–surgical management, and nursing care for the bleeding situations in pregnancy.
- Describe the development, medical–surgical management, and nursing care of a client with gestational hypertension.
- Describe the nursing care for a client with a chronic medical problem: diabetes, hypertension, heart disease, maternal PKU.
- Discuss the effects of infection on a pregnant woman and her fetus and ways of preventing the infections.
- Compare and contrast the etiology, medical–surgical management, nursing care, and effect on the fetus of Rh incompatibility and ABO incompatibility.
- Explain the effects of multiple pregnancies on the mother, fetuses, and family.
- Describe the effects of addiction on the mother and fetus.
- Summarize the needs of a woman in preterm labor.

## KEY TERMS

| | | |
|---|---|---|
| abortion | HELLP syndrome | miscarriage |
| abruptio placenta | hydatidiform mole | modified biophysical profile |
| amniocentesis | hydramnios | oligohydramnios |
| biophysical profile | hyperemesis gravidarum | placenta previa |
| early deceleration | incompetent cervix | preeclampsia |
| eclampsia | kernicterus | surfactant |
| ectopic pregnancy | late deceleration | tocolysis |
| euglycemia | macrosomia | variable deceleration |

## INTRODUCTION

It is truly impressive that most pregnancies have no complications. For those clients who do have complications, it can be a very frightening and guilt-ridden situation. Regular prenatal care is the best way to identify clients who have high-risk factors. These clients are assessed and monitored more closely, and signs and symptoms of complications are detected as early as possible. Medical–surgical management and effective nursing care can then be implemented. Many of the high-risk factors in pregnancy are listed in Table 2-1.

This chapter covers the common complications of pregnancy including etiology, medical–surgical management, and the nursing process.

## ASSESSMENT OF FETAL WELL-BEING

When complications arise in a pregnancy, more intense and specific assessments of the fetus are required.

### ULTRASOUND

Two-dimensional (2D) ultrasound allows visualization of the uterine contents. The fetal assessments described in

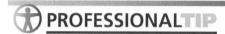

## PROFESSIONAL TIP

### Ultrasound

After more than 40 years of use, no studies have confirmed harmful effects from ultrasound use in pregnancy. The Power Doppler or pulsed Doppler emits more power signals than the 2-D ultrasound scan or flow velocity waveform Doppler. Therefore, cautious use of the pulsed Doppler is recommended in the first trimester until safety is proven (Woo, 2009).

the Prenatal Care chapter are also used. High-frequency, inaudible sound waves are directed toward the uterus. The sound waves reflected back are converted into a visual image (Figure 2-1).

Ultrasound provides the following information.

*First Trimester*
- Early positive diagnosis of pregnancy about 5 or 6 weeks after LMP.
- Identification of more than one fetus.

**TABLE 2-1 High-Risk Factors in Pregnancy**

| GENERAL | OBSTETRICAL | MEDICAL | OTHER |
|---|---|---|---|
| Age (under 15 or over 35 years) | Previous problems | Chronic diseases | Smoking |
| Unmarried | Abortion | Diabetes | Drug abuse |
| Low socioeconomic group, little education | Excessive size of infant | Hypertension | Alcohol abuse |
| Prenatal care begun 27 weeks or later | Cesarean birth | Sickle-cell anemia | Nutritional deficit |
| | Preterm/Postterm birth | Thyroid disease | Obesity |
| | Incompetent cervix | Sexually transmitted infection | |
| | Abnormal fetal presentation | Cervical neoplasia | |
| | Rh negative and sensitized | Urinary tract infection | |
| | Preeclampsia | Neurological problem | |
| | Multiple pregnancy | Psychiatric problem | |

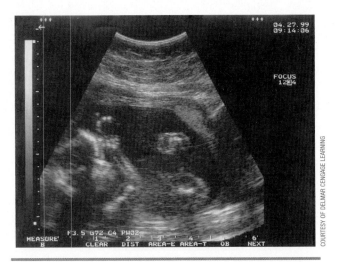

**FIGURE 2-1** Ultrasound provides a visual image of uterine contents.

- Observation of cardiac activity at 21 days and respiratory movements about 11th week of gestation.
- Diagnosis of an ectopic pregnancy.
- Diagnosis of a molar pregnancy.
- Visualization of ultrasonic "soft" markers indicating chromosomal abnormalities (Woo, 2009).

*Second and Third Trimester*
- Location of pockets of amniotic fluid for retrieval of fluid for testing.
- Measurement of biparietal diameter, femur length, overall length (crown-heel and crown-rump), gestational age, and intrauterine growth restriction (IUGR), formerly intrauterine growth retardation.
- Detection of some fetal anomalies, especially anencephaly and hydrocephalus.
- Detection of amniotic fluid volume, including hydramnios, also known as polyhydramnios, (excessive amniotic fluid) or **oligohydramnios** (deficiency of amniotic fluid), either of which is frequently associated with fetal anomalies.
- Identification of amniotic fluid pockets; a vertical pocket of 2 cm is associated with normal fetal status.
- Location of the placenta, which is necessary before an amniocentesis and to determine placenta abnormalities.
- Determination of fetal position and presentation.
- Detection of fetal death; fetal heart beating is not visualized, and the bones in the fetal head separate.
- Evaluation of cervical length.

Three- and four-dimensional (3-D and 4-D) ultrasound is currently used to improve visualization of fetal anatomic structures and to promote parental bonding. Pictures are obtained with sound waves similar to 2-D, but 3-D images are more life-like in appearance. 4-D ultrasounds are 3-D images shown in rapid succession to view the image as if it is moving. 2-D ultrasound is the standard, and benefits of 3- and 4-D images will be determined with more research (Lee & Simpson, 2007; NIH, 2009).

## Transabdominal Ultrasound

The mother is asked to have a full bladder when the ultrasound is performed. This allows the other structures to be assessed in relation to the bladder. The transducer is moved slowly over the abdomen while the client lies on her back. This position may cause shortness of breath or supine hypotension syndrome. The procedure takes about 20 to 30 minutes.

## Transvaginal Ultrasound

During a transvaginal ultrasound or endovaginal ultrasound, a probe is inserted into the vagina and placed close to the structures being imaged. This produces a clearer image. The client is in the lithotomy position and has an empty bladder. These scans assist with early detection of ectopic pregnancies, fetal abnormalities in the first trimester, and diagnosing congenital anomalies in the second trimester (Woo, 2009).

## NONSTRESS TEST

A nonstress test (NST) assesses the well being of the fetus by recording the fetal heart rate (FHR) and determining increased heart rate with fetal movement. Fetal movement indicates a well oxygenated fetus with a healthy central and autonomic nervous system. An NST requires an electronic fetal monitor to record fetal movement and FHR accelerations (short-term increases in FHR caused by fetal movement). Specific equipment may vary. The mother reclines in a chair or in bed in semi-Fowler's or side-lying position. This noninvasive test is used every day or once weekly as needed after 30 weeks gestation in high-risk clients (Figure 2-2).

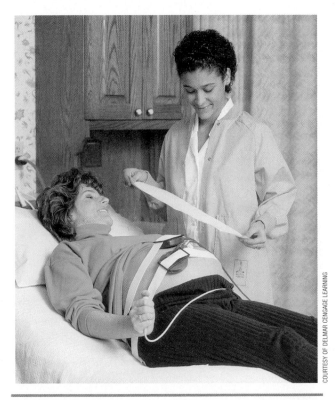

**FIGURE 2-2** Nonstress Test (NST) to Assess Fetal Well-Being

The test is reactive if there are two accelerations of 15 beats/min, lasting 15 seconds in a 20-minute period. This indicates that the fetus has adequate oxygenation and an intact central nervous system.

The test is nonreactive if the criteria for reactive are not met. This may indicate that the fetus is asleep or there are problems with fetal oxygenation, and the health care provider is notified. A repeat NST or additional testing is ordered to determine fetal status.

An unsatisfactory test is identified if there is inadequate fetal activity or the data cannot be interpreted. If decelerations of the FHR are noted, the health care provider is notified promptly.

## VIBROACOUSTIC STIMULATION TEST

The vibroacoustic stimulation (VAS) test, also called the fetal acoustic stimulation test (FAST) is used in conjunction with the NST. A small, battery-operated device is placed on the mother's abdomen over the fetal head. A low-frequency vibration and a buzzing sound are emitted from the device to stimulate the fetus who had a nonreactive NST. The sounds emitted last no more than 3 seconds and are repeated every minute if no accelerations occur.

## BIOPHYSICAL PROFILE

The fetal biophysical profile (BPP) assesses five biophysical variables: fetal breathing movement, fetal movements of body or limbs, fetal tone (extension/flexion of extremities), amniotic fluid volume, and reactive NST (Table 2-2). The first four are assessed by ultrasound. A score of 8 or more shows probable fetal well-being.

### TABLE 2-2 Biophysical Profile

|  | SCORE 2 | SCORE 0 |
|---|---|---|
| Fetal breathing | One or more episodes lasting 30 seconds in 30 minutes | Not present or not lasting 30 seconds |
| Fetal movement | Three or more body/limb movements in 30 minutes | Two or fewer body/limb movements in 30 minutes |
| Fetal tone | One or more episodes of active flexion/extension | Slow extension with return to partial flexion, or movement absent |
| Fluid assessment | One or more pockets of amniotic fluid 1 cm in two perpendicular planes | No pocket, or no pocket 1 cm in two perpendicular planes |
| Fetal reaction | Reactive NST | Nonreactive NST |

COURTESY OF DELMAR CENGAGE LEARNING

## MODIFIED BIOPHYSICAL PROFILE

The modified biophysical profile (MBPP) assesses only two of the variables of the BPP; the NST and the amniotic fluid volume. The MBPP indicates positive fetal well-being if the NST is reactive and the amniotic fluid volume is greater than 5 cm. If either of these two assessments is abnormal, the complete BPP is completed. The MBPP saves time and decreases the cost of fetal surveillance.

## FETAL MOVEMENTS

From the time of quickening (16 to 20 weeks), fetal movement is reassuring to the mother. Counting fetal movement daily provides evidence that the fetus is not having difficulty.

One method is to count fetal movements for 10 minutes three times a day. Another, which is the Cardiff method, requires the mother to count fetal movements at the same time each day until 10 movements are felt. The start and stop times are recorded.

The health care provider should be contacted if there are:

- fewer than 10 movements in 12 hours
- no movements for 8 hours
- sudden violent movements followed by reduced movements

## BIOCHEMICAL ASSESSMENTS

Three tests include maternal serum alpha-fetoprotein, estriol, and human placental lactogen.

### Maternal Serum Alpha-Fetoprotein

Maternal serum alpha-fetoprotein (MSAFP) identifies some birth defects and chromosomal anomalies during the antepartum period. AFP is found in maternal serum about 7 weeks' gestation and rises steadily until the last trimester. Women should have the test between 16 and 18 weeks' gestation. Because there is a normal range for each week of pregnancy, a correct gestational age is important to the interpretation of the test.

If the MSAFP level is high, it indicates a fetal open neural tube defect, multiple gestation, Rh isoimmunization, maternal diabetes mellitus, or fetal distress and death. If the MSAFP level is low, the fetus may have Down syndrome or there may be a maternal hypertensive state.

### Estriol

Maternal estriol level indicates fetoplacental function. Essential precursors from the fetal adrenal glands are converted by the placenta to estriol. The level in maternal serum and urine usually increases throughout pregnancy, so there must be a series of tests throughout pregnancy. Gradual increase in the maternal estriol level indicates that the fetal adrenal glands and the placenta are functioning normally.

### Human Placental Lactogen

Human placental lactogen (hPL) increases throughout pregnancy correlating with increased fetal weight.

## AMNIOCENTESIS

Amniocentesis is a procedure in which a needle is inserted through the abdomen into the amniotic sac. Amniotic fluid

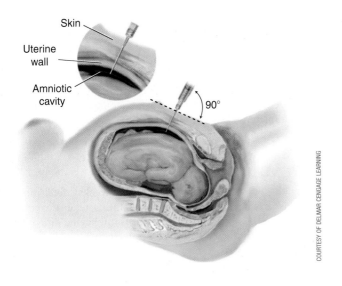

FIGURE 2-3  **Amniocentesis: 15 to 20 mL of amniotic fluid is withdrawn for study.**

is withdrawn and sent to the laboratory for testing. At 14 to 16 weeks' gestation, an amniocentesis may be performed for diagnosis of genetic diseases or birth defects if the mother is older than 35 or either parent has a family history of genetic disease (Figure 2-3).

Later in pregnancy, amniocentesis is most often used to determine fetal lung maturity. In a high-risk pregnancy when preterm delivery of the fetus is a possibility, the physician will often try to maintain the pregnancy until the lungs are mature.

An ultrasound is used to determine the location of pockets of fluid so the fetus, placenta, and cord are not damaged. The nurse assists the physician performing the amniocentesis and provides emotional support to the client.

### Tests on Amniotic Fluid

Both the fluid and the cells in the amniotic fluid are used for testing. The fluid should be clear, colorless, and may have flecks of vernix caseosa floating in it.

**Lecithin/Sphingomyelin Ratio** **Surfactant** is phospholipids in the lungs that lower surface tension and stabilize the alveoli so they do not collapse on exhalation. The ratio of two phospholipids, which are components of surfactant, lecithin and sphingomyelin (L/S ratio), determines the maturity of the lungs.

Early in pregnancy, the lecithin level is low and the sphingomyelin level is high. At about 32 weeks' gestation, this relationship begins to change. By 35 weeks' gestation, the lecithin level is twice as high as the level of sphingomyelin. An L/S ratio of 2:1 is considered indicative of lung maturity.

Some conditions may accelerate lung maturation, such as severe pregnancy-induced hypertension (PIH), chronic maternal hypertension, or prolonged rupture of membranes. Diabetes and Rh isoimmunization seem to delay fetal lung maturity.

**Phosphatidylglycerol**  Another phospholipid in surfactant, phosphatidylglycerol (PG), appears in the amniotic fluid when the lungs are mature, about 35 weeks' gestation.

**Bilirubin**  In clients with Rh incompatibility, there is bilirubin in the amniotic fluid. The level of bilirubin corresponds to the degree of fetal anemia.

**Sex Determination**  The sex of the fetus can be accurately determined by cell studies. This is important in sex-linked genetic abnormalities.

## CHORIONIC VILLI SAMPLING

In chorionic villi sampling (CVS), samples of chorionic villi from the developing placenta are obtained to assess for the same genetic disorders as in amniocentesis. CVS is performed between 8 and 10 weeks' gestation. Either a vaginal or abdominal approach is used (Figure 2-4).

## CONTRACTION STRESS TEST

A contraction stress test (CST) evaluates the respiratory function of the placenta. During a uterine contraction, blood flow to the intervillous spaces is momentarily reduced, thus decreasing oxygen available to the fetus. A healthy fetus tolerates this well. Fetal hypoxia, myocardial depression, and a decrease in FHR occur if the placenta's reserve is not sufficient.

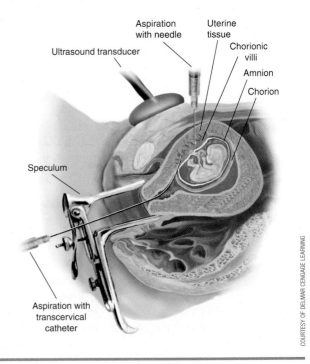

FIGURE 2-4  **Chorionic Villi Sampling (Performed between 8 and 10 Weeks' Gestation)**

---

### ▼ SAFETY ▼

### Amniocentesis

- Wash hands.
- Wear goggles or face mask, splash apron, and disposable gloves.
- Label specimen clearly so laboratory personnel can use appropriate precautions.
- Wash hands after removal of gloves.

This test is used with clients who have heart disease, hypertension, gestational hypertension, sickle-cell anemia, previous stillbirths, Rh sensitization, or a nonreactive NST. It is most often performed on the client with diabetes (chronic or gestational).

The vascular changes that take place in diabetes also affect the placenta. Vascular changes in the placenta cause placental insufficiency, so the fetus will not tolerate a CST well. Contraindications for use of this test are placenta previa, abruptio placenta, premature rupture of membranes, a history of preterm labor, or previous cesarean birth.

The uterine contractions are induced by either intravenous oxytocin or breast self-stimulation. An electronic fetal monitor provides continuous information of the FHR and uterine contractions. The FHR is observed for decelerations with the contractions. A 15-minute baseline recording on the fetal monitor is obtained before contractions are stimulated. Intravenous oxytocin is given piggyback to another IV so it can be stopped when necessary. When three uterine contractions lasting 40 to 60 seconds occur in 10 minutes, the oxytocin is stopped. If three late decelerations occur, the oxytocin is stopped.

For nipple stimulation, warm washcloths are applied to the breasts and/or one nipple is manually rolled by the client. When three uterine contractions lasting 40 to 60 seconds occur in 10 minutes, the stimulation is discontinued. If a decrease in FHR occurs with a contraction, the nipple stimulation is stopped.

A negative CST with no late decelerations indicates the fetus is well-oxygenated. The fetus is able to tolerate the hypoxia of uterine contractions. A CST with late decelerations that occur with at least 50% of contractions is considered a positive CST, which indicates fetoplacental exchange may be compromised. The CST is more invasive and time consuming, so the BPP or MBPP is the preferred method of determining fetal well-being.

# ELECTRONIC FETAL MONITORING

Electronic fetal monitoring (EFM) provides a visual record of the FHR in relation to the uterine contractions. It allows early detection of fetal distress and abnormal uterine activity. High-risk clients and clients with a problem in their pregnancy are candidates for EFM. Most birthing places routinely have all clients on EFM.

## External (Indirect) Monitoring

A tocodynamometer (tocotransducer) that records uterine activity is placed on the mother's abdomen, on the fundus of the uterus. The least amount of tissue is between the dynamometer and fundus at this location so activity is recorded more accurately. With this device, contraction frequency, the amount of time between the beginning of one contraction to the beginning of the next contraction, is determined. The nurse palpates the client's abdomen during a contraction to determine the contraction strength.

An ultrasound transducer that records the FHR is placed over the maternal abdomen in a location where the fetal heart is heard. When the head is the presenting part, the fetal heart is usually best heard just below the umbilicus on one side or the other. With this device, sound waves are bounced off the fetal heart and picked up and displayed as a

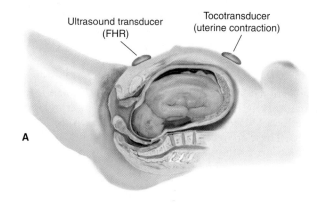

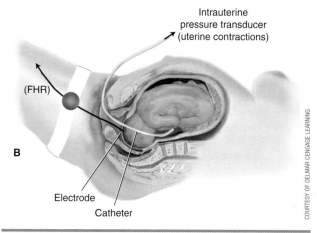

COURTESY OF DELMAR CENGAGE LEARNING

**FIGURE 2-5** Fetal Monitoring: *A*, External (indirect). The top transducer picks up the fetal heart tones and transmits the signal as an electrical impulse to the monitor where they are recorded; *B*, Internal (direct). The EKG electrode on the fetus's scalp picks up the fetal heart tones and the intrauterine catheter picks up uterine contractions.

rate by the monitor. FHR baseline and periodic/nonperiodic changes of the FHR are determined. Elastic bands are placed around the maternal abdomen to hold the transducers in place (Figure 2-5A).

## Internal (Direct) Monitoring

This is a more reliable method then external monitoring. An EKG electrode to directly monitor FHR is attached to the fetal presenting part (head) (Figure 2-5B). For this to be initiated, the membranes must be ruptured, the cervix must be dilated at least 2 cm, the presenting part must be down against the cervix, and the presenting part must be known. Only a person specially trained for this procedure should perform it.

Either the external tocodynamometer or an intrauterine catheter may be used to assess uterine contractions. A thin, flexible polyethylene catheter filled with sterile, distilled water is inserted into the amniotic fluid in the uterus. Other catheters used are solid and flexible. In either case, the catheter is inserted between the fetus and the uterine wall into a pocket of amniotic fluid.

The increased pressure on the fluid during a contraction is translated into an electrical signal. This provides reliable information about the contractions. Sterile technique is used when inserting both the scalp electrode and the catheter.

## Interpretations

The National Institute of Child Health and Human Development (NICHD) recommended EFM interpretations as follows (Macones, Hankins, Spong, Hauth, & Moore, 2008). These are recommended for use in labor and delivery units across the nation to achieve a more consistent use of terms.

**Baseline Rate** Baseline rate is the average FHR during a 10-minute period. The normal rate is 110 to 160 beats/minute. A rate greater than 160 beats/minute is tachycardia, and a rate below 110 beats/minute is bradycardia.

**Baseline Variability** Variability is determined by the irregular fluctuations of the FHR, quantified as the peak to trough amplitude noted in beats per minute (bpm) that occurs during a 10-minute period. These are classified into one of four categories: absent (no difference), minimal (> 0 to </=5 bpm), moderate (6 to </=25 bpm) or marked (>25 bpm).

**Accelerations** Accelerations are short-term increases in FHR and are usually caused by fetal movement. There is a change in FHR that is a visible abrupt increase: (onset of acceleration to peak less than 30 seconds) by at least 15 bpm, lasting at least 15 seconds. The presence of accelerations indicates the fetus has a pH of at least 7.2, which is normal. The fetus is not in an acidotic state.

**Early Deceleration** **Early decelerations** are gradual reductions in FHR that begin early with the contraction and typically mirror the contraction. Head compression during contractions causes a decrease in cerebral blood flow, which stimulates a vagal response and causes the heart rate to decrease. The decreased heart rate displays on the monitor as an early deceleration. As pressure is relieved, the FHR returns to normal by the end of the contraction. No intervention is required (Figure 2-6).

**Late Deceleration** **Late decelerations** are reductions in FHR that begin at or after the peak of the contraction and increase to the baseline level after the contraction has ceased, caused by uteroplacental insufficiency. When a timing discrepancy exists and early versus late decelerations are in question, the nadir (the lowest point) of the deceleration and the peak of the contraction will differentiate early from late. Oxygen administered to the mother may be started. Late decelerations should be reported to the health care provider (Figure 2-6).

**Variable Deceleration** **Variable decelerations** are abrupt reductions in FHR that have no relationship to contractions of the uterus. They occur when compression of the umbilical cord reduces blood flow between fetus and placenta. A change in the mother's position may take pressure off the cord. When pressure is relieved, the FHR abruptly returns to the baseline. These should also be reported immediately (Figure 2-6).

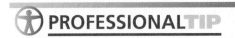

## PROFESSIONALTIP

### Electronic Fetal Monitoring

The NICHD agreed upon 3 categories of FHR patterns to help guide obstetrical health care providers in providing consistent care in relation to the pattern observed. The categories are listed as follows (Macones, Hankins, Spong, Hauth, & Moore, 2008).

*Category I –* **Normal** There is no acidosis and there are no interventions necessary.

FHR baseline rate is 110 to 160 bpm

Moderate variability

Absence of variable or late decelerations

Presence or absence of accelerations or early decelerations

*Category II –* **Indeterminate** In this category, patterns from categories I or III are not found. These patterns do not indicate compromised acid-base balance but necessitate close observation and reevaluation. Health care providers may perform fetal scalp stimulation (gentle rubbing of the presenting part to elicit an acceleration) to determine if fetal oxygenation has been compromised. Other actions may be indicated if there is no positive response.

*Category III –* **Abnormal** In this category, any one of the following FHR patterns in the absence of FHR variability indicate probable abnormal fetal acid-base balance.

Recurrent late decelerations

Recurrent variable decelerations

Bradycardia

Also considered abnormal is the sinusoidal pattern. This is a wavy pattern of regular variability occurring at 3-5 cycles per minute with an amplitude of 5 to 40 bpm. This pattern resembles a "sine wave" and may indicate a serious condition in the fetus, such as anemia.

Category III patterns require that the health care provider be present to determine timing and mode of delivery. The cause of the pattern is determined, if possible, and the following measures are implemented to correct the problem. These interventions may also be used in Category II patterns that do not respond to scalp stimulation with an acceleration.

Change maternal position

Increase the rate of the mainline intravenous infusion

Administer oxygen to the mother

Discontinue oxytocin if infusing

Resolve maternal hypotension

If the interventions do not improve fetal status, delivery is immediate.

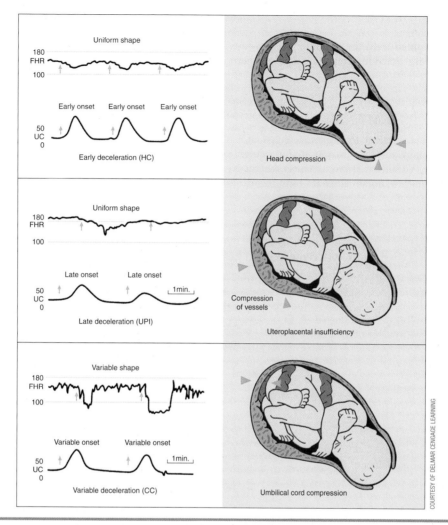

**FIGURE 2-6** Fetal Heart Rate Patterns from Continuous Electronic Fetal Monitoring

# HYPEREMESIS GRAVIDARUM

Hyperemesis gravidarum is a severe form of nausea and vomiting occurring during pregnancy that usually persists beyond the first trimester. The cause is unknown but may be related to an increased estrogen level, gonadotropin production, or trophoblastic activity. Psychological factors may also be involved. The excessive secretion of saliva (ptyalism) may contribute to the feeling of nausea. The nausea and vomiting does not subside at about 12 weeks' gestation as does "morning sickness." If untreated, the vomiting causes nutritional deficiencies and dehydration.

Dehydration leads to fluid and electrolyte imbalance and alkalosis from the loss of hydrochloric acid. As the situation becomes worse, the client experiences tachycardia and may have hypovolemia, hypotension, an increase in hematocrit and blood urea nitrogen (BUN), and a decrease in urine output.

The starvation situation causes protein and vitamin deficiencies. Cardiac functioning may be disrupted by severe potassium loss. Untreated, the client may experience metabolic changes or death. Embryonic or fetal death may occur.

The treatment goals are to control vomiting, correct dehydration, restore electrolyte balance, and maintain adequate nutrition.

## MEDICAL–SURGICAL MANAGEMENT

### Medical

The client is usually hospitalized and intravenous fluids containing glucose, vitamins, and electrolytes are started immediately. IV therapy is continued until all vomiting has stopped for 48 hours. Psychotherapy may be recommended.

### Pharmacological

A sedative may be given, but medications are kept to a minimum because of potential teratogenic (harmful) effects to the fetus.

### Diet

The client is kept NPO until all vomiting has stopped for 48 hours. Small amounts of dry foods are then offered with slow progression to a regular diet. If the client is unable to eat without vomiting, total parenteral nutrition may be initiated through a peripherally inserted central catheter (i.e., PICC) or other IV access.

## Activity

Bed rest is usually maintained until the condition begins to improve. Visitors may be restricted for a few days to allow the client to rest.

## NURSING MANAGEMENT

Provide opportunities for the client to express feelings and perceptions of the pregnancy and the fetus. Maintain a quiet environment. Administer IV fluids as ordered. Assess skin turgor and mucous membranes. Maintain accurate I&O record. Ensure good oral hygiene.

## NURSING PROCESS

### ASSESSMENT

#### Subjective Data

Especially important is the client's emotional state and her feelings about the pregnancy, the fetus, and her mate. Ask what triggers her nausea and vomiting.

#### Objective Data

Check the amount and character of all emesis, intake and output, and FHR. Note signs of jaundice and vaginal bleeding.

### Nursing diagnoses for a client with hyperemesis gravidarum include the following:

| NURSING DIAGNOSES | PLANNING/OUTCOMES | NURSING INTERVENTIONS |
|---|---|---|
| *Imbalanced Nutrition: Less Than Body Requirements* related to persistent vomiting | The client will cease vomiting. | Maintain relaxed, quiet environment. |
| | | Monitor amount and character of all emesis, and maintain accurate I&O record. |
| | | Ensure good oral hygiene after each vomiting episode. |
| | | When vomiting stops, provide dry foods, then bland foods and oral fluids as ordered. |
| | | Maintain cheerful, optimistic attitude. |
| *Deficient Fluid Volume* related to decreased fluid intake and excessive fluid loss | The client will have fluid balance. | Administer IV fluids as ordered. |
| | | Monitor laboratory reports for electrolyte levels. |
| | | Assess skin turgor and mucous membranes. |
| | | Provide small amounts of oral fluids when tolerated. |
| | | Maintain accurate I&O record. |
| *Fear* related to fetal well-being | The client will discuss fears with health caregivers. | Provide opportunities for client to express concerns. |
| | | Show acceptance of client's perceptions. |
| | | Assist client to identify personal strengths. |
| | | Listen to the client's concerns. |
| | | Help client identify sources of support. |

**Evaluation:** Evaluate each outcome to determine how it has been met by the client.

## BLEEDING

**B**leeding disorders include abortion, ectopic pregnancy, hydatidiform mole, placenta previa, abruptio placenta, and disseminated intravascular coagulation.

## ABORTION

**A**bortion is the spontaneous (natural) or induced (elective) termination of a pregnancy before viability of the fetus. A fetus is considered viable at 20 weeks' gestation. With medical intervention, a fetus between 20 and 24 weeks' gestation may survive. Some states have defined viability as 20 weeks' gestation and a weight of 500 g.

A spontaneous abortion is often called a **miscarriage**. Spontaneous abortions may be related to chromosomal abnormalities, faulty implantation, teratogenic substances, placental abnormalities, incompetent cervix, chronic maternal diseases, maternal infections, and endocrine imbalances. Clinically, spontaneous abortions are classified as:

- *Threatened*: Unexplained bleeding and cramping. The cervix is closed and membranes are intact (Figure 2-7A).
- *Inevitable*: Increased bleeding and cramping. The cervix begins to dilate and the membranes may rupture (Figure 2-7B).
- *Incomplete*: Some of the products of conception are expelled. Most often the placenta is not expelled. Bleeding is heavy and cramping severe (Figure 2-7C).
- *Complete*: All products of conception are expelled.

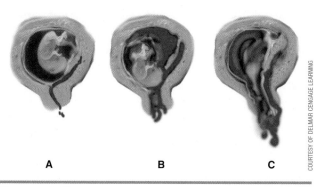

COURTESY OF DELMAR CENGAGE LEARNING

**FIGURE 2-7** Types of Spontaneous Abortions; *A*, Threatened; *B*, Inevitable; *C*, Incomplete

- *Missed*: Embryo or fetus dies but is retained. The cervix is closed. If the fetus is not expelled within 6 weeks, disseminated intravascular coagulation (DIC) may develop.
- *Recurrent spontaneous*: Any of the above occurring in three consecutive pregnancies. Most commonly, the cervix begins to dilate in the second trimester. This is called an **incompetent cervix**.

## MEDICAL–SURGICAL MANAGEMENT

### Medical

For threatened abortion, the client is usually told to limit activities for 24 to 48 hours. If the bleeding is going to stop, it will usually do so in 48 hours. If the bleeding stops, the client is advised to avoid stress, fatigue, strenuous activity, and sexual intercourse. Having one or two rest periods during the day is also recommended until the pregnancy seems to be progressing normally.

### Surgical

A client with an inevitable or incomplete abortion generally is hospitalized to remove the products of conception from the uterus. A dilation and curettage (D & C) or suction evacuation is performed. Depending on the amount of blood loss, the client may be given blood transfusions.

When the products of conception, in a missed abortion, are not expelled in 4 to 6 weeks, the client is hospitalized. For 12 weeks' gestation or less, a D & C is performed. If more than 12 weeks' gestation, induction of labor with oxytocin may be used.

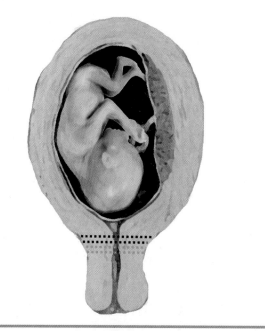

COURTESY OF DELMAR CENGAGE LEARNING

**FIGURE 2-8** Shirodkar or McDonald Procedure. Purse-string sutures keep the cervix closed in an incompetent cervix.

When recurrent spontaneous abortions are caused by an incompetent cervix, a treatment option is surgical cerclage (Shirodkar or McDonald procedure, Figure 2-8). The cervix is stitched with a heavy suture in a purse-string fashion at the level of the internal os at about 13 to 17 weeks' gestation. The difference between the Shirodkar and the McDonald method is the height on the cervix and method of suture placement. The Shirodkar suture can be left in for future pregnancies and a cesarean birth planned, or the suture may be removed at term and a vaginal birth occurs (Trofatter, 2009). If the mother goes into labor or the membranes rupture, she must call her health-care provider and go to the hospital immediately.

## NURSING MANAGEMENT

Frequently assess the amount of bleeding, presence of clots, and any expelled tissue. Provide a calm environment and actively listen to the client. Provide information about the situation and prepare client for procedures and treatments.

## NURSING PROCESS

### ASSESSMENT

### Subjective Data

The client may describe abdominal cramping and vaginal bleeding, and may have feelings of fear and guilt.

### Objective Data

Note the amount of bleeding, presence of clots, and any tissue expelled. Expelled tissue is sent to pathology as ordered for analysis. Vital signs may indicate excessive blood loss (hypovolemia). Assess location, quality, and intensity of pain.

---

### 🧍 PROFESSIONALTIP

**Spontaneous Abortion**

The client who has a miscarriage may experience a wide spectrum of emotions from shock, disbelief, and guilt, to anger and despair. She may have difficulty managing these feelings as well as responding to the reactions of her partner, family, and friends. The nurse can assist by answering the woman's questions, allowing her to express her emotions, and respecting her need to grieve.

Nursing diagnoses for a client having an abortion include the following:

| NURSING DIAGNOSES | PLANNING/OUTCOMES | NURSING INTERVENTIONS |
|---|---|---|
| *Situational Low Self-esteem* related to feelings of guilt for doing something to cause abortion | The client will maintain usual level of self-esteem. | Provide information about causes of a spontaneous abortion.<br>Assist client to identify personal strengths.<br>Actively listen to the client. |
| *Aute Pain* related to contractions (cramping) of uterine muscle | The client will describe having less pain. | Administer analgesic as ordered.<br>Monitor effect of analgesic. |
| *Fear* related to potential loss of pregnancy | The client will discuss fear with family. | Provide opportunities for the client to express fears.<br>Help client identify sources of support.<br>Show acceptance of client's perceptions. |

**Evaluation:** Evaluate each outcome to determine how it has been met by the client.

## SAMPLE NURSING CARE PLAN

## The Client Having a Spontaneous Abortion

P.C., age 25, G4, P3, T2, P1, A0, L3, is admitted to the hospital with some bleeding and cramping. She states, "I'm scared, I don't understand what's happening." Vital signs are BP 108/66, T 98.6, P 86, R 24. Her skin is cool. At her first prenatal visit, 3 weeks ago, the fetus was 12 weeks' gestation. Crying, she says, "I don't know what I did to cause this to happen."

Two hours later, P.C.'s cramping is severe and the bleeding heavy, bright red. Vital signs are BP 88/60, P 100, and R 28. Her skin is cold and clammy.

**NURSING DIAGNOSIS 1** *Deficient Fluid Volume* related to heavy bleeding as evidenced by hypotension and decreased pulse pressure

**Nursing Outcomes Classification (NOC)**
*Fluid Balance*

**Nursing Interventions Classification (NIC)**
*Fluid Monitoring*

| PLANNING/OUTCOMES | NURSING INTERVENTIONS | RATIONALE |
|---|---|---|
| P.C. will have vital signs return to baseline values. | Administer IV fluids and/or blood as ordered. | Replaces fluid volume lost by bleeding. |
| | Monitor P.C.'s vital signs every 15 minutes or less. | Clinical indicators of fluid volume. |
| | Save all vaginal pads and clots or tissue passed for physician to see. | Allows physician to estimate blood loss and identify any tissue passed. |
| | Administer analgesic as ordered. | Relieving pain will make P.C. more comfortable. |
| | Prepare P.C. for surgery as ordered. | Most likely, a D & C will be performed. |

## EVALUATION

After a D & C, P.C.'s vital signs returned to baseline values.

**NURSING DIAGNOSIS 2** *Anxiety* related to changes in her pregnancy as evidenced by statement "I'm scared, I don't understand what's happening."

**Nursing Outcomes Classification (NOC)**
*Anxiety Reduction*
*Coping*

**Nursing Interventions Classification (NIC)**
*Anxiety Reduction*

*(Continues)*

## SAMPLE NURSING CARE PLAN (Continued)

| PLANNING/OUTCOMES | NURSING INTERVENTIONS | RATIONALE |
|---|---|---|
| P.C. will verbalize her feelings about bleeding and cramping while pregnant. | Speak slowly and calmly to P.C. | Conveys calmness and sense of security. |
| | Evaluate P.C.'s understanding of what is happening and possible treatment options. | Provides information for educational needs. |
| | Involve spouse/significant other in discussion. | Gives family information and a feeling of control. |
| | Be direct and focus on the specific topic. | Anxiety decreases ability to concentrate. |
| | Help P.C. identify coping methods used in the past. | Reviewing past coping mechanisms helps P.C. find effective coping mechanisms to use now. |

## EVALUATION

P.C. shared feelings of fear and guilt about the bleeding and cramping.

### NURSING DIAGNOSIS 3

*Anticipatory Grieving* related to probable loss of pregnancy as evidenced by crying and statement "I don't know what I did to cause this to happen."

**NOC:** *Coping, Family Coping, Grief Resolution*
**NIC:** *Family Support, Grief Work Facilitation, Coping Enhancement, Emotional Support*

### CLIENT GOAL

P.C. will verbalize what losing a pregnancy means to her.

| NURSING INTERVENTIONS | SCIENTIFIC RATIONALES |
|---|---|
| 1. Allow P.C. to express her feelings. | 1. Releases energy and is calming. |
| 2. Assess P.C.'s coping skills. | 2. Coping skills may need reinforcing or adapting. |
| 3. Assist P.C.'s to identify personal resources and strengths. | 3. Promotes integrity of self. |
| 4. Provide privacy for P.C. and her family. | 4. Allows them a chance to discuss the situation and make plans. |
| 5. Refer to local pregnancy loss support group. | 5. Referral assists family to find encouragement and support from others. |

### EVALUATION

Have P.C.'s vital signs returned to baseline values?
Is P.C. expressing her feelings about losing the pregnancy?

# ■ ECTOPIC PREGNANCY

An **ectopic pregnancy** occurs when a fertilized ovum implants outside the uterine cavity. The most common site is in the fallopian tube. This generally happens when the fertilized ovum is unable to move through the tube. Figure 2-9 illustrates other possible sites of implantation in an ectopic pregnancy.

In the United States, an ectopic pregnancy occurs in 2% of all pregnancies (Sepilian & Wood, 2009). Risk factors include pelvic inflammatory disease, in utero exposure to diethylstilbestrol (DES), sexually transmitted infections, pharmacologic treatment of infertility, endometriosis, smoking, advanced maternal age, and prior abdominal surgery (Sepilian & Wood, 2009).

The pregnancy appears normal at first with the usual signs and symptoms, including the presence of hCG in the blood and urine. Symptoms of ectopic pregnancy begin gradually about 3 to 5 weeks after the first missed menstrual period. Pain is noted as the fallopian tube stretches with the growing embryo. The tube finally ruptures (a severe pain occurs) and bleeds into the peritoneal cavity. Some vaginal bleeding

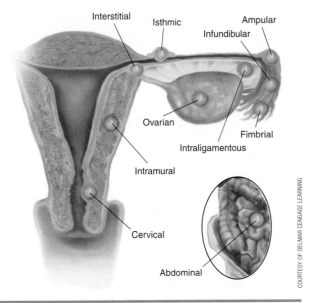

**FIGURE 2-9** **Possible Sites of Implantation in Ectopic Pregnancy**

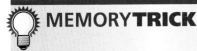

## MEMORY **TRICK**

To remember the 3 classic symptoms of an ectopic pregnancy, recall **VAP**:

**V** = Vaginal bleeding

**A** = Amenorrhea

**P** = Pain

(Sepilian & Wood, 2009)

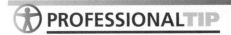

## PROFESSIONAL**TIP**

### Treatment Alternative for Ectopic Pregnancy

A viable alternative to surgery that is just as successful as laparoscopic salpingostomy is now available. Methotrexate (Mexate, Folex) works by interfering with DNA synthesis and cell multiplication. The actively proliferating trophoblastic tissue is sensitive to methotrexate.

Women who desire future fertility and have an unruptured ectopic pregnancy 3.5 cm or less in size and have no symptoms of bleeding are candidates for methotrexate therapy. The treatment is a single dose of methotrexate (Mexate, Folex) 50 mg/m² IM in a single injection or as a divided dose injected into each hip.

Potential drug side effects are photosensitivity, nausea and vomiting, stomatitis, gastris, diarrhea, and dizziness. Effects to expect from methotrexate treatment are increased abdominal pain 2 to 3 days after the injection, an increase in bhCG for 1 to 3 days, and vaginal bleeding or spotting.

Stress the importance of follow-up visits with the health care provider until the weekly monitored levels of bhCG levels are not present. If the client is Rh negative, administer Rh immune globulin (RhoGAM) (Sepilian & Wood, 2009).

may be apparent. The client may rapidly show signs of hypovolemic shock. The signs of shock are out of proportion to the apparent blood loss. Ectopic pregnancy is nearly always fatal to the embryo.

## MEDICAL–SURGICAL MANAGEMENT

### Medical

The menstrual history is reviewed and a pelvic examination performed to identify abnormal pelvic masses and tenderness. Severe pain occurs when the cervix is moved. A transvaginal ultrasound is also done. Serial testing of hCG shows a slower increase than in a normal pregnancy, in which the hCG level doubles every 48 to 72 hours. A serum progesterone level of 25 ng/mL strongly suggests a normal pregnancy, whereas a level of 5 ng/mL or less indicates a nonviable pregnancy. A level between 5 ng/mL and 25 ng/mL is uncertain, and a transvaginal ultrasound is needed.

### Surgical

Rapid surgical treatment is generally necessary to remove the products of conception and to control bleeding. Laparotomy is seldom used unless the client has orthostatic hypotension, tachycardia, or a falling hematocrit.

Laparoscopic salpingostomy or salpingectomy are preferred. The procedure of choice is salpingostomy when future fertility is desired (Sepilian & Wood, 2009). If the fallopian tube is badly damaged, a salpingectomy is performed. The ovary is left in place if not damaged. Blood transfusions are often required.

## Pharmacological

Methotrexate (Mexate, Folex) may be given to resolve an ectopic pregnancy.

## Diet

If the client has surgery, she will be NPO before and after surgery.

## Activity

The client is usually on bed rest until the situation is resolved.

## NURSING MANAGEMENT

Administer analgesics as ordered. Provide information about an ectopic pregnancy. Actively listen to client. Encourage client to express feelings. Monitor vital signs. Prepare for surgery as ordered and begin preoperative teaching.

# NURSING PROCESS
## ASSESSMENT
### Subjective Data

The client describes amenorrhea, nausea, breast tenderness, and a dull ache on one side that has increasingly become more severe. When the tube ruptures, the client will describe a single excruciating pain in the abdomen and may also have referred shoulder pain.

### Objective Data

Some vaginal bleeding may be apparent. Laboratory reports may show a low hemoglobin and hematocrit, a rising leukocyte level, and a slowly rising hCG level. The red blood count (RBC) count is low and sedimentation rate elevated. The abdomen may be rigid and tender. Vital signs may indicate hypovolemic shock.

### Nursing diagnoses for a client with an ectopic pregnancy include the following:

| NURSING DIAGNOSES | PLANNING/OUTCOMES | NURSING INTERVENTIONS |
|---|---|---|
| *Anticipatory Grieving* related to the loss of the pregnancy | The client will understand that grieving may last several months. | Encourage client and family to talk about their feelings. Allow them privacy to grieve. Listen actively to concerns about this and future pregnancies. Provide information about causes of ectopic pregnancy. Refer to other professionals for help as needed. |
| *Impaired Tissue Integrity* related to the rupture of a fallopian tube | The client will regain tissue integrity of the fallopian tube or it will be removed. | Prepare client for surgery as ordered. Begin preoperative teaching. |
| *Acute Pain* related to tubal rupture and blood in the abdomen | The client will express less pain. | Administer analgesics as ordered and evaluate its effectiveness. Provide information about cause of pain. |

**Evaluation:** Evaluate each outcome to determine how it has been met by the client.

## ■ HYDATIDIFORM MOLE

**H**ydatidiform mole (trophoblastic disease), or molar pregnancy, is an abnormality of the placenta. The chorionic villi become fluid-filled, grapelike clusters; the trophoblastic tissue proliferates; and there is no viable embryo. In effect, the fertilized ovum dies and the chorion develops into vesicles. There is a possibility of developing choriocarcinoma (malignant, metastaic, potentially fatal trophoblastic disease).

Two types of hydatidiform moles are the complete and the partial. The complete mole has only paternal genetic material. There is no embryonic tissue, only the fluid-filled cystic villi. A large amount of hCG is produced because the chorionic villi are proliferating. The classic signs are bleeding (usually brownish but may be red), uterine enlargement greater than would be expected for the gestation, and no fetal heart tones (FHT) heard (Figure 2-10). If any of the grapelike clusters are passed, it is diagnostic. There is greater potential of developing a choriocarcinoma with the complete than the partial mole.

The partial mole has only focal areas of the fluid-filled cystic villi; some chorionic villi are formed normally. There is a fetus with multiple chromosomal anomalies and little chance for survival. A partial mole may not be recognized until

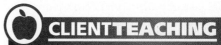

the products of conception are examined after a spontaneous abortion.

The client may experience hyperemesis gravidarum because of the higher serum hCG level. If symptoms of pregnancy-induced hypertension appear before 24 weeks' gestation, a molar pregnancy is very probable. The primary diagnostic tool is ultrasound.

## MEDICAL–SURGICAL MANAGEMENT
### Medical

After surgery to remove the mole, the client must be followed for 1 to 2 years. The care includes chest x-rays to detect metastases, physical examinations with a pelvic examination, and regular (usually weekly) laboratory measurement of hCG level. The client is advised not to become pregnant during the follow-up time.

### Surgical

The desire of the client for future fertility influences the surgical procedure used to empty the uterus. A D & C may be performed, but it is difficult to make certain that no fragment of the molar pregnancy is left in the uterus. A hysterotomy, cutting the uterus open (like cesarean birth), allows visual determination that the uterus is completely emptied. If the client is older and no future pregnancy is desired or there is excessive bleeding, a hysterectomy is performed.

### Pharmacological

If the hCG level remains high or rises after the uterus is evacuated, methotrexate (Mexate, Folex) is given. Oxytocin is given to keep the uterus contracted to control bleeding. Typed and cross-matched blood must be available.

### Activity

Bed rest is maintained until after surgery, then ambulation is progressively increased.

## NURSING MANAGEMENT

Monitor vaginal bleeding. Assess uterine size and FHT (none heard). Prepare for ultrasound. Prepare for surgery as ordered.

## NURSING PROCESS
### ASSESSMENT
#### Subjective Data

The client may describe severe nausea and vomiting and may have some brownish vaginal discharge.

#### Objective Data

There is vaginal bleeding, usually brownish but may be bright red. Uterine enlargement is greater than expected for gestational age. Ultrasound reveals a characteristic molar pattern. The client may have symptoms of gestational hypertension (BP 140/90 mm Hg or an increase of 30/15, proteinuria, and edema measured by sudden weight gain). The lack of FHTs when the client has other signs of pregnancy is a classic symptom of a hydatidiform mole. The client has very low levels of serum alpha-fetoprotein.

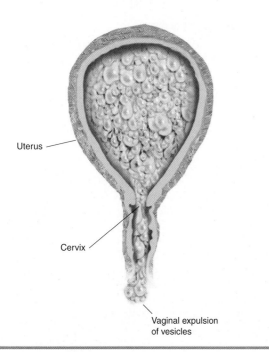

Uterus

Cervix

Vaginal expulsion of vesicles

FIGURE 2-10  **Hydatidiform Mole**

COURTESY OF DELMAR CENGAGE LEARNING

**Nursing diagnoses for a client with hydatidiform mole include the following:**

| NURSING DIAGNOSES | PLANNING/OUTCOMES | NURSING INTERVENTIONS |
|---|---|---|
| *Fear* related to the possible development of choriocarcinoma | The client will discuss fears with health care provider or other professional. | Provide opportunities for client to express fears. Help client identify sources of support. Refer to other professionals as needed. |
| *Deficient* **Knowledge** related to lack of understanding for regular monitoring of hCG level and delaying pregnancy | The client will discuss reasons for regular monitoring of hCG level and reasons for delaying pregnancy. | Explain that the hCG level indicates whether choriocarcinoma is developing. Provide reasons for delaying another pregnancy. Allow client to express feelings about regular laboratory testing of blood. |

**Evaluation:** Evaluate each outcome to determine how it has been met by the client.

## ■ PLACENTA PREVIA

**P**lacenta previa occurs when implantation is in the lower uterine segment with the placenta lying over or very near the internal cervical os, the opening into the uterus (Figure 2-11). The cause is unknown, but predisposing factors may be multiparity, uterine scarring from D & C or cesarean birth, endometritis, maternal advancing age, and smoking.

The classic symptom is *painless bleeding* in the last half of pregnancy. There may be occasional bright red spotting or intermittent gushes of blood. Rarely is bleeding continuous. The uterus is relaxed and not tender. Bleeding is unrelated to maternal activity. Placenta previa is classified in three ways:

- *Low-lying or Marginal*: Placenta is near the internal cervical os but does not cover any part of the opening
- *Partial*: Placenta covers part of internal cervical os opening
- *Complete or Total*: Placenta completely covers internal cervical os opening

Toward the last part of pregnancy, the cervix effaces (thins). This movement of the cervix pulls away from the placenta, and the exposed placental sinuses begin to bleed. The earlier this happens, the more serious the situation.

## EFFECTS ON THE FETUS/NEONATE

The gestational age of the fetus and the amount of bleeding determine the effects on the fetus/neonate. During profuse bleeding, the fetus may suffer from hypoxia. After delivery, the neonate is assessed to see whether the bleeding resulted in anemia.

## MEDICAL–SURGICAL MANAGEMENT

### Medical

The goal is to maintain the pregnancy until the fetus is mature enough to survive outside the uterus. Fetal maturity is assessed by checking the lecithin/sphingomyelin ratio for lung maturity. The mother is usually hospitalized. Hemoglobin and hematocrit (H & H) is usually determined every 12 hours. The laboratory will type and cross-match, and two units of blood is kept on call in the event of severe blood loss.

Diagnosis is made with an ultrasound. Once the diagnosis is made, no vaginal examinations are performed because of the risk of causing more bleeding by disturbing the placenta. If an ultrasound is unavailable, vaginal bleeding profuse, and the pregnancy near term, the health care provider may examine the client vaginally. This is done in the delivery room with a setup for both a vaginal delivery and a cesarean delivery. An IV is started in case the client starts bleeding profusely. Urinary output decreases as the bleeding increases.

### Surgical

If the maternal situation becomes worse or there are signs of fetal distress, a cesarean birth is begun immediately.

### Pharmacological

In an attempt to accelerate fetal lung maturity, a drug such as betamethasone (Celestone) may be given to the mother.

### Activity

The client is on bed rest with bathroom privileges as long as no bleeding occurs. If the client has bathroom privileges, place a graduated container or commode "hat" in the toilet

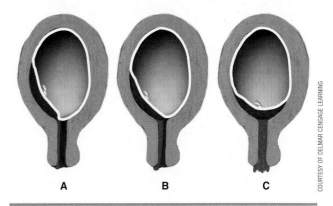

A          B          C

**FIGURE 2-11** Placenta Previa; *A,* Low Implantation (**Marginal**); *B,* Partial Placenta Previa; *C,* Total Placenta Previa

COURTESY OF DELMAR CENGAGE LEARNING

to collect urine and any products of conception passed by the woman. If bleeding begins, the client is on complete bed rest.

## NURSING MANAGEMENT

Maintain the client on bed rest. Monitor vital signs and FHR. Prepare for ultrasound. Maintain a calm environment.

### CRITICAL THINKING

**Placenta Previa**

A client is admitted with a placenta previa.
1. What assessments does the nurse do to monitor for blood loss?
2. What is the most important assessment the nurse does throughout the labor process?

Assess for uterine contractions. Administer IV solutions as ordered. Monitor urinary output. Be prepared for a possible C-section.

## NURSING PROCESS

### ASSESSMENT

#### Subjective Data

The client describes painless bleeding.

#### Objective Data

Vaginal bleeding may range from spotting to profuse bleeding. The uterus remains soft and relaxes fully between contractions if labor begins. FHR generally remains stable unless bleeding is profuse and maternal shock occurs.

**Nursing diagnoses for a client with placenta previa include the following:**

| NURSING DIAGNOSES | PLANNING/OUTCOMES | NURSING INTERVENTIONS |
|---|---|---|
| *Deficient Fluid Volume* related to blood loss | The client will maintain perfusion to placenta and vital organs. | Observe, report, and record blood loss (count and/or weigh pads). |
| | | Monitor client's vital signs, FHR, I&O, and laboratory reports. |
| | | Maintain comfortable environment to prevent diaphoresis. |
| | | Inspect skin for pallor, cyanosis, clamminess, and coldness. |
| | | Encourage client to maintain fluid intake. |
| *Impaired Gas Exchange, Fetal* related to decreased maternal blood volume and hypotension | FHR will remain within normal limits. | Monitor FHR, baseline variability, and decelerations. |
| | | Observe amniotic fluid for meconium. |
| | | Instruct client in positions to promote placental perfusion. |
| | | Administer IV fluids to mother to promote placental perfusion. |

**Evaluation:** Evaluate each outcome to determine how it has been met by the client.

## ABRUPTIO PLACENTA

The premature separation from the wall of the uterus of a normally implanted placenta is called **abruptio placenta**. It occurs spontaneously after the 20th week of gestation in approximately 1% of all pregnancies (Bougere, 1998; Deering, 2008). The cause is unknown. Contributing factors include maternal hypertension, multiple pregnancy, abdominal trauma, smoking, use of alcohol, or use of cocaine. Generally, it occurs late in pregnancy or during labor. There are three types of abruptio placenta (Figure 2-12).

- *Central*: Center of the placenta separates with blood trapped between placenta and uterine wall; there is no apparent bleeding
- *Marginal*: Edge of placenta separates and bright red bleeding is apparent vaginally

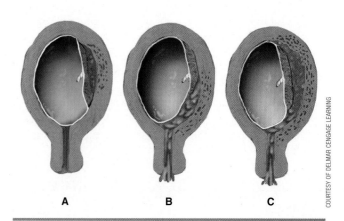

**FIGURE 2-12** Abruptio Placenta; *A*, Central Abruption, Concealed Hemorrhage; *B*, Marginal Abruption, External Hemorrhage; *C*, Complete Abruption, External Hemorrhage (Could also Be Concealed)

**TABLE 2-3  Comparison of Placenta Previa and Abruptio Placenta**

| CONDITION | BLEEDING | ABDOMEN | PAIN | BP |
|---|---|---|---|---|
| **Placenta Previa** | Bright red | No rigidity | None | Depends on amount of bleeding |
| **Abruptio Placenta** | | | | |
| Central | None | Rigid | Acute | Decreased |
| Marginal | Dark red | No rigidity | Uterine tenderness | Decreased |
| Complete | Profuse or concealed | Rigid | Acute | Shock |

- *Complete*: Entire placenta separates with profuse bleeding apparent vaginally or concealed

A central abruption may progress to a complete abruption. In central and complete, blood invades the uterine muscle (bruising called *Couvelaire uterus*), causing a rigid, painful abdomen. After delivery, the uterus contracts poorly and the client may require a hysterectomy to control the bleeding. The damage to the uterine muscle and the retroplacental clotting can cause a large release of thromboplastin. This can trigger the development of disseminated intravascular coagulation (DIC). Maternal mortality is relatively low. Problems after the delivery depend on the severity of the bleeding. Table 2-3 compares placenta previa and the various types of abruptio placenta.

## EFFECTS ON THE FETUS/ NEONATE

Perinatal mortality occurs in 0.12% (1:830) of pregnancies (Deering, 2008). The outcome depends on fetal maturity and severity of the abruption. Preterm labor, hypoxia, and anemia are the most serious complications. Irreversible brain damage or fetal death occurs if hypoxia is not reversed quickly.

## MEDICAL–SURGICAL MANAGEMENT

### Medical

Intravenous fluids, generally lactated Ringer's solution, are given to prevent or reverse hypovolemia. Laboratory tests to evaluate client's status and the clotting mechanism are ordered: H & H, platelet count, fibrinogen level, fibrin split products, thrombin time, prothrombin time, partial thromboplastin time, and bleeding time. Also, a type and cross-match for three to four units of blood or packed cells is requested (Bougere, 1998). If the mother is Rh negative, she is checked for Rh sensitization. An indwelling urinary catheter is inserted.

If separation is small and the pregnancy near term, induction of labor and vaginal delivery may be possible. If labor is not progressing, a cesarean birth is performed. If separation is moderate or severe, a cesarean birth is performed as soon as possible.

### Surgical

Cesarean delivery is performed in many cases to prevent fetal demise. A hysterectomy may be required to control hemorrhage.

### Pharmacological

Rh immune globulin (RhoGAM) is given to the nonsensitized Rh-negative mother. Cryoprecipitate or plasma is given to treat hypofibrinogenemia. Analgesics are given as ordered.

### Diet

No special diet or restrictions are required, although the client will be NPO if surgery is necessary.

### Activity

The client will remain on bed rest until the situation is resolved.

## NURSING MANAGEMENT

Monitor the client's bleeding, pain, vital signs, FHR, and fetal activity. Administer blood products or blood as ordered. Provide oxygen as ordered. If a cesarean delivery is to be performed, prepare the client for surgery. Maintain the client on bed rest. Accurately record I&O and insert indwelling urinary catheter as ordered. Have client lie on her side (left preferred) but not on her back.

## NURSING PROCESS

### ASSESSMENT

#### Subjective Data

The client may describe moderate to severe pain in the abdomen. Fetal movement may become hyperactive and then may cease.

#### Objective Data

Vaginal bleeding is assessed. External fetal monitor will show uteroplacental insufficiency, baseline changes, late decelerations, and reduced variability. The contraction pattern will change and the resting tone will increase. Vital signs show indications of shock.

**Nursing diagnoses for a client with abruptio placenta include the following:**

| NURSING DIAGNOSES | PLANNING/OUTCOMES | NURSING INTERVENTIONS |
|---|---|---|
| *Impaired **G**as Exchange, Fetal* related to altered uteroplacenta oxygen transfer due to placental separation | The fetus will have a normal baseline FHR, variability with no decelerations. | Observe external fetal monitor for decelerations, decreased baseline variability, and FHR. Provide oxygen to mother via mask. Have mother lie on left side. |
| ***A**nxiety* related to vaginal bleeding and possible fetal loss | The client will be able to verbalize feelings about bleeding and possible loss of pregnancy. | Explain pathophysiology of bleeding and status of fetus. Encourage client and family to talk about their feelings. Allow them some privacy to grieve. Contact minister, priest, or rabbi as requested by the client. |
| *Acute **P**ain* related to retroplacental bleeding and possibly contractions | The client will verbalize an understanding of the cause of the pain. | Provide simple explanation for cause of pain. Encourage and assist client to relax. Prepare for cesarean delivery. |
| *Deficient **F**luid Volume* related to blood loss | The client will regain fluid balance. | Monitor vital signs and assess for cold, clammy, cyanotic skin. Administer IV fluids as ordered and accurately record I&O. Evaluate client's state of consciousness. |

**Evaluation:** Evaluate each outcome to determine how it has been met by the client.

## DISSEMINATED INTRA-VASCULAR COAGULATION

Disseminated intravascular coagulation (DIC) is an overstimulation of the normal clotting process. Rapid, massive fibrin formation causes small thrombi to form throughout the circulatory system, depleting the clotting factors and platelets. Generalized bleeding may then occur, leading to anemia or ischemia to vital organs because of the clots in the blood vessels.

DIC occurs as a complication of a primary problem. It is not only a complication of obstetrical situations, but also of many medical–surgical situations such as neoplasms, blood transfusion reaction, traumas, and infections. Men can also experience DIC. Obstetrical problems that may precipitate DIC include abruptio placenta, placenta previa, hydatidiform mole, gestational hypertension, retained products of conception, amniotic fluid embolism, and infections.

## EFFECTS ON THE FETUS/NEONATE

The primary problem may require immediate delivery of the fetus, even if preterm. The fetus may experience hypoxia to varying degrees. Fetal death can occur.

## MEDICAL–SURGICAL MANAGEMENT

### Medical

Symptom onset is sudden. The client may have spontaneous bleeding from the gums, nose, or any orifice. The client may experience dyspnea or chest pain and become very restless and cyanotic with frothy, blood-tinged mucus. A catheter is anchored to monitor urinary output and to observe for hematuria. The mother may have tachycardia and diaphoresis.

The underlying cause must be identified and corrected. If the fetus is not yet born, delivery should be facilitated. Diagnostic tests are hemoglobin, hematocrit, fibrinogen level, fibrin split, or degradation products, platelet count, prothrombin time, and partial thromboplastin time. The laboratory tests reveal a prolonged PT and PTT, a decreased platelet count and fibrinogen level, and fibrin split products are present. Administer intravenous fluids to replace fluid loss from bleeding and to maintain an output of 30 mL/hr.

### Pharmacological

Intravenous administration of blood, fibrinogen, or cryoprecipitate is begun. Heparin given by continuous-infusion pump inhibits thrombin activity and thus prevents formation of microemboli. There is no effect on already existing clots. Oxygen therapy is often begun.

## NURSING MANAGEMENT

Closely monitor all clients with an obstetrical problem that may precipitate DIC for sudden onset of dyspnea or chest pain, restlessness, cyanosis, and spitting frothy blood-tinged mucus. Maintain a calm, positive manner. Administer IV fluids, blood, or other substance to help restore normal clotting. Give heparin as ordered. Provide oxygen as ordered. Place the client in a semi-Fowlers side-lying position to increase blood flow to the uterus. Continuously monitor vital signs, lung sounds, and fetus (if not yet delivered) with an electronic fetal monitor. Monitor urinary output for an output of a least 30 mL/hr.

# NURSING PROCESS

## ASSESSMENT

### Subjective Data

The client may describe dyspnea or chest pain.

### Objective Data

The client may be extremely restless or cyanotic and be expectorating blood-tinged frothy mucus. Bleeding gums, epistaxis (nose bleed), hematuria, petechiae under the blood pressure cuff around the client's arm, or bleeding from injection sites may also be present.

**Nursing diagnoses for a pregnant client with DIC include the following:**

| NURSING DIAGNOSES | PLANNING/OUTCOMES | NURSING INTERVENTIONS |
|---|---|---|
| **A**nxiety related to the sudden change in health status | The client will express understanding of what is happening to her and will feel less anxious. | Maintain a calm, positive manner. Explain to client what is happening, procedures, and treatment to be implemented. Remain with client. Allow client to express her anxiety. Answer client's questions. |
| *Impaired* **G**as Exchange related to reduced oxygen-carrying capacity and ischemia of lung tissue | The client will maintain adequate gas exchange to prevent tissue death. | Administer $O_2$ by mask. Place the client in a semi-Fowlers side-lying position. Administer IV fluids, blood, or other substance to help restore a normal clotting mechanism. Administer heparin and provide oxygen as ordered. Monitor lung sounds and respiratory rate. If fetus not yet delivered, monitor continuously with electronic fetal monitor. |

**Evaluation:** Evaluate each outcome to determine how it has been met by the client.

# GESTATIONAL HYPERTENSION

Gestational hypertension, also known as pregnancy-induced hypertension, is the most common hypertensive disorder in pregnancy that appears after 20 weeks' gestation. The classic symptoms are hypertension, edema, and proteinuria. It is seen most often in primigravidas, especially those younger than 20 or older than 35 years of age, who are in the lower socioeconomic group and have poor nutritional status. Diabetes, multiple pregnancy, or a family history of gestational hypertension also increase a client's risk.

Peripheral arteriole vasoconstriction and vasospasm lead to increased blood pressure and decreased perfusion of the uterus and placenta. Blood vessels are constricted and there is less circulating blood volume. Renal blood flow is decreased as well as the glomerular filtration rate. Wide spread vasospasm may cause capillary damage and leakage. If this occurs in the kidneys, proteinuria results. Cerebral edema causes headaches and visual disturbances. Deep tendon reflexes become hyperactive. The liver enlarges, putting pressure on the liver capsule, which causes epigastric pain. The condition may progress to **eclampsia**, or convulsions.

Despite decades of research, the cause remains unknown. It was previously called *toxemia* because it was thought that a toxin was produced in a pregnant woman's body. This term is no longer used. The only cure is delivery of the baby. Gestational hypertension may progress from mild to severe **preeclampsia** to eclampsia.

## EFFECTS ON THE FETUS/NEONATE

Abruptio placenta and placental infarction may occur. IUGR may occur as well as acute hypoxia and intrauterine death. A preterm infant may be born either because of spontaneous labor or obstetrical intervention.

### CRITICAL THINKING

**Noncompliance**

How would you counsel a client with severe gestational hypertension who tells you that she just cannot stay in bed and gets up when no one is around?

# MILD PREECLAMPSIA

In mild preeclampsia, the blood pressure is 140/90 mm Hg *or* increases 30 mm Hg systolic *or* 15 mm Hg diastolic over the client's baseline blood pressure on two occasions at least 6 hours apart. For example, a client with a baseline BP of 92/64 would be considered hypertensive at 122/80. Thus it is very important to have a baseline BP early in pregnancy.

Edema (1+) may be noted in the face and hands. It is objectively defined as weight gain of more than 1 pound per week.

Proteinuria shows as 1+ (300 mg/L) or 2+ (1 g/L) albumin on a dipstick in 24 hours. Proteinuria is usually the last of the three classic symptoms to appear.

# SEVERE PREECLAMPSIA

Blood pressure increases to 160/110 mm hg or higher on two occasions 6 hours apart in severe preeclampsia. Generalized edema is easily noted in the face, hands, sacral area, lower extremities, and abdomen. Weight gain may be more than 2 pounds/week.

Urinary albumin is 3+ or 4+ on dipstick. Urine output may drop to less than 500 mL/24 hours. Hematocrit, uric acid, and serum creatinine levels are elevated. The client may exhibit other symptoms such as continuous headache, blurred vision, scotomata (spots before the eyes), nausea, vomiting, irritability, hyperreflexia, cerebral disturbances, pulmonary edema, dyspnea, cyanosis, and epigastric pain. Epigastric pain indicates the condition is worsening and is often the last symptom identified before the client moves into eclampsia.

# ECLAMPSIA

The grand mal seizure experienced by the client has a tonic phase (pronounced muscular contractions) and a clonic phase (alternate contraction and relaxation of muscles). Then the client slips into a coma lasting from minutes to hours. With no treatment, the seizure/coma sequence may be repeated one or more times and death may follow.

Seizure activity may trigger uterine contractions, but the client in a coma is unaware of them and unable to let anyone know.

## CLIENT TEACHING
### Home Management of Mild Preeclampsia

- Bed rest is essential.
- Lie on either side but not on the back.
- Reduce anxiety.
- Take medications as prescribed.
- Eat a high-protein, moderate-sodium diet.
- Keep all prenatal appointments (may be two per week).
- Report immediately headache, visual disturbances, edema of face or hands, severe nausea and vomiting, and epigastric pain.

# HELLP SYNDROME

**HELLP syndrome** is a complication of preeclampsia/eclampsia that includes liver damage. The syndrome occurs in 20% of women with gestational hypertension (Ruddy & Kearney, 2000). It is characterized by hemolysis, elevated liver enzymes, and low platelet count (See Memory Trick: HELLP).

HELLP syndrome is a multisystem condition with widespread coagulation abnormalities characterized by weak vessel tone, vasospasm, and a coagulation defect. The exact pathophysiology of HELLP syndrome is unknown, but there seems to be an underlying activation of the coagulation cascade/mechanism (clot formation process). HELLP is a complication of gestational hypertension, but there is no common factor that causes HELLP except for the final group of symptoms that causes endothelial damage in small vessels and platelet activation within the vessels. RBCs are damaged and break as they pass through the damaged endothelium. With the activation of the platelets in the clotting mechanism, thromboxane A and serotonin are released, leading to vasospasm and platelet agglutination (clumping). Vasospasms, triggered from the clotting mechanism, force RBCs through the fibrin mesh formed by the clotting mechanism potentially causing the destruction of the RBCs (hemolysis). The RBC lyses produces a large drop in hematocrit (Padden, 1999).

Hemorrhaging occurs in the liver and the clotting mechanism stimulates the formation of microemboli in the vessels of the liver, causing ischemia. The damaged liver tissue causes the elevated liver enzymes (AST and ALT). Thrombocytopenia (low platelet count) of less than 100,000/mm³ results as the platelets are depleted attempting to control the hemorrhaging or by being trapped in the fibrin mesh (Padden, 1999).

Weak vessel tone leads to capillary leakage causing edema and pulmonary edema (Sibai & Stella, 2009).

The client presents with malaise, epigastric pain, nausea and vomiting, and headache usually in the third trimester. They also may have right upper quadrant tenderness, edema, hypertension, and proteinuria. With these last 4 symptoms, a

## MEMORY TRICK

**HELLP** is characterized by **h**emolysis, **e**levated liver enzymes, and **l**ow **p**latelet count:

**H** = Hemolysis – caused when intra-arterial lesions develop as a result of vasospasm, causing platelets to aggregate and a fibrin network to form. The RBCs are forced through the fibrin network and lysed, resulting in a large drop in hematocrit.

**E** = Elevated.

**L** = Liver enzymes – may be caused by microemboli in the vessels of the liver, causing ischemia.

**L** = Low.

**P** = Platelet count – results when the platelets are entrapped at the intra-arterial lesions.

complete blood count and liver functions are done to confirm the diagnosis of HELLP syndrome.

A low platelet count and a positive D-dimer test are the most reliable indicators to diagnose HELLP syndrome. If the platelet count drops below 40,000 per mm3, the client is prone to hemorrhaging. If the client has severe right upper quadrant pain, neck pain, or shoulder pain, the health care provider orders a liver scan to assess for a liver hematoma or liver rupture.

The main treatment is seizure prophylaxis, blood pressure control in clients with hypertension, and prompt delivery of the fetus. The administration of corticosteroids (dexamethasone [Decadron]) is controversial. Magnesium sulfate is given intravenously to prevent seizures and is titrated according to urine output and magnesium blood level. If magnesium toxicity occurs, calcium gluconate is given intravenously. A hypertensive crisis is treated with nitroprusside (Nipride). HELLP laboratory tests worsen after delivery but begin to return to normal by the third to fourth day postpartum.

## MEDICAL–SURGICAL MANAGEMENT

### Medical

The goals of treatment are to lower blood pressure, prevent convulsions, and deliver a healthy baby.

A client with mild preeclampsia may be allowed to stay home but is advised to stay in bed, lying on either side. This increases renal and placental blood flow. The client generally feels well, so education is very important to improve compliance with the plan of care.

Laboratory tests may include hematocrit, platelet count, electrolytes, liver function (AST and ALT), estriol level, 24-hour urine for protein and creatinine, and serum creatinine.

### Surgical

If the mother's condition continues to deteriorate or the environment within the uterus becomes harmful to fetal well-being, a cesarean birth may be necessary.

### Pharmacological

Magnesium sulfate ($MgSO_4$) is a central nervous system depressant that decreases the possibility of convulsions. It also relaxes smooth muscles and may decrease blood pressure to some degree. $MgSO_4$ is given intravenously. It is excreted by the kidneys and may reach a toxic level if the client has impaired renal function. Magnesium sulfate toxicity may lead to cardiac arrest. Common side effects are flushing, sweating, hypotension, bradycardia, respiratory depression, hypothermia, muscle weakness, constipation, nausea, and vomiting. An indwelling catheter is generally inserted to accurately measure output.

Calcium gluconate, the antidote for $MgSO_4$ must be kept in a syringe at the bedside ready to be given if signs of magnesium toxicity are noted. $MgSO_4$ is usually given for 24 to 48 hours after delivery to ensure that convulsions do not occur.

An antihypertensive drug may be given. Hydralazine (Apresoline) is the drug of choice except for clients with cardiac dysfunctions, who are given labetalol hydrochloride (Normodyne, Trandate).

A sedative such as phenobarbital or diazepam (Valium) may be given to help the client rest quietly.

### PROFESSIONALTIP

**Magnesium Sulfate Administration**

- Respirations must be at least 14 per minute.
- Deep tendon reflexes must be kept at normal response. The deep tendon reflex is obtained by giving a brisk tap with the blunt end of a reflex hammer to the patellar tendon just below the patella. The reflex response is a contraction of the quadriceps muscle and an extension of the lower leg. The reflex is graded as 0 - no response, 1+ - sluggish, 2+ - normal, 3+ - brisk, or 4+ - hyperreflexic.
- Urine output must be at least 30 mL/hr.
- Serum magnesium level must be monitored (therapeutic level 4.0 to 8.0 mEq/dL).

Oxytocin may be given to induce labor. It may be given along with magnesium sulfate.

### Diet

A well-balanced, high-protein, moderate-sodium diet is provided. Excessively salty foods are not eaten, but sodium restriction is no longer recommended. If the client is nauseated or there are signs of impending convulsions, the diet is withheld.

### Activity

The client is on bed rest, lying preferably on the left side but not on the back.

## NURSING MANAGEMENT

Frequently monitor vital signs and FHT. Assess for edema (hands and face), proteinuria, headache, blurred vision, irritability, hyperreflexia (deep tendon reflexes), dyspnea, cyanosis, nausea, and epigastric pain. Involve client and family in decisions when possible. Assist client and family to identify sources of support. Encourage the client to express feelings about her situation. Assess for toxicity when magnesium sulfate is administered. Keep environmental stimuli at a minimum.

## NURSING PROCESS

### ASSESSMENT

#### Subjective Data

Ask the client about headache, visual disturbances, epigastric pain, swelling of hands and face, nausea, and dyspnea.

#### Objective Data

Check vital signs and weight and compare to previous figures, and check urine for protein. Edema may be found in the face, hands, sacral area, lower extremities, or abdomen. Check laboratory reports of electrolytes, platelet count, liver enzymes, and hematocrit. Monitor I&O.

**Nursing diagnoses for a client with gestational hypertension include the following:**

| NURSING DIAGNOSES | PLANNING/OUTCOMES | NURSING INTERVENTIONS |
|---|---|---|
| Interrupted **F**amily Processes related to illness and bed rest or hospitalization of mother | The family will work together to maintain family functioning. | Involve client and family in decisions when possible. Encourage client and family to verbalize feelings about situation. Encourage family to visit client as client's condition allows. Assist family in discussions regarding how they will manage the household while the client is hospitalized or on bed rest at home. Help client and family identify sources of support. Refer to social service or local community resources as necessary. |
| Deficient **K**nowledge related to lack of information about gestational hypertension, its treatment, and implications for mother and baby | The client will verbalize an understanding of gestational hypertension, its treatment, and implications for herself and her baby. | Teach symptoms of gestational hypertension, importance of following care guidelines, and what to report to the health care provider. Explain the purpose and importance of each aspect of the plan of care. Encourage client to express feelings about her situation. |
| Deficient **F**luid Volume related to shift in fluids from intravascular to interstitial | The client will maintain intravascular fluid volume. | Assess BP and FHT every 1 to 4 hours. Weigh daily. Maintain client on bed rest, lying on side, especially the left side. Assess for edema. Accurately record I&O. Test urine for protein as ordered. Monitor laboratory test results. |

**Evaluation:** Evaluate each outcome to determine how it has been met by the client.

# CHRONIC MEDICAL PROBLEMS

Conditions in this section include diabetes mellitus, chronic hypertension, heart disease, and maternal phenylketonuria.

## ■ DIABETES MELLITUS

Diabetic clients who wish to become pregnant should have their diabetes well under control before conception. Gestational diabetes mellitus (GDM) is an abnormal glucose metabolism that appears only during pregnancy. Many women with GDM will have diabetes later in life. Whether the mother has chronic diabetes or GDM, the effects during pregnancy are the same.

## PREGNANCY AND CARBOHYDRATE METABOLISM

Insulin production is increased in early pregnancy because of the stimulation of the mother's pancreas by the increased levels of estrogen, progesterone, and other hormones. The tissue response to insulin is also increased along with increased storage of glycogen in the liver and muscles. An increased resistance to insulin develops in the last half of pregnancy because of hPL (an insulin antagonist), prolactin, and elevated levels of cortisol and placental enzymes called insulinases, which destroy insulin. This diabetogenic effect of pregnancy occurs after about 20 weeks' gestation. The result is a catabolic state after a meal is absorbed and also during the night. Fat, at this time, is more readily metabolized, and ketones may be found in the mother's urine. Glucose from the mother provides the growing fetus with energy, thus putting stress on the balance of glucose production and utilization. Diabetes already present is more difficult to control. In cases in which the pancreas has little insulin reserve, gestational diabetes occurs.

## EFFECTS OF PREGNANCY ON DIABETES

The insulin requirements change throughout pregnancy. The need for insulin may decrease during the first trimester. The risk of hypoglycemia or hyperinsulinemia is increased if nausea and vomiting are present. Placental maturation and the increasing production of hPL cause the insulin requirements to rise during the second trimester, and they may even be four times higher by the end of pregnancy. After the placenta is passed, removing the source of hPL, there is generally an immediate decrease in the amount of insulin required.

There is a physiological decrease in the renal threshold for glucose. The risk of ketoacidosis is greater during pregnancy, as is an acceleration of vascular disease.

## EFFECTS OF DIABETES ON PREGNANCY

Pregnancy in a diabetic client has a higher risk of complications than for a nondiabetic client. If vascular changes already exist, the chance for gestational hypertension is greater.

**Hydramnios**, an excessive amount of amniotic fluid, may occur. This may lead to preterm labor or premature rupture of the membranes.

Hyperglycemia can result in ketoacidosis caused by increased fat metabolism. Often, ketoacidosis develops slowly, but it can result in maternal and fetal death if untreated. Maternal complications are directly related to the degree of blood glucose control.

## EFFECTS ON THE FETUS/ NEONATE

**Macrosomia**, excessive fetal growth, results from maternal hyperglycemia. The hyperglycemia stimulates fetal insulin production to utilize the available glucose. After birth, there is no more maternal glucose, but the fetal pancreas continues to produce a high level of insulin. In 2 to 4 hours, the neonate is hypoglycemic. Fetal insulin production gradually decreases to an appropriate level.

IUGR may result when the mother has vascular changes, which also occur in the placenta. This decreases perfusion of the placenta, and the fetus does not receive adequate amounts of nutrients.

A high fetal insulin level inhibits the production of surfactant in the lungs, making the possibility of respiratory distress syndrome very high. The decreased ability of maternal glycosylated hemoglobin (hemoglobin with glucose attached) to release oxygen causes the fetus to have polycythemia (excessive number of red blood cells). Polycythemia is a direct cause of hyperbilirubinemia in the infant because the immature liver is unable to metabolize the increased amount of bilirubin.

Congenital anomalies are several times higher in diabetic pregnancies and may be caused by hyperglycemia in early pregnancy. Many anomalies involve the heart, central nervous system, and skeletal system.

## MEDICAL–SURGICAL MANAGEMENT

### Medical

The goals of care are to maintain **euglycemia** (normal blood glucose level) between 70 mg/dL and 105 mg/dL, and to have a healthy mother and baby. The client is usually followed by both her endocrinologist and obstetrician.

Clients are taught to monitor their blood glucose level and give themselves insulin according to a sliding scale. For clients with GDM, this may be very difficult because diabetes is new to them.

Fetal status is evaluated throughout the pregnancy. AFP screening is performed because diabetic pregnancies have an increased risk of fetal neural tube defects. Gestational age is established by ultrasound at about 18 weeks' gestation and repeated every 4 to 6 weeks to monitor fetal growth and assess for congenital abnormalities. The mother monitors fetal activity daily beginning about 28 weeks' gestation. An NST is scheduled weekly beginning also at about 28 weeks. A BPP may be performed at about 32 weeks and may be scheduled weekly. According to research, insulin lispo (Humalog) does not cross the placenta at low dose concentrations (Holcberg, Tsadkin-Tamir, Sapir, Wiznizer, Segal, Polacheck, & Ben Zvi, 2004). The American Diabetes Association (2009) also states insulin does not cross the placenta to the fetus (ADA, 2009).

Many clients with diabetes are hospitalized several times during the pregnancy. The timing of birth is based mainly on fetal well-being but should never be past 40 weeks' gestation. The L/S ratio and presence of PG in the amniotic fluid is usually checked about 38 weeks or earlier if indicated by fetal status.

### Surgical

If fetal well-being is deteriorating, a cesarean birth is often performed.

### Pharmacological

To monitor fetal well-being, humalin is generally used because it is unlikely to cause an allergic reaction. Insulin is given, most commonly, by multiple injections. This may be scheduled twice a day or four to six times per day after a blood glucose check. Some oral hypoglycemics should be discontinued, with the physician's knowledge, when the client plans to become pregnant, or immediately when she becomes pregnant, to prevent teratogenic effects on the fetus. Glyburide (Diabeta, Micronase) is an oral hypoglycemic that is often administered safely during pregnancy.

### Diet

Pregnant women increase their caloric intake about 300 kcal/day (35 to 40 kcal/Kg/day of ideal weight is recommended). Total kilocalories for the day are divided among three meals and three snacks. The bedtime snack, eaten as late as possible, has complex carbohydrates and protein to prevent hypoglycemia during the night. There should be no more than 10 hours between the bedtime snack and breakfast. A dietician assists the pregnant diabetic client with meal plans based on food preferences, lifestyle, and culture.

### Activity

Activity is maintained throughout pregnancy unless contraindicated by complications. Activity level is taken into account when the diet and insulin are prescribed.

## NURSING MANAGEMENT

Listen actively to the client. Answer questions and provide support. Teach glucose monitoring and insulin self-injection as needed. Monitor fetal status through results of AFP screening, ultrasound, NST, BPP, and amniocentesis. Emphasize the importance of keeping all scheduled prenatal visits and testing appointments.

# NURSING PROCESS

## ASSESSMENT

### Subjective Data

Ask questions regarding a family history of diabetes, congenital abnormalities, neonatal deaths, or unexplained stillbirths. At each prenatal visit, ask about diet, activity, and medication compliance. After 28 weeks, record maternal evaluation of fetal activity.

### Objective Data

Check blood sugar per fingerstick as ordered, and also measure vital signs and weight. Evaluate NST results and results of laboratory tests. Note signs of infection.

| Nursing diagnoses for a client with diabetes during pregnancy include the following: | | |
| --- | --- | --- |
| **NURSING DIAGNOSES** | **PLANNING/OUTCOMES** | **NURSING INTERVENTIONS** |
| *Deficient Knowledge* related to disease process of diabetes, control of diabetes, and implications for pregnancy | The client will verbalize an understanding of the disease process of diabetes, control of diabetes, and implications for the pregnancy. | Present to or review with the client the pathophysiology of diabetes and clarify client misconceptions. Teach how to monitor blood glucose level, the desired range, and importance of good control. Teach self-administration of insulin (if applicable) to client and significant other. Review effects of diabetes on client and fetus. Teach danger signs and whom to notify. Refer to diabetic support group in the community. Refer to dietitian for diet instructions. |
| *Risk for Injury, Fetus* related to decreased uteroplacental functioning | The client will verbalize an understanding of the various antepartal tests and what to expect during the procedures. | Teach client the possible effects of inadequate glucose control and uteroplacental functioning. Explain purpose of periodic ultrasound, fetal activity record, weekly NST, amniocentesis for L/S ratio and PG level, and biophysical profile. |
| *Noncompliance* related to need for close monitoring and extra prenatal visits | The client will perform blood glucose testing on schedule and attend all scheduled prenatal visits. | Review the importance of maintaining euglycemia. Assist client in making a chart on which to record results of blood glucose testing. Review importance of attending all scheduled prenatal visits. Schedule prenatal visits when most convenient for the client. |

**Evaluation:** Evaluate each outcome to determine how it has been met by the client.

## CHRONIC HYPERTENSION

Chronic hypertension is a BP of 140/90 mm Hg or higher before pregnancy or before the 20th week of gestation that lasts longer than 6 weeks after delivery. A diastolic pressure of more than 80 mm Hg in the second trimester may indicate chronic hypertension.

A client with untreated or poorly controlled hypertension may show signs of hypertensive vascular disease such as arteriosclerosis and retinal hemorrhage. Renal, disease may be present. The placenta may have infarcts, and placenta abruptio may occur.

### EFFECTS ON THE FETUS/ NEONATE

A placenta with infarcts has reduced perfusion. This may cause IUGR and fetal hypoxia.

## GESTATIONAL HYPERTENSION SUPERIMPOSED ON CHRONIC HYPERTENSION

Clients who have moderate-to-severe chronic hypertension are most at risk to develop gestational hypertension. In these women, gestational hypertension develops rapidly and moves to a crisis state faster than in women without chronic hypertension. More stillbirths, abruptio placenta, and severe renal failure are found in clients with chronic hypertension. These clients are hospitalized for medical management and nursing care.

### MEDICAL–SURGICAL MANAGEMENT

#### Medical

The goals of care are to prevent development of preeclampsia and to ensure a healthy fetus. Prenatal visits are generally scheduled every 2 weeks. An ultrasound is performed early to establish, or verify, the EDB. Around 22 and 32 weeks' gestation, an ultrasound checks for IUGR. If renal disease is suspected, creatinine clearance is determined early and repeated every 2 months.

## Pharmacological

Antihypertensive medication, such as methyldopa (Aldomet), nifedipine (Procardia), or labetalol (Trandate) is continued throughout the pregnancy. Dosage is adjusted according to maternal needs.

## Diet

A well-balanced diet providing 1.5 g/kg/day of protein is recommended. Salt intake should remain as it was before pregnancy.

## Activity

Daily rest periods, with the client preferably lying on her left side (never on the back), are important to maintain adequate perfusion to the placenta and relieve dependent edema.

## NURSING MANAGEMENT

Provide information about hypertension and how it may affect a pregnancy. Answer client's questions. Encourage client to plan rest periods (lying on the side) throughout the day. Emphasize the importance of keeping all scheduled prenatal visits and testing appointments.

## NURSING PROCESS
### ASSESSMENT
#### Subjective Data

Most clients have no symptoms of hypertension until it becomes severe. Then headaches or visual disturbances may occur.

#### Objective Data

Blood pressure will be 140/90 mm Hg or higher.

**Nursing diagnoses for a pregnant client with chronic hypertension include the following:**

| NURSING DIAGNOSES | PLANNING/OUTCOMES | NURSING INTERVENTIONS |
|---|---|---|
| *Risk for Injury, Fetus* related to placental infarcts and poor placental perfusion | The client will verbalize an understanding of possible placental changes leading to fetal injury and interventions to prevent this. | Teach client the possible placental changes related to hypertension. Assist client to plan for rest periods throughout the day. Administer antihypertensive medications as ordered. |
| *Deficient Knowledge* related to disease process and effects on pregnancy | The client will verbalize an understanding of the disease process and effects on pregnancy. | Provide the client with information about the disease process and how pregnancy may be affected. Allow opportunity for client to ask questions. |

**Evaluation:** Evaluate each outcome to determine how it has been met by the client.

## HEART DISEASE

The normal physiological increase in blood volume that peaks about 28 to 32 weeks' gestation, and the increased cardiac output and heart rate, may cause problems in the client with heart disease. The heart compensates at first by tachycardia, and ventricular dilation and hypertrophy. When these mechanisms fail, the heart is no longer able to compensate and congestive heart failure occurs.

The results of having had rheumatic fever often restrict cardiac output and cause pulmonary congestion. The effects of congenital heart disease on pregnancy depend on the specific defect. Hypertension may cause cardiac insufficiency.

## EFFECTS ON THE FETUS/NEONATE

IUGR and hypoxia may occur.

## MEDICAL–SURGICAL MANAGEMENT
### Medical

Many clients are cared for by both their cardiologist and obstetrician. Early diagnosis and ongoing management is assessed by the use of chest x-rays, auscultation of heart sounds, EKG, echocardiogram, and sometimes cardiac catheterization. Prenatal care appointments may be increased to two or three per week between 28 and 32 weeks' gestation, when blood volume is highest. Sometimes hospitalization is necessary.

### Pharmacological

Antibiotics are often used as a prophylaxis for all pregnant women with heart disease. Enoxaparin sodium (Lovenex) may be used if coagulation problems develop because enoxaparin sodium does not cross the placenta. Thiazide diuretics and furosemide (Lasix) may be used for congestive heart failure.

## Diet

The diet should be high in iron and protein but low in sodium. Adequate kilocalories for normal weight gain should be provided.

## Activity

Physical activity is restricted depending on the client's symptoms. Eight to 10 hours of sleep and frequent rest periods throughout the day are important. The side-lying position is best to prevent compression of the inferior vena cava.

## Nursing Management

Monitor vital signs, lung and heart sounds, and FHT. Emphasize the importance of keeping all scheduled prenatal visits and testing appointments. Encourage the client to eat a diet high in iron and protein, but low in sodium. Stress importance of side lying during daytime rest periods and during the night.

Assist client to identify a support system to help with household chores.

## NURSING PROCESS

### Assessment

#### Subjective Data

Ask about activity level, amount of rest, increasing fatigue with activity, dyspnea, palpitations, cough, and anxiety. Inquire about the availability of household help and her support system, to ascertain the client's ability to rest and relax.

#### Objective Data

These data include weight gain (fluid retention), edema, vital signs, signs of infection, anemia, heart murmurs, or crackles in the lungs.

| Nursing diagnoses for a pregnant client with heart disease include the following: | | |
|---|---|---|
| **NURSING DIAGNOSES** | **PLANNING/OUTCOMES** | **NURSING INTERVENTIONS** |
| *Impaired Gas Exchange* related to pulmonary edema | The client will maintain adequate gas exchange. | Monitor and accurately record I&O. Assess vital signs frequently. Administer medications as ordered. |
| *Activity Intolerance* related to generalized decreased perfusion | The client will be able to tolerate some activity. | Assess activity tolerance frequently. Promote activity level established by the physician. Discuss activity limitations and the need for sleep and rest periods. |
| *Fear* related to effects of maternal cardiac condition on fetal well-being | The client will express her fears about fetal well-being. | Provide information on how fetal well-being may be affected by maternal cardiac condition. Listen to the client express her fears about fetal well-being. |

**Evaluation:** Evaluate each outcome to determine how it has been met by the client.

## ■ MATERNAL PHENYLKETONURIA

Phenylketonuria (PKU) is an inborn error of metabolism in which there is a deficiency of the enzyme necessary to metabolize the amino acid phenylalanine. It is genetically inherited by a recessive gene. Accumulation of this amino acid and its metabolites leads to irreversible brain damage.

Since 1967, all newborns in the United States have had a screening blood test for PKU. The infants diagnosed with PKU were put on a phenylalanine-free diet. For years, it was thought that the child treated with a phenylalanine-free diet outgrew the problem by about age 9. Research has shown that dietary therapy throughout childhood and adolescence preserves intelligence. Some researchers recommend lifelong dietary therapy (Saal, Braddock, Bull, Enns, Gruen, Mendelsohn, & Saul, 2008). According to research, the best outcomes of pregnancy occur when the woman with PKU maintains a phenylalanine level between 2 and 6 mg/dL before conception, or at least by 8 weeks of gestation, and continuing throughout pregnancy (Koch, Azen, Friedman, et al, 2003).

### Effects on the Fetus/Neonate

A poorly regulated maternal phenylalanine level causes an increase in the incidence of IUGR, mental retardation, microcephaly, and heart defects.

### Medical–Surgical Management

#### Medical

The mother's blood phenylalanine level is checked every 2 to 4 weeks during the first half of pregnancy. It is checked every week in the last half of pregnancy.

Research indicates that the restricted intake of protein in the phenylalanine-free diet results in lower blood levels of iron and zinc (Acosta, 1996). Therefore, the iron and zinc blood levels are also checked every week in the last half of pregnancy. Low levels of iron may lead to anemia.

#### Diet

A very expensive modified protein supplement is used before and during pregnancy. Fruits, vegetables, fats, and some low-protein cereals make up the rest of the diet.

## NURSING MANAGEMENT

Encourage client to maintain a phenylalanine-free diet and to have her blood level checked throughout the pregnancy. Refer the client to dietary and genetic counseling.

# INFECTIONS

Any infection is a risk factor during pregnancy and should be diagnosed and treated promptly. Untreated infections may cause abortion, congenital anomalies, fetal infections, IUGR, preterm labor, mental retardation, or death.

## ■ TORCH GROUP

The TORCH group of congenital (passed from the mother to her fetus) infections include toxoplasmosis, rubella, cytomegalovirus, and herpesvirus type 2. The TORCH panel is a laboratory test used to screen for infections in the TORCH group (AACC, 2009).

## TOXOPLASMOSIS

Toxoplasmosis is caused by the protozoan *Toxoplasma gondii*. This disease goes almost unnoticed by adults because the symptoms are mild, vague, and flu-like. The organism may be ingested by eating undercooked, raw, or cured meat or by contact with contaminated soil or cat litter (Hokelek, 2009). Maternal toxoplasmosis before pregnancy seems to offer protection against fetal infection.

### EFFECTS ON THE FETUS/NEONATE

There is an increased incidence of abortion, preterm birth, stillbirth, and neonatal death if the mother contracts toxoplasmosis when she is pregnant. The time, within the pregnancy that a mother has the primary infection, determines the severity of symptoms in the fetus (Rorman, Zamir, Rilkis, Ben-David, 2006). Damage to the fetus is generally more severe if the disease is acquired before 20 weeks' gestation. The neonate may have microcephaly, hydrocephaly, and convulsions. Many infants die soon after birth. Those who survive may be blind, deaf, or severely retarded.

### MEDICAL–SURGICAL MANAGEMENT

#### Medical

The goals are to identify the pregnant client at risk and treat the disease promptly when diagnosed. The incubation period is 10 days. Tests that confirm the diagnosis of congenital toxoplasmosis is T cell proliferation and CD25 expression (Ciardelli, Meroni, Avanzini, Bollani, Tinelli, Garofoli, Gasparoni, & Stronati, 2008).

#### Pharmacological

The client is treated with sulfadiazine (Microsulfon) or pyrimethamine (Daraprim). Spiramycin (Rovamycine) may also be used to treat toxoplasmosis (Hokelek, 2009).

#### Diet

No raw or partially cooked meats are eaten. Fruits and vegetables are washed before they are eaten.

#### Activity

Gloves are worn when gardening because contact with soil is a significant risk factor. Travel outside the United States, Canada, and Europe is also a significant risk factor (Hokelek, 2009).

### NURSING MANAGEMENT

Encourage the client to eat only well-done meats, to wash all fruits and vegetables before eating them, and to wear gloves when gardening.

### CRITICAL THINKING

#### Toxoplasmosis

In Figure 2-13, the, pregnant woman is keeping the cat indoors and feeding it "canned" food. If the cat were an outside cat eating birds and rodents, it could acquire the parasite, *Toxoplasmia gondii*. The pregnant woman would be placing herself at risk for Toxoplasmosis and potentially causing harm to her unborn child. The cat is also kept off of any countertops where food is prepared. What other precautions should she take in caring for her cat?

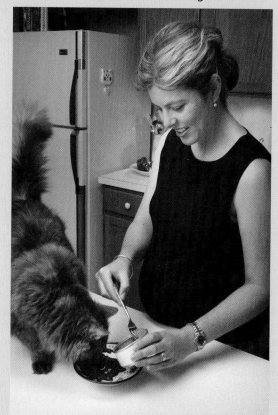

FIGURE 2-13  Preventing Toxoplasmosis (*Courtesy of the CDC/Photo by James Gathany.*)

# NURSING PROCESS

## ASSESSMENT

### Subjective Data

The client may have no symptoms or may have malaise and/or myalgia.

### Objective Data

A rash may be evident as well as splenomegaly and enlarged cervical lymph nodes.

**Nursing diagnoses for a pregnant client with toxoplasmosis include the following:**

| NURSING DIAGNOSES | PLANNING/OUTCOMES | NURSING INTERVENTIONS |
| --- | --- | --- |
| *Deficient Knowledge* related to lack of knowledge about toxoplasmosis disease process | The client will verbalize an understanding of toxoplasmosis disease process. | Provide information about toxoplasmosis, incubation period, how acquired, and ways to prevent it. Allow time for client to ask questions and clarify misconceptions. |
| *Anticipatory Grieving* related to effects of toxoplasmosis on fetus/neonate | The client will express feelings about possible effects on fetus/neonate. | Encourage client to discuss feelings about possible effects of toxoplasmosis on her fetus. Provide a private place for client and family to discuss the situation. |

**Evaluation:** Evaluate each outcome to determine how it has been met by the client.

# RUBELLA

Rubella, German measles, and 3-day measles are all names for the same disease. After an incubation period of 14 to 21 days, a maculopapular rash appears and then vanishes in 3 days. Rubella is highly contagious and is spread by airborne droplets.

## EFFECTS ON THE FETUS/NEONATE

The earlier in pregnancy the infection occurs, the more severe the fetal effects. Congenital rubella syndrome occurs in many of the infections that occur before 8 weeks' gestation. It is characterized by cataracts, deafness, and patent ductus arteriosus. The infant may also have IUGR, mental retardation, and hyperbilirubinemia. Sometimes a petechial rash may be seen. These infants are infectious and may shed the virus for months.

## MEDICAL–SURGICAL MANAGEMENT

### Medical

Prevention is the best cure. The prenatal laboratory screening includes the hemagglutination inhibition. A titer of 1:16 or greater signifies immunity, while a titer of less than 1:8 signifies a susceptibility to rubella. The client who is susceptible should avoid exposure to rubella while pregnant.

A pregnant woman who becomes infected with rubella during the first trimester has a 90% chance of fetal infection with the accompanying anomalies (Schweon, 2001).

### Pharmacological

All children should be immunized with the live attenuated vaccine by age 1. Susceptible pregnant women should be immunized very soon after delivery, and they should avoid becoming pregnant at least for 1 month after immunization to avoid the chance of infecting a fetus.

## NURSING MANAGEMENT

Identify clients who are susceptible to rubella and provide information about avoiding exposure while pregnant. Encourage susceptible clients to receive the immunization very soon after delivery and then delay another pregnancy at least for 1 month. Encourage parents to have infants receive all immunizations as scheduled.

RhoGAM may prevent the effectiveness of the measles, mumps, and Rubella vaccine (MMR) if the two medications are administered at the same time. Therefore, the client returns to the health care providers' office in 2 months for a blood test to check for immunity against rubella. The MMR vaccine administration is repeated if the client has no immunity to rubella (Hamilton Health Sciences, 2008).

# NURSING PROCESS

## ASSESSMENT

### Subjective Data

There may be no symptoms or the client may describe muscle aches and joint pain.

### Objective Data

Temperature may be slightly elevated, and a maculopapular rash and lymphadenopathy may be present.

**Nursing diagnoses for a pregnant client with rubella include the following:**

| NURSING DIAGNOSES | PLANNING/OUTCOMES | NURSING INTERVENTIONS |
|---|---|---|
| *Ineffective Health Maintenance* related to lack of knowledge about her need for rubella immunization before becoming pregnant | The client will receive rubella vaccine soon after delivery. | Provide information about the implications of rubella when the hemagglutination inhibition results are known. Provide information about rubella immunization. Answer client questions and clarify any misunderstandings. |
| *Interrupted Family Processes* related to the probability of fetal anomalies caused by maternal rubella | The client and family will verbalize understanding of the probability of fetal anomalies. | Discuss with client and family the probability and types of fetal anomalies that generally occur with maternal rubella. Provide a private place for client and family to discuss the situation. Answer questions and clarify misconceptions. |

**Evaluation:** Evaluate each outcome to determine how it has been met by the client.

# CYTOMEGALOVIRUS

Cytomegalovirus (CMV) is a member of the herpesvirus group. More than half of all adults have antibodies for CMV, which is found in saliva, breast milk, cervical mucus, urine, and semen. It spreads by close contact. It is asymptomatic in adults and children but can affect the fetus in utero or during delivery.

## EFFECTS ON THE FETUS/NEONATE

The fetus may have extensive damage leading to fetal death; however, the fetus may survive with hydrocephaly, microcephaly, mental retardation, cerebral palsy, or with no noticeable damage. An infected newborn is usually small for gestational age (SGA). Mental retardation, auditory deficits, or learning disabilities may not be immediately apparent.

## MEDICAL–SURGICAL MANAGEMENT

### Medical

Diagnosis is made when CMV is found in the maternal urine and an elevated IgM level with CMV antibodies identified in the blood. There is no treatment for the mother or neonate.

# HERPES GENITALIS (HERPES SIMPLEX VIRUS TYPE 2)

Genital herpes is one of the three most common sexually transmitted infections with approximately 22% of pregnant women having HSV-2 (Perozzi, Zalice, Howard, Skariot, 2007). Herpes simplex virus type 2 (HSV-2) causes painful, vesicular genital lesions. The lesions appear within a few hours to 20 days after exposure. The primary episode is the most severe. Women who have their first infection close to the time of delivery have a greater chance of transmitting the infection to the neonate during a vaginal birth. After the membranes rupture, the virus ascends from active lesions to the fetus, or the fetus comes in contact with the lesions during a vaginal delivery. HSV-2 is not found in breast milk, so the mother may breast-feed.

## EFFECTS ON THE FETUS/NEONATE

When there is an active HSV-2 infection in the first trimester, about one-half will end in spontaneous abortion or stillbirth. Most infected infants have no symptoms at birth. Symptoms of poor feeding, jaundice, and seizures develop after a 2- to 12-day incubation period. Many of these infants will also have the vesicular lesions.

## MEDICAL–SURGICAL MANAGEMENT

### Medical

Diagnosis is made by culturing active lesions. Treatment is mainly to relieve pain. When no lesions are visible at the time of delivery, a vaginal birth is acceptable. Pregnancy is one of many causes of recurrence. There is no known cure.

### Surgical

When active lesions are visible at the time of delivery, a cesarean birth is best to prevent fetal contact with the lesions (virus).

### Pharmacological

Antiviral therapy for HSV-2 is acyclovir (Zovirax), famciclovir (Famvir), and valacyclovir hydrochloride (Valtrex). The use of acyclovir has been studied in pregnant women and does not increase birth defects or harm the neonate (Brown, Gardella, Wald, Morrow, & Corey, 2005). The use of acyclovir in the third trimester has decreased symptoms and viral shedding, thus decreasing the need for cesarean births (Watts, Brown, Money, Selke, Huang, Sacks, et al., 2003). Burow's solution may relieve discomfort.

## NURSING MANAGEMENT

Inquire whether client has ever had a herpes infection. Provide information regarding possible effect on the fetus/neonate, preventing spread of infection, and how to care for active lesions.

# NURSING PROCESS

## ASSESSMENT

### Subjective Data

Ask whether the client or her partner have ever had a herpes infection. Client may describe pain and discomfort from the lesions if she has a herpes infection.

### Objective Data

Lesions may be seen when infection is active. A cervical culture may indicate presence or absence of the virus.

**Nursing diagnoses for the pregnant client with HSV-2 infection include the following:**

| NURSING DIAGNOSES | PLANNING/OUTCOMES | NURSING INTERVENTIONS |
|---|---|---|
| *Acute Pain* related to local, open vulvar lesions | The client will describe a decrease in pain after treatment is begun. | Administer medications as ordered. Suggest a sitz bath several times a day followed by air-drying of the vulva and wearing cotton underwear. |
| *Ineffective Sexuality Patterns* related to unwillingness to engage in sexual intercourse | The client will maintain sexuality patterns. | Provide client with information about disease process, and the method of transmission. Refer client to community resources. Encourage client to engage in forms of sexual expression that do not involve genital contact. |
| *Ineffective Coping* related to depression about risk to fetus if herpes lesions are present at birth | The client will verbalize an understanding about how decision is made regarding the type of delivery when herpes lesions are present. | Provide client with information about the factors relative to type of delivery performed. Encourage client to have appropriate cultures run as recommended by her health care provider. Encourage client to report any changes that may indicate a recurrence of lesions. |

**Evaluation:** Evaluate each outcome to determine how it has been met by the client.

## ■ HIV/AIDS

Weight gain or even maintenance of weight during pregnancy is a challenge for an HIV-infected client. Counseling is provided regarding optimum nutrition, exercise, rest, and sleep.

Pregnancy is considered to be a somewhat immunosuppressive state and may theoretically speed up the process of going from being HIV positive to an AIDS diagnosis.

## EFFECTS ON THE FETUS/NEONATE

HIV may be transmitted to the fetus through the placenta, at the time of birth when exposed to maternal blood and vaginal secretions, or through breast milk. Infants often have a positive antibody titer for as long as 15 months after birth because of the transfer of maternal antibodies. Those infants who are not infected with HIV will seroconvert to a negative antibody titer.

## MEDICAL–SURGICAL MANAGEMENT

### Medical

There is no cure for HIV or AIDS. Routine prenatal testing includes a CD 4 lymphocyte count and serologic testing for changes indicating that AIDS is progressing. NST and ultrasound are performed at 32 weeks' gestation. NST is continued weekly, and ultrasound is performed every few weeks to monitor for fetal status.

### Diet

Nutritional counseling and support regarding food handling, food preparation, and diet choices is often necessary.

## NURSING MANAGEMENT

Follow Standard Precautions at all times. Discuss how HIV/AIDS affects the pregnancy. Encourage an adequate food intake for fetal development. Emphasize the importance of attending all scheduled prenatal visits and testing appointments.

# NURSING PROCESS

## ASSESSMENT

### Subjective Data

The client may be asymptomatic or may describe having fatigue, malaise, loss of appetite, or diarrhea.

### Objective Data

Signs of anemia, cell-mediated immunodeficiency, progressive weight loss, lymphadenopathy, and neurologic dysfunction may be present. Purplish lesions may also be noted during assessment.

**Nursing diagnoses for a pregnant client who has HIV/AIDS include the following:**

| NURSING DIAGNOSES | PLANNING/OUTCOMES | NURSING INTERVENTIONS |
|---|---|---|
| *Risk for Infection* related to altered immune status | The client will not develop infections during pregnancy. | Use Standard Precautions at all times. Monitor client for signs of infection (fever, cough, sore throat). Teach client to report changes that may indicate infection. Teach client to avoid large crowds or known cases of infectious diseases. |
| *Fear* related to outcome of pregnancy and disease | The client will verbalize fears about her pregnancy and HIV/AIDS. | Discuss HIV/AIDS disease process and how it can affect pregnancy and fetus. Provide opportunities for client to ask questions and clarify misconceptions. Assess client's support system and refer to community resources. |
| *Imbalanced Nutrition: Less Than Body Requirements* related to lack of appetite | The client will maintain weight or gain weight. | Monitor client's weight. Obtain 24-hour diet recall from client. Provide information about nutritional needs. Assist client in planning a high-protein, high-calorie diet. |

**Evaluation:** Evaluate each outcome to determine how it has been met by the client.

# OTHER INFECTIONS

Maternal infections may result in spontaneous abortion, a preterm infant, or an infected infant. Table 2-4 provides a summary of other infections affecting pregnancy.

# HEMOLYTIC DISEASES

There are two types of hemolytic diseases: Rh incompatibility and ABO incompatibility. Rh incompatibility can be devastating to the fetus, but it can be prevented. ABO incompatibility is naturally occurring and much less severe, but it cannot be prevented.

# RH INCOMPATIBILITY

Rh incompatibility can happen only when the mother is Rh negative and the fetus is Rh positive. That is, the mother does not have the Rh factor and the fetus does have the Rh factor. In this case, the father is Rh positive for the fetus to be Rh positive. If the father is Rh negative, there is no problem because the fetus will also be Rh negative.

The placenta keeps the mother's blood and the fetus's blood separated. In cases of ectopic pregnancy, abortion, infection of the placenta, abruptio placenta, birth, or at the time of placental separation, small tears occur in the placenta and fetal blood enters maternal circulation. The mother is then sensitized by the fetal Rh-positive blood. She also is sensitized by having a transfusion of Rh-positive blood, even the smallest amount.

Fetal (Rh-positive) blood in maternal (Rh-negative) circulation stimulates maternal production of Rh antibodies. The Rh antibodies, like many other antibodies, pass through the placenta and destroy fetal RBCs (Figure 2-14). Because this usually occurs at the time of birth, the first infant is usually not affected.

## EFFECTS ON THE FETUS/NEONATE

If a placental tear occurred and there was no treatment, the next Rh-positive fetus will have red blood cells destroyed by the maternal Rh antibodies. This causes anemia, which in turn causes fetal edema (hydrops fetalis).

The next step is congestive heart failure and severe jaundice, which can cause neurologic damage called **kernicterus**. This entire syndrome, the most severe of the two hemolytic diseases of the newborn, is called erythroblastosis fetalis.

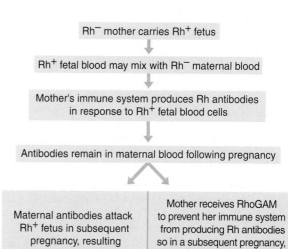

FIGURE 2-14 **Rh Sensitization and Prevention**

COURTESY OF DELMAR CENGAGE LEARNING

**TABLE 2-4  Selected Infections and Pregnancy**

| INFECTION | TREATMENT | MATERNAL EFFECTS | FETAL EFFECTS |
|---|---|---|---|
| **Sexually Transmitted** | | | |
| Syphilis | penicillin G benzathin (Bicillin L-A) or doxycycline (Vibramycin) Sexual partner should also be treated | Chancre, slight fever, malaise Progresses through secondary and tertiary stages if untreated | Spontaneous abortion, stillbirth, congenital syphilis, sniffling, peeling of soles and palms |
| Gonorrhea | ceftriaxone (Rocephin) plus erythromycin (Erythrocin Lactobionate) Partners must be treated | Often no symptoms; may have purulent vaginal discharge, dysuria, or urinary frequency | Ophthalmia neonatorum |
| Chlamydia | erthromycin ethyl succinate (ABO-Erythro-ES) | Often no symptoms; may have purulent or thin vaginal discharge, burning on urination, preterm labor | Conjunctivitis, chlamydial pneumonia, fetal death |
| Condylomata acuminata (venereal warts) | Cryosurgery, laser surgery, electrocautery, or trichloroacetic acid | Soft, grayish, raised lesions | Laryngeal papillomatosis if infection is present at birth |
| Hepatitis B (HBV) | Supportive; vaccine available | Often no symptoms | Most become carriers |
| **Vaginal Infections** | | | |
| Monilia | miconazole (Monistat), clotrimazole (Gyne-Lotrimin) | Thick, white, cheesy discharge Itching, dysuria | Thrush |
| Trichomoniasis | clotrimazole (Gyne-Lotrimin) in early pregnancy, metronidazole (Flagyl) | Foamy, green-gray discharge, prutitus | |
| **Urinary Tract Infection** | | | |
| Cystitis | Oral sulfonamides in early pregnancy, nitrofurantoin (Furadantin) in late pregnancy | Dysuria, urgency, low-grade fever; if not treated, may result in acute pyelonephritis | Hyperbilirubinemia if sulfonamides taken in last few weeks of pregnancy |

## MEDICAL–SURGICAL MANAGEMENT

### Medical

One of the screening tests performed at the first prenatal visit determines the mother's Rh factor. When the mother is found to be Rh negative and the father is Rh positive or unknown, additional tests are run. An indirect Coombs' test detects Rh antibodies in maternal serum. The Rh antibody titer monitors what is happening when an Rh-negative woman is carrying an Rh-positive fetus. A rising titer indicates the need for immediate intervention.

Ultrasound is performed at about 15 weeks to determine gestational age. It is repeated several times throughout the pregnancy to measure fetal growth, assess fetal heart size, and check for hydramnios.

Amniocentesis may also be performed several times to determine the bilirubin (product of RBC breakdown) level and lung maturity. A fetal intrauterine blood transfusion may be indicated to maintain the fetus in the uterus until the lungs are more mature. The fetus is given Rh-negative erythrocytes to replace those destroyed by the Rh-positive antibodies. The erythrocytes are put into the peritoneal cavity, where they are absorbed. Rh-positive antibodies will not harm the Rh-negative blood given to the fetus.

### Pharmacological

RhoGAM is given to an Rh-negative mother who is not sensitized (has a negative indirect Coombs' and antibody titer) and whose Rh-positive infant has no antibodies on the infant's RBCs (negative direct Coombs'). RhoGAM must be administered within 72 hours of the infant's birth. It prevents the mother's body from making the Rh antibodies by providing temporary passive immunity.

It is recommended that RhoGAM be given at 28 weeks' gestation and after the delivery. RhoGAM is also given to an Rh-negative woman after an abortion (spontaneous or induced), an ectopic pregnancy, and amniocentesis. It is never given to an Rh-positive woman.

## NURSING MANAGEMENT

Ensure that the client's Rh factor is known. If the client is Rh-negative and the father is Rh-positive or unknown, ensure that the client keeps all appointments to have her Rh antibody titer checked. At 28 weeks' gestation and after the delivery, administer RhoGAM as ordered.

## TABLE 2-5 Possible Combinations for ABO Incompatibility

| MOTHER | FETUS |
| --- | --- |
| A | B |
| B | A |
| O | A, B, AB |

# ABO INCOMPATIBILITY

In ABO incompatibility, the way in which a tear in the placenta may occur and fetal and maternal blood mix is the same as for Rh incompatibility. In this situation, the problem occurs when maternal blood enters fetal circulation. Possible combinations for ABO incompatibility are given in Table 2-5. The most common type of ABO incompatibility occurs when the mother is type O and the fetus is either type A, B, or AB. The mother's plasma naturally contains anti-A and anti-B antibodies. These antibodies have a weaker hemolytic effect than Rh antibodies, and they only affect mature RBCs. The number of antibodies is limited to the amount of maternal blood that entered fetal circulation. There is not a continuous supply of antibodies. Because ABO incompatibility is naturally occurring, it may affect the fetus of the first pregnancy. The affected newborn will have a positive direct Coombs' and will become jaundiced in the first 3 days of life.

## NURSING MANAGEMENT

Ensure that the client's blood type is known. Observe the newborn for jaundice within the first 3 days of life.

# MULTIPLE PREGNANCY

The twin birth rate has increased 42% since 1990 (CDC, 2007). Women having children after 30 years of age have a higher risk of delivering multiples than younger women. The use of fertility stimulating drugs and assisted reproductive technology (infertility treatment) has increased a woman's chance of carrying multiple fetuses.

A multiple pregnancy is suspected when the fundal height is greater than expected for the weeks of gestation. An ultrasound will verify two or more fetuses. Two or more heartbeats that differ by 10 bpm may be heard. The alpha fetoprotein level may be elevated. The first trimester proceeds much the same as with a single fetus except that maternal blood volume has a greater increase. Some women have more severe nausea and vomiting as well as shortness of breath on exertion, dyspnea, and backache.

As the uterus grows, there is greater pressure on and displacement of the internal organs. Pressure on the ureters causes urinary stasis and possible infection. Digestive problems and constipation is more disturbing, dependent edema more marked, and varicose veins more prominent. Gestational hypertension is more frequent than with a single fetus.

## EFFECTS ON THE FETUS/ NEONATE

Each fetus may have a decreased intrauterine growth rate (low birthweight). There is a greater risk of fetal anomalies, abnormal presentations, and preterm birth. Perinatal mortality is much greater for twins than for a single fetus.

## MEDICAL–SURGICAL MANAGEMENT

### Medical

The goals are to promote normal fetal development for all fetuses and to prevent delivery of preterm infants. Prenatal visits are more frequent, and serial ultrasounds assess the growth of each fetus. NST and BPP testing usually begin about 30 weeks' gestation and are repeated as indicated by fetal condition.

### Surgical

The method of birth may not be determined until the mother is in labor. Depending on complications that may occur, a cesarean birth may be required.

### Pharmacological

A prenatal vitamin/mineral preparation is doubly important with a multiple pregnancy. An extra calcium supplement and folic acid is required.

### Diet

A well-balanced diet of 4,000 kcal with 135 g of protein is recommended. A weight gain of 40 to 50 pounds is acceptable, with 15 to 20 pounds being gained by 20 weeks' gestation.

### Activity

Frequent rest periods are planned during the day. Resting in the side-lying position increases uteroplacental blood flow. The legs and feet are elevated to reduce edema. Good posture is maintained and good body mechanics used when lifting or moving objects.

## NURSING MANAGEMENT

Actively listen to the client. Provide anticipatory guidance regarding the discomforts of pregnancy because they may be more intense with a multiple pregnancy. Encourage keeping scheduled prenatal visits and testing appointments. Emphasize the importance of taking the prescribed prenatal vitamin/mineral supplements and eating a well-balanced, high-protein diet. Assist the client to plan for rest periods in the side-lying position.

# SUBSTANCE ABUSE

Drugs commonly abused include tobacco, alcohol, cocaine, crack, marijuana, methamphetamine, and heroin. The use of any of these substances is a threat to pregnancy. Substance abusers may not seek prenatal care, or they seek prenatal care very late in pregnancy. Most substance abusers do not voluntarily admit their addiction. These mothers may have an increased rate of gestational hypertension, abruptio placenta, poor nutrition, and sexually transmitted infections. They often use available money for the drug habit instead of food.

## EFFECTS ON THE FETUS/NEONATE

Maternal smoking causes placenta previa, abruption placenta, premature rupture of membranes, premature birth, intrauterine growth restriction, and sudden death syndrome (Andres & Day, 2000).

Alcohol may result in fetal alcohol syndrome, which manifests as both physical and mental abnormalities. Cocaine/crack increases the risk for IUGR, short body length, small head circumference, preterm birth, irritability, and low Apgar scores (an assessment of infant at 1 and 5 minutes after birth). Marijuana causes fine tremors and irritability. Methamphetamine causes low birth weight, microencephaly, premature birth, and heart defects (March of Dimes, 2009). Heroin increases the risk for IUGR, hypoxia, preterm birth, irritability, and meconium aspiration. Irritability and poor consolability may interfere with maternal–infant bonding and attachment and increase the risk of infant abuse and neglect.

## MEDICAL–SURGICAL MANAGEMENT

### Medical

When a client is known or discovered to be a substance abuser, a multidisciplinary approach is best to manage the medical, legal, and socioeconomic considerations, and provide a safe labor and delivery. The client may require hospitalization for detoxification. "Cold turkey" withdrawal is not recommended during pregnancy because of possible fetal risks. Urine and blood screening is performed regularly.

## NURSING MANAGEMENT

Maintain a calm, nonjudgmental manner. Actively listen to the client. Provide information and care as needed. Know the

---

### CRITICAL THINKING

**Substance Abuse**

How would you handle the situation if you knew a client was a substance abuser, but she would not tell anyone at the prenatal clinic?

---

state laws regarding prenatal drug use, as some states require a referral to child protective services.

## NURSING PROCESS

### ASSESSMENT

### Subjective Data

Ask questions about the use of caffeine, tobacco, and over-the-counter drugs, and then about alcohol use and drug use. The client may have altered perceptions, so validation through other sources, if possible, is desirable.

### Objective Data

Assess for irritability, psychomotor problems, poor nutrition, and possible infections.

---

**Nursing diagnoses for a pregnant client who is a substance abuser include the following:**

| NURSING DIAGNOSES | PLANNING/OUTCOMES | NURSING INTERVENTIONS |
|---|---|---|
| *Imbalanced Nutrition: Less than Body Requirements* related to inadequate intake of food | The client will gain appropriate weight during pregnancy. | Refer client to WIC (women, infant, and children) nutrition program. Monitor weight gain. Collect 24-hour diet recall from client. Explain the rationale for a nutritious diet, listing foods the client could eat for her health and the fetus. Assist the client to plan meals. |
| *Deficient Knowledge* related to not understanding how substance abuse affects the fetus | The client will verbalize how substance abuse can affect the fetus. | Explain how substance abuse affects the fetus. Provide written materials regarding effects of the client's drug of choice on the fetal development. Allow time for client questions and for clarification of misconceptions. |
| *Risk for Infection* related to use of dirty needles and syringes | The client will not have an infection from dirty needles and syringes. | Explain how client may pick up an infection from dirty needles and syringes. Refer client to community resources where clean syringes and needles are available. Refer client to drug counseling program. |

**Evaluation:** Evaluate each outcome to determine how it has been met by the client.

# PRETERM LABOR

Preterm labor is labor that begins after viability but before 37 weeks' gestation. The causes of preterm labor may be maternal, fetal, or placental. Maternal factors that may cause preterm labor include gestational hypertension, diabetes, heart or renal disease, an incompetent cervix, premature rupture of membranes, and maternal infection. Fetal factors include fetal infection, multiple pregnancy, and hydramnios. Placental factors are placenta previa and abruptio placenta.

## EFFECTS ON THE FETUS/NEONATE

Preterm labor may produce a neonate who is not able to cope well with extrauterine life.

## MEDICAL–SURGICAL MANAGEMENT

### Medical

Preterm labor is confirmed by documented uterine contractions, ruptured membranes, and cervical dilation and effacement. No attempt is made to stop labor if any of the following conditions exist: the cervix dilated 4 cm or more, severe gestational hypertension, prolonged rupture of membranes, hemorrhage, abruptio placenta, fetal complications, or fetal death.

### Pharmacological

The process of stopping labor with medications is called **tocolysis**. The drugs used in an attempt to stop preterm labor are called *tocolytics*. Tocolytics include beta-adrenergic agonists, magnesium sulfate, calcium-channel blockers, and prostaglandin inhibitors.

Ritodrine hydrochloride (Yutopar) is a beta-adrenergic agonist that inhibits contractility of the uterus. Maternal pulse, BP, lung sounds, and FHR must be closely monitored.

Terbutaline sulfate (Brethine) is also a beta-adrenergic agonist that relaxes the uterine muscle. It is used frequently, although the Food and Drug Administration has not approved it for tocolysis.

Magnesium sulfate ($MgSO_4$) has fewer side effects than the beta-adrenergic agonists and is being used more in preterm labor. A loading dose is given and then continued at the lowest rate necessary to maintain a noncontracting uterus.

## PROFESSIONAL TIP

### Progesterone

Progesterone may not delay preterm birth by decreasing uterine contractility but may reduce preterm birth by preventing the softening of the cervix (Bernstein, 2008).

Tocolysis is usually maintained with a maternal serum level of 5 to 8 mg/dL.

Nifedipine (Procardia) and nicardipine hydrochloride (Cardene), calcium channel blockers, are used to delay delivery. Indomethacin (Indocin), sulindac (Clinoril), and ketorolac tromethamine (Toradol), prostaglandin inhibitors, also delay delivery.

A research study by Murphy and MACS Collaborative Group (2007) recommended that women who are at risk for preterm delivery be given a single injection of corticosteroids to enhance fetal lung maturity. Weekly injections gave no better results.

## NURSING MANAGEMENT

Explain all treatments and procedures and keep the client informed of responses to them. Allow client time to ask questions. Monitor vital signs, FHT, and contractions. Administer medications as ordered.

# NURSING PROCESS

## ASSESSMENT

### Subjective Data

Client may describe having contractions or that "my water broke." The client expresses concern about what is happening.

### Objective Data

Contractions may be documented, cervix dilating and effacing, or membranes ruptured. The client may experience tension, restlessness, or vital sign changes.

### Nursing diagnoses for a client in preterm labor include the following:

| NURSING DIAGNOSES | PLANNING/OUTCOMES | NURSING INTERVENTIONS |
|---|---|---|
| *Anxiety* related to perception of what is happening and not having time to prepare for labor | The client will express less anxiety about being in preterm labor. | Explain what is happening to client and all tests and procedures before beginning them. Spend time with client so she can express her anxieties and ask questions. Keep client informed about how the preterm labor is responding to treatment. |
| *Deficient Knowledge* related to lack of information about preterm labor causes, determination, and treatment | The client will verbalize an understanding about preterm labor and treatments. | Explain what preterm labor is, possible/probable causes, and treatment. Allow client time to ask questions. Clarify any misunderstandings. |

*(Continues)*

| Nursing diagnoses for a client in preterm labor include the following: (Continued) | | |
|---|---|---|
| **NURSING DIAGNOSES** | **PLANNING/OUTCOMES** | **NURSING INTERVENTIONS** |
| *Fear* related to risk for fetus | The client will express her fears for fetal welfare. | Encourage client to express fears related to fetal well-being. Keep client informed about fetal status. Encourage family to spend time with client. |

**Evaluation:** Evaluate each outcome to determine how it has been met by the client.

## CASE STUDY

**Part A:** M.J., age 32, is G 3, P 2, T 1, P 1, A 0, L 2. The children are ages 1-1/2, and 3. B.J., her husband, works 8 to 5. She is 32 weeks' gestation. Her BP has been 104/68 mm Hg at her prenatal visits. Today, her BP is 136/84. She has gained 6-1/2 pounds in the 4 weeks since her last visit. There is edema in both feet.

**Part B:** Two weeks later, M.J.'s BP is 140/90 mm Hg, and she has gained 4 more pounds. She states that she had to take her rings off because they were too tight. The physician admits her to the hospital with orders for bed rest in side-lying position, $MgSO_4$ IV drip, and a high-protein diet.

**Part C:** The electronic fetal monitor shows a sustained increase in the baseline FHR. M.J.'s deep tendon reflexes are very reactive.

The following questions will guide your development of a nursing care plan for the case study:

**Part A:**
1. What other assessments should be made?
2. What advice would you anticipate the physician giving M.J.?
3. How can you assist M.J. to implement the physician's advice?

**Part B:**
4. What are the goals for M.J.'s care?
5. What nursing assessments must now be obtained?
6. What diagnostic tests might be ordered?

**Part C:**
7. Identify three nursing diagnoses and goals for M.J.
8. Identify nursing interventions for each nursing diagnosis.

## SUMMARY

- High-risk factors can often be identified early in prenatal care.
- Continuing prenatal care allows for signs of complications to be identified as early as possible.
- Many procedures and tests are available to assess fetal well-being.
- When bleeding occurs in pregnancy, mothers often feel guilty that they may have done something to cause the bleeding.
- Mothers with chronic medical conditions are often cared for by both the medical physician and the obstetrician during pregnancy.
- Complications of pregnancy add to the emotional and financial stress for the client and family.

## REVIEW QUESTIONS

1. J.S. is a 16-year-old primigravida at 38 weeks, whose membranes ruptured spontaneously. Her chart indicates that she was seen by a physician for the first time 2 weeks ago. She is having contractions 10 to 12 minutes apart. The assessment finding indicating a high-risk pregnancy is:
   1. lack of prenatal care and age.
   2. she is not considered high risk.
   3. the membranes rupturing spontaneously.
   4. the contractions being 10 to 12 minutes apart.

2. The maturity of which organ is based on the ratio of lecithin to sphingomyelin?
   1. Placenta.
   2. Fetal lungs.
   3. Acini glands.
   4. Fetal kidneys.
3. In planning the care of a client with DIC, the nurse would include:
   1. giving coagulants.
   2. turning every 2 hours.
   3. watching for signs of bleeding.
   4. massaging the fundus frequently.
4. A pregnant client is receiving magnesium sulfate. The nurse observes that the client's respirations are 8 and her patellar reflexes have decreased. The nurse recognizes that these observations should be:
   1. considered to be the desired result.
   2. recorded and monitored to see if they continue.
   3. brought to the attention of the charge nurse immediately.
   4. considered as an indication that a higher dose of medication is needed.
5. A pregnant woman's blood is found to be Rh negative. Which of the following must be true for Rh incompatibility to be possible?
   1. Father's blood is found to be Rh positive.
   2. Father's blood is found to be Rh negative.
   3. Mother does not develop a secondary anemia during pregnancy.
   4. Mother has at least 2 blood transfusions during pregnancy.
6. A client is admitted at 18 weeks' gestation with a probable diagnosis of hydatidiform mole. For the nursing diagnosis, **F**ear related to the possible development of choriocarcinoma, which of these nursing interventions is appropriate?
   1. Educate the client regarding the need for weekly blood tests.
   2. Explain the need for follow-up physical examinations and chest x-rays.
   3. Stress the importance of delaying another pregnancy until her baby is one year old.
   4. Allow the client to express her feelings and refer her to support sources.
7. A client at 28 weeks' gestation is Rh negative. The nurse determines that the client understands what the nurse has taught her about Rh sensitization when the client states:
   1. "I know I can never have another child."
   2. "I may have to have a shot after delivery if my baby's blood type is Rh positive."
   3. "I will have to have an injection once per month until the baby is born."
   4. "I'm glad I won't have to receive RhoGam if I have another child."
8. A nurse is monitoring a pregnant client with gestational hypertension who is at risk for preeclampsia. The nurse asks the client about subjective signs of preeclampsia, which include:
   1. headache and scomato.
   2. nausea and weight gain of 3 pounds in the last week.
   3. epigastric pain and hypertension.
   4. hypertension and proteinuria.
9. A nurse is assigned to a client with abruption placenta who is experiencing vaginal bleeding. The nurse collects data from the client, knowing that abruption placenta is often accompanied by which additional finding?
   1. A soft abdomen.
   2. No complaints of abdominal pain.
   3. Lack of uterine contractions.
   4. A rigid, board-like abdomen.
10. A client is admitted to the labor suite complaining of painless vaginal bleeding. The nurse assists with the examination of the client, knowing that a routine procedure contraindicated with this client's situation is:
    1. Leopold's maneuvers.
    2. external electronic fetal monitoring.
    3. a manual pelvic examination.
    4. hemoglobin and hematocrit evaluation.

## REFERENCES/SUGGESTED READINGS

Acosta, P. (1996). Nutrition studies in treated infants and children with phenylketonuria: Vitamins, minerals, trace elements. *European Journal of Pediatrics, 155*(1), S136–S139.

Acosta, P., & Wright, L. (1992). Nurses' role in preventing birth defects in offspring of women with phenylketonuria. *JOGNN, 21*(4), 270.

American Association for Clinical Chemistry (AACC). (2009). Pregnancy and prenatal testing. Retrieved August 21, 2009 from http://www.labtestonline.org/understanding/wellness/pre_torch.html

American Diabetes Association (ADA). (2009). Gestational diabetes. Retrieved August 20, 2009 from http://www.diabetes.org/gestational-diabetes.jsp

Andres, R, & Day, M. (2000). Perinatal complications associated with maternal tobacco use. *Seminars in Fetal and Neonatal, 5*(3), 231–241.

Atassi, K., & Harris, M. (2001). Disseminated intravascular coagulation. *Nursing2001, 31*(3), 64.

Barton, J. B., & Sibai, B. M. (2001). HELLP syndrome. In B. M. Sibai (Ed.). *Hypertensive disorders in women.* Philadelphia: W. B. Saunders.

Berstein, P. (2008). Highlights of the 2008 annual clinical meeting of the society of maternal-fetal medicine. Retrieved August 22, 2009 from http://www.medscape.com/viewarticle/570338_print

Bougere, M. (1998). Action stat: Abruptio placenta. *Nursing98, 28*(2), 47.

Brown, Z., Gardella, C., Wald, A., Morrow, R., & Corey, L. (2005). Genital herpes complicating pregnancy. *Obstetrics and Gynecology, 106,* 845–856.

Bulechek, G., Butcher, H., McCloskey, J., & Dochterman, J., eds. (2008). *Nursing Interventions Classification (NIC)* (5th ed.). St. Louis, MO: Mosby/Elsevier.

Carpenter, T. (2003). Is it morning sickness or something worse? *RN, 66*(10), 34–37.

Centers for Disease Control and Prevention (CDC). (2007). *Births: Final data for 2005. National Vital Statistics Reports (NVSS), 56*(6), 1–104. Retrieved August 22, 2009 from http://www.cdc.gov/nchs/data/nvsr/nvsr56/nvsr56_06.pdf

Ciardelli, L., Meroni, V., Avanzini, A., Bollani, L., Tinelli, C., Garofoli, F., Gasparoni, A., & Stronati, M. (2008). Early and accurate diagnosis of congenital toxoplasmosis. *The Pediatric Infectious Disease Journal, 27,* 125–129.

Cook, A., Gilbert, R., Buffolano, W., Zufferey, J., Petersen, E., et al. (2000). Sources of toxoplasma infection in pregnant women: European multicentre case-control study. European Research Network on Congenital Toxoplasmosis. *BMJ, 321*(7254), 142–147.

Davidson, M., London, M., & Ladewig, P. (2008). *Old's maternal-newborn nursing and women's health across the lifespan* (8th ed.). Upper Saddle River, NJ: Pearson Prentice Hall.

Deering, S. (2008). Abruptio placentae. Retrieved August 20, 2009 from http://emedicince.medscape.com/article/252810-overview

Dickason, E., Silverman, B., & Kaplan J. (1998). *Maternal-infant nursing care* (3rd ed.). St. Louis: MO: Mosby–Year Book.

Farrell, M. (2003). Improving the care of women with gestational diabetes. *MCN, 28*(5), 301–305.

Feig, D., Briggs, G., & Koren, G. (2007). Oral antidiabetic agents in pregnancy and lactation: a paradigm shift? *The Annuals of Pharmacotherapy, 41*(7), 1174–1180.

Friedman, S.A., Lubarsky, S.L., & Lim, K.H. (2001). Mild gestational hypertension and preeclampsia. In B. M. Sibai (Ed.). *Hypertensive disorders in women.* Philadelphia: W. B. Saunders.

Guinn, D., Atkinson, M. ., Sullivan, L., Lee, M., MacGregor, S., et al. (2001). Single vs weekly courses of antenatal corticosteroids for women at risk of preterm delivery: A randomized controlled trial. *JAMA, 286*(13), 1581–1587.

Hamilton Health Sciences. (2008). Are you immune to rubella? Retrieved August 21, 2009 from http://www.hhsc.ca/documents/Patient%20Education/Rubella-th.pdf

Harvey, C. (1997). A look at electronic fetal monitoring update; the new terms. *Lifelines, 1*(6), 49–51.

Hokelek, M. 2009. Toxoplasmosis. Retrieved August 21, 2009 from http://emedicine.medscape.com/article/229969-print

Holcberg, G., Tsadkin-Tamir, M., Sapir, O., Wiznizer, A., Segal, D., et al. (2004). Transfer of insulin lispro across the human placenta. *European Journal of Obstetrics and Gynecology and Reproductive Biology, 115*(1), 117–118.

Irgens, J.U., Reisaeter, L. Irgens, L.M., & Lie, R.T. (2001). Long-term mortality of mothers and fathers after preeclampsia: Population-based cohort study. *BMJ, 323*(7323), 1213–1217.

Katz, V., Farmer, R., & Kuller, J. (2000). Preeclampsia into eclampsia: Towards a new paradigm. *American Journal of Obstetrics & Gynecology, 182*(6), 1389–1396.

Koch, R., Azen, C., Friedman, E., Hanley, W., Kevy, H., et al. (2003). Research design, organization, and sample characteristics of the maternal PKU collaborative study. *Pediatrics, 112*(6), 1519–1522.

Lachat, M., Scott, C., & Refl, M. ( 2006). HIV and pregnancy: Considerations for nursing practice. *The American Journal of Maternal Child Nursing, 31*(4), 233–241.

Ladewig, P., Moberly, S., Olds, L., & London, M. (2001). *Contemporary maternal-newborn nursing care* (5th ed.). Menlo Park, CA: Addison-Wesley.

Lee, Y., & Simpson, L. (2007). Major fetal structural malformations: The role of new imaging modalities. *American Journal of Medical Genetics Part C (Seminars in Medical Genetics), 145C,* 33–44.

Littleton, L., & Engebretson, J. (2004). *Maternity nursing care.* Clifton Park, NY: Delmar Cengage Learning.

Lu, J., & Nightengale, C. (2000). Magnesium sulfate in eclampsia and preeclampsia: Pharmokinetic principles. *Clinical Pharmacology, 38*(4), 305–314.

Macones, G., Hankins, G., Spong, C., Hauth, J., & Moore, T. (2008). The 2008 National Institute of Child Health and Human Development Research Workshop Report on electronic fetal heart rate monitoring. *Obstetrics and Gynecology, 112,* 661–666.

Mandeville, L.K., & Troiano, N.H. (1999). *High risk and critical care intrapartum nursing* (2nd ed.). Philadelphia: Lippincott Williams & Wilkins.

March of Dimes. (2009). Illicit drug use during pregnancy. Retrieved August 22, 2009 from http://www.marchofdimes.com/professionals/14332_1169.asp#head3

Minnick-Smith, K., & Cook, F. (1997). Current treatment options for ectopic pregnancy. *MCN, 22*(1), 21–25.

Montgomery, K. (2003). Health promotion for pregnant adolescents. *Lifelines, 7*(5), 432–444.

Moorhead, S., Johnson, M., Maas, M., & Swanson, E. (2007). *Nursing outcomes classification (NOC)* (4th ed). St. Louis, MO: Elsevier–Health Sciences Division.

Morgan, E. (2002). Eclampsia. *Nursing2002, 32*(3), 104.

Murphy, K., & MACS Collaborative Group. (2007). Multiple courses of antenatal corticosteroids for preterm birth study. *American Journal of Obstetrics and Gynecology, 197,* S2.

National Heart, Lung, and Blood Institute. (2000). *Working group report on high blood pressure in pregnancy.* Washington, DC: National Institutes of Health.

National Institute of Child Health and Human Development Research Planning Workshop. (1997). Electronic fetal heart rate monitoring: Research guidelines for interpretation. *American Journal of Obstetrics and Gynecology, 177,* 1385–1390.

National Institutes of Health (NIH). (2009). Use of 3D/4D Ultrasound in the Evaluation of Fetal Anomalies. Retrieved August 17, 2009 from http://clinicaltrials.gov/ct2/show/NCT00826917

Neal, J. (2001). RhD isoimmunization and current management modalities. *JOGNN, 30*(6), 589–606.

Neuman, M., & Graf, C. (2003). Pregnancy after age 35: Are these women at high risk? *Lifelines, 7*(5), 422–430.

NICHD (1997). Electronic fetal heart monitoring: Research guidelines for interpretation. The National Institute of Child Health and Human Development Research Planning Workshop. *JOGNN, 26*(6), 635–640.

Nick, J. (2003). Deep tendon reflexes: The what, why, where, and how of tapping. *JOGNN, 32*(3), 297–306.

North American Nursing Diagnosis Association International. (2010). *NANDA-I nursing diagnoses: Definitions and classification 2009–2011.* Ames, IA: Wiley-Blackwell.

Padden, M. (1999). HELLP syndrome: Recognition and pernatal management. *American Family Physician.* Retrieved August 22, 2009 from http://www.aafp.org/afp/990901ap/829.html

Perozzi, K., Zalice, K., Howard, V., & Skariot, L. (2007). What you need to know to care for your pregnant patient. *The American Journal of Maternal Child Nursing, 32*(6), 345–352.

Reis, P., Sander, C., & Pearlman, M. (2000). Abruptio placentae after auto accidents: A case control study. *Journal of Reproductive Medicine, 45*(1), 6–10.

Rorman, E., Zamir, C., Rilkis, I., & Ben-David, H. (2006). Congenital toxoplasmosisprenatal aspects of Toxoplasma gondii infection. *Reproductive Toxicology, 21*(4), 458–472.

Ruddy, L. (2000). Preeclampsia. *AJN, 100*(8), 45–46.

Ruddy, L., & Kearney, K. (2000). Preeclampsia. *American Journal of Nursing, 100*(8), 45–46.

Saal, H., Braddock, S., Bull, M., Enns, G., Gruen, J., et al. (2008). Maternal phenylketonuria. *Pediatrics, 122*, 445–449.

Schweon, S. (2001). Protecting yourself during pregnancy. Nursing2001, 31(3), 72.

Sepilian, V., & Wood, E. (2009). Ectopic pregnancy. Retrieved August 18, 2009 from http://emedicine.medscape.com/article/258768-print

Sibai, B., & Stella, C. (2009). Diagnosis and management of atypical preeclampsia-eclampsia. *American Journal of Obstetrics and Gynecology, 200*, 481.e1–481.e7.

Simpson, K., & Creehan, P. (2007). *AWHONN's Perinatal nursing: Co-published with AWHONN* (3rd ed.). Philadelphia: Lippincott Williams & Wilkins.

Spratto, G., & Woods, A. (2008). *2009 PDR for nursing.* Clifton Park, NY: Delmar Cengage Learning.

Tenore, J. (2000). Ectopic pregnancy. *American Family Physician, 61*(4), 1080–1088.

Trofatter, K. (2009). Cervical incompetence and cerclage-8-Shirodkar vs McDonald cerclage. Retrieved August 18, 2009 from http://www.healthline.com/blogs/pregnancy_childbirth/2008/09/cervical-incompetence-and-cerclage-8.html

Urbanski, T., Higgins, P., Murray, M., & Joffe, G. (1996). Caring for a woman with a hydatidiform mole and coexisting pregnancy. *MCN, 21*(2), 85–89.

Watts, D., Brown, Z., Money, D., Selke, S., Huang, M., Sacks, S., & Corey, L. (2003). A double-blind, randomized, placebo-controlled trial of acyclovir in late pregnancy for the reduction of herpes simplex virus shedding and cesarean delivery. *American Journal of Obstetrics and Gynecology, 188*, 836–843.

Woo, J. (2009). Obstetric ultrasound: A comprehensive guide to ultrasound scans in pregnancy. Retrieved August 15, 2009 from http://www.ob-ultrasound.net/

# RESOURCES

Association of Women's Health, Obstetric, and Neonatal Nurses (AWHONN), http:// www.awhonn.org

National Organization of Mothers of Twins Clubs, Inc. (NOMOTC), http://www.nomotc.org

The Society of Obstetricians and Gynaecologists of Canada (SOGC), http://www.sogc.org

# CHAPTER 3
## The Birth Process

## MAKING THE CONNECTION

*Refer to the following chapters to increase your understanding of the birth process:*

*Maternal & Pediatric Nursing*

- *Prenatal Care*
- *Complications of Pregnancy*

## LEARNING OBJECTIVES

Upon completion of this chapter, you should be able to:

- Explain key terms.
- Describe possible causes of labor.
- Identify premonitory signs of labor.
- Differentiate between true labor and false labor.
- Discuss the maternal systemic responses to labor.
- Identify the variables that affect the progress of labor.
- Explain the four stages of labor.
- Describe the mechanisms of labor.
- Show nursing actions necessary when admitting a woman to the labor unit.
- Demonstrate the specific assessments used when caring for a woman in labor: fetopelvic relationships, fetal assessment, contractions, Leopold's maneuvers, vaginal examination.
- Explain possible nursing diagnoses and nursing interventions for a client during labor and delivery.
- Identify the most common complications of labor—dystocia and fetal distress.
- Identify possible medical—surgical interventions for labor: cesarean birth, induction and augmentation of labor, amniotomy, episiotomy, forceps, vacuum extractor, and analgesia/anesthesia.
- Provide care for a client during labor and delivery.

## KEY TERMS

acme
amniotomy
augmentation of labor
bloody show
Braxton Hicks contractions
cardinal movements
cephalopelvic disproportion (CPD)
cervical dilation
cesarean birth
crowning
decrement
duration
dysfunctional labor
dystocia
effacement
engagement
episiotomy

external version
false labor
Ferguson's reflex
fetal attitude
fetal lie
fetal position
fetal presentation
fontanelle
forceps
frequency
fundus
increment
induction of labor
intensity
interval
lightening
macrosomic

molding
nuchal cord
precipitate birth
precipitate labor
presenting part
preterm birth
preterm labor
prolapsed cord
pudendal block
restitution
rupture of membranes (ROM)
station
suture
tocolytic agent
uterine retraction

# INTRODUCTION

The past decade has brought great changes in birthing practices. For hospital births, the concept of labor, delivery, recovery, postpartum (LDRP) rooms has given the expecting couple a more homelike environment, and the mother is not moved from the labor room to the delivery room, to the recovery room, to the postpartum room during the birthing process (Figure 3-1). Family and friends, even the baby's siblings, may be present in the LDRP room during the birth process.

Community birthing centers and other settings offer alternatives for the laboring couple. Many clients attend childbirth classes and have in mind a birthing plan or expectations of what they anticipate the birthing process will be like.

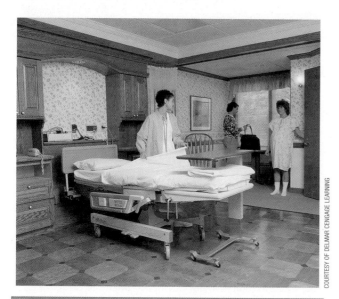

COURTESY OF DELMAR CENGAGE LEARNING

FIGURE 3-1 The LDRP concept allows the laboring couple to remain in the same room throughout the birth experience.

Some clients hire a midwife or doula to assist them through the process of labor, birth, and postpartum. Midwives are classified as either a certified midwife (CM) or a certified nurse-midwife (CNM) depending on their education and training. Midwives provide health care to women throughout the life span (American College of Nurse-Midwives, 2009). The CNM is trained to independently manage the care of low-risk pregnancy, birth, and postpartum care for healthy woman and newborns.

Doulas are trained and experienced childbirth support persons who continuously attend to the physical, emotional, and informational needs of the laboring woman and family through the entire birthing process. According to the Doulas of North America International (2009) when a doula attends the birth, the labor is shorter with fewer complications, and the infants are healthier and breastfeed more easily. The doula is an adjunct and can be an asset to the health care team (London, Ladewig, Ball, & Bindler, 2007).

This chapter outlines the birth process, from the onset of labor through the birth of the infant.

# ONSET OF LABOR

For 38 to 40 weeks, the pregnancy has been advancing and the fetus developing. Now, as the fetus reaches maturity, the birth process begins. Researchers are still trying to determine exactly what causes the onset of true labor; however, there are two theories relative to why labor begins.

## THEORIES REGARDING ONSET OF LABOR

The mechanical theory is based on the principle that as a hollow organ in the body becomes filled and distended, the organ tends to empty itself. Examples of this phenomenon are the bladder and sigmoid colon. This mechanism alone is not enough to fully explain the onset of labor because a woman can have a full-term 6 ½ lb baby with one pregnancy and full-term twins each weighing 5-½ lb with the next pregnancy.

The hormonal theory of the onset of labor relates to the changes in maternal progesterone and estrogen levels, the maternal production of oxytocin and prostaglandin, and the increase in fetal production of cortisol. There seems to be a highly integrated relationship among these hormones.

As the pregnancy nears its end, the placental production of progesterone decreases, thus decreasing the relaxing effect of progesterone on the uterus. The estrogen level rises, causing an increased sensitivity of the myometrium to oxytocin. Oxytocin, now produced by the mother's posterior pituitary gland, stimulates uterine contractions. As the pregnancy nears 40 weeks of gestation, the uterus becomes more sensitive to oxytocin. Fetal cortisol production increases as the pregnancy nears term. It is believed to decrease the placental production of progesterone and stimulate the precursors of prostaglandin.

## PREMONITORY SIGNS OF LABOR

Several signs indicate that labor will soon begin. The signs are lightening, Braxton Hicks contractions, cervical changes, bloody show, rupture of membranes, gastrointestinal disturbance, and a sudden burst of energy.

### Lightening

Lightening is the descent of the fetus into the pelvis. This may occur as early as 2 weeks before labor begins in the primigravida client but may not occur until a multigravida client is already in labor. The downward movement of the fetus and thus the uterus makes the upper part of the abdomen flatter. This relieves pressure on the diaphragm, allowing the mother to breathe easier, but she may experience:

• Leg cramps from pressure now on pelvic nerves.
• Urinary frequency from pressure now on the bladder.

• Increased venous stasis from pressure now on the veins, resulting in edema of the lower extremities.
• Increased vaginal secretions.

### Braxton Hicks Contractions

Braxton Hicks contractions are irregular, intermittent contractions felt by the pregnant woman toward the end of pregnancy. The tightening sensation in the abdomen may become fairly regular and uncomfortable. The woman may go to the care provider's office or the hospital thinking she is in labor. If the cervix is not dilated and then the contractions stop, this is called false labor. Table 3-1 compares false labor and true labor.

### Cervical Changes

At about 34 weeks of gestation, because of the changing ratio of estrogen to progesterone and the production of prostaglandin, the cervix begins to "mature" or "ripen." That is, the cervix becomes softer and spongier. Effacement, thinning and shortening of the cervix, may begin, especially when the woman is a primigravida. Cervical changes of dilation and effacement progress during labor to allow delivery of the fetus.

### Bloody Show

Bloody show consists of cervical secretion, blood-tinged mucus, and the mucous plug that blocked the cervix during pregnancy. Labor often begins within 24 to 48 hours after the bloody show is noticed; however, a vaginal examination that includes cervical manipulation may result in a blood-tinged discharge. This may be confused with bloody show.

### Rupture of Membranes

Rupture of membranes (ROM), the rupture of the amniotic sac, usually occurs after labor has begun; however, in about 12% of women, the amniotic membranes rupture

| TABLE 3-1 Comparison of False Labor and True Labor | |
|---|---|
| **FALSE LABOR** | **TRUE LABOR** |
| Contractions often irregular but may be regular for a short time (1 to 2 hours). | Contractions occur at regular intervals. |
| Interval between contractions stays the same. | Interval between contractions gradually shortens. |
| Contraction intensity and duration remain the same. | Contractions increase in intensity and duration. |
| Contractions frequently stop when the client ambulates or changes position. | Contractions continue and often become stronger when the client ambulates. |
| Contractions eventually cease with controlled breathing, relaxation techniques, comfort measures, or hydration. | Contractions are usually not stopped with controlled breathing, other relaxation techniques, sedation, comfort measures, or hydration. |
| Cervix may soften but does not efface or dilate. | Cervix softens, effaces, and dilates. |
| Contractions felt above navel. | Contractions felt in lower back and radiate to abdomen. |
| No change in cervical dilation and effacement. | Produces cervical dilation and effacement. |

before the onset of labor (London, Ladewig, Ball, & Bindler, 2007). Spontaneous rupture of membranes (SROM) occurs naturally with a gush of amniotic fluid out of the vagina. Artificial rupture of membranes (AROM) is a procedure known as an amniotomy (discussed later in chapter) in which a physician or certified nurse-midwife uses an amnihook instrument to rupture the amniotic membranes. If engagement (when the widest diameter of the fetal presenting part [head] enters the inlet to the true pelvis) has not yet occurred, there exists the danger that the umbilical cord will wash out with the amniotic fluid (prolapsed cord).

If labor does not begin spontaneously within 12 to 24 hours after the membranes rupture and the pregnancy is near term, labor is often induced to avoid infection.

It is sometimes difficult for the woman to determine whether the membranes have ruptured or whether urine has escaped from her bladder. A simple test with nitrazine paper is helpful. When moistened in the discharge, the nitrazine paper will turn a deep blue (react) if the discharge is amniotic fluid; the paper will usually not react if the membranes are still intact. The health-care provider may also test for "ferning." When amniotic fluid is placed on a microscope slide, it dries in the shape of fern leaves. Newer testing devices for detecting rupture of the amniotic membrane in pregnant women include the Amnisure and Amnioswab. Both of these testing methods are convenient swab screenings that are rapid and less invasive.

## Gastrointestinal Disturbance

Some women report having one or more of the following near the time of labor: indigestion, nausea, vomiting, and diarrhea. They may experience a 1- to 3-pound weight loss.

## Sudden Burst of Energy

Approximately 24 to 48 hours before labor begins, some women will have a sudden burst of energy. The reason for this is unknown. The prospective mother should be careful not to tire herself. She will need the energy when labor begins. Encourage the client to eat frequent small nutritious meals during this time.

# MATERNAL SYSTEMIC RESPONSES TO LABOR

Knowing how the various systems of the mother's body respond to labor is important when making assessments and performing nursing interventions.

## CARDIOVASCULAR SYSTEM

Cardiac output increases because 300 to 500 mL of blood is squeezed from the uterus into maternal circulation with each contraction (London, et al., 2007). The client's blood pressure increases during the first and second stages of labor due to contractions. Blood pressure is highest during a contraction, so blood pressure should be taken *between* contractions. Anxiety and pain may also make the blood pressure increase. Women in labor may experience supine hypotensive syndrome, or decreased blood pressure when in a supine position due to the vessels being compressed by the fetal weight (Leifer, 2008).

## RESPIRATORY SYSTEM

Oxygen consumption during labor is equal to that of moderate to strenuous exercise. As long as the respiratory center is not depressed by medication, the increased respiratory rate continues with oxygen consumption almost double the normal amount. If the mother develops hypoxia or acidosis, the fetus may be compromised. Hyperventilation may decrease the level of carbon dioxide in the mother's blood.

## RENAL SYSTEM

When engagement occurs, the bladder, now an abdominal organ, is pushed forward and upward. A distended bladder may impede fetal descent. Pressure from the presenting part, especially during a contraction, may cause edema of the tissues because of impaired blood and lymph drainage (Cunningham, Leveno, Gilstrap, Bloom, Hauth, & Wenstrom, 2005). Urinary flow is decreased, especially when the woman is supine, because the uterus compresses the ureters. Often there is a lessened urge to void, so the client must be encouraged to do so.

## GASTROINTESTINAL SYSTEM

During labor, peristalsis and absorption decrease. Gastric emptying time is prolonged and gastric contents increase in acidity (Blackburn, 2007). The client in labor should not eat solid food because there is always a possibility of an obstetrical emergency requiring surgery. Eating solid food would increase the risk of aspirating vomitus. The absorption of liquid is unchanged during labor. The lips and mouth become dry as a result of mouth breathing.

## FLUID AND ELECTROLYTE BALANCE

Because of the muscular activity of labor, the mother's body temperature increases and she perspires profusely. The normal increase in respiratory rate and the tendency of women in labor to hyperventilate both cause an increase in fluid loss. The hyperventilation also affects electrolyte balance. To prevent dehydration, it is routine for intravenous fluids such as lactated ringers to be administered to women during labor and delivery.

## IMMUNE SYSTEM

The white blood count (WBC) increases, sometimes up to 25,000/mm³, during labor and stays elevated during the early postpartum period. The natural increase makes it difficult to identify any infectious process the woman may have.

## INTEGUMENTARY SYSTEM

The vagina and perineum have a great ability to stretch. The degree of stretching varies with each client; however, minute tears may occur in the vagina and/or perineum during the birth of the baby.

## MUSCULOSKELETAL SYSTEM

The marked increase in muscle activity during labor is accompanied by increased body temperature, diaphoresis, fatigue, and some proteinuria (1+) (Lowdermilk & Perry,

## PROFESSIONALTIP

### Mother to Infant HIV Transmission

A mother can pass HIV to her infant during pregnancy, childbirth delivery, or through breast milk. According to the CDC (2007), mother-to-infant transmission is the most common way that children become infected with HIV. Antiretroviral medications work well to stop the transmission of HIV if the mother takes these drugs before and during childbirth and if the newborn is given the drugs after birth. Without breastfeeding or treatment, approximately 25% of pregnant women with HIV will transmit HIV to the infant. By following this protocol of antiviral medication administration, mother-to-infant HIV transmission is reduced from 25% to less than 2% (CDC, 2007).

| Severe discomfort | Moderate discomfort | Mild discomfort |

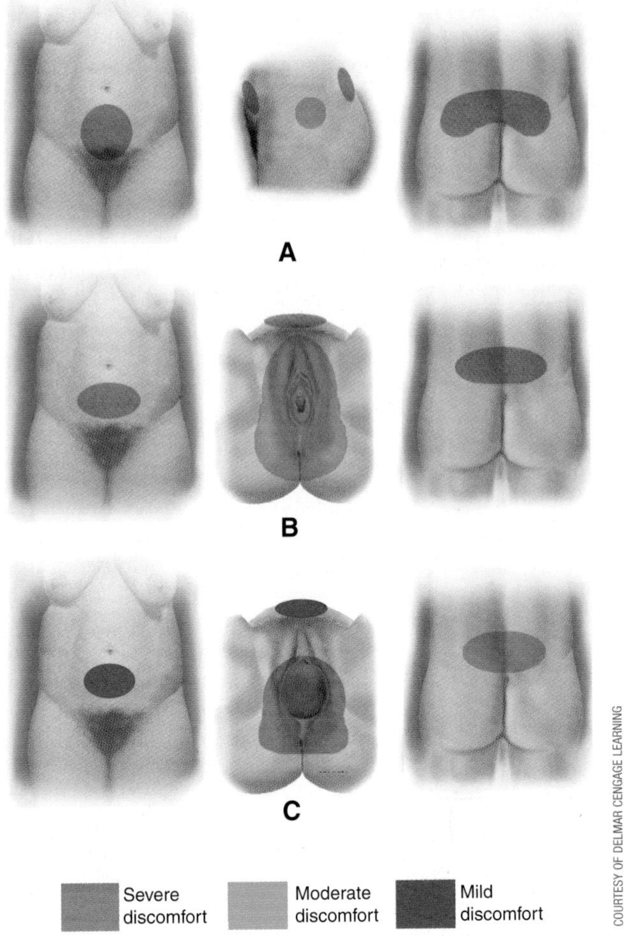

FIGURE 3-2 Intensity and Distribution of Discomfort during Various Stages of Labor; *A*, First Stage; *B*, Early Second Stage; *C*, Late Second Stage and Birth

2006). The relaxation of pelvic joints, caused by the influence of relaxin, may result in backache. Leg cramps also may be experienced.

## NEUROLOGICAL SYSTEM

The client may be euphoric at the beginning of labor. This often changes to seriousness and then to amnesia between contractions during the second stage of labor. Endogenous endorphins (a morphine-like chemical produced naturally by the body) increase the client's pain threshold and have a sedative effect. Pressure on the perineum, by the fetus descending through the birth canal, causes physiologic anesthesia in the perineal tissues.

## Pain

The discomfort and pain of labor and birth are individual, subjective, very personal, and have a wide range of expression. Visceral pain usually predominates the first stage of labor, with the stimuli originating in the uterus, cervix, adnexa, and pelvic ligaments. With fetal descent increasing during the late first stage and beginning second stage of labor, the traction and distention on the pelvic structures around the vagina are the primary stimuli for pain. The distention of the perineum is the stimulus for pain during the remainder of the second stage of labor and is transmitted primarily by the pudendal nerves. Figure 3-2 illustrates the intensity and distribution of discomfort during various stages of labor. Stages of labor are discussed later in this chapter.

The softness of pelvic tissues in parous women (women who have delivered at least one child) seems to cause less nociceptive stimuli than in nulliparous women (women who have never delivered a child) during the first stage of labor; however, during the second stage of labor, parous women have increased nociceptive stimuli because of the speed and the intensity of fetal descent. As with pain from any other cause, individuals respond in ways that are acceptable in their culture. Health-care providers must be sensitive to the fact that expression of pain is rooted in cultural heritage.

## VARIABLES AFFECTING LABOR

There are five major variables that affect labor. They are known as the five Ps: passageway, passenger, position, powers, and psychological response.

### PASSAGEWAY

The passageway consists of the bony pelvis, uterus, cervix, vagina, and perineum.

### Pelvis

The size and shape of the true pelvis must be adequate for the fetal head to pass through for a vaginal birth. The CNM/physician uses several methods to determine the adequacy of the true pelvis, such as:

- *Palpation*—Internally, the bony prominences are felt; externally, the distance between the ischial tuberosities is measured and then the distance between the ischial spines estimated.
- *Ultrasound*—An ultrasound is used to estimate pelvic adequacy as well as fetal growth, multiple pregnancy, placenta location, and **fetal presentation**.
- *Pelvimetry*—X-ray of the pelvis is seldom performed during pregnancy because of the radiation involved.

## Uterus

The upper part of the uterus (fundus) becomes thicker with contractions and the lower section becomes thinner, forming a tube.

## Cervix

The uterine contractions put pressure on the fetus, which in turn puts pressure on the cervix, causing the cervix to efface and dilate. The cervix must dilate and efface sufficiently for the fetus to descend into the vagina.

## Vagina

The vagina sustains many changes throughout pregnancy. Various hormones cause an increase in vascularity, loosening of connective tissue, and hypertrophy of the smooth muscle cells. These changes allow the vagina to stretch enough for the fetus to pass through.

## Perineum

The pressure of the fetus on the perineum causes stretching and thinning of the perineum.

## PASSENGER

The size of the fetus as well as the fetal attitude, fetal lie, fetal presentation, and fetal position affects how easily the fetus can advance through the passage.

## Size

The largest part of the fetal body is usually the head. Because the bones of the fetal skull are not fused, the bones can move, sometimes even overlap, as the fetus moves through the mother's bony pelvis. The shaping of the fetal head to adapt to the mother's pelvis during labor is called **molding**.

The major bones of the skull are two frontal bones, two temporal bones, two parietal bones, and the occiput. The bones are joined by thin, fibrous, membrane-covered spaces called

**sutures**. Where the sutures meet, there are larger membranous areas called **fontanelles** (Figure 3-3). The largest is the diamond-shaped anterior fontanelle. The posterior fontanelle is triangular and smaller. The care providers can palpate the two fontanelles and the suture connecting them through the cervix and determine fetal position.

## Fetal Attitude

**Fetal attitude** is the relationship of fetal body parts to one another. The ideal attitude of the fetus at term is flexion, with the head flexed onto the chest, the arms flexed over the chest, and the hips and knees flexed on the abdomen. If any part of the fetus is extended, especially the head or the legs, labor is usually more difficult. The attitude is then called extension.

## Fetal Lie

The relationship of the cephalocaudal (head to foot) axis of the fetus to the cephalocaudal axis of the mother is called the **fetal lie**. When the fetal cephalocaudal axis is parallel to the mother's, it is called a longitudinal lie. When the fetal cephalocaudal axis is at a right angle to the mother's, it is called a transverse lie (Figure 3-4).

## Fetal Presentation

Fetal presentation is determined by the fetal lie and the part of the fetus that enters the pelvis first. The part of the fetus in contact with the cervix is called the **presenting part**. The most common type of presentation is cephalic (head), in 95% of deliveries, with breech (buttocks) being 4%, and shoulder 1% of deliveries (Leifer, 2008) (Figure 3-5).

**Cephalic Presentations** Cephalic presentations may be further differentiated by the part of the head entering the pelvis first. They may be:

- Vertex—with the occiput as the presenting part
- Brow—with the sinciput as the presenting part
- Face—with the face as the presenting part

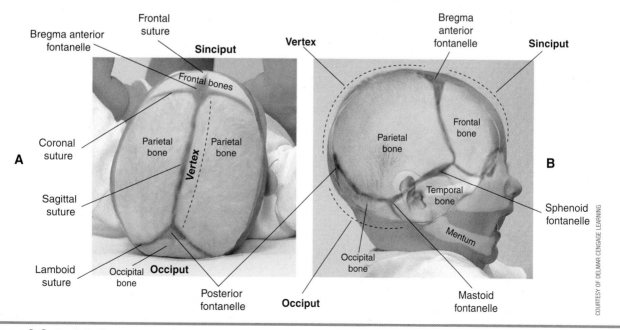

FIGURE 3-3  Fetal Skull—Sutures and Fontanelles; *A*, Superior View; *B*, Lateral View

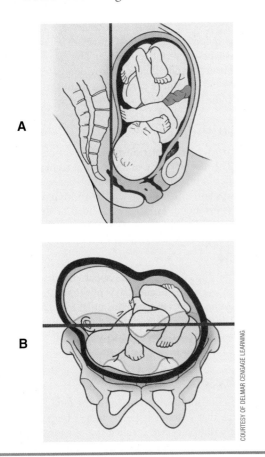

FIGURE 3-4 **Fetal Attitude and Fetal Lie;** *A*, **Fetal Attitude Flexion, Fetal Lie Longitudinal;** *B*, **Fetal Attitude Flexion, Fetal Lie Transverse**

**Breech Presentations** Breech presentations are differentiated by the attitude of the fetus's legs. The various breech presentations are as follows:

- *Complete breech*: Hips and knees are flexed on the abdomen in an attitude of flexion, with the buttocks as the presenting part
- *Frank breech*: The hips are flexed, but the knees are extended with the buttocks as the presenting part
- *Footling breech*: The hips and knees are extended with the foot as the presenting part (may be single footling or double footling)

**Shoulder Presentation** A shoulder presentation occurs in a transverse lie. The presenting part is usually the shoulder but may be the arm, back, abdomen, or side.

## POSITION

### Engagement

Engagement is fixation of the fetal presenting part in the maternal true pelvis in which the widest diameter of the presenting part is at or below the level of the ischial spines.

### Station

**Station** is the relationship of the fetal presenting part to the ischial spines. It is measured in centimeters above (−) or below (+) the ischial spines (Figure 3-6).

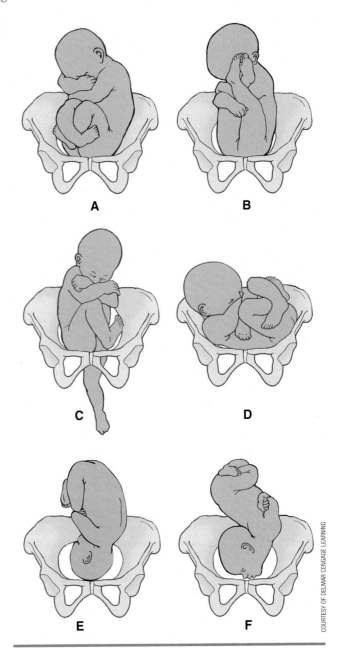

FIGURE 3-5 **Fetal Presentation;** *A*, **Complete breech;** *B*, **Frank breech;** *C*, **Footling breech;** *D*, **Shoulder;** *E*, **Vertex;** *F*, **Face**

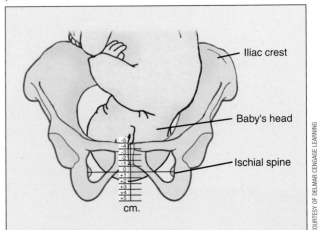

FIGURE 3-6 **Station: Relationship of the fetal presenting part to the ischial spines. The station illustrated is +2.**

## Fetal Position

**Fetal position** refers to the relationship of the identified landmark on the presenting part of the four quadrants of the mother's pelvis (Figure 3-7). The identified landmarks on various presenting parts are shown in Table 3-2.

The brow presentation does not have an identified landmark. The brow usually changes either to a vertex or face presentation. Although the shoulder presentation cannot be delivered vaginally, there is still a landmark designated for it, which is SC (scapula).

There are six possible positions for each presenting part as follows:

- Right occiput anterior (ROA) mentum (RMA) sacrum (RSA)
- Right occiput transverse (ROT) mentum (RMT) sacrum (RST)
- Right occiput posterior (ROP) mentum (RMP) sacrum (RSP)
- Left occiput anterior (LOA) mentum (LMA) sacrum (LSA)
- Left occiput transverse (LOT) mentum (LMT) sacrum (LST)
- Left occiput posterior (LOP) mentum (LMP) sacrum (LSP)

Figure 3-8 illustrates the six positions of a vertex presentation. The same six positions apply to the face and breech presentations. The most common position is LOA, which is considered to be the most favorable for the welfare of both mother and baby.

## POWERS

The primary power during labor is the involuntary contractions of the uterus, which cause cervical effacement and dilatation during the first stage of labor. The secondary power is the voluntary use of the abdominal muscles by the mother to push or "bear-down" during the second stage of labor to expel the fetus.

| TABLE 3-2 Identified Landmarks on Various Presenting Part | |
|---|---|
| **PRESENTING PART** | **IDENTIFIED LANDMARK** |
| Vertex | Occiput (O) |
| Face | Mentum (M) |
| Breech (all) | Sacrum (S) |

## Uterine Contractions

The smooth muscle of the uterus has the ability to contract and relax rhythmically. The relaxation period between contractions allows the muscles and the mother to rest. Uterine relaxation also restores uteroplacental circulation, which is important to fetal oxygenation and effective circulation in the uterus. Contractions begin in the **fundus**, top of the uterus, and spread over the uterus in about 15 seconds (Leifer, 2008).

The muscle fibers of the uterus have the unique property of remaining permanently shortened to a small degree after

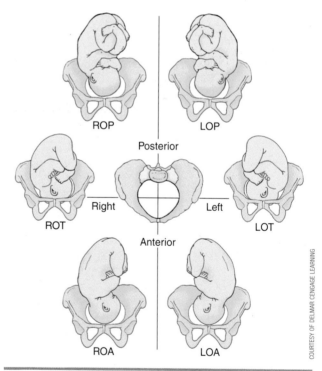

**FIGURE 3-8** Various Positions of a Vertex Presentation

## ⊕ PROFESSIONALTIP

### Fetal Positions

- The right or left and anterior, posterior, or transverse always refer to the mother's pelvis.
- The middle word or letter refers to the identified landmark on the fetus, either occiput, mentum, or sacrum.

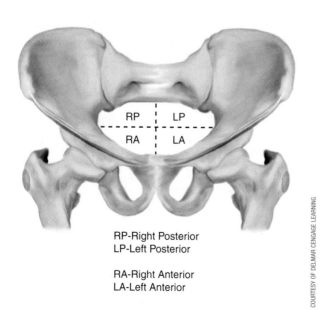

RP-Right Posterior
LP-Left Posterior

RA-Right Anterior
LA-Left Anterior

**FIGURE 3-7** Pelvic Quadrants

each contraction. This is called **uterine retraction**. The shortening of the muscle fibers results in a gradual decrease in the uterine cavity size and a thickening of the muscle in the fundus. As the muscle fibers in the fundus retract, the lower uterine segment is pulled up. These two actions efface and dilate the cervix (Figure 3-9).

Each contraction has three phases:

1. **Increment:** increasing intensity of a contraction
2. **Acme:** peak of a contraction
3. **Decrement:** decreasing intensity of a contraction

Contractions are described in terms of frequency, duration, and intensity. **Frequency** is the time from the beginning of one contraction to the beginning of the next contraction. It includes one contraction and one resting period between contractions (**interval**). **Duration** is the length of one contraction, from the beginning of the increment to the conclusion of the decrement. **Intensity** is the strength of the contraction at the acme. Figure 3-10A illustrates these aspects of a contraction while B shows the mother's abdomen before and during a contraction.

The duration of a contraction should not be longer than 90 seconds nor should the interval be less than 60 seconds.

The uterus should completely relax between contractions. Contractions lasting longer than 90 seconds reduce uterine and placental circulation because of the prolonged compression of the blood vessels. This in turn compromises the fetus.

Contractions are affected by the mother's position. When the mother lies on her back, the contractions are often more frequent but have less intensity. When she lies on her side, the contractions are usually less frequent but have greater intensity. Thus, a side-lying position improves progress in labor. Lying on the side also prevents supine hypotension syndrome in the mother and improves oxygenation of the uterus, placenta, and fetus because the heavy uterus is not compressing the inferior vena cava.

## Maternal Pushing Efforts

Once the cervix has dilated completely, it is time for the fetus to navigate through the remaining mechanisms of labor. The accepted procedure has been for the mother to take a deep breath at the beginning of a contraction, hold her breath, and voluntarily push in a Valsalva-type bearing down throughout a contraction. This pushing technique is directed by the nurses and/or the CNM/physician.

The spontaneous onset of the urge to bear down is triggered when the presenting part reaches the pelvic floor where stretch receptors in the posterior vagina cause the release of oxytocin, which spontaneously increases the pushing sensation. This spontaneous, involuntary urge to bear down is known as **Ferguson's reflex**.

## PSYCHOLOGICAL RESPONSE

Psychological response refers to the mother's attitude toward labor and her preparation for labor. The mother's attitude toward labor is shaped by her experiences and expectations. Culture shapes values about and responses to childbirth.

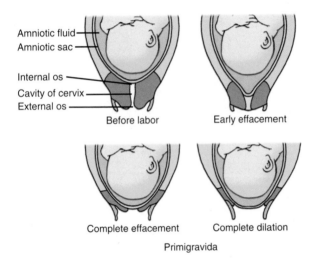

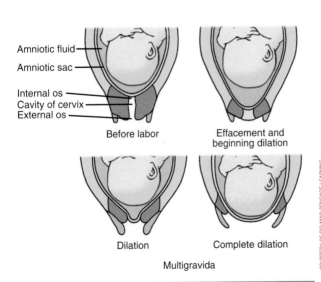

**FIGURE 3-9** **Examples of Effacement and Dilation;** *A*, **Primigravida;** *B*, **Multigravida**

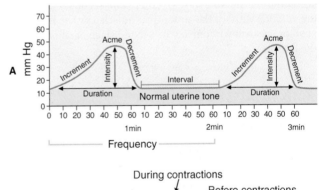

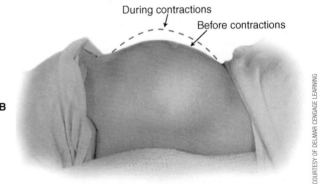

**FIGURE 3-10** *A*, **Aspects of a contraction (frequency 2 minutes, duration 60 seconds, intensity moderate);** *B*, **Abdominal contour before and during a contraction.**

COURTESY OF DELMAR CENGAGE LEARNING

It provides the mother with ideas about how to behave during labor and how to interact with her baby.

Anxiety or fear causes the mother's body to secrete catecholamines, which can suppress uterine contractions and restrict placental blood flow. Relaxation increases the progress of labor. Childbirth preparation classes enhance the mother's ability to work with her body rather than working against it. When a woman has realistic expectations about childbirth, she is more likely to have a positive experience.

## STAGES OF LABOR

For many years, labor was divided into three stages. In each of these three stages, specific events can be identified. A fourth stage has been acknowledged as being critical to the birth process: the recovery period after the birth of the baby. This chapter discusses four stages of labor. Table 3-3 presents an overview of the average duration of the first two stages. Stages 1 and 2 vary in average length for primigravida clients and multigravida clients. Stages 3 and 4 are approximately the same length for all clients and are not included in this table.

### FIRST STAGE: DILATION AND EFFACEMENT

The first stage of labor begins with the onset of regular contractions and ends when **cervical dilation**, the enlargement of the cervical opening (os), is complete (10 cm). This is usually the longest stage of labor and is divided into three phases: latent, active, and transition.

### Latent Phase

The latent phase of the first stage of labor ends when the cervix is dilated 3 cm and is the longest phase. Contractions occur every 10 to 20 minutes. The duration of the contractions lasts 15 to 30 seconds. The contraction intensity begins as mild and gradually becomes moderate.

The client is usually alert and often talkative. She is often relieved that labor has started yet anxious about what is ahead of her. This is a good time to review the client's preparations for labor and expectations of how labor and delivery will be handled (e.g., medications, persons present). Any needed teaching, especially breathing techniques, should be

undertaken at this time. If the membranes have not ruptured, many women prefer to walk during this time.

### Active Phase

The active phase of the first stage of labor begins when the cervix is dilated 4 cm and ends when the cervix is dilated 8 cm. Contractions occur every 3 to 5 minutes with a duration of 30 to 60 seconds. They are of moderate intensity, progressing to strong. Clients perceive varying degrees of discomfort. The client now focuses more on the breathing techniques during contractions and is less talkative.

### Transition Phase

The transition phase of the first stage of labor begins when the cervix is dilated 8 cm and ends when the cervix is dilated 10 cm. Contractions occur every 2 to 3 minutes with a duration of 60 to 90 seconds. There is little rest for the client between contractions. The intensity of the contractions is strong. The client usually needs to be reminded to focus, relax, and breathe with each contraction. She is very aware of the increasing intensity of the contractions, may become very restless, and may fear being left alone. Requests for medication often accompany statements like "I can't take it anymore." Following are characteristics of the transition phase:

- Restlessness
- Hyperventilation
- Bewilderment and sometimes anger
- Difficulty following directions
- Focus on self
- Irritability
- Statements like "Don't touch me"
- Nausea, occasionally vomiting
- Very warm feeling
- Perspiration on upper lip
- Increasing rectal pressure

### SECOND STAGE: BIRTH OF BABY

The second stage of labor begins when cervical dilation is complete (10 cm) and ends with the birth of the baby. Contractions continue at a frequency of every 1 to 2 minutes, duration of 60 to 90 seconds, and strong intensity. Now that the

| | FIRST STAGE | | | |
|---|---|---|---|---|
| CHARACTERISTIC | LATENT PHASE | ACTIVE PHASE | TRANSITION PHASE | SECOND STAGE |
| Primigravida | 8 to 20 hours | 6 hours | 2 hours | 1 hour |
| Multigravida | 5-14 hours | 4 hours | 1 hour | 15 minutes |
| Cervical dilation | 0 to 3 cm | 4 to 8 cm | 8 to 10 cm | 10 cm (full dilation) |
| **Contractions** | | | | |
| Frequency | 10 to 20 minutes | 3 to 5 minutes | 2 to 3 minutes | 1 to 2 minutes |
| Duration | 15 to 30 seconds | 30 to 60 seconds | 60 to 90 seconds | 60 to 90 seconds |
| Intensity | Mild progressing to moderate | Moderate progressing to strong | Strong | Strong |

**TABLE 3-3 Average Length of Labor Stages 1 and 2**

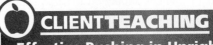

cervix is completely dilated, the mother can actively assist in the descent of the fetus by contracting the abdominal muscles and bearing down with each contraction. This active participation in the process often gives her a sense of control.

As the fetal head descends, it puts pressure on the pelvic nerves and the mother has a greater desire to push. Pressure from the fetal head makes the perineum bulge, then flatten and move anteriorly. With each contraction, the labia begin to separate and the baby's head is seen, but the head recedes between contractions. When the largest diameter of the fetal head is past the vulva (head can be seen between contractions), **crowning** has occurred and the birth is imminent (Figure 3-11). At this time, an **episiotomy**, an incision in the perineum to facilitate passage of the baby, may be performed (Figure 3-12). Routine episiotomies are no longer considered necessary, but in some cases, it is still warranted (CDC, 2008). The health-care provider may recommend an episiotomy if the baby is in an abnormal position, needs to be delivered quickly, or it appears that extensive vaginal tearing is going to occur. A few more contractions will push the head out, and a few more will deliver the body.

As the fetus moves through the pelvis and birth canal, several changes in position must occur. This series of movements is collectively called the mechanisms of labor or **cardinal movements**.

## Mechanisms of Labor

The mechanisms of labor are engagement, descent, flexion, internal rotation, extension, external rotation, and expulsion

(Figure 3-13). The first three generally occur during the first stage of labor.

**Engagement** As explained earlier, engagement occurs when the presenting part of the fetus (usually head) fully enters the true pelvis. It generally happens before labor begins in primigravidas and after labor begins in multigravidas.

**Descent** Descent begins with engagement and continues with each contraction throughout the labor process.

**Flexion** The fetal head is bent forward as it meets resistance during descent, causing the chin to rest on the sternum. This allows the narrowest part of the head to enter the pelvic outlet.

**Inernal Rotation** Internal rotation takes place mainly during the second stage of labor. The head rotates so the occiput is next to the symphysis pubis.

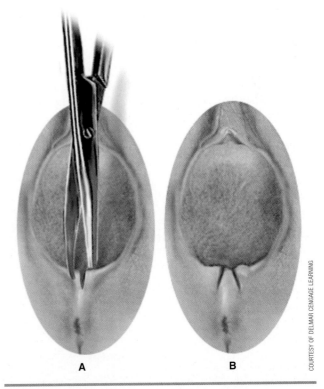

COURTESY OF DELMAR CENGAGE LEARNING

**A**    **B**

**FIGURE 3-12** Episiotomy; *A*, Midline, most common, directly toward anus; *B*, Right and left mediolateral, diagonal cut toward the side to prevent tearing into the rectum

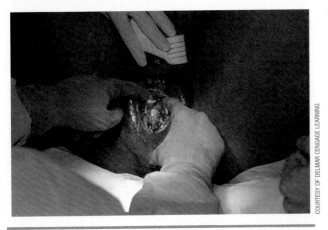

COURTESY OF DELMAR CENGAGE LEARNING

**FIGURE 3-11** Crowning

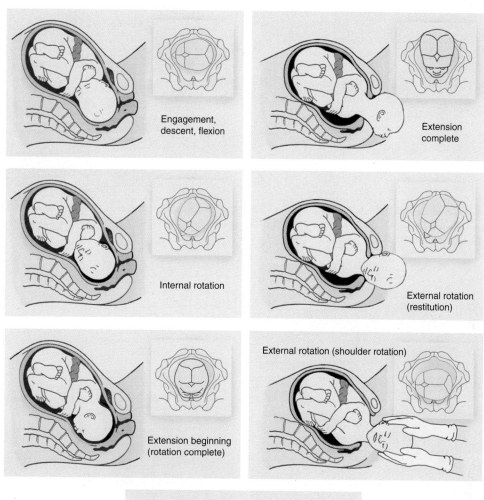

Engagement, descent, flexion

Extension complete

Internal rotation

External rotation (restitution)

Extension beginning (rotation complete)

External rotation (shoulder rotation)

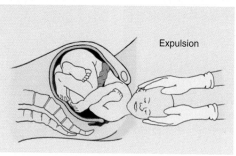

Expulsion

COURTESY OF DELMAR CENGAGE LEARNING

**FIGURE 3-13**  **Mechanisms of Labor**

**Extension**  As the fetal head continues to descend, the occiput pivots under the symphysis pubis and the fetal head becomes extended and pushes upward out of the vagina. The head is actually born at this time.

**Restitution and External Rotation**  Once the head has emerged, it rotates back to be in normal alignment with the shoulders. This is called **restitution**. Fetal position in the uterus can be identified by observing this turning of the head. The shoulders now rotate to be in an anteroposterior position under the symphysis pubis.

**Expulsion**  The health-care provider assisting with the birth applies gentle downward pressure on the baby's head to allow the anterior shoulder to emerge. Then the baby's head is gently raised so the posterior shoulder can be delivered. The rest of the baby's body then just slides out. This is called expulsion (Figure 3-14).

## THIRD STAGE: DELIVERY OF PLACENTA

The third stage of labor begins with the birth of the baby and ends with the delivery of the placenta. This should occur in 5 to 30 minutes. After the baby is born, the uterus continues contracting, decreasing its capacity and thereby reducing the surface area of placental attachment. The reduced surface area causes the placenta to separate from the uterine wall. As it separates, bleeding occurs, causing the formation of a retro-placental (behind the placenta) hematoma. This hematoma facilitates the separation process. The membranes are peeled from the uterine wall as the placenta slides into the vagina.

Signs that the placenta has separated should be observed about 5 to 10 minutes after the birth of the baby. These signs are:

- Globular shape of the uterus.

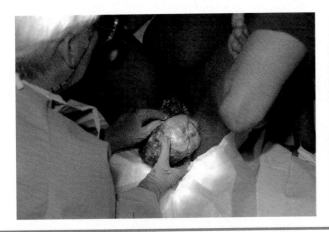
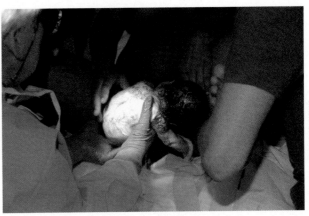

**FIGURE 3-14** Birth of an Infant

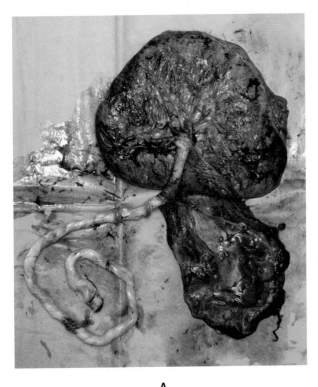
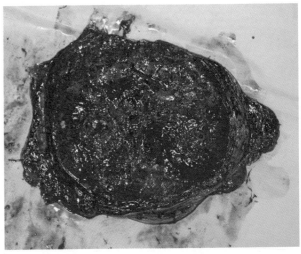

A                                          B

**FIGURE 3-15** *A,* Fetal Side (note empty amniotic sac); *B,* Maternal Side

- Gush of blood from the vagina.
- More of the cord protrudes from the vagina (is visible).

When these signs of placental separation have appeared, the client is asked to push one last time to deliver the placenta. Figure 3-15 shows a placenta.

The birthing facility disposes of the placenta after the delivery. Occasionally, a client may request to have the placenta to uphold cultural expectations.

## FOURTH STAGE: RECOVERY

The fourth stage of labor is the first 4 hours after the birth of the baby when the mother's body begins its physiological readjustments. Blood loss is usually between 250 mL and 500 mL. There is a moderate decrease in the systolic and diastolic blood pressure and an increase in pulse rate. The uterus should remain contracted to control bleeding and be

### CRITICAL THINKING

#### Care Throughout Labor

How and why does the care of the client change as she moves through the phases and stages of labor?

positioned in the midline of the abdomen about level with the umbilicus.

The new mother may be very hungry and thirsty. A shaking chill may be experienced in response to the ending of the physical work of labor. The bladder may be hypotonic due either to trauma during the second stage of labor and/or to decreased sensation from anesthesia. This may result in urinary retention. Mother–infant bonding is important in this stage.

## PROFESSIONAL TIP

### Prenatal Care and Childbirth Classes

- The client who has not had prenatal care or has not attended childbirth classes deserves the same care, support, and respect as the client who has had prenatal care and is prepared for childbirth.
- Nurses must be careful not to be judgmental toward clients who have not participated in prenatal care or childbirth classes.

## CULTURAL CONSIDERATIONS

### Client Beliefs

Most people believe that their own cultural beliefs are the best. The birth experience is given meaning by the client's cultural beliefs and practices. Incorporate cultural practices into care as much as possible as long as they are not detrimental to mother or fetus.

# ADMISSION OF CLIENT IN LABOR

Admission of a client in labor may be different for each person. Although there are standard nursing assessments and interventions for a woman in labor, each client must be cared for individually based on her particular situation. The priorities of establishing a nurse– client relationship and assessing the condition of mother and fetus may be undertaken in a sequential order or may need to be performed simultaneously.

It is important to determine which stage of labor the mother may be in at the time of admission. A few specific questions might include the following:

- When did your labor begin?
- How frequent are the contractions and how long do they last?
- Have the membranes ruptured? (Has your water broken?)
- What time did the membranes rupture?
- What was the color was the fluid?
- How many times have you been pregnant?
- How long were your other labors (if this is not the first pregnancy)?

Depending on the answers to these questions, a determination is made about how to proceed with the admission. When a woman is admitted in early labor, time can be taken to establish the nurse–client relationship by:

- Making the woman and her partner or family feel welcome
- Determining their expectations about the birth (did they attend childbirth classes?)
- Determining if a birth plan has been developed

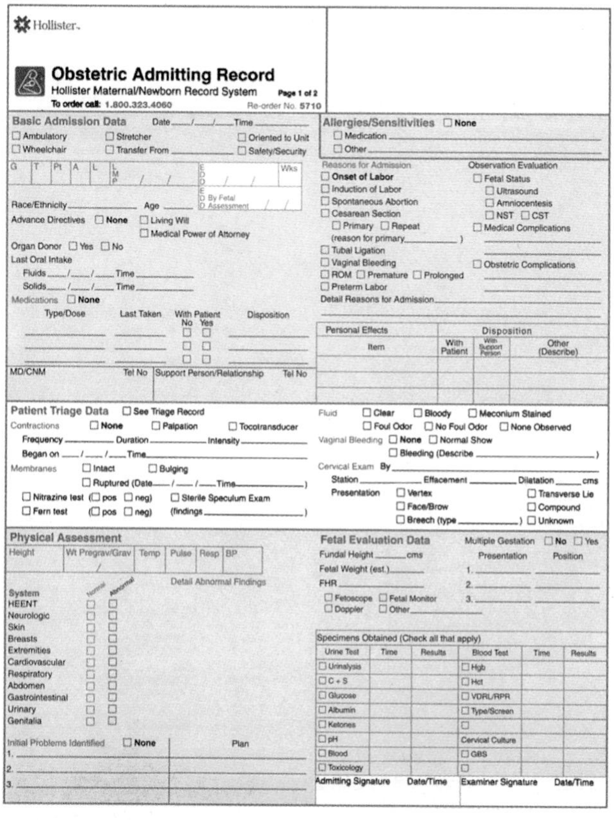

Hollister.
Obstetric Admitting Record
Hollister Maternal/Newborn Record System Page 1 of 2
To order call: 1.800.323.4060 Re-order No. 5710

Basic Admission Data Date ___/___/___ Time ___
☐ Ambulatory ☐ Stretcher ☐ Oriented to Unit
☐ Wheelchair ☐ Transfer From ___ ☐ Safety/Security
G T Pt A L LMP EDD Wks By Fetal Assessment
Race/Ethnicity ___ Age ___
Advance Directives ☐ None ☐ Living Will ☐ Medical Power of Attorney
Organ Donor ☐ Yes ☐ No
Last Oral Intake: Fluids ___/___/___ Time ___; Solids ___/___/___ Time ___
Medications ☐ None — Type/Dose, Last Taken, With Patient (No / Yes), Disposition
MD/CNM Tel No / Support Person/Relationship Tel No

Allergies/Sensitivities ☐ None ☐ Medication ___ ☐ Other ___
Reasons for Admission: ☐ Onset of Labor ☐ Induction of Labor ☐ Spontaneous Abortion ☐ Cesarean Section ☐ Primary ☐ Repeat (reason for primary ___) ☐ Tubal Ligation ☐ Vaginal Bleeding ☐ ROM ☐ Premature ☐ Prolonged ☐ Preterm Labor; Detail Reasons for Admission ___
Observation Evaluation: ☐ Fetal Status ☐ Ultrasound ☐ Amniocentesis ☐ NST ☐ CST ☐ Medical Complications ☐ Obstetric Complications
Personal Effects: Item, With Patient, With Support Person, Other (Describe)

Patient Triage Data ☐ See Triage Record
Contractions ☐ None ☐ Palpation ☐ Tocotransducer; Frequency ___ Duration ___ Intensity ___; Began on ___/___/___ Time ___
Membranes ☐ Intact ☐ Bulging ☐ Ruptured (Date ___/___/___ Time ___)
☐ Nitrazine test (☐ pos ☐ neg) ☐ Sterile Speculum Exam
☐ Fern test (☐ pos ☐ neg) (findings ___)
Fluid ☐ Clear ☐ Bloody ☐ Meconium Stained ☐ Foul Odor ☐ No Foul Odor ☐ None Observed
Vaginal Bleeding ☐ None ☐ Normal Show ☐ Bleeding (Describe ___)
Cervical Exam By ___ Station ___ Effacement ___ Dilatation ___ cms
Presentation ☐ Vertex ☐ Face/Brow ☐ Breech (type ___) ☐ Transverse Lie ☐ Compound ☐ Unknown

Physical Assessment: Height, Wt Pregrav/Grav, Temp, Pulse, Resp, BP
System (Normal / Abnormal), Detail Abnormal Findings: HEENT, Neurologic, Skin, Breasts, Extremities, Cardiovascular, Respiratory, Abdomen, Gastrointestinal, Urinary, Genitalia
Initial Problems Identified ☐ None — Plan: 1. 2. 3.

Fetal Evaluation Data — Multiple Gestation ☐ No ☐ Yes; Fundal Height ___ cms; Fetal Weight (est.) ___; FHR ___; Presentation, Position 1. 2. 3.; ☐ Fetoscope ☐ Fetal Monitor ☐ Doppler ☐ Other ___
Specimens Obtained (Check all that apply): Urine Test, Time, Results — ☐ Urinalysis ☐ C+S ☐ Glucose ☐ Albumin ☐ Ketones ☐ pH ☐ Blood ☐ Toxicology; Blood Test, Time, Results — ☐ Hgb ☐ Hct ☐ VDRL/RPR ☐ Type/Screen ☐ Cervical Culture ☐ GBS
Admitting Signature Date/Time Examiner Signature Date/Time

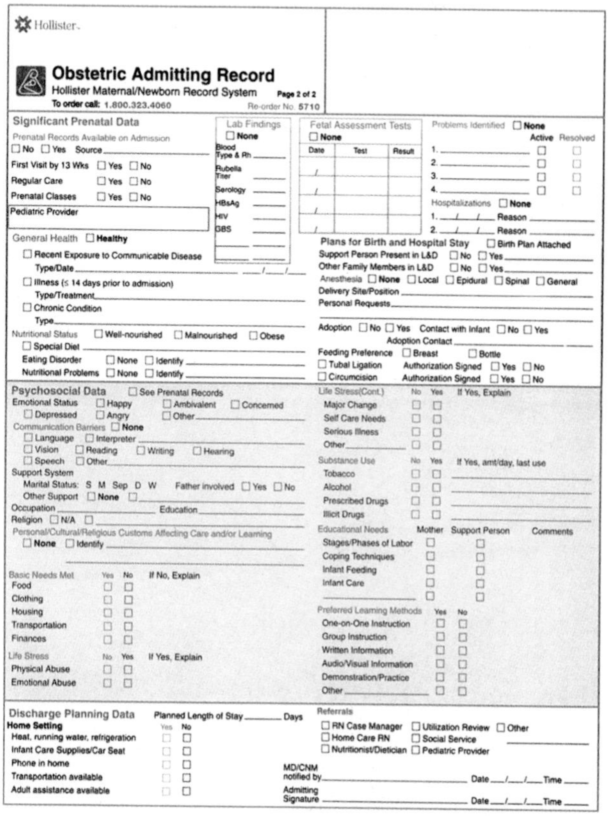

Hollister.
Obstetric Admitting Record
Hollister Maternal/Newborn Record System Page 2 of 2
To order call: 1.800.323.4060 Re-order No. 5710

Significant Prenatal Data
Prenatal Records Available on Admission ☐ No ☐ Yes Source ___
First Visit by 13 Wks ☐ Yes ☐ No; Regular Care ☐ Yes ☐ No; Prenatal Classes ☐ Yes ☐ No
Pediatric Provider
Lab Findings ☐ None: Blood Type & Rh, Rubella Titer, Serology, HBsAg, HIV, GBS
Fetal Assessment Tests ☐ None: Date, Test, Result
Problems Identified ☐ None — Active, Resolved 1. 2. 3. 4.
Hospitalizations ☐ None 1. ___/___/___ Reason 2. ___/___/___ Reason
General Health ☐ Healthy ☐ Recent Exposure to Communicable Disease Type/Date ☐ Illness (≤ 14 days prior to admission) Type/Treatment ☐ Chronic Condition Type
Nutritional Status ☐ Well-nourished ☐ Malnourished ☐ Obese ☐ Special Diet; Eating Disorder ☐ None ☐ Identify; Nutritional Problems ☐ None ☐ Identify
Plans for Birth and Hospital Stay ☐ Birth Plan Attached
Support Person Present in L&D ☐ No ☐ Yes; Other Family Members in L&D ☐ No ☐ Yes
Anesthesia ☐ None ☐ Local ☐ Epidural ☐ Spinal ☐ General
Delivery Site/Position; Personal Requests
Adoption ☐ No ☐ Yes Contact with Infant ☐ No ☐ Yes; Adoption Contact
Feeding Preference ☐ Breast ☐ Bottle
☐ Tubal Ligation Authorization Signed ☐ Yes ☐ No
☐ Circumcision Authorization Signed ☐ Yes ☐ No

Psychosocial Data ☐ See Prenatal Records
Emotional Status ☐ Happy ☐ Ambivalent ☐ Concerned ☐ Depressed ☐ Angry ☐ Other
Communication Barriers ☐ None ☐ Language ☐ Interpreter ☐ Vision ☐ Reading ☐ Writing ☐ Hearing ☐ Speech ☐ Other
Support System: Marital Status S M Sep D W; Father involved ☐ Yes ☐ No; Other Support ☐ None ☐
Occupation ___ Education ___; Religion ☐ N/A ☐
Personal/Cultural/Religious Customs Affecting Care and/or Learning ☐ None ☐ Identify
Basic Needs Met (Yes / No, If No, Explain): Food, Clothing, Housing, Transportation, Finances
Life Stress (No / Yes, If Yes, Explain): Physical Abuse, Emotional Abuse
Life Stress (Cont.) (No / Yes, If Yes, Explain): Major Change, Self Care Needs, Serious Illness, Other
Substance Use (No / Yes, If Yes, amt/day, last use): Tobacco, Alcohol, Prescribed Drugs, Illicit Drugs
Educational Needs (Mother, Support Person, Comments): Stages/Phases of Labor, Coping Techniques, Infant Feeding, Infant Care
Preferred Learning Methods (Yes / No): One-on-One Instruction, Group Instruction, Written Information, Audio/Visual Information, Demonstration/Practice, Other

Discharge Planning Data — Planned Length of Stay ___ Days
Home Setting (Yes / No): Heat, running water, refrigeration; Infant Care Supplies/Car Seat; Phone in home; Transportation available; Adult assistance available
Referrals ☐ RN Case Manager ☐ Utilization Review ☐ Other ☐ Home Care RN ☐ Social Service ☐ Nutritionist/Dietician ☐ Pediatric Provider
MD/CNM notified by ___ Date ___/___/___ Time ___
Admitting Signature ___ Date ___/___/___ Time ___

FIGURE 3-16 Representative Obstetric Admitting Record (*Permission to use this copyright material has been granted by the owner, Hollister Incorporated.*)

- Identifying cultural values and preferences related to the birth process

## INITIAL ASSESSMENT

After the nurse–client relationship has been established on admission, more specific assessments are made. Figure 3-16 shows a sample obstetric admitting record. Many facilities are changing to electronic client records. These records may be initiated in the health-care provider's office and are transferred to the nursing unit upon admission to the hospital. A copy of the prenatal record is generally sent to the birthing facility and is added to the client's record when she is admitted. Information can be obtained from the prenatal record. Clients who have not received prenatal care will need a more extensive assessment.

A physical examination is performed, including the following:

- Vital signs.
- Auscultation of heart and lungs.
- Leopold's maneuvers (described in Prenatal Care chapter) to determine fetal lie and presentation.
- Fetal heart rate (FHR) (described in Prenatal Care chapter), continuous electronic fetal monitoring may be used during the birthing process (described in Complications of Pregnancy chapter).
- Contractions for frequency, duration, and intensity.
- Nitrazine test, ferning test, Amnisure, or Aminoswab test if mother is not sure whether the membranes have ruptured.
- Vaginal examination (Figure 3-17) to determine cervical effacement and dilation, fetal position, and station; usually done by the registered nurse (RN) or CNM/physician.
- Inspection for signs of edema of face, hands, legs, and sacrum.

The FHR may be heard in various places on the mother's abdomen depending on the position of the fetus (Figure 3-18).

Contractions are assessed by placing the fingers of one hand on the fundus of the uterus, and using light pressure to

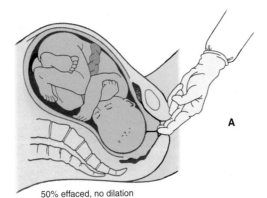

50% effaced, no dilation

A

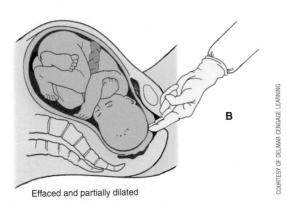

Effaced and partially dilated

B

COURTESY OF DELMAR CENGAGE LEARNING

**FIGURE 3-17** Vaginal Examination; *A*, 50% Effaced, No Dilation; *B*, 100% Effaced, Partly Dilated

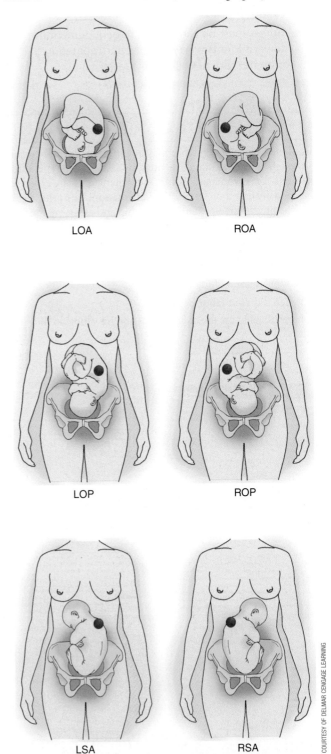

LOA   ROA

LOP   ROP

LSA   RSA

COURTESY OF DELMAR CENGAGE LEARNING

**FIGURE 3-18** Based on Leopold's maneuvers, FHR will best be heard in the marked areas for the various positions.

keep the fingers still. Contractions begin in the fundus and spread down the uterus. The person assessing the contractions can feel the tightening of the uterus before the mother is aware of it.

At least three contractions in a row should be assessed. The time each contraction begins and ends and the time lapse between contractions should be noted. The intensity can be estimated by how easily the uterus can be indented during a contraction.

- *Mild contraction*: Uterus is easily indented with the fingertips; feels like the tip of the nose.
- *Moderate contraction*: Uterus is more difficult to indent with the fingertips; feels similar to the chin.

**PROFESSIONAL**TIP

**Intrapartum Care for Obese Women**

Obesity in pregnant women during the intrapartum period can challenge nursing management. Special nursing care and preparation during birthing for obese clients includes:
- Maintaining a nonjudgmental attitude.
- Assessing the client for underlying medical conditions.
- Coordinating multidisciplinary care involving CNM/physicians, anesthesia providers, and nursing staff.
- Determining if the unit's furniture and equipment are appropriate and safe for obese clients.
- Evaluating equipment for size and weight limits (beds, operating tables, commodes, blood pressure cuffs, gowns, walkers, scales, wheel chairs, transfer devices, external fetal monitoring equipment and belts, and intermittent pneumatic compression devices).
- Assessing availability of extra staff nurses to assist in moving and positioning of client during certain procedures (amniotomy, analgesia, and pushing).

(James & Maher, 2009)

- *Strong contraction*: Uterus unable to be indented with the fingertips; feels like the forehead.

# NURSING PROCESS

The nurse is an important member of the team that helps the mother successfully progress through the birth experience.

## ASSESSMENT

The nurse's role begins with a thorough assessment of the laboring woman and her progress.

### Subjective Data

Subjective data to be gathered throughout labor and birth of the infant include the comfort of the mother, her ability to cope, and her desire to urinate or defecate.

### Objective Data

Objective data include vital signs; FHR; frequency, duration, interval, and intensity of contractions; fetopelvic relationships, including fetal attitude, fetal lie, fetal presentation, and station; condition of membranes; maternal behavior, including tone of voice and facial expressions; and maternal verbalizations. Table 3-4 provides suggested time frames for selected assessments.

## NURSING DIAGNOSES

Many different nursing diagnoses may be appropriate for a client during labor and the birthing process. Selected nursing diagnoses appropriate for the first three stages of labor are listed.

- *Anxiety*
- *Impaired Verbal Communication*
- *Ineffective Coping*
- *Interrupted Family Processes*
- *Fatigue*
- *Fear*
- *Risk for Deficient Fluid Volume*
- *Gas Exchange Impaired (fetal)*
- *Risk for Infection*
- *Risk for Injury*
- *Deficient Knowledge*
- *Acute Pain*

**PROFESSIONAL**TIP

**Station**

- It is often a challenge to remember the notations of station.
- Remember, plus (+) is what is desired; the presenting part is below the level of the ischial spines. Minus (–) means the presenting part is not yet to the level of the ischial spines.

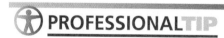

**TABLE 3-4 Suggested Time Frames for Selected Assessments**

| ASSESSMENT | LATENT PHASE | ACTIVE PHASE | TRANSITION PHASE | SECOND STAGE |
|---|---|---|---|---|
| BP, P, R | every 1 h | every 1 h | every 30 min | every 5 min |
| Temperature | every 4 h | every 4 h | every 4 h | |
| (if ROM) | every 2 h | every 2 h | every 2 h | |
| FHR | every 1 h | every 30 min | every 15 min | every 15 min |
| Contractions | every 1 h | every 30 min | every 15 min | continuously |

- *Impaired **P**hysical Mobility*
- *Social Isolation*
- *Impaired **U**rinary Elimination*

## PLANNING/OUTCOME IDENTIFICATION

Based on the client's expectations of labor and the birthing process and the assessments performed by the facility staff, the planning and goals can be mutually set by the client and the nurse. Examples of possible goals may include that the client will:

- Demonstrate expected progress through labor
- Express satisfaction with the assistance provided by her support person and facility staff
- Maintain adequate hydration with oral and/or IV intake
- Void at least every 2 hours to prevent bladder distention
- Actively participate in the labor process
- Not experience any injury during the labor and birthing process

## NURSING INTERVENTIONS

Nursing interventions focus on continuing assessment of labor progress and fetal well-being, providing maternal physical care, assisting the client and her support person, and providing or assisting with pharmacologic comfort measures.

### Continuing Assessment of Labor and Fetal Well-Being

Continuing assessment of labor progress and fetal well-being is performed as previously discussed. Any changes outside the normally expected changes must be reported immediately. Some facilities use continuous electronic fetal monitoring on all clients; however, the nurse should still personally assess and time contractions and listen to the FHR at regular intervals. Figure 3-19 presents a sample labor in progress record.

### Providing Maternal Physical Care

Maternal physical care includes comfort measures, hygiene measures, ambulation and position, food and fluid intake, and elimination.

**Comfort Measures** Many comfort measures can be used with the client in labor. Some may work with one client and not the next, or may work for a while with one client and then she will not want that comfort measure used any more. Comfort measures include the following:

- Offer the client fluids and ice chips as ordered per institutional policy
- Provide oral care
- Assist the client with frequent position changes, encouraging side-lying or upright positions
- Encourage voluntary relaxation of specific muscle groups and the use of effleurage
- Suggest the use of a cold washcloth on the forehead or nape of the neck
- Provide encouragement and praise
- Keep the client informed of progress
- Palpate for bladder distention and encourage urination every 2 hours
- Give a back rub or apply counterpressure to the sacrococcygeal area
- Assist the client in walking and using a shower or Jacuzzi
- Offer the client analgesics as ordered
- Offer the client complementary therapies such as aromatherapy, massage, use of birth balls, hydrotherapy, and music therapy (Zwelling, Johnson, & Allen, 2006)

**Hygiene Measures** If showers or jacuzzis are available and are not contraindicated for the client, their use should be offered to the client. The discomfort of labor is often reduced by these measures. Bed linens should be kept clean and dry. Linen savers should be changed frequently.

**Ambulation and Position** Ambulation may increase uterine activity, provide distraction from the discomforts of labor, and enhance maternal control of the situation. The client should be encouraged to walk only if the membranes are still intact, the presenting part is engaged after ROM, and if she has not had pain medication.

The side-lying position promotes utero-placental blood flow (and thus fetal oxygenation) and renal blood flow. If the client wants to lie on her back, a pillow can be placed under one hip to keep the uterus from compressing the aorta and vena cava. Both the squatting position and the hands-and-knees position seem to facilitate an occiput posterior fetal position to rotate to an anterior position.

**Food and Fluid Intake** Clear liquids and ice chips are usually all that is offered to clients in labor. Because regional anesthesia has almost replaced general anesthesia in childbirth, the risk of aspiration is also almost eliminated, and the practice of giving clear liquids only is being challenged (Lowdermilk & Perry, 2006).

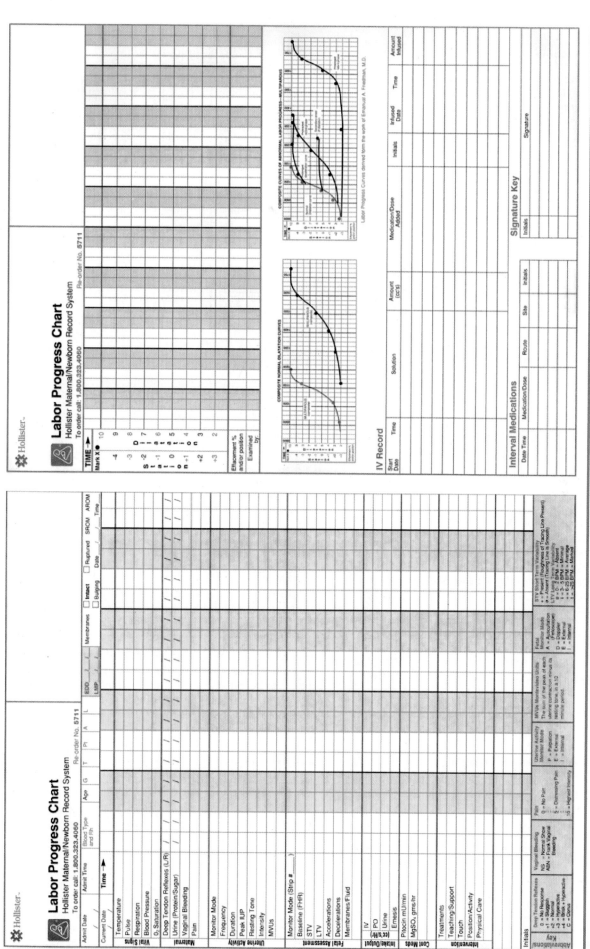

FIGURE 3-19   Representative Labor Progress Record (*Permission to use this copyright material has been granted by the owner, Hollister Incorporated.*)

In some facilities, IV fluids are started on every client. It is very important to keep an accurate I&O when IV fluids are infusing because of the danger of hypervolemia.

Elimination The client should be encouraged to void every 2 hours. A distended bladder may impede descent of the presenting part, cause undue discomfort, and lead to bladder atony after the birth.

If allowed, getting up to go to the bathroom may be the easiest for the client. Sitting on a bedpan at the edge of the bed with feet on a chair may be the next best option.

Catheterization may be required if the client cannot void and the bladder is distended. The vulva and perineum must be thoroughly cleaned to remove any amniotic fluid and bloody show before catheterization. If the catheter cannot be inserted, the presenting part is probably compressing the urethra. The procedure must be discontinued and the CNM/physician notified.

Because of the decrease in intestinal motility, most women do not have a bowel movement during labor; however, the pushing and birth of the infant during the second stage of labor may cause some stool to be expelled from the rectum. This should be cleaned immediately and the client reassured that this is a normal and expected outcome.

## Assisting Client and Support Person

The support person many times is the father, but it may be another woman or man. The person the mother has chosen to be the support person should be treated with the same respect as the mother, regardless of the relationship to the mother or the fetus.

The client who has participated in childbirth preparation classes with a support person already has some skills and a plan for coping with labor and birth. The nurse should determine what that plan is and assist, as needed, in carrying out that plan.

The client and support person who have not attended childbirth preparation classes should be taught the various techniques of coping with labor during the latent phase of labor. The nurse may actually provide more of the supportive care in this situation.

Breathing Techniques Three different breathing patterns are used. The first pattern is used until it is no longer effective, then the next pattern is used. Each breathing pattern begins and ends with a deep cleansing breath, with inhalation through the nose and exhalation through pursed lips, moving only the chest. The breathing techniques:

- Provide adequate oxygenation of mother and fetus
- Provide a focus of attention
- Decrease anxiety
- Increase mental and physical relaxation

These breathing patterns are used only during a uterine contraction. Between contractions, breathing returns to the woman's regular breathing pattern. The client is encouraged to rest between contractions.

*Slow, Deep Chest Breathing* For this pattern, the client takes a cleansing breath, then inhales through the nose and exhales through pursed lips, 6 to 9 breaths per minute. At the end of the contraction, she takes another cleansing breath. It takes concentration to breathe this slowly.

*Shallow Breathing* A cleansing breath is taken first. The client inhales and exhales through the mouth about 4 times every 5 seconds. This may be increased to 2 breaths per second, usually at the peak of a contraction. The client should take another deep cleansing breath at the end of the contraction.

*Pant-Blow Breathing* The pant-blow breathing is generally used when the contractions become very intense. This pattern is very similar to the shallow breathing except that every three or four breaths a forceful exhalation (blow) is made through pursed lips. A cleansing breath is taken at the beginning and end of the contraction. It takes great concentration to maintain this pattern during a contraction.

All clients should be kept informed of their progress in labor. Positive feedback to the client and support person regarding how they are coping with the labor process is also important.

If siblings are to be present for labor and the birth, another person should be there to watch over the children and provide them with explanations, diversions, and comfort as needed. Neither the support person nor the nurses should be responsible for the children. Their focus should be on the client.

## Providing Pharmacological Comfort Measures

The nonpharmacological comfort measures may be all that is needed for some women in labor. For other women, the increasing discomfort interferes with their ability to relax, use the breathing techniques appropriately, and maintain a sense of control. Pharmacological comfort measures include systemic medications, regional blocks, and general anesthesia.

Systemic Medications Systemic medications should be administered only if:

- The client is willing to receive them and her vital signs are stable.
- The fetus is at term, exhibits regular movement, has a FHR between 110 and 160 with no late or variable decelerations and average variability.
- Contractions are well established with the cervix dilated at least 4 to 5 cm in a nullipara or 3 to 4 cm in a multipara, the presenting part is engaged, and no complications are identified.

Effect on the fetus depends on the dosage given, timing and route of administration, and the pharmacokinetics of the drug. The intravenous (IV) route is generally preferred over the intramuscular (IM) route because the drug's effect is faster and more reliable. Table 3-5 lists drugs commonly used for pain management during labor.

### CRITICAL THINKING

#### Pushing in Labor

A client gravida 1 para 0 in labor is 7 cm dilated, station +1, and says that she wants to push. Her grandmother told her that she would have to push hard to have a baby, so the client wants to push and get it over with. How should the nurse respond?

**TABLE 3-5 Pain-Management Drugs Commonly Used During Labor**

| DRUG | ROUTE | ONSET | PEAK EFFECT | LASTING |
|---|---|---|---|---|
| **Narcotic Analgesics** | | | | |
| meperidine | IV | 30 sec | 5 to 10 min | 2 to 4 hr |
| (Demerol) | IM | 10 to 15 min | 40 to 50 min | 2 to 4 hr |
| fentanyl citrate | IV | 1 to 2 min | 3 to 5 min | 1/2 to 1 hr |
| (Sulimaze) | IM | 7 to 10 min | 20 to 30 min | 1 to 2 hr |
| **Narcotic Agonist-Antagonists** | | | | |
| nalbuphine hydrochloride | IV | 2 to 3 min | 30 min | 3 to 4 hr |
| (Nubain) | IM | 15 min | 60 min | 3 to 6 hr |
| butorphanol tartrate | IV | 2 to 3 min | ½ to 1 hr | 2 to 4 hr |
| (Stadol) | IM | 10 to 30 min | ½ to 1 hr | 3 to 4 hr |
| pentazocine lactate | IV | 2 to 3 min | 15 to 30 min | 2 to 3 hr |
| (Talwin) | IM | 15 to 20 min | 30 to 60 min | 2 to 3 hr |
| **Narcotic Antagonist** | | | | |
| Naloxone | IV | 1 to 2 min | unknown | depends on dose |
| (Narcan) | IM | 2 to 5 min | unknown | longer than IV |
| **Analgesic Potentiators** | | | | |
| promethazine hydrochloride | IV | 3 to 5 min | unknown | 12 hr |
| (Phenergan) | IM | 20 min | unknown | 12 hr |
| hydroxyzine hydrochloride Z-track (Atarax, Vistaril) | IM only | unknown | unknown | 4 to 6 hr |

**Regional Blocks** Several types of regional blocks may be used during labor and/or birth, including epidural block, intrathecal block, local infiltration, and pudendal block.

**Epidural Block** An epidural block may be used for pain control during labor and birth. It may be a continuous or intermittent infusion of a local anesthetic drug through a catheter placed in the epidural space. A very small dose of fentanyl (Sublimaze) or sufentanil (Sufenta) is often added to the local anesthetic drug for faster and longer-lasting relief of pain. Advantages

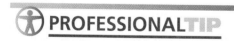

## PROFESSIONALTIP

### Pain-Relief Medications

Before receiving a medication, the client should understand the following:

- Type of medication
- Route of administration
- Expected effects of the medication
- Possible side effects of the medication
- Implications for the fetus/neonate
- Safety measures to be followed (e.g., stay in bed, have siderails up)
- Duration of effects of the medication

are good pain control, yet the client can participate in the birth process and interact with her infant and support person. Disadvantages may include maternal hypotension, bladder distention, epidural catheter migration, nausea and vomiting, pruritis, and delayed respiratory depression.

**Intrathecal Block** Intrathecal injection of an opioid analgesic such as fentanyl (Sublimaze), sufentanil (Sufenta), or morphine (Duramorph) is a pain management option for labor. A much smaller dose than is given systemically is injected into the subarachnoid space. Advantages are rapid onset yet no sedation, no hypotensive effect, and no motor block, so the client may walk during labor. Disadvantages may include the short duration of action so that the client may require another injection and the inadequate relief of pain in late labor and during birth so that another pain relief measure is required.

**Local Infiltration** Local infiltration anesthesia of the perineum is achieved by injecting a local anesthetic into the perineum. This is used just before the time of birth in preparation for performing an episiotomy, suturing a laceration, or when a pudendal block cannot be performed. Local anesthetics such as procaine hydrochloride (Novocain), chloroprocaine hydrochloride (Nesacaine), and tetracaine hydrochloride (Pontocaine), which metabolize rapidly, and bupivacaine hydrochloride (Marcaine), lidocaine hydrochloride (Xylocaine), and mepivacaine hydrochloride (Carbocaine), which are more powerful and longer-acting, are often used. Advantages are that the procedure is technically uncomplicated

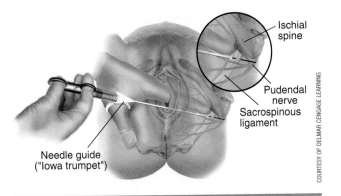

FIGURE 3-20 Pudendal block provides anesthesia to the perineum, external genitalia, and lower vagina.

and practically free of complications. A disadvantage is that a large amount of local anesthetic may be required.

***Pudendal Block*** A **pudendal block** is not commonly used today. It is the injection of a local anesthetic into the pudendal nerve to provide perineal, external genitalia, and lower vaginal anesthesia (Figure 3-20). The pudendal block may be performed during the transition phase of the first stage or the second stage of labor. The advantage is that there are no changes in maternal vital signs or the FHR. Disadvantages may include rectal puncture, sciatic nerve block, or a hematoma.

**General Anesthesia** Because general anesthesia involves loss of consciousness, it is rarely used in vaginal births. It is used for cesarean births only in extreme emergency situations. The greatest danger is fetal depression because most general anesthetics reach the fetus in about 2 minutes.

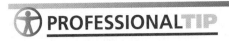

### Meperidine (Demerol) Use in Labor

When meperidine (Demerol) is given IM during labor, the birth of the infant should ideally occur in less than 1 hour after administration or more than 4 hours after administration (time of peak affect) to minimize respiratory depression of the neonate.

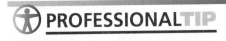

### Narcotic Agonist-Antagonists and Narcotic Antagonists Administration

The drugs nalbuphine hydrochloride (Nubain), butorphanol tartrate (Stadol), pentazocine lactate (Talwin), and naloxone (Narcan) should not be given to substance-dependent clients because these drugs may precipitate withdrawal symptoms.

# RISKS OF LABOR AND BIRTH

Most labors and births proceed as expected; however, there are complications that may be anticipated and some that happen unexpectedly. The most common risks—preterm labor and birth, premature rupture of membranes, dystocia, abnormal duration of labor, and prolapsed cord—are discussed.

## PRETERM LABOR AND BIRTH

**Preterm labor** is the onset of regular contractions of the uterus that cause cervical changes between 20 and 37 weeks of gestation. **Preterm birth** is a birth that takes place before the end of the 37th week of gestation. Only about half of the time can a precipitating cause be identified. The single most important factor predisposing to preterm labor and birth is having already had a preterm birth. Other factors often associated with preterm labor and birth include premature rupture of the membranes (PROM), multiple gestation, bacterial vaginosis, intraamniotic infection, bleeding, and uterine/cervical abnormalities.

Most women in preterm labor are admitted to the hospital for further evaluation. A urine specimen is examined for evidence of a urinary tract infection. Cervical or vaginal secretions are obtained during a sterile speculum examination to culture for Chlamydia trachomatis, group B streptococcus, or gonococcus infections.

If contractions are continuing and cervical changes are occurring, tocolytic agents may be prescribed. **Tocolytic agents** are medications that inhibit contractions. The most commonly used are terbutaline (Breathine) and magnesium sulfate. A corticosteroid may also be given to accelerate fetal lung maturation. There is greater fetal benefit if at least 24 hours elapse between the first dose and the birth.

If contractions subside and cervical dilation and effacement remain the same, the client may be discharged with instructions to limit activities and medication to prevent labor.

## PREMATURE RUPTURE OF MEMBRANES

When the membranes rupture before labor begins, it is called premature rupture of membranes (PROM). This is the most common cause of preterm labor. Contractions usually begin

### LIFE SPAN CONSIDERATIONS

#### Risks of Labor and Birth

- Adolescents (younger than age 15) have a greater risk of preterm labor, prolonged labor, and dystocia related to the small size of the pelvis because they have not yet reached bone growth maturity, which results in cephalopelvic disproportion (CPD).
- Mature women (older than age 35) have a greater risk of preterm labor, longer labor, cesarean birth, and dystocia related to fetal anomalies.

(Lowdermilk & Perry, 2006)

within 24 hours when the client is at term. In pregnancies of 28 to 34 weeks' gestation, labor may not start for a week or more. If the amniotic membranes rupture before labor begins in a client who is less than 37 weeks gestation, it is called preterm premature rupture of membranes (PPROM). African American mothers are more at risk for occurrence and reoccurrence of PPROM than Caucasian mothers, with the greatest risk at less than 28 weeks gestation (Shen, DeFranco, Stamilio, Chang, & Muglia, 2008).

In most cases of PROM, the cause is unknown. New evidence suggests that a contributing factor to preterm delivery is intrauterine infection (Hutzal, Boyle, Kenyon, Nash, Winsor, Taylor, & Kirpalani, 2008).

Besides preterm labor and birth, PROM can result in prolapse of the cord and intrauterine infection. A positive identification of amniotic fluid is made by observation of amniotic fluid escape from the cervix during a sterile speculum examination, a positive nitrazine test, a positive Amnisure or Amnioswab test, or the presence of ferning when the fluid is viewed under a microscope. The client may be hospitalized until after the birth of the infant, or if there are no signs of infections or fetal distress, she may be sent home. If hospitalized, continuing assessments include maternal vital signs; FHR; fetal movements; vaginal discharge for odor, color, and amount; and palpation of the uterus for tenderness.

## DYSTOCIA

**Dystocia** is a long, difficult, or abnormal labor caused by any of the five major variables (5 Ps) that affect labor. The following may be causes:

- Dysfunctional labor: ineffective contractions or maternal pushing efforts (powers).
- Pelvic structure variations (passageway).
- Fetal variations: anomalies, abnormal presentation, very large size, or number of fetuses (passenger).
- Mother's responses: related to preparation for childbirth, past experiences, culture, and support persons (psychological response).
- Engagement of the presenting part, station, and fetal position (position).

## Dysfunctional Labor

**Dysfunctional labor** is a labor with problems of the contractions or with maternal bearing-down efforts. The contractions may be hypertonic or hypotonic.

**Hypertonic Uterine Contractions** Hypertonic uterine contractions, usually occurring in the latent phase of labor, are very frequent and uncoordinated and have an increased resting tone. The mother has discomfort out of proportion to the intensity of the contractions, which do not dilate or efface the cervix. The excessive pain results from anoxia of the uterine muscle cells. A prolonged latent phase is generally the result.

The client may become fatigued and dehydrated and may express fear that she is losing control with the lack of progress. The fetus may experience distress because the hypertonic contractions and increased resting tone of the uterus interfere with uteroplacental blood flow. The increased and prolonged pressure on the fetal head may cause excessive molding, caput succedaneum, or cephalhematoma (discussed in Newborn chapter).

Bed rest and analgesics such as morphine sulfate or meperidine hydrochloride (Demerol) are given to relieve pain, promote relaxation, and induce sleep. When the client awakens, uterine contractions are often normal and labor proceeds.

**Hypotonic Uterine Contractions** Hypotonic uterine contractions, also called uterine inertia, usually occur in the active phase of labor. After normal progress through the latent phase of labor, the contractions become weak and inefficient in the active phase and may even cease. Common causes are cephalopelvic disproportion (CPD) (discussed later), malposition of the fetus, an overstretched uterus from multiple fetuses, a fetus of very large body size, hydramnios, or grandmultiparity (having delivered more than six infants).

The risks for the mother include intrauterine infection, especially if the membranes are ruptured and labor is prolonged; postpartum hemorrhage caused by inefficient uterine contractions

---

### ::|:: COMMUNITY/HOME HEALTH CARE

#### Preterm Labor

- Follow instructions regarding activity limitation.
- Monitor uterine contractions 2 to 3 times a day for 30 minutes to 1 hour.
- Count fetal movements as instructed.
- Practice relaxation techniques.
- Drink 8 to 10 (8 oz) glasses of fluids each day.
- Empty bladder frequently.
- Avoid smoking, alcohol, and nontherapeutic drugs.
- Limit caffeine intake (colas, coffee, tea, chocolate).
- Avoid activities that can stimulate labor (e.g., nipple stimulation, any sexual activity that causes orgasm).
- Take medications as prescribed.
- Keep appointments with CNM/physician.

---

### ::|:: COMMUNITY/HOME HEALTH CARE

#### Premature Rupture of Membranes

- Stay in bed, lying on either side, except to go to the bathroom (or as instructed).
- Take temperature every 4 hours when awake.
- Count fetal movements daily (report if less than 4 in 1 hour or an abnormal increase).
- Be aware of uterine contractions; if frequency is less than 10 minutes, notify CNM/physician.
- Use good perineal hygiene (e.g., wipe from front to back).
- Report any foul-smelling vaginal discharge or uterine tenderness.
- Take showers or sponge baths, not a tub bath.
- Avoid breast stimulation, sexual stimulation, and sexual intercourse.

after birth; exhaustion; and decreased coping ability. The fetus may experience distress because of the length of labor and sepsis from maternal pathogens ascending the birth canal.

An ultrasound is usually performed to rule out CPD. If all factors are normal, one or more measures for augmentation of (increasing) labor are instituted, including ambulation, amniotomy, nipple stimulation, and oxytocin infusion (discussed later).

***Amniotomy*** An **amniotomy**, artificial rupture of membranes (AROM), is performed by the CNM/physician. Several linen savers and a folded bath towel are placed under the client to absorb the amniotic fluid. A disposable plastic hook (amnihook) is generally used (Figure 3-21). A vaginal examination is performed to determine dilation, effacement, presenting part, and station, and FHR is assessed to determine fetal well-being. If the presenting part is not engaged or if the presentation is not cephalic, the risk of a prolapsed cord is high and the amniotomy is generally not performed.

After an amniotomy, the FHR must be assessed for 1 full minute. A monitor pattern that is nonreassuring or has any significant changes must be promptly reported to the CNM/physician. Amniotic fluid odor, color, and quantity are documented. The fluid should be clear (sometimes flecks of vernix are present) with a mild odor. Greenish meconium-stained fluid may indicate placental insufficiency. Foul-smelling fluid or fluid with a strong odor with a cloudy appearance or yellow color often indicates chorioamnionitis. Maternal temperature should be taken every hour after ROM and any elevation above 38°C (100.4°F) reported to the CNM/physician.

**Maternal Bearing-Down Efforts** Analgesia and/or anesthesia may block Ferguson's reflex and thus decrease the effectiveness of maternal bearing down. Lack of sleep, a long labor, inadequate hydration, and maternal position may also have an adverse effect on the mother's bearing-down efforts.

## Pelvic Structure Variations

A woman with a small or abnormally shaped pelvis may experience a long and difficult labor. Only about 50% of women have the pelvic shape (gynecoid) most conducive to labor, fetal descent, and birth (Murray et al., 2001).

A distended bladder reduces the space available in the pelvis and is an obstruction to fetal descent. This greatly increases the client's discomfort. Other, less common obstructions are uterine fibroids or pelvic cysts.

## Fetal Variations

Variations of the fetus that may cause dystocia include the following:

- Anomalies
- Abnormal presentation or position
- Size
- Number of fetuses

**Anomalies** Fetal anomalies such as hydrocephalus may prevent descent of the fetus. Anomalies are often discovered by an ultrasound during pregnancy. If a vaginal birth is not advisable or not possible, a cesarean birth is scheduled.

**Abnormal Presentation or Position** A cephalic presentation other than vertex makes a larger diameter of the fetal head move through the birth canal. Labor generally takes longer and is more difficult.

In a breech presentation, cervical effacement and dilatation are often slower because the buttocks are softer than the head and do not put firm pressure on the cervix to aid in dilation. Following are risks to the fetus born in a breech presentation:

- Prolapsed cord
- Cord compression
- Aspiration of fluids in the vagina
- Head becoming stuck

**External version** (manipulation of the fetus through the mother's abdomen to a presentation facilitating birth) may be tried to change the presentation to cephalic.

It is not always possible to change the presentation of the fetus. Figure 3-22 illustrates the birth of a fetus in a complete breech presentation.

A position of occiput posterior or occiput transverse can contribute to dysfunctional labor. Labor is generally longer and causes more discomfort because the head has farther to rotate during internal rotation. Many women describe severe back pain and have leg pain on the side where the head is positioned. A change in the mother's position may promote rotation of the fetal head. When the mother's abdomen is dependent to her spine, as in the hands-and-knees position, fetal rotation is encouraged (Figure 3-23).

**Size** An infant weighing more than 4,000 g (8.8 lb) is said to be **macrosomic**—having a very large body size. This may cause problems for a vaginal birth. As long as the mother's pelvis is of a size and shape to accommodate an infant this size, there is no problem. When the fetal head will not fit through the mother's pelvis, it is called **cephalopelvic disproportion (CPD)**. The cause can be either fetal or maternal. The fetal head may be abnormally large and the mother's pelvis of normal size and shape, or the fetal head may be of average size and the mother's pelvis small or abnormally shaped. Whatever the cause, a cesarean birth is required.

**Number of Fetuses** When more than one fetus is present, the uterus is overdistended. One or more of the fetuses may be

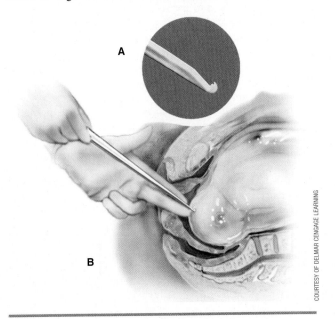

COURTESY OF DELMAR CENGAGE LEARNING

**FIGURE 3-21** *A,* Disposable Plastic Hook to Rupture Membranes; *B,* Technique for Rupturing Membranes

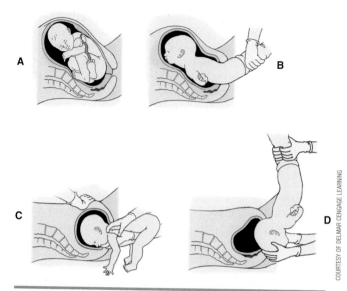

FIGURE 3-22  **Birth of Fetus in Complete Breech Presentation; _A_, Descent and Internal Rotation; _B_, Extension of Fetal Back Under Symphysis (Towel on Legs Used for Traction); _C_, CNM/Physician Maintains Head Flexion by Putting Pressure on Lower Face with Fingers of Left Hand (Suprapubic Pressure is Applied by Assistant to Keep Fetal Head Flexed); _D_, Assistant Holds Fetal Legs with Towel while CNM/Physician Assists the Face and Head Over the Perineum**

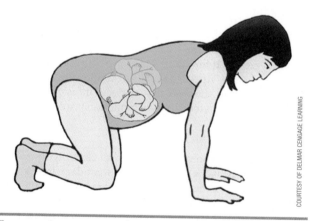

FIGURE 3-23  **Fetus tends to rotate from occiput posterior to occiput anterior when mother is in a hands-and-knees position.**

in a presentation less desirable than vertex. Twins often have a cesarean birth, and when there are three or more fetuses, birth is almost always cesarean.

## Mother's Responses

The mother's perception of labor is more important than her actual experience in labor. Tales from family and friends, a bad experience with a previous labor, and cultural expectations can add to the stress of labor. Excessive or prolonged stress experienced by the woman in labor may interfere with the progress of labor in several ways:

- Secretion of catecholamines (epinephrine and norepinephrine) by the adrenal glands in response to stress inhibits uterine contractions and decreases blood supply to the uterus and placenta while increasing blood supply to the skeletal muscles.

- Tense abdominal and pelvic muscles make contractions less effective.
- Contractions working against tense abdominal muscles increase pain, which adds stress to the situation and makes the mother more anxious.

The nurse can help allay the client's fears by offering encouragement, answering her questions honestly, and offering tips on how to make labor more successful. For instance, the nurse might suggest a change of position to a squatting bar to aid in fetal descent, or may offer a mirror so the mother can see the baby crown and be encouraged by her progress.

## ABNORMAL DURATION OF LABOR

Labor may be prolonged or abnormally short (precipitate).

### Prolonged Labor

Many of the conditions previously discussed, such as hypotonic uterine contractions, CPD, abnormal fetal presentations or positions, or early use of analgesics may cause prolonged labor. Labor progress in either the first or second stage may be prolonged or arrested (stopped). The plotting of cervical dilation on a labor graph, as found in Figure 3-19, helps in identifying these situations. Once the cause of the prolonged labor is identified, the CNM/physician can take steps to remedy the situation. A possible course of action might be induction of labor, a forceps- or vacuum-assisted birth, or cesarean birth (all discussed later).

When the active phase of the first stage of labor lasts more than 15 hours, the risk of fetal death increases (Lowdermilk & Perry, 2006). With prolonged labor, maternal morbidity and mortality may result from infection, uterine rupture, serious dehydration, and postpartum hemorrhage.

### Precipitate Labor/Precipitate Birth

A labor lasting less than 3 hours from the onset of contractions to the birth of the infant is considered a **precipitate labor**. Although a precipitate labor may end with a precipitate birth, they are not the same. Possible maternal complications during a precipitate labor include a loss of coping ability; an increased risk of uterine rupture; lacerations of the cervix, vagina, and perineum; and postpartum hemorrhage. Possible fetal complications include hypoxia, distress, and cerebral trauma.

A **precipitate birth** is a birth occurring suddenly and unexpectedly without a CNM/physician to assist. When a client says "the baby's coming" or words to that effect, the health care provider should always inspect to see whether she is correct. Most of the time a large part of the fetal head is visible, if not already crowning. In this situation the nurse should do the following:

- Stay with the mother.
- Call for assistance or send support person to get assistance. Other staff members can notify the CNM/ physician.
- Remain calm and reassure mother.
- Open emergency birth pack.
- If time permits, scrub hands, put on sterile gloves, and place sterile drape under mother's buttocks.
- As the head crowns, instruct mother to pant.
- If membranes are still intact, tear the sac, allowing amniotic fluid to flow out.
- Apply gentle pressure to the fetal head with one hand to prevent it from popping out. _Do not hold the head back with force enough to prevent it from being born._

- With the mother still panting, check at the back of the fetal head for the umbilical cord. If there is a **nuchal cord** (umbilical cord around the neck) and it is loose enough, slip the cord over the baby's head. If it is too tight, place two clamps on the cord, cut the cord between the clamps, and unwind the cord from the neck.
- Suction the baby's mouth and throat first and then the nose to prevent the infant from aspirating amniotic fluid.
- With one hand on each side of the head, push gently downward until the anterior shoulder comes under the symphysis. Then gently raise the baby's head so the posterior shoulder is born.
- Ask the mother to push gently to assist in the birth of the rest of the infant's body.
- Hold the infant at the level of the uterus, being careful not to drop the slippery infant.
- Again, suction the mouth, throat, and nose of the infant.
- Dry the infant to prevent heat loss and place the infant on the mother's abdomen. Cover with a dry blanket.
- If not already completed, clamp the cord in two places and cut it between the two.
- Document on the birth record the fetal position, nuchal cord, time of birth, Apgar scores (addressed later in this chapter) at 1 and 5 minutes after birth, gender, time and method of placental expulsion, and mother's condition.

## PROLAPSED CORD

When the umbilical cord lies below the presenting part of the fetus, it is termed a **prolapsed cord**. Prolapse of the cord may occur anytime and may be hidden (occult, not visible) or visible (Figure 3-24). It most commonly occurs with ROM, either spontaneous rupture of membranes (SROM) or AROM, as the cord washes down with the amniotic fluid.

A cord below the presenting part is compressed between the fetus and the mother's pelvis, resulting in decreased blood flow to the fetus. The fetus will have bradycardia with variable decelerations during uterine contractions. Contributing factors include a long cord (greater than 100 cm or 40 in), unengaged presenting part, breech presentation, or transverse lie.

When a prolapsed cord is identified, pressure on the cord must be relieved immediately. The provider must call for assistance, don a sterile glove, insert two fingers into the vagina, and put pressure on the presenting part to relieve the compression of the cord. The client can then be assisted into a modified Sims' position with her hips up on pillows, the knee-chest position, or place the bed in Trendelenburg position. In these positions, gravity keeps the pressure of the presenting part off the cord (Figure 3-25). Generally a cesarean birth is necessary.

## INDUCTION/AUGMENTATION OF LABOR

Induction of labor and augmentation of labor both relate to the stimulation of uterine contractions, but at different times in the labor process.

### INDUCTION OF LABOR

**Induction of labor** is the stimulation of uterine contractions *before* they begin spontaneously for the purpose of birthing an infant. Both chemical and mechanical methods can be used to induce labor. The most common methods used in the United States are intravenous oxytocin and amniotomy. Induction of labor is considered in situations of preexisting maternal disease, maternal diabetes mellitus, gestational hypertension (PIH), preeclampsia/eclampsia, PROM, intrauterine fetal growth restriction, postterm pregnancy, fetal demise, and chorioamniotis (Moleti, 2009). Fetal maturity, especially lung maturity, must also be considered. Contraindications to induction are the same as those to spontaneous labor and vaginal birth (e.g., hydrocephaly, transverse lie).

If the cervix is "ripe" (soft), the probability of induction success is greater. If the cervix is not "ripe," prostaglandins are often used first to "ripen" the cervix. Dinoprostone (Prepidil) is often used, and the next day oxytocin infusion is begun. Frequently, oxytocin infusion and amniotomy are both used.

### Oxytocin Infusion

A primary IV infusion of 1,000 mL of an electrolyte solution (e.g., lactated Ringer's) is started. A secondary infusion of 1,000 mL of the same solution is prepared with 20 units of oxytocin (Pitocin). The secondary infusion (with the oxytocin) is regulated by an infusion pump. The rate is very slow at

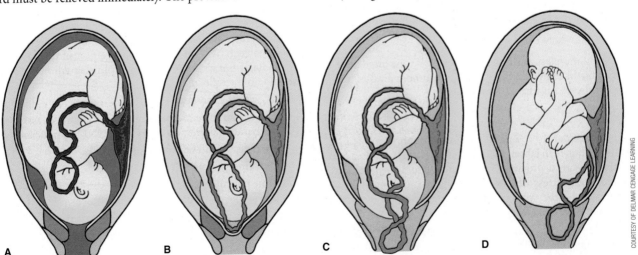

**FIGURE 3-24** Prolapsed Cord; *A,* Hidden (Occult, Not Visible); *B,* Prolapse with Membranes Still Intact; *C,* Cord May Be Seen in Vagina; *D,* Breech with Prolapsed Cord

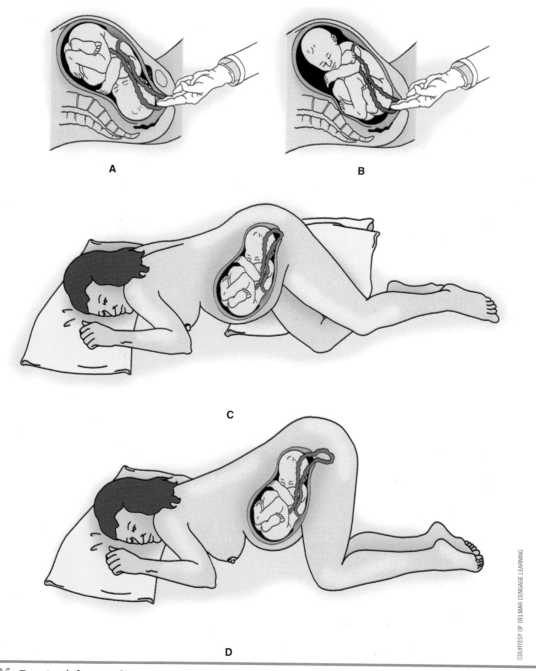

A

B

C

D

COURTESY OF DELMAR CENGAGE LEARNING

**FIGURE 3-25** Examiner's fingers relieve pressure on prolapsed cord in; *A*, vertex presentation and *B*, breech presentation. Gravity relieves pressure on prolapsed cord with mother in *C*, modified Sim's position and *D*, knee-chest position.

the beginning with very small increases at regular intervals according to agency protocol or CNM/physician orders. The goal is to have contractions with a frequency 2 to 3 minutes, duration less than 80 to 90 seconds, and moderate intensity (Clark, Simpson, Knox, & Garite, 2009).

A fetal monitor is used to provide continuous data about FHR and contractions. Before each increase of the infusion rate, assessments of maternal blood pressure and pulse, FHR (bradycardia or decelerations), and contractions should be made and documented. An intake and output record is maintained throughout the induction process.

## AUGMENTATION OF LABOR

**Augmentation of labor** is the stimulation of uterine contractions *after* spontaneously beginning but the progress of

labor is unsatisfactory. Intravenous oxytocin is used in the same manner as for induction of labor.

## OBSTETRIC PROCEDURES

Sometimes a special obstetric procedure is needed to assist with the birth of an infant. These procedures are cesarean birth, forceps-assisted birth, and vacuum-assisted birth.

### CESAREAN BIRTH

**Cesarean birth** is the birth of an infant through an incision in the abdomen and uterus. Indications for cesarean birth include placenta previa, placenta abruptio, CPD, prolapsed cord, breech presentation, active genital herpes, dystocia,

▼ **SAFETY** ▼

### Oxytocin Infusion

Discontinue the secondary infusion with the oxytocin if the following occur:

- Contractions are more frequent than every 2 minutes or the duration is more than 90 seconds.
- Uterine resting tone is more than 20 mm Hg.
- Fetal monitor shows:

  repeated late decelerations

  prolonged decelerations

  no variability

And then:

- Keep mother in side-lying position.
- Increase rate of primary IV fluid.
- Administer oxygen by face mask.
- Notify CNM/physician.

The Institute for Safe Medication Practices in 2007 added intravenous oxytocin to the list of high-alert medications (Simpson & Knox, 2009).

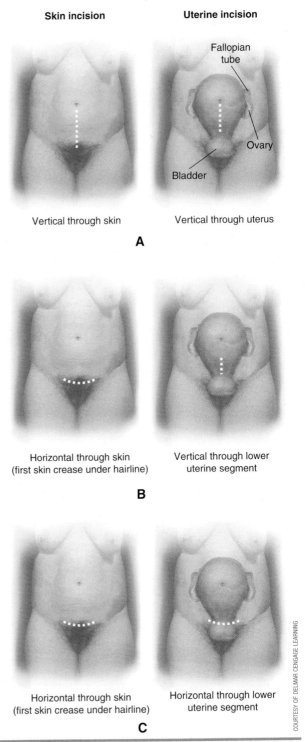

**A**

Vertical through skin          Vertical through uterus

**B**

Horizontal through skin        Vertical through lower
(first skin crease under hairline)      uterine segment

**C**

Horizontal through skin        Horizontal through lower
(first skin crease under hairline)      uterine segment

COURTESY OF DELMAR CENGAGE LEARNING

**FIGURE 3-26** Cesarean Birth—Skin and Uterine Incisions; *A,* Classic, Vertical Skin Incision with High Uterine Incision; Seldom used Except in Emergency Situation; *B,* Horizontal Skin Incision with Low Vertical Uterine Incision; *C,* Horizontal Skin Incision with Horizontal Uterine Incision

gestational hypertension, hydrocephaly, multifetal pregnancy, and repeat cesarean birth. Globally, the rate of cesarean births is escalating, and birthing is becoming surgery for more than ⅓ of pregnant women (Callister, 2008).

## Incisions

The skin incision and uterine incision are not necessarily the same. The skin incision may either be transverse (Pfannenstiel) or vertical. The uterine incision may be vertical in either the upper uterus (classic) or lower uterine segment or transverse in the lower uterine segment (Figure 3-26). Which incisions are used are determined by the client and physician depending on the time factor, reason for the cesarean birth, client's desire for future pregnancies, and physician preference.

## Anesthesia

Regional block, epidural, or spinal anesthesia are the most popular because the mother is awake and aware of the birth of her infant. When time is of the essence or when an epidural or spinal cannot be used, general anesthetic is used.

## Scheduled or Unscheduled Cesarean Birth

A cesarean birth may either be scheduled or unscheduled.

**Scheduled Cesarean Birth** A cesarean birth is scheduled if it is to be a repeat cesarean birth, if labor is contraindicated (e.g., complete placenta previa, hydrocephaly), or if labor cannot be induced and birth is necessary. These clients have some time to prepare for the cesarean birth.

**Unscheduled Cesarean Birth** Unscheduled cesarean births are usually the result of some difficulty in the labor process. Besides concern about the situation causing the need for a

cesarean birth, the client and her support person often experience a sense of failure at not being able to have the baby "normally." The client is generally tired from the labor process and forgets or misunderstands any explanations given. After the infant's birth, it is important for the client to review with the nurse the events before the cesarean birth to ensure the client's understanding of what happened.

Preoperative procedures must be performed quickly. Generally, a urinary catheter is inserted to keep the bladder empty; an abdominal-mons surgical shave prep is completed; abdomen is scrubbed with a solution such as betadine; intravenous fluids are started (if not already running); blood and urine tests are ordered; and, if time is available, preoperative teaching may be instituted. The support person is encouraged to remain with the mother even in surgery to provide emotional support.

When the mother is awake during the cesarean birth, she is involved in seeing and holding her infant just as in a vaginal birth, unless infant resuscitation is required. A pediatrician is usually present to care for the infant. It is extremely important to keep the mother informed about what is happening. Some facilities allow the mother to breastfeed the newborn on the operating table after delivery.

## Vaginal Birth after Cesarean

When the reason for the initial cesarean birth is a nonrecurring situation such as placenta previa, prolapsed cord, or breech presentation, the client may be able to have a vaginal birth with the next pregnancy. If a low transverse uterine incision was made for the cesarean birth, a trial of labor is often recommended. If a classic uterine incision was made in the uterus, a trial of labor is contraindicated because the possibility of uterine rupture is very great. The possibility of a vaginal birth after cesarean (VBAC) is discussed throughout the pregnancy with the obstetrician.

## FORCEPS-ASSISTED BIRTH

**Forceps** are metal instruments used on the fetal head to provide traction or to provide a method of rotating the fetal head to an occiput-anterior position. There are several types of forceps. Some forceps have fenestrated (open) blades and some solid blades, but they all have a locking mechanism that prevents the blades from compressing the fetal skull (Figure 3-27).

Forceps may be applied as:

- *Outlet forceps*—when head is crowning (Figure 3-28).
- *Low forceps*—when head is at +2 station or lower but not yet crowning.
- *Midforceps*—when head is engaged but above +2 stations.

## Indications

Any situation that threatens the mother or fetus that can be relieved by a vaginal birth is an indication for forceps use. Examples are an exhausted mother or one who has heart disease and a fetus in distress, in arrested rotation, or breech position (after coming head).

## Application of Forceps

Before forceps are applied, the cervix must be completely dilated, membranes must be ruptured, and position and station of the fetal head must be known. The FHR must be checked, reported, and recorded *before* forceps are applied and again *after* forceps are applied to make sure the cord is not being compressed by the forceps. It may help the mother to understand about the forceps if it is explained that the forceps blades fit around the baby's head like two teaspoons fit around an egg (Lowdermilk & Perry, 2006). Traction is applied to the forceps only during contractions. Rotation is performed between contractions.

After the birth of the infant, the mother must be assessed for vaginal and cervical lacerations, hematoma, and bruising. The newborn infant may have facial bruising or edema.

## VACUUM-ASSISTED BIRTH

A cup connected to suction is placed over the occiput on the fetal head. After the suction (negative pressure) is attained, traction downward and outward is applied during contractions (Figure 3-29). Indications are the same as for forceps-assisted birth.

Maternal risks include vaginal and rectal lacerations. Fetal risks include cephalhematoma, brachial plexus palsy, retinal and intracranial hemorrhage, and hyperbilirubinemia.

## IMMEDIATE INFANT / MOTHER CARE

During the first 20 to 30 minutes after the infant's birth, specific care is given to the infant and the mother.

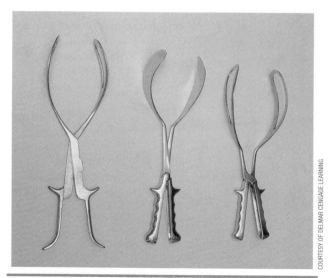

FIGURE 3-27  **Types of Forceps**

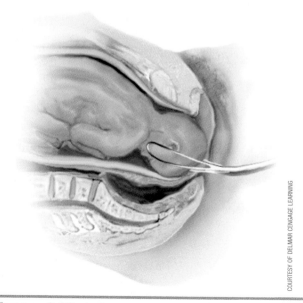

FIGURE 3-28  **Outlet Forceps. Traction is applied downward and outward during contractions.**

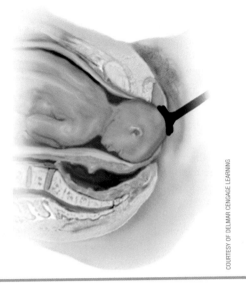

FIGURE 3-29 **Vacuum-Assisted Birth**

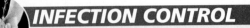

## INFECTION CONTROL

### Standard Precautions

Disposable gloves should be worn when:
- Caring for the newborn until after the infant has received the initial bath
- Assessing the amount of lochia and the perineum
- Cleansing the perineum

## CARE OF THE INFANT

Following are the immediate needs of the newborn infant:
- A—airway
- B—breathing
- C—circulation
- W—warmth

Infants born by cesarean delivery are at greater risk for respiratory distress because they do not receive the "vaginal squeeze" that aids in expelling amniotic fluid from the lungs.

Identification of the infant is the top priority after the immediate needs are met.

### Airway

The CNM/physician suctions secretions from the mouth and nose of the infant at the time of birth. Shortly thereafter, the infant takes the first breath and may begin to cry. The mouth and nose of the infant are suctioned by the nurse as needed to maintain an open airway. The bulb syringe must be compressed before inserting into the mouth or nose of infant.

### Breathing/Circulation

The infant's cardiopulmonary adaptation to extrauterine life is assessed by using the Apgar score (Table 3-6).

Each of the five items are assessed at 1 and 5 minutes after birth, providing a quick evaluation of how the heart and lungs are adapting. The five items to be assessed are arranged in priority from most important (heart rate) to least important (color). The infant is given a score, from 0 to 2, for each item. The five scores are then totaled.

The Apgar score indicates how the infant is transitioning at 1 and 5 minutes. Caregivers should not wait for Apgar scores to determine the next step in neonatal resuscitation. When the Apgar score is less than 6, it is an indication that the neonate is in distress. A nurse or physician who is skilled in neonatal resuscitation must take action to assist the newborn in their transition process. It must be determined whether and when the mother received a narcotic for pain management during labor. Naloxone (Narcan) may be administered if the mother received a narcotic during labor.

### Warmth

The infant must be dried to prevent heat loss by evaporation. A prewarmed radiant warmer is used while giving initial care. Skin-to-skin contact with a parent can also be used to provide warmth. A stockinette cap on the infant's *dry head* also helps prevent heat loss.

### Identification

A set of four identification bands, two long and two short, imprinted with the same number are used. The mother's name, sex of infant, time of birth, and CNM/physician's name are written on each band. The two small bands are put on the infant (both ankles or a wrist and an ankle).

### TABLE 3-6 APGAR Score

| | SCORE | | |
|---|---|---|---|
| **ITEM ASSESSED** | **0** | **1** | **2** |
| Heart rate | Absent | Slow (<100) | Over 100 |
| Respiratory rate | Absent | Slow, weak cry | Good cry |
| Muscle tone | Flaccid | Some flexion of extremities | Well flexed |
| Reflex irritability | No response | Grimace | Cry, cough, or sneeze |
| Color | Blue, pale | Body pink, extremities blue | Completely pink (light skinned); absence of cyanosis (dark skinned) |

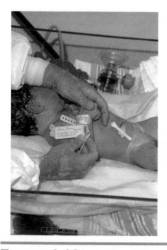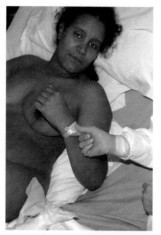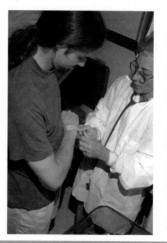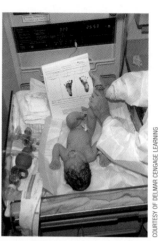

**FIGURE 3-30** Matching identification bands are placed on infant, mother, and partner; infant is foot printed.

The bands must fit the infant snugly but not too tightly (Figure 3-30).

A long band is applied to the mother's wrist. The other long band is usually applied to the father's wrist or other person serving as primary support. In multiple births, the mother and father have a band for each infant. Barcode technology on wrist and ankle bands is currently being used in some hospitals for newborn and mother identification. A small two-dimensional barcode fits perfectly on a newborn's identification band and can be scanned through an Isolette (McCartney, 2008).

Most hospitals also footprint the newborn infant and either fingerprint or thumbprint the mother. The soles of the infant's feet must be dried and any vernix caseosa removed before footprinting.

## CARE OF THE MOTHER

If an oxytocic medication is to be given when the placenta is delivered, the blood pressure is taken both before and after the medication is administered. Maternal blood pressure is monitored every 5 to 15 minutes. The oxytocic medication may increase the BP. Excessive blood loss will cause the BP to fall.

The fundus of the uterus is palpated for firmness. It should be firm, about the size of a grapefruit, in the midline, below the umbilicus. The proper method of palpating the uterus is illustrated in Figure 3-31.

After the CNM/physician has completed repairing the episiotomy (if one was made) and/or any lacerations, the perineum is washed with warm, sterile water and dried with a sterile towel. Maternity vaginal pads are then applied.

The mother may remain in the same bed (LDRP) or be moved to a recovery room bed. If the client is cold and begins to shiver, she should be covered with a warmed blanket, and a second blanket placed over it.

Mother, infant, and father or other support person are allowed time together to further the bonding and attachment process.

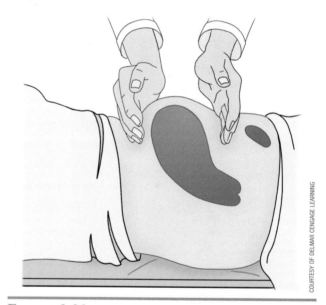

**FIGURE 3-31** Palpation of Uterus after Delivery of Placenta

### ▼ SAFETY ▼

**Removing Legs from Stirrups**

If legs were in stirrups during the birth:
- Two persons are needed to remove them.
- Each person places one hand under the knee and one under the heel (the mother generally has little control over leg movement).
- At the same time, both legs are lowered to the bed.
- If the legs are numb, they may be bicycled to aid circulation return.

# The Client in Labor

A.L., a 23-year-old gravida 1, para 0, is admitted in early labor. Her cervix is dilated 3 cm and is completely effaced. The fetus is at station 0. Contractions are every 5 minutes, duration 50 seconds, and of mild intensity. Her husband, J.L., is with her. They attend only the first two of the six childbirth preparation classes due to J.L.'s work schedule. A.L. is tightly holding J.L.'s hand. Her voice is quivering as she says, "My water just broke. I'm scared. I don't know if I can do this. I've never done this before."

**NURSING DIAGNOSIS 1** *Anxiety* related to the situational crisis of labor and the birthing process at evidenced by gravida 1, para 0, attended only first 2 childbirth classes, voice quivering, statement that she is scared and doesn't know if she can do this

**Nursing Outcomes Classification (NOC)**
*Anxiety Control*
*Coping*

**Nursing Interventions Classification (NIC)**
*Anxiety Reduction*
*Coping Enhancement*

| PLANNING/OUTCOMES | NURSING INTERVENTIONS | RATIONALE |
| --- | --- | --- |
| A.L. will express less anxiety within an hour. | Maintain calm and confident manner. | Provides verbal and nonverbal message that labor is a normal process. |
| | Orient A.L. and J.L. to birthing room and explain admission procedure. | Allays feelings of anxiety regarding unfamiliar environment. |
| | Determine A.L.'s and J.L.'s knowledge and expectation of labor. | Establishes a baseline for intervention and enhances their sense of control. |
| | Discuss the expected progress of labor and what will happen during the process. | Lessens anxiety associated with the unknown. |
| | Involve A.L. and J.L. in decisions about care and share information on progress of labor. | Increases their sense of control. |
| | Involve J.L. in the care of A.L. | Strengthens A.L.'s ability to cope. |

## EVALUATION
A.L. states that she feels a little better and is now gently holding J.L.'s hand.

**NURSING DIAGNOSIS 2** *Risk for Infection* related to rupture of membranes as evidenced by statement "My water just broke."

**Nursing Outcomes Classification (NOC)**
*Treatment Behavior: Illness or Injury*

**Nursing Interventions Classification (NIC)**
*Infection Protection*
*Labor Induction*

| PLANNING/OUTCOMES | NURSING INTERVENTIONS | RATIONALE |
| --- | --- | --- |
| A.L. will show no evidence of infection. | Assess amniotic fluid's color, odor, amount, and presence of meconium. | May indicate intrauterine infection or fetal distress. |

## SAMPLE NURSING CARE PLAN (Continued)

| PLANNING/OUTCOMES | NURSING INTERVENTIONS | RATIONALE |
|---|---|---|
| | Monitor maternal vital signs and the FHR. | Evaluates for signs of infection and fetal distress. |
| | Maintain Standard Precautions by following good hand hygiene, wearing gloves when providing perineal care to A.L., and using aseptic technique when indicated. | Prevents spread of microorganisms. |

### EVALUATION

There are no signs of intrauterine infection or fetal distress.

A.L.'s vital signs are normal: T 98.6°F, P 84, R 20, and BP 114/70 mm Hg. FHR is 138. A.L. reports back pain. Contractions are now every 3 to 4 minutes, duration 60 seconds, and of moderate intensity. The cervix is dilated 5 cm with station +1.

**NURSING DIAGNOSIS 3** *Acute Pain* related to increasing frequency, duration, and intensity as evidenced by contraction assessment

| **Nursing Outcomes Classification (NOC)** | **Nursing Interventions Classification (NIC)** |
|---|---|
| *Pain Level* | *Pain Management* |
| *Pain: Disruptive Effects* | *Anxiety Reduction* |

| PLANNING/OUTCOMES | NURSING INTERVENTIONS | RATIONALE |
|---|---|---|
| A.L. will be able to cope with the discomfort. | Encourage A.L. to change position frequently (every 30 minutes), using such positions as leaning forward when sitting or standing, side-lying, and hands and knees. | Shifts weight of fetus away from the back, relieving back pain; relieves strain and constant pressure; and helps fetus descend through pelvis. |
| | Instruct A.L. and J.L. to use focused breathing, effleurage, massage, sacral pressure, and conscious relaxation. | Increases relaxation and counteracts some of the discomfort. |
| | Offer the use of shower, jacuzzi, or hydrotherapy. | Increases ability to relax. Heat interferes with transmission of pain impulses. |
| | Palpate for distended bladder and encourage regular voiding (at least every 2 hours). | Prevents discomfort and the impediment of fetal descent. |
| | Share with A.L. and J.L. about the progress in labor. | Increases willingness to continue when A.L. knows efforts are having desired results. |
| | Provide comfort measures such as oral care; ice chips; and cool, damp cloth to head or neck, and change damp gown and bed linens. | Relieves discomforts of dry mouth, diaphoresis, and leaking amniotic fluid. |

*(Continues)*

## SAMPLE NURSING CARE PLAN (Continued)

| PLANNING/OUTCOMES | NURSING INTERVENTIONS | RATIONALE |
|---|---|---|
| | Inform A.L. about the pharmacologic pain relief measures available to her. | Gives A.L. a sense of control when she can choose when to use medication for pain. |
| | Administer pain medication as ordered. | Provides pain relief and increases the ability to relax. |

### EVALUATION

A.L. is able to handle the discomfort with J.L.'s help with focused breathing and by applying counterpressure to her back.

### NURSING DIAGNOSIS 4 *Risk for Impaired Urinary Elimination*, related to sensory impairment as evidenced by progress of labor, station 11

**Nursing Outcomes Classification (NOC)**
*Neurological Status: Autonomic*

**Nursing Interventions Classification (NIC)**
*Urinary Catheterization*

| PLANNING/OUTCOMES | NURSING INTERVENTIONS | RATIONALE |
|---|---|---|
| A.L.'s bladder will not exhibit signs of distention. | Palpate A.L.'s bladder at least every 2 hours. | Identifies a full bladder when A.L. is unable to feel the urge to void. |
| | Encourage frequent voiding; catheterize if necessary. | Avoids bladder distention that may impede descent of fetus and result in trauma to bladder. |

### EVALUATION

A.L. voids every 2 hours.

A.L.'s cervix is now 8 cm dilated, station is +2. Contractions are every 2 to 3 minutes, duration 70 seconds, and strong intensity. She is very uncomfortable, requests the pain medication, and says, "I can't take it anymore." J.L. is concerned and asks, "Is she alright?" FHR and maternal vital signs remain close to the admission assessment. A.L. is given meperidine (Demerol) 50 mg IV. She is now resting well between contractions. In 30 minutes A.L.'s cervix is completely dilated, station is +3. She pushes spontaneously several times during each contraction. When she pushes her back stiffens, her arms push on the bed, and she holds her breath. A.L. prefers a semi-Fowler's position.

### NURSING DIAGNOSIS 5 *Deficient Knowledge (effective pushing technique)* related to lack of exposure to information since only attended first 2 prenatal classes, as evidenced by posture during pushing and breath holding

**Nursing Outcomes Classification (NOC)**
*Knowledge: Labor and Delivery*

**Nursing Interventions Classification (NIC)**
*Teaching: Individual*

| PLANNING/OUTCOMES | NURSING INTERVENTIONS | RATIONALE |
|---|---|---|
| A.L. will push more effectively after instructions. | Teach A.L. techniques to push more effectively. | Makes pushing more effective. |
| | During each contraction, A.L. should do the following:<br>• Sit upright or squat | • Takes advantage of gravity; squatting slightly enlarges the pelvic outlet |

## SAMPLE NURSING CARE PLAN (Continued)

| PLANNING/OUTCOMES | NURSING INTERVENTIONS | RATIONALE |
|---|---|---|
| | • Flex chin on chest and curl over uterus | • Directs force of push into pelvis |
| | • *With elbows bent*, pull on her flexed knees | • Provides more force to push |
| | • Exhale and vocalize when she pushes | • Prevents Valsalva maneuver, which causes a decrease in palcenta blood flow and thus oxygenation to the fetus |
| | Observe A.L.'s perineum for crowning. | Keeps everyone informed of progress. |
| | Allow A.L. to rest between contractions (no unnecessary talking). | Allows A.L. to gain strength for next contraction. |

### EVALUATION

In 30 minutes A.L. and J.L. have a 6 lb 10 oz (3,005 g) baby girl. The baby's Apgar scores are 8 at 1 minute and 9 at 5 minutes.

### CASE STUDY

P.K., a 30-year-old gravida 4, para 3, has been in labor 3 hours. Her cervix is 7 cm dilated, station is −1. The fetus is in a vertex presentation, LOA position. When the membranes rupture during a strong contraction, the umbilical cord prolapses from the vagina, and the head is making the perineum bulge. P.K. begins to cry and asks, "What is happening? I feel something hanging out of me."

The following questions will guide your development of a nursing care plan for the case study.
1. What are the first actions the nurse should take?
2. What assessments should be made?
3. Identify two nursing diagnoses and goals for P.K.
4. Identify appropriate nursing interventions for the diagnoses.

### SUMMARY

- There are two theories relative to why labor begins: the mechanical theory and the hormonal theory.
- Signs of impending labor are lightening, Braxton Hicks contractions, cervical softening, bloody show, rupture of membranes, and a sudden burst of energy.
- The five major variables that affect labor are known as the 5 Ps: passageway, passenger, position, powers, and psychological response.
- Labor is divided into four stages, which include first stage (dilation and effacement), second stage (birth of baby), third stage (delivery of placenta), and fourth stage (recovery).
- The mechanisms of labor describe how the fetus moves through the maternal pelvis and birth canal.
- There are many cultural aspects of labor and birth for the nurse to consider when caring for a client from another culture.
- Standard Precautions must be kept in mind when caring for a client during labor and birth because of the many opportunities for contact with body fluids and blood.
- Contractions are assessed for frequency, duration, interval, and intensity.
- Pain management is an important nursing intervention with both nonpharmacological and pharmacological measures.
- The most common risks of labor and birth are preterm labor and birth, premature rupture of membranes, dystocia, abnormal duration of labor, and prolapsed cord.
- Obstetric procedures that may be required to assist with the birth of an infant are cesarean birth, forceps-assisted birth, and vacuum-assisted birth.

# REVIEW QUESTIONS

1. Which of the following measures should the nurse take when supporting a prepared couple during labor?
   1. Verbally encouraging them.
   2. Staying with them all the time.
   3. Taking FHR after each contraction.
   4. Leaving them alone to do "their own thing."

2. It is important for the nurse caring for a client in labor to make sure the bladder is kept empty because a full bladder may:
   1. cause glucosuria.
   2. cause proteinuria.
   3. impede the progress of labor.
   4. make the mother's back ache more.

3. After rupture of the membranes, the most appropriate action for the nurse is to:
   1. listen to the FHR.
   2. remove the wet linen.
   3. time the contractions.
   4. report the color and odor of the fluid.

4. A client is admitted for induction of labor with an oxytocic drug. She is 2 weeks past her EDB. Which of the following findings, if present, would it be essential to report to the CNM/physician before the oxytocic infusion is started?
   1. Low back ache.
   2. Regular contractions of 60 seconds' duration.
   3. Irregular contractions of 20 seconds' duration.
   4. An increase in blood pressure from 122/80 to 130/84 mm Hg.

5. A client is having a precipitate birth. The most appropriate nursing action is to:
   1. stay with her and call for help.
   2. quickly move her to the delivery room.
   3. carefully monitor the FHR and contractions.
   4. assist her to change her position and breathe deeply.

6. The client's membranes have just ruptured. The nurse's initial action is to:
   1. listen to the FHR.
   2. remove the wet linen.
   3. time the contractions.
   4. report the color and odor of the amniotic fluid.

7. A client comes to the hospital at 38 weeks gestation thinking she is in labor, but after several hours of observation, she is sent home. The student nurse asks how she can tell the difference between true and false labor. Which of the following responses should the nurse indicate will occur in true labor?
   1. A sudden burst of energy.
   2. Discomfort with uterine contractions.
   3. Bloody show with a vaginal exam.
   4. Cervical dilation.

8. A client is admitted to the labor and delivery unit stating she has not felt her baby move in several hours. Which of the following is the nurse's initial assessment?
   1. Cervical dilation and effacement.
   2. Status of amniotic membranes.
   3. Contraction pattern.
   4. Fetal heart rate.

9. The client is 5 cm dilated and is having back pain. She is asked to rest on her hands and knees because this position:
   1. keeps her from being bored in one position.
   2. prevents pressure sores from developing during labor.
   3. may rotate the fetus from occiput posterior to anterior.
   4. better allows the nurse to determine cervical dilation.

10. The nurse is assessing whether or not the client's membranes are ruptured. Which of the following findings would indicate her water has broken?
    1. The nitrazine tape turns green.
    2. There is clear fluid on the client's peripad.
    3. The client says her water broke.
    4. There is ferning on the microscope slide.

# REFERENCES/SUGGESTED READINGS

Adams, E., & Bianchi, A. (2008). A practical approach to labor support. *Journal of Obstetric, Gynecological, & Neonatal Nursing, 37,* 106–115.

Ahmed, S. (1994, December). *Culturally sensitive caregiving for Pakistani women.* Lecture presented at the Medical College of Virginia Hospitals, Richmond, VA.

American College of Nurse-Midwives. (2009). Become a midwife. Retrieved August 19, 2009, from http://www.midwife.org/become_midwife.cfm.

Bergstrom, L., Seidel, J., Skellman-Hull, L., & Roberts, J. (1997). "I gotta push. Please let me push!": Social interactions during the change from first to second stage labor. *Birth, 24,* 173–180.

Blackburn, S. (2003). *Maternal, fetal, and neonatal physiology.* Philadelphia: W. B. Saunders.

Bulechek, G., Butcher, H., McCloskey, J., & Dochterman, J., eds. (2008). *Nursing Interventions Classification (NIC)* (5th ed.). St. Louis, MO: Mosby/Elsevier.

Burst, H. (2004). *Varney's midwifery* (4th ed). Sudberry, MA: Jones & Barlett.

Callister, L. (2008). Cesarean birth rates: global trends. *MCN: The American Journal of Maternal/Child Nursing, 33*(2), 129.

Callister, L., & Vega, R. (1998). Giving birth: Guatemalan women's voices. *JOGNN, 27*(3), 289–295.

Centers for Disease Control and Prevention. (2007). Pregnancy and childbirth. Retrieved August 20, 2009, from http://www.cdc.gov/hiv/topics/perinatal/.

Centers for Disease and Prevention. (2008). Episiotomy: can you deliver a baby without one? Retrieved August 20, 2009, from http://www.mayoclinic.com/health/episiotomy/HO00064.

Cesario, S. (2001). Care of the Native American woman: Strategies for practice, education, and research. *JOGNN, 30*(1), 13–19.

Chapman, L. (2000). Expectant fathers and labor epidurals. *MCN, 25*(3), 133–138.

Clark, S., Simpson, K., Knox, E., & Garite, T. (2009). Oxytocin: new perspectives on an old drug. *American Journal of Obstetrics & Gynecology*, 200, 35-37.

Cunningham, F., Leveno, K., Gilstrap, L., Bloom, S., Hauth, J., & Wenstrom, K. D. (2005). *Williams obstetrics* (22nd ed). New York, NY: McGraw-Hill.

D'Arcy, Y. (1999). Managing discomfort with a walking epidural. *Nursing99, 29*(6), 22.

DeSeve, M. (1997). Keeping the faith: Jewish traditions in pregnancy & childbirth. *Lifelines, 1*(4), 46–49.

Dickason, L., Silverman, B., & Kaplan, J. (1998). *Maternal–infant nursing care* (3rd ed.). St. Louis, MO: Mosby–Year Book.

Doulas of North America International. (2009). What is a doula? Retrieved August 19, 2009, from http://www.dona.org/mothers/index.php.

Dwyer, D., & Swayze, S. (2002). Problems after vacuum-assisted childbirth. *Nursing2002, 32*(1), 74.

Ferri, R., & Sofer, D. (2003). Do vaginal births need a good push? *AJN, 103*(4), 19.

Gennaro, S., Kamwendo, L., Mbweza, E., & Kershbaumer, R. (1998). Childbearing in Malawi, Africa. *JOGNN, 27*(2), 191–196.

Gilbert, E., & Harmon, J. (1998). *Manual of high risk pregnancy and delivery* (2nd ed.). St. Louis, MO: Mosby–Year Book.

Howard, J., & Berbiglia, V. (1997). Caring for childbearing Korean women. *JOGNN, 26*(6), 665–671.

Hutchinson, M., & Baqi-Aziz, M. (1994). Nursing care of the childbearing Muslim family. *JOGNN, 23*(9), 767–771.

Hutzal, C., Boyle, E., Kenyon, S., Nash, J., Winsor, S., Taylor, D., & Kirpalani, H. (2008). Use of antibiotics for the treatment of preterm parturition and prevention of neonatal morbidity: a metaanalysis. *American Journal of Obstetrics & Gynecology, 199*(6), 115-121.

James, D., & Maher, M. (2009). Caring for the extremely obese woman during pregnancy and birth. *MCN: The American Journal of Maternal/Child Nursing, 34*(1), 24-30.

Jordan, B. (1978). *Birth in four cultures*. St. Albans: Eden Press Women's Publications.

Lambert, P. (2003). Laboring Lessons. *AWHONN Lifelines, 7*(2), 184.

Leifer, G. (2008). *Maternity nursing: an introductory text* (10th ed) St. Louis, MO: Saunders Elsevier.

Littleton, L., & Engebretson, J. (2002). *Maternal, neonatal, and women's health nursing*. Clifton Park, NY: Delmar Cengage Learning.

London, M., Ladewig, P., Ball, J., & Bindler, R. (2007). *Maternal & child nursing care* (2nd ed). Upper Saddle River, NJ: Pearson Education, Inc.

Lowdermilk, D., & Perry, S. (2006). *Maternity nursing* (7th ed.). St. Louis, MO: Mosby–Year Book.

Lowe, N. (1996). The pain and discomfort of labor and birth. *JOGNN, 25*(1), 82–92.

Martin, P., & Leaton, M. (2001). Amniotic fluid embolism. *AJN, 101*(3), 43–44.

Mattson, S. (1995). Culturally sensitive perinatal care for Southeast Asians. *JOGNN, 24*(4), 335–341.

McCartney, P. (1998a). The birth ball—Are you using it in your practice setting? *MCN, 23*(4), 218.

McCartney, P. (1998b). Caring for women with epidurals using the "laboring down" technique. *MCN, 23*(5), 274.

McCartney, P. (2008). Newborn identification and barcodes. *MCN: The American Journal of Maternal/Child Nursing, 33*(2), 128.

Moleti, C. (2009). Trends and controversies in labor induction. *MCN: The American Journal of Maternal/Child Nursing, 34*(1), 41–47.

Moorhead, S., Johnson, M., Maas, M., & Swanson, E. (2008). *Nursing Outcomes Classification (NOC)* (4th ed.). St. Louis, MO: Elsevier-Health Sciences Division.

Murray, S., McKinney, E., & Gorrie, T. (2001). *Foundations of maternal–newborn nursing* (3rd ed.). Philadelphia, W. B. Saunders.

North American Nursing Diagnosis Association International. (2010). *NANDA-I nursing diagnoses: Definitions and classification 2009–2011*. Ames, IA: Wiley-Blackwell.

O'Brian, W.F., & Cefalo, R.C. (1996). Labor and delivery. In S. G. Gabbe, J. R. Niehyl, & J. L. Simpson (Eds.). *Obstetrics: Normal and problem pregnancies* (3rd ed.). New York: Churchill Livingstone.

Payant, L., Davies, B., Graham, I., Peterson, W., & Clinch, J. (2008). Nurses' intentions to provide continuous labor support to women. *Journal of Obstetric, Gynecological, & Neonatal Nursing, 37*, 405–414.

Perez, P., & Herrick, L. (1998). Doulas: Exploring their roles with parents, hospitals & nurses. *Lifelines, 2*(2), 54.

Petersen, L., & Besuner, P. (1997). Pushing techniques during labor: Issues and controversies. *JOGNN, 26*(6), 719–726.

Romano, A., & Lothian, J. (2008). Promoting, protecting, and supporting normal birth: a look at the evidence. *Journal of Obstetric, Gynecological, & Neonatal Nursing, 37*, 94–105.

Schneiderman, J. (1998). Rituals of placenta disposal. *MCN, 23*(3), 142–143.

Scott-Ramos, I. (1995, January). *Culturally sensitive care giving for Latino women*. Lecture presented at the Medical College of Virginia Hospitals. Richmond, VA.

Sharts-Hopko, N. (1995). Birth in the Japanese context. *JOGNN, 24*(4), 343–351.

Shen, T., DeFranco, E., Stamilio, D., Chang, J., & Muglia, L. (2008). A population-based study of race-specific risk for preterm premature rupture of membranes. *American Journal of Obstetrics & Gynecology, 199*, 373–375.

Shrestha, N. (2007). Nuchal cord and perinatal outcome. *Kathmandu University Medical Journal, 5*(19), 360–363.

Simpson, K., & Creehan, P. (2001). *AWHONN perinatal nursing* (2nd ed.). Philadelphia: Lippincott Williams & Wilkins.

Simpson, K., & Knox, G. (2009). Oxytocin as a high-alert medication: implications for perinatal patient safety. *MCN: The American Journal of Maternal/Child Nursing, 34*(1), 8-15.

Stark, M., Rudell, B., & Haus, G. (2008). Observing position and movements in hydrotherapy: a pilot study. *Journal of Obstetric, Gynecological, & Neonatal Nursing, 37*, 116–122.

Stremler, R., Halpren, S., Weston, J., Yee, J., & Hodnett, E. (2009). Hands-and-knees positioning during labor with epidural analgesic. *Journal of Obstetric, Gynecological, & Neonatal Nursing, 38*, 391–398.

Suplee, P., Dawley, K., & Bloch, J. (2007). Tailoring peripartum nursing care for women of advanced maternal age. *Journal of Obstetric, Gynecological, & Neonatal Nursing, 36*, 616–623.

Tennyson, M. (2000). Labor at 20,000 feet. *AJN, 100*(9), 49–52.

Usta, M., Merier, B.M., & Sibai, B.M. (1999). Current obstetrical practice & umbilical cord prolapse. *AWHONN Lifelines, 5*(6), 10–13.

Weber, S. (1996). Cultural aspects of pain in childbearing women. *JOGNN, 25*(1), 67–72.

World Health Organization. (2008). Adolescent pregnancy fact sheet. Retrieved August 20, 2009, from http://www.who.int/making_pregnancy_safer/events/2008/mdg5/adolescent_preg.pdf.

World Health Organization. (2008). Maternal mortality fact sheet. Retrieved August 20, 2009, from http://www.who.int/making_pregnancy_safer/events/2008/mdg5/factsheet_maternal_mortality.pdf.

Zwelling, E. (2008). The emergence of high-tech birthing. *Journal of Obstetric, Gynecological, & Neonatal Nursing, 37*, 85–93.

Zwelling, E., Johnson, K., & Allen, J. (2006). How to implement complementary therapies for laboring women. *MCN: The American Journal of Maternal/Child Nursing, 31*(6), 364–370.

## RESOURCES

**American College of Nurse-Midwives (ACNM),**
http://www.midwife.org

**American College of Obstetricians and Gynecologists (ACOG),** http://www.acog.com

**Association of Women's Health, Obstetric, and Neonatal Nurses (AWHONN),**
http://www.awhonn.org

**Childbirth Graphics,**
http://www.childbirthgraphics.com

**Doulas of North America (DONA) International,**
http://www.dona.org

**InterNational Association of Parents & Professionals for Safe Alternatives in Childbirth (NAPSAC),**
http://www.napsac.org

**Midwives Alliance of North America,**
http://www.mana.org

**National Association of Childbearing Centers,**
http://www.BirthCenters.org

# CHAPTER 4
## Postpartum Care

## MAKING THE CONNECTION

*Refer to the following chapters to increase your understanding of postpartum care:*

*Maternal & Pediatric Nursing*

- *Prenatal Care*
- *Complications of Pregnancy*
- *The Birth Process*

## LEARNING OBJECTIVES

Upon completion of this chapter, you should be able to:

- Define key terms.
- Describe the various aspects of family adaptation.
- Discuss the mother's physiologic changes after the birth of her baby.
- Describe the expected and unexpected emotional/behavioral changes in the new mother.
- Demonstrate the postpartum assessments for every new mother and the additional assessments for a mother who has had a cesarean birth.
- Discuss the possible postpartum complications of hemorrhage and puerperal infection, including endometritis, mastitis, and thrombophlebitis.
- Explain the advantages and disadvantages of the various methods of family planning.
- Plan and provide the care of a woman who has had a baby.

## KEY TERMS

afterpains
attachment
bonding
claiming process
colostrum
disseminated intravascular
   coagulation (DIC)
dyspareunia
engorgement

engrossment
entrainment
involution
let-down reflex
lochia
mastitis
metritis
neonate
oophoritis

postpartum blues
postpartum depression
postpartum hemorrhage
postpartum psychosis
puerperal (postpartum) infection
puerperium
salpingitis
subinvolution
thrombophlebitis

# INTRODUCTION

Postpartum period, or **puerperium**, is the term for the first 6 weeks after the birth of an infant. During this time, the mother and family will experience many changes, including changes in the structure and function of a family. The mother and, if she has one, her partner begin to establish a relationship with their newborn infant and adjust their lives to include the newborn. The mother and partner must also redefine their own relationship. If there are siblings, they must adjust to their new place in the family structure and the newborn's claim on the time and love of the parents.

Many factors influence family adaptation, including previous experience with a newborn and the convenience of a support system. Previously, postpartum care was focused on the mother and newborn, but now the father or partner, siblings, and sometimes grandparents are included. This chapter explores the events of the postpartum period, including the various ways a family adapts to the newborn; the physiologic and psychosocial changes the mother experiences; preparation for discharge; health promotion; postcesarean section care; and possible postpartum complications.

# FAMILY ADAPTATION

Family roles and relationships must be reorganized with the birth of a baby. Bonding and attachment are the terms used to describe this process of becoming acquainted with the **neonate** (a newborn from birth to 28 days of life). The terms bonding and attachment are often used interchangeably, although they do have different meanings.

**Bonding** refers to a rapid process of attachment, parent to child only, taking place during the sensitive period—the first 30 to 60 minutes after the birth. The bonding is enhanced when parent and infant touch and interact with each other (Figure 4-1). Immediately after birth, the neonate generally is in a quiet, alert state and is ready for bonding and closeness. It is very important that the nurse facilitate quiet time for mother and her new infant. This might mean that the nurse may have to delay bathing the infant so mom has adequate time to bond. It is a good time to initiate breast-feeding.

**Attachment**, a long-term process that begins during pregnancy and intensifies during the postpartum period, establishes an enduring bond between parent and child and develops through reciprocal (parent-to-child and child-to-parent) behaviors. Becoming acquainted with the neonate is an important part of attachment. Touching, exploring, talking to, and using eye contact are all methods used to become acquainted.

The family identifies the infant's "likeness" to and the infant's "differences" from family members, and then the infant's unique qualities. This is often referred to as the **claiming process**.

## MOTHER'S ADAPTATION TO NEONATE

A mother's touch changes as she moves through a discovery phase with her infant. The mother usually begins by using her fingertips to explore her infant's face, fingers, and toes. This is called finger-tipping. The mother may then change to using her palm to stroke her infant's back, chest, arms, and legs. The mother uses her arms to enfold and bring her infant close to her body (Figure 4-2). She may smooth her infant's hair and rub her cheek on the infant's cheek or head. A parent's intense interest and preoccupation in the newborn is termed **engrossment**.

Most mothers speak in a high-pitched voice spontaneously to their infants, seeming to know intuitively that infants respond to higher-pitched voices. Soon after birth, infants can distinguish their mother's voice from others.

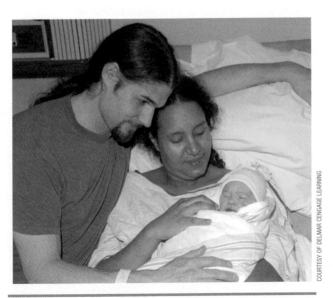

**FIGURE 4-1** **Bonding Between Parents and Infant after the Birth**

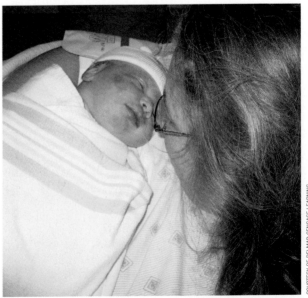

**FIGURE 4-2** **Mother Enfolding and Cuddling Her Infant**

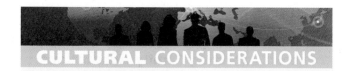

## CULTURAL CONSIDERATIONS

### Touching an Infant

Nurses should be aware that in some cultures (Southeast Asian, Vietnamese, Cambodian, and Laotian), it is considered offensive to pat an infant on the head because the head is viewed as a sacred place where the soul resides (Mattson, 1995).

## FATHER/PARTNER'S ADAPTATION TO NEONATE—NURSE'S ROLE IN ASSESSING WITH ADAPTATION

A father or partner may also exhibit engrossment and display an intense interest in how the baby looks and responds (Figure 4-3). The father also has a desire to touch and hold his baby.

Research has shown that, for fathers and partners, variables other than being an active participant in the birth process are important in developing attachment to the newborn. They include the father or partner's relationship with his own parents, relationship with the infant's mother, and previous experience with children.

Montigny & Lacharité (2003) found that a father's interaction in the immediate postpartum period can have an effect on the ability to bond with their newborns. The study also found that nurses played a big role in this process. The fathers in the study gave specific examples of situations that helped in the bonding experience with their new infant, "obtaining a response from nurses in regard to father's emotional and physical needs" (333). Fathers also stated that being able to talk with the nurse and "sharing needs, preoccupations, and

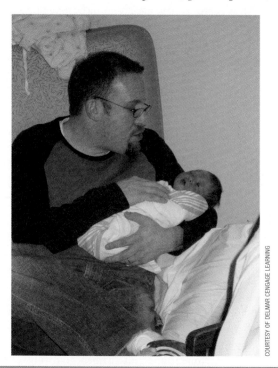

**FIGURE 4-3** Father Displaying Engrossment

COURTESY OF DELMAR CENGAGE LEARNING

## LIFE SPAN CONSIDERATIONS

### Neonates' Reciprocal Behaviors

Neonates have the ability to:
- Make eye contact and move eyes to follow parent's face.
- Engage in intense, prolonged mutual gazing.
- Grasp parent's finger and hold on.
- Move in rhythm to the parent's voice. This is called **entrainment**.

Studies have shown that the infant's vision goes from the mother's breast to her face. For bottle feeding infants, it is from the crook of the mothers arm to her face. Encourage the mother to look at her infant and talk to the infant while the infant is feeding (Staff, 2008).

worries with nurses" helped them feel involved in the infant process. A few things that were noted as having a negative effect on paternal bonding were nurses who humiliated new fathers when they were helping to care for their new infant and nurses who gave contradictory information to new fathers on infant care.

The study also looked at the level of involvement of the father in the postpartum period and found the following results:

- Fathers who were less involved reported very few incidents positive or negative in the postpartum period.
- Fathers who were moderately involved reported the highest number of negative incidents and reported that the highlight of their experience was feeding their infant.
- The fathers who were highly involved in the postpartum period were most likely to report positive interactions between new infant, spouse, and staff.
- The highly involved fathers were interested in all aspects of infant care and took an active role in learning (Montigny & Lacharité, 2003).

It is important for the nurse to recognize the important role that the father/partner has in the postpartum period. The nurse should understand that by helping to facilitate positive experiences for the new father they may help build stronger family bonds in the future.

## SIBLINGS' ADAPTATION TO NEONATE

The response of a sibling to the birth of a new sister or brother depends on the age and developmental level of the older sibling. The adaptation is probably most difficult for toddlers, who often view the new baby as competition, someone who takes the parent's time and love. Negative behavioral changes may occur in the toddler, such as a return to thumb sucking or bed wetting; sleep problems; or hostility toward the mother, especially when she is caring for the new baby. Positive behavioral changes may be increased independence and taking an interest in the care of the newborn.

Parents' attitudes toward the newborn and their preparation of the siblings for the new arrival guide the older children's reactions. Parents can include each child in the care of the baby according to their capabilities. For example, toddlers may be able to bring a clean diaper to the parent; preschoolers may help prepare for the baby's bath; and older children may hold, carry, or feed the baby (Figure 4-4). Parents need to ensure that siblings are not left out. In addition to allowing the sibling to help with the new baby, parents should provide quality time with the older children.

## GRANDPARENTS' ADAPTATION TO NEONATE

Grandparents go through a transition to grandparenthood just as parents go through a transition to parenthood. Practices and attitudes about childbirth and childrearing change from one generation to another, as do the roles of men and women. The extent to which grandparents understand and accept the current practices and attitudes affects their relationship with their children and how supportive they may be (Figure 4-5). It is important for the nurse to take into consideration that some pregnancies are not always a joyous occasion in some families, especially in the case of a teenage pregnancy. As the nurse, you should encourage the new grandparent to hold the baby and help the family with any resources that they might need.

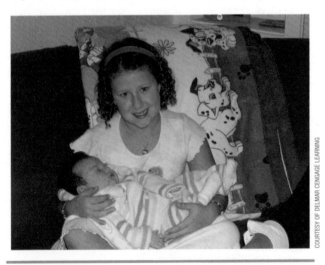

**FIGURE 4-4** An older sibling can help hold the baby.

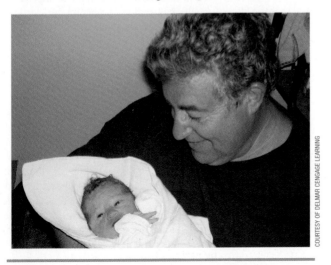

**FIGURE 4-5** Grandparent Enjoying New Grandchild

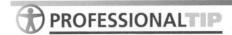

## PROFESSIONALTIP

### Factors Affecting Family Adaptation

Many factors affect family adaptation to the newborn:

- *Parental fatigue*: Not being able to sleep uninterrupted through the night may affect the caregivers' energy level.
- *Previous experience with a newborn*: First-time parents and parents with children will progress at different rates through the attachment process.
- *Parental expectations of the newborn*: The newborn's appearance, gender, and behaviors in relation to parental expectations may influence the attachment process.
- *Knowledge of and confidence in providing for newborn needs*: Parents have varying levels of experience in feeding, consoling, and providing care in general to newborns.
- *Temperament of the newborn*: Some infants are calm, easily consoled, and cuddly, whereas others are irritable, difficult to console, and do not like cuddling.
- *Temperament of parents*: Anxious, insecure, excitable parents have more difficulties than calm, secure, less anxious parents.
- *Age of parents*: Teenage, middle-age, and older parents will all react differently to the new family structure based on their life experiences.
- *Available support system*: Help with household tasks and help and encouragement with infant care can ease family adaptation to the newborn.
- *Unexpected events*: Cesarean birth may add stress and increase recovery time, therefore limiting time and energies available for newborn care.

## MATERNAL PHYSIOLOGIC CHANGES

Many of the physiologic changes postpartum (following birth) are a reversal of the changes in the various body systems that occurred during pregnancy. The initiation of lactation and reestablishment of normal menstrual cycles also occur.

### REPRODUCTIVE SYSTEM

Changes occur in the uterus, cervix, vagina, and perineum.

### Uterus

**Involution** is the return of the uterus to its prepregnancy size and condition. There are three processes involved in involution:

- *Muscle fiber contraction*: With the uterus now empty, it firmly contracts to control bleeding from the area of placental attachment; the muscle fibers gradually regain their former size and shape.

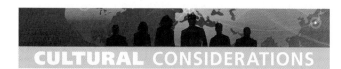

### Lochia

Cultural norms may affect interpretation of postpartum events. For instance, women in Malawi, Africa, are considered "dirty" as long as they have a lochia discharge; sexual intercourse is therefore prohibited for 6 months after birth (Gennaro, Kamwendo, Mbweza, & Kershbaumer, 1998). In Judaism, husbands may not touch their wives during the postpartum period, as the wives are considered unclean when they are bleeding. The nurse should recognize this and assist by passing the newborn back and forth between parents if they are in the room.

- *Catabolism*: The enlarged muscle cells of the uterus experience catabolic changes in protein cytoplasm that reduce the size of each cell. Catabolic products are excreted as nitrogenous wastes in the urine.
- *Regeneration*: The endometrium is regenerated within 2 to 3 weeks, except for the placental site, which is healed and regenerated by approximately 6 weeks.

**Uterine Fundal Descent** Immediately after the birth, the uterus is about the size of a grapefruit, with the fundus about halfway between the umbilicus and symphysis pubis. The fundus then rises to the umbilicus and stays there about 12 hours. Then the fundus descends about 1 cm, 1 finger breadth, each day for about 10 days, when it is once again in the pelvis and unable to be palpated abdominally (Figure 4-6). A full bladder will push the uterus upward.

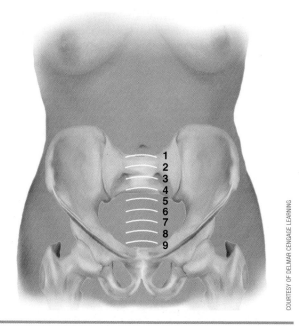

**FIGURE 4-6** Uterine Involution. Uterine fundal descent is approximately 1 cm/day.

COURTESY OF DELMAR CENGAGE LEARNING

### Postpartum Vaginal Bleeding

- All vaginal bleeding in the postpartum period is not necessarily lochia. Lochia usually trickles from the vagina, although a gush of bright red blood may result when the fundus is massaged or when blood pooled in the vagina is expelled when the mother stands up.
- Ambulation and breastfeeding usually increases the amount of lochia.
- If blood spurts from the vagina or the amount is excessive when the uterus is firmly contracted, suspect cervical or vaginal tears.

Even a slow trickle of blood should be cause for further investigation in the postpartum period. Some postpartum hemorrhages start out very slowly. It is important to teach clients the difference in normal lochia flow versus a hemorrhage. A good time for teaching is the first time the client ambulates to the bathroom for pericare.

The contracting uterus may be a source of discomfort for some women after the infant's birth, especially for multiparas and those who are breastfeeding. Breastfeeding stimulates the release of oxytocin from the posterior pituitary, which stimulates strong uterine contractions as well as the "let-down" reflex. These contractions are known as **afterpains**.

**Lochia** Lochia is the uterine/vaginal discharge after childbirth. It is initially bright red, then changes to a pink or pinkish brown, and then to a yellowish white. The odor of lochia is like a normal menstrual flow. A foul odor indicates infection.

For the first 3 days, the lochia is mostly blood with small pieces of decidua and mucus. This is called lochia rubra. About the 4th day, the amount decreases and the color changes to a pink or pinkish brown called lochia serosa. It is mostly a serous exudate with cervical mucus, erythrocytes, and leukocytes. After the 10th day, the erythrocyte level decreases and the discharge becomes yellowish white, lochia alba. Now the lochia consists of leukocytes, epithelial cells, decidua, mucus, serum, and bacteria. This discharge may last for 6 weeks or more (Lowdermilk & Perry, 2007).

### Cervix

Within 18 hours after birth, the cervix has become firm, has shortened, and has regained its form (Lowdermilk & Perry, 2007). By the end of 2 weeks, the cervical os (cervical opening) is closed, but after delivery, the opening appears as a horizontal slit. The cervical os of a nulliparous woman is round or oval, but a parous woman's cervical os is a horizontal slit.

### Vagina and Perineum

The vagina was greatly stretched during labor. It takes 6 weeks for the vagina to complete involution and regain the contour it had before pregnancy. It never does regain the size it had before pregnancy. The vaginal mucosa is atrophic in lactating women, at least until menstruation returns. The reduced level of estrogen causes a decrease in vaginal lubrication, which may cause **dyspareunia**, or coital discomfort.

The stretching and thinning of the perineum during labor may cause edema and bruising of the perineum after the birth. Many women have an episiotomy (surgical incision of the perineum) before the infant's birth. Lacerations of the perineum also may occur. Both lacerations and episiotomies are classified according to the tissues involved and will take time to heal:

> *First degree*: skin and mucous membrane.
>
> *Second degree*: skin, mucous membrane, and muscle.
>
> *Third degree*: skin, mucous membrane, muscle, and anal sphincter.
>
> *Fourth degree*: skin, mucous membrane, muscle, anal sphincter, and rectal mucosa.

Even when the episiotomy or laceration is small, it can cause a great deal of discomfort because the muscles of the perineum are used when sitting, stooping, bending, squatting, walking, and defecating.

## ENDOCRINE SYSTEM

After the expulsion of the placenta, the levels of the placental hormones estrogen, progesterone, human placental lactogen (hPL), human chorionic gonadotropin (hCG), and relaxin rapidly decline. The decrease in hPL, estrogen, and cortisol causes a reversal of the diabetogenic effect of pregnancy. This rapid change necessitates frequent assessment of the diabetic mother's blood glucose level.

## Lactation

The rapid decrease of the estrogen and progesterone levels allows the prolactin to initiate milk production within 2 to 3 days after the infant's birth. Oxytocin, a posterior pituitary hormone, causes the milk to be expressed from the alveoli into the lactiferous ducts. This is called "let down." The **let-down reflex** is a neurohormonal reflex; that is, either neuro (the mind) or the hormone (oxytocin) may initiate "let down." A breastfeeding mother hearing a baby cry or thinking about feeding her infant often stimulates the let-down reflex, and milk will drip from the nipples (neuro). The release of oxytocin in response to the infant's sucking also stimulates the let-down reflex (hormonal). Many women describe a tingling/burning feeling in the breasts when the milk is "let down."

## Menstrual Cycle

There is a great difference when ovulation and menstruation are reestablished based on whether the mother is breastfeeding or not breastfeeding. The level of follicle-stimulating hormone (FSH) is the same in both breastfeeding and nonbreastfeeding mothers. It is believed that the increased level of prolactin in breastfeeding mothers causes the ovaries to not respond to the FSH and ovulation does not occur (Bowes, 2001). The prolactin level remains high in breastfeeding women for approximately 6 weeks. The prolactin level is influenced by three factors: frequency and duration of feedings, supplemental feedings, and possibly the strength of the infant's sucking (Lowdermilk & Perry, 2007). In nonbreastfeeding mothers, the prolactin level returns to the prepregnant level within 2 weeks.

Ovulation in nonbreastfeeding mothers takes place as early as 27 days after the birth and usually has resumed by

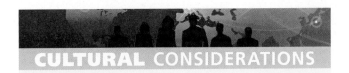

## CULTURAL CONSIDERATIONS

### Breastfeeding

- Some Hispanic, Southeast Asian, Vietnamese, Cambodian, and Laotian women may choose not to breastfeed until the milk comes in (Mattson, 1995).
- Rural Indian women discard the colostrum because they think it harms the child's health. The child is not breastfeed until the milk comes in (Bandyonpadhyay, 2009).
- Many women will breastfeed until the child is 2 years old, based on cultural practices and expectations (Hutchinson & Baqi-Aziz, 1994).
- African-American women have the lowest rate of breastfeeding at 6 months of age in the postpartum period, currently ranking at 52.9% (Oyeku, 2003). It is important for the nurse to encourage breastfeeding initiation if wanted in the postpartum period.

2 months (Bowes, 2001). Most nonbreastfeeding mothers resume menstruating within 3 months after the birth.

The average time for ovulation to take place in breastfeeding mothers is approximately 190 days (Bowes, 2001). The return of ovulation and menstruation in breastfeeding mothers is determined, to a large measure, by the breastfeeding pattern. This underscores the fact that breastfeeding is not a reliable form of birth control.

## BREASTS

During the last few weeks of pregnancy, the breasts begin to fill with a fluid called colostrum. **Colostrum** is a yellowish fluid rich in antibodies and high in protein. As milk production begins, 2 to 3 days after birth, the breasts feel firm, warm, and may be tender. This lasts about 48 hours. By day 3 or 4 after the birth, **engorgement** may occur; the breasts become quite distended (swollen), tender, and warm. This is caused mainly by vasocongestion, especially of the veins and lymphatics.

The changes in the breasts after the birth of a baby are partly determined by whether the mother is breastfeeding or not. For the nursing mother, frequent breastfeeding sessions encourage milk production and sustain lactation.

If the mother does not intend to breastfeed, although milk is present it should not be expressed because this causes more milk to be produced. Engorgement spontaneously disappears and discomfort decreases in 24 to 48 hours if the breasts are not emptied of milk. If breastfeeding is never begun or is stopped, lactation ceases within a week. Encourage the mother to wear a tight-fitting sports bra to help with the pain during this period.

## GASTROINTESTINAL SYSTEM

Most new mothers are hungry and thirsty after giving birth because of the energy expended during labor. Following

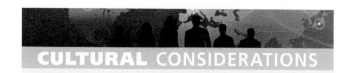

## Foods in the Postpartum Period

A nurse must be sensitive to the fact that a new mother's food choices and preferences may have cultural or ethnic foundations. For instance:

- Women of Southeast Asia are taught that any food or drink must be hot in temperature for at least 1 month. Foods are mainly rice and boiled chicken (Davis, 2001).
- Muslim women may request a vegetarian or kosher diet following childbirth (Hutchinson & Baqi-Aziz, 1994).
- Rural Indian women avoid high-fiber foods, acidic foods, cold foods of foods considered hot and cold. Instead, they eat milk, ghee, butter and some types of fish. Garlic is believed to cause uterine contraction (Bandyopadhyay, 2009).

recovery from any analgesia or anesthesia the mother may have received, she may request extra food.

Mothers may encounter difficulty in having a bowel movement after giving birth. There are several reasons, including:

- Peristalsis has been decreased by the effects of the increased progesterone level during pregnancy; this may take several days to become normal again.
- Prelabor diarrhea.
- Lack of food during labor.
- Dehydration.
- Perineal trauma, episiotomy repair, or hemorrhoids.
- Mother's anticipation of discomfort.
- Certain pain medications can cause constipation.

## CARDIOVASCULAR SYSTEM

The increase in blood volume during pregnancy allows a significant loss of blood without any ill effects to the mother. In a vaginal birth, blood loss averages 500 mL, whereas a cesarean birth averages a 1,000 mL blood loss.

### Vital Signs

The new mother's temperature may increase to 100.4°F (38°C) during the first 24 hours because of dehydration during labor and the trauma of delivery. After 24 hours, the temperature returns to normal, although it may rise again when milk production begins.

The pulse, which increased during pregnancy, remains elevated or may even rise for up to 24 to 48 hours, but it should not exceed 100 beats per minute. Periods of bradycardia may also be experienced. The pulse returns to the prepregnant rate in approximately 8 weeks (Bowes, 2001).

The diaphragm descends when the uterus is emptied, making respirations much easier. In 6 to 8 weeks, respiratory function returns to the prepregnant rate. The blood pressure may have a small increase in both the systolic and diastolic aspects

that lasts about 4 days (Bowes, 2001). The rapid decrease in intra-abdominal pressure after birth results in visceral blood vessel dilation, which may cause orthostatic hypotension.

### Cardiac Output

Cardiac output that increased during pregnancy, may increase even higher for up to 60 minutes following delivery. This increase occurs following both vaginal and cesarean births (Bowes, 2001). Cardiac output remains elevated for at least 48 hours, and then rapidly decreases in the first 2 weeks postpartum. The return of cardiac output to the prepregnancy level takes about 24 weeks (Simpson & Creehan, 2007).

### Blood Volume

The changes in blood volume are rapid and dramatic. Three physiologic changes protect from excessive blood loss:

- Loss of the uteroplacental circulation (when the placenta is expelled) reduces the maternal vascular bed by 10% to 15%.
- Stimulus for vasodilation is removed with the loss of placental endocrine function.
- Movement of extravascular water, stored during pregnancy, into the blood vessels increases blood volume.

The excess plasma volume is eliminated from the body by both diuresis and diaphoresis. Diuresis (excessive urine excretion) results from a decrease in aldosterone, which was increased during pregnancy. It is not uncommon for a new mother to have a urinary output of 3,000 mL per day for 2 to 3 days (Murray, McKinney, & Gorrie, 2005). Diaphoresis (profuse perspiration), while not clinically significant relative to fluid elimination, may be uncomfortable for the mother, especially if she is not expecting it to occur. It often occurs at night for 2 to 3 nights after delivery.

### Blood Values

The white blood cell count, which increased slightly during pregnancy (to 12,000/mm$^3$), now increases to 20,000 or even 30,000/mm$^3$ during the first 10 to 12 days after the infant's birth (Cunningham, Grant, Leveno, Gilstrap, & Cox, 2005). The neutrophil level increases the most for protection against invading organisms.

The large loss of plasma volume during the first 3 days after the birth results in a rise in both the hemoglobin and hematocrit levels by the seventh day, unless excessive blood loss has occurred.

### Coagulation

The increased levels of clotting factors and fibrinogen during pregnancy remain elevated for a few days as protection against postpartum hemorrhage. Thus, there is an increased risk for thrombus (clot) formation. Mothers having varicose veins, a cesarean birth, or a history of thrombophlebitis are at greater risk for thrombus formation.

### Varicosities

Varices of the legs, anus (hemorrhoids), and vulvar area empty rapidly immediately after the birth. For clients who have residual hemorrhoids, try to encourage them to eat a diet high in fiber. Diets that are high in fiber will make softer stool, which will reduce straining and pressure on the hemorrhoids. Sitz baths offer a client temporary relief of hemorrhoid symptoms such as pressure, pain, and itching (Harvard.edu, 2008).

# URINARY SYSTEM

Physical changes take place in the structures of the urinary system; there are also chemical changes in the urine.

## Physical Changes

The hypotonia of the bladder and dilation of the ureters during pregnancy take approximately 2 to 8 weeks to return to the prepregnant state (Cunningham et al., 2005). Also, the bladder, urethra, and tissue around the urinary meatus may have been traumatized and become edematous during labor and birth, which may result in difficulty in urination.

The mother may have a problem with overdistention and incomplete emptying of the bladder and residual retention of urine because the diuresis causes the bladder to fill quickly. Those mothers who received a regional anesthesia are especially at risk for bladder distention and difficulty voiding until the anesthesia wears off.

Postpartum hemorrhage and urinary tract infection are two complications related to urinary retention and bladder overdistention. Urinary stasis provides the bacteria with enough time to multiply and cause an infection. A full bladder displaces the uterus up and to the side, resulting in uterine atony (inability of the uterus to contract). This is the primary cause of excessive bleeding. Adequate emptying of the bladder helps the bladder regain its tone in 5 to 7 days after the birth (Lowdermilk & Perry, 2003).

## Chemical Changes

The catabolic processes of uterine involution cause a mild proteinuria for 1 to 2 days in approximately 50% of new mothers (Simpson & Creehan, 2007). Ketonuria and elevated blood urea nitrogen (BUN) may also be present.

# MUSCULOSKELETAL SYSTEM

The musculoskeletal changes that occur during pregnancy are reversed during the postpartum period.

## Joints, Ligaments, and Cartilage

As the level of the hormone relaxin decreases, the ligaments and cartilage, especially of the pelvis, begin to revert to their prepregnant positions. Hip or joint pain may be noticed as these changes take place. Joints, cartilage, and ligaments are stabilized by 6 to 8 weeks after the birth.

All joints return to their normal prepregnant state, except those in the feet. The new mother may discover a permanent increase in her shoe size (Lowdermilk & Perry, 2007).

## Abdominal Muscles

Many new mothers, when they stand up, are dismayed when the abdominal muscles protrude, giving a still-pregnant appearance. It usually takes 6 weeks for the abdominal muscles to return almost to their prepregnant state (Lowdermilk & Perry, 2007). Previous muscle tone, proper exercise, and the amount of adipose tissue all influence the return of muscle tone.

# INTEGUMENTARY SYSTEM

The level of melanocyte-stimulating hormone (MSH) declines rapidly after the birth, and the areas of hyperpigmentation begin to lighten in color. In some women, however, the linea nigra and the darkened nipple areola may remain dark. Most of

the skin's elasticity returns, but some striae may still be visible as small or large silver streaks on the breasts, abdomen, buttocks, or thighs.

Spider angiomas (nevi) and palmar erythema usually fade with the decrease in the estrogen level. In some women, however, they do stay.

Any fine hair appearing during pregnancy usually disappears; however, any coarse or bristly hair appearing during pregnancy may remain.

# NEUROLOGIC SYSTEM

Any pregnancy-induced neurologic discomforts usually lessen after birth (Lowdermilk & Perry, 2003); however, fatigue, afterpains, muscle aches, episiotomy or abdominal incision pain, and breast engorgement all may create maternal discomfort. If the mother received an analgesic or anesthesia, she may experience a temporary loss of feeling in her legs and dizziness.

The mother who has a headache must be carefully assessed. If the mother had a regional anesthesia (epidural or spinal), the headache may be caused by a leakage of cerebrospinal fluid into the extradural space during needle placement; this is known as a spinal headache. This headache is generally more severe when the mother sits or stands and is relieved when she lies down. If the mother has blurred vision, photophobia, and abdominal pain with a headache, it may indicate that she is developing pregnancy-induced hypertension (PIH), or if she had PIH during pregnancy, that it is getting worse.

# WEIGHT LOSS

Immediate weight loss is the sum of the infant's weight, placenta, amniotic fluid, and blood loss. Typically, this is approximately 13 lbs. During the next 6 weeks, an additional 8 to 9 lbs is lost as the result of diuresis, diaphoresis, and the involution of the reproductive organs. It takes most mothers approximately 6 months to return to their prepregnant weight, and some may take an entire year. The energy required for breastfeeding may assist in the weight-loss process.

# MATERNAL PSYCHOSOCIAL CHANGES

Both expected and unexpected emotional/behavioral changes may be encountered. The effects of early discharge must also be considered.

## EXPECTED CHANGES

Expected emotional/behavioral changes include those restorative/adaptive phases described by Reva Rubin, postpartum "blues," and those related to a cesarean birth.

### Rubin's Restorative/Adaptive Phases

Rubin (1961) described three phases of maternal restoration/adaptation: *taking-in, taking-hold,* and *letting-go.*

**Taking-In Phase** This phase is focused mainly on the mother's need for food, fluid, and sleep. The mother's behavior is passive as she takes in the physical care and attention from others. She depends on others to meet her needs. Rubin (1961) described this as the phase of nurturing and protective care lasting 2 to 3 days. Studies by Ament (1990) and Wrasper (1996) confirmed the behavior described by Rubin but noted that the behavior was present only during the first 24 hours after birth.

Integration of the labor and birth experience into reality is the major task of the mother at this time. It is important for her to discuss the details of the labor and birth, especially with the nurse(s) who cared for her. She is thus able to clarify details about her experience that she may not remember because of the effects of medication or the natural sleep and amnesia between contractions, especially in the second stage of labor. By describing to family and friends the birth experience, the mother realizes that the pregnancy is past and the infant is now a separate individual.

The father or partner may also experience a taking-in phase as he is congratulated on the birth of the infant. Family members often treat him in a special way.

**Taking-Hold Phase** In the taking-hold phase, the mother becomes more independent as she takes an interest in and responsibility for her own physical care. Her focus shifts to the care of her infant. She welcomes opportunities to learn about the behavior of infants and to practice caring for her infant. Martell (1996) and Wrasper (1996) believe that childbirth preparation classes, pain management practices, early newborn contact, rooming-in, and early discharge enhance taking-hold behaviors. Because most mothers are discharged during this phase, which lasts approximately 10 days, continued coping with the physical and emotional/behavioral changes at home is required.

The father or partner's interest in infant behaviors and care is similar to the mother's in the taking-hold phase. He may also be anxious but is usually willing to learn.

**Letting-Go Phase** If this is a first baby, the mother and father/partner must give up the role and carefree lifestyle of being only a couple. They are now a couple with a child. The expected birth experience may not have been realized. For example, a planned vaginal birth with no anesthesia may have changed to a cesarean birth and/or use of regional anesthesia. The parents must let go of the planned experience and accept what really happened.

For some mothers and/or fathers, the newborn infant does not fit the expected baby they dreamed of and talked about during pregnancy. They may be disappointed in the gender, size, or other characteristics of the infant. Now they must let go of their expectations and accept the reality of their infant.

The mother and father let go of their role of "expecting" and move forward as a unit with a new member. They establish

## COMMUNITY/HOME HEALTH CARE

### Coping with Taking-Hold Phase

- Acknowledge parents' anxiety about caretaking abilities.
- Provide information about infant behaviors.
- Allow parents to provide infant care (nurse should not take over) even if performed awkwardly.
- Praise parents' caregiving efforts.
- Provide parents with a contact and phone number in the event they have questions.

a lifestyle that includes the child and their role as parents. Time must be made for sharing adult activities and interests.

## Postpartum Blues

**Postpartum blues** or "baby blues" is a mild, transient condition of emotional lability and crying for no apparent reason that affects women who have just given birth and lasts about 2 weeks. Other symptoms include fatigue, anxiety, restlessness, let-down feeling, headache, and sadness. The etiology is unknown. This is a self-limiting situation that begins about 3 days, peaks about 5 days, and disappears approximately 10 days after birth.

## Cesarean Birth

When a cesarean birth is an emergency (unplanned), the taking-in phase may last longer because these mothers also need to accept and understand the events that made the cesarean birth necessary. It is important for the nurse to understand that these mothers are surgical clients requiring immediate physical care to restore or maintain physiologic health. When pain, bleeding, and incision care are under control, the nurse can help the mother understand the birth and incorporate the experience into her reality.

Some mothers have feelings of frustration, anger, low self-esteem, or disappointment that they could not have their baby the "normal way" (vaginal birth). At the same time, they are relieved, happy, and filled with gratitude that the infant had a safe birth and is healthy. It may be a time of many, often opposing, emotions. The nurse offers encouragement and support to the client and her family. The nurse helps the patient understand that she did not fail just because her birth did not go as planned. The client needs to talk through the birth again and again to help gain a better understanding of the situation. The nurse demonstrates patience and tries to help the client reach a level of comfort with the situation.

## UNEXPECTED CHANGES

Unexpected emotional/behavioral changes include postpartum depression, postpartum psychosis, and reaction to an infant with problems.

## Postpartum Depression

**Postpartum depression** (PPD) is similar to postpartum blues but is more serious, intense, and persistent. Approximately 12% of new mothers experience a syndrome more severe than postpartum blues (Lowdermilk & Perry, 2007). PPD may be mild, moderate, or severe, with symptoms becoming more numerous and intense as the severity increases.

The mother with mild PPD cares lovingly for her infant but is unable to feel the love. She may express feelings of irritability, guilt, shame, unworthiness, and a sense of loss of self. Symptoms persist past the first few weeks after the infant's birth.

Moderate PPD is characterized by spontaneous crying, insomnia or hypersomnia, fatigue, decreased concentration, and sometimes food cravings.

With severe PPD, the irritability of the mother may explode into violent outbursts or uncontrollable crying often directed toward significant others. She often will not discuss her symptoms or negative feelings toward the infant, which may include disinterest, annoyance with care demands, or even thoughts of harming the infant.

Psychotherapy and pharmacological interventions are generally required. Sometimes, hospitalization is necessary.

## Postpartum Psychosis

**Postpartum psychosis** is the most dangerous form of depression in a new mother. Postpartum psychosis occurs in 1 to 2/1000 births usually within the first 2 to 4 weeks after delivery but can happen as early as 2 to 3 days postpartum. The psychosis is marked by "paranoid, grandiose, or bizarre delusions, mood swings, confused thinking, and grossly disorganized behavior that represent a dramatic change from her previous functioning" (Sit, Rothchild, & Wisner, 2006). Postpartum psychosis is the least common form of postpartum depression, affecting approximately 10 to 13% of new mothers as compared with the 50 to 75% who are affected by milder forms of depression/baby blues.

Postpartum psychosis is a medical emergency. Many women will require a psychiatric evaluation and, in many cases, hospitalization, until they are no longer a threat to themselves or others. The initial medical evaluation will include "thorough history, physical examination, and laboratory investigations" (Sit, Rothchild, & Wisner, 2006). It is very important for the nurse to educate new mothers and their families about the signs and symptoms of postpartum depression so it can be caught early and treated.

## Infant with a Problem

It may be difficult for the mother and/or father to bond with and attach to an infant born preterm or with physical or functional anomalies (Figure 4-7). The parents may have feelings of guilt that they, somehow, caused the infant's problem. Either or both of the parents may not be able to accept an infant who does not look like a normal, healthy infant. When one parent's reaction to the infant with a problem is opposite that of the other's, there may be a terrific strain on their relationship.

## DISCHARGE

In an effort to reduce health care costs and meet consumer demand for a more family-centered experience with less medical intervention, the short hospital stay came into existence. In the 1950s, most new mothers remained in the hospital 5 days for a vaginal birth and 7 days for a cesarean birth. The stays were gradually reduced to 3 days for a vaginal birth and 5 days for a cesarean birth. For several years in the early 1990s, third-party payers (health plans and insurance companies) mandated discharge within 24 hours for a vaginal birth and 72 hours or less for a cesarean birth.

Health-care professionals became concerned about client (mother and infant) safety because many problems do not show up in the first 24 hours after birth. The time for assessing bonding/attachment and parenting behaviors was almost eliminated. Parents were barely acquainted with their infant and client teaching about newborn care, and identifying health problems such as dehydration, jaundice, and breastfeeding difficulties had to be rushed.

The federal government passed the Newborns' and Mothers' Health Protection Act of 1996, which requires all health plans to allow a stay of 48 hours following vaginal birth and 96 hours following a cesarean birth (Health Care Financing Administration, 2002). Self-insured health plans must comply with this act. Group insurance plans and individual insurance may not have to comply if the client lives in a state having a law with certain protections for hospital stays after childbirth. More than 40 states and the District of Columbia have such laws (Health Care Financing Administration, 2002).

Follow-up home care is being used in many areas. This may be a telephone call or two to see how the mother and infant are doing, or it may include actual home visits. Research has shown that women who receive follow-up care at home by phone or in person did better overall in the postpartum period. Unfortunately, the United States lags behind in this area. This area of more efficient postpartum care is part of a nationwide initiative to improve care of women and children in this period (Chang, Fowles, & Walker, 2006).

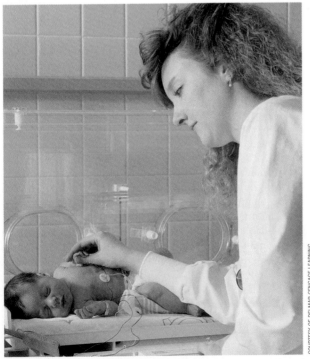

COURTESY OF DELMAR CENGAGE LEARNING

**FIGURE 4-7** Parents of an infant who requires special medical care should be encouraged to spend as much time with their child as possible.

### INFECTION CONTROL

**Standard Precautions in Postpartum Care**

Gloves should be worn when:
- Assessing the breasts if there is leakage of colostrum or milk
- Handling used breast pads
- Assessing lochia and the perineum
- Changing peripads or chux
- Handling anything on which there is lochia (bed linen, towels, washcloth, clothing, peripads, chux)

## CLIENTTEACHING
### Breast Assessment

- Explain the characteristics of the breast and what to expect depending on whether the mother is breastfeeding or not.
- Describe how to recognize problems such as mastitis and nipple fissures or cracks.

# NURSING PROCESS

## ASSESSMENT

Assessments specific to the first few days postpartum include breasts, uterus, bladder, bowel, lochia, and episiotomy; vital signs; lower extremities and Homans' sign; bonding/attachment; parenting; activity; comfort; and self-care. These assessments are usually performed, at least once a shift, until the mother is discharged. A sample initial postpartum profile sheet is shown in Figure 4-8.

## Subjective Data

Ask the mother whether the milk has come in or whether there is any breast discomfort; whether the bladder feels empty after urination; whether the mother is able to pass gas rectally or has the urge to have a bowel movement; whether any clots are passed vaginally and when the peripad was last changed; whether there is dizziness when getting up; whether

contractions are felt during breastfeeding; or whether there is discomfort or pain, especially in the perineal area.

## Objective Data

### Breasts

Note the size and shape of the breasts and any abnormalities or reddened areas. The breasts should be gently palpated for softness, firmness, engorgement, warmth, or tenderness. Check the nipples for cracks, fissures, soreness, and inversion.

### Uterus

Palpate the abdomen to find the top (fundus) of the uterus by pressing in and down with the side of one hand, and placing the other hand above the symphysis to support the uterus. The size, consistency, and placement (midline or off to one side) of the uterus is noted. It should be firm (not boggy) and in the midline. Each day it should descend approximately 1 cm (1 finger breadth). Fundal descent is documented in relation to the umbilicus (Figure 4-9).

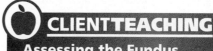

## CLIENTTEACHING
### Assessing the Fundus

- Explain why it is important for the uterus to be firmly contracted.
- Demonstrate how to palpate the uterine fundus.
- Demonstrate the way to gently massage the fundus.

**FIGURE 4-8 Representative Initial Postpartum Profile** (*Permission to use this copyrighted material has been granted by the owner, Hollister Incorporated.*)

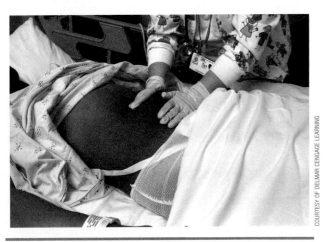

FIGURE 4-9 The nurse supports the uterus with her left hand held beneath it while palpating the uterus to determine if it is firm or boggy and its position, midline, or displaced.

---

## MEMORY TRICK
### Postpartum Assessment

Remember **BUBBLE** for the order of the Post-Partum Assessment:

**B** = Breasts

**U** = Uterus

**B** = Bowels

**B** = Bladder

**L** = Lochia

**E** = Episiotomy/laceration/C-section incision

---

## CLIENT TEACHING
### Bladder and Bowel Elimination

Encourage the new mother to:

• Drink plenty of fluids.

• Ambulate frequently and use the bathroom, not a bedpan.

• Eat a well-balanced diet with increased fiber and fluids.

• Promptly answer nature's call to urinate or defecate.

---

## Bladder

When the abdomen is palpated for the uterine fundus, the bladder can also be palpated for distention. A full, distended bladder is very often the cause for the fundus to be higher than it should be and to be positioned off to one side (not in the midline) (Figure 4-10). An intake and output (I&O) record is kept during the first 24 hours, at least, to assist in identifying urine retention.

---

## CLIENT TEACHING
### Lochia Assessment

• Describe the expected changes in the color and amount of lochia.

• Advise the mother that if the lochia changes from serosa back to rubra, she is either doing too much heavy work or the uterus is not firmly contracted. The mother should check fundal firmness and rest for a while.

• Instruct mother to notify her certified nurse-midwife (CNM)/physician if clots are passed or if the lochia has an unusual or unpleasant odor.

---

## Bowels

Inspect the abdomen for distention and auscultate for the presence of bowel sounds. The client's labor record should be reviewed to check whether she received an enema. The anus can be inspected when the episiotomy is checked. Make sure to check for hemorrhoids at this point.

## Lochia

Ask the mother to lie on her back with knees flexed so the peri-pad can be lowered in the front. Lochia is assessed for color, amount, odor, and presence of clots. Then, ask the mother to turn to her side to see whether any lochia has pooled under her buttocks.

**Amount** It is difficult to estimate the amount of lochia on a perineal pad. Luegenbiehl, Brophy, Artigue, Phillips, and Flack (1990) identified a method to estimate the amount of lochia discharged in 1 hour (Figure 4-11).

The mother who has had a cesarean birth will have less lochia after the first 24 hours than a mother who had

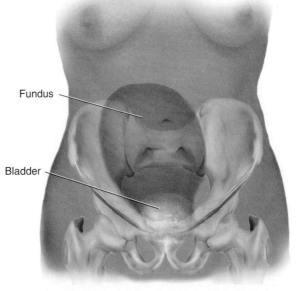

Fundus

Bladder

FIGURE 4-10 A full bladder displaces the uterus and prevents its contractions.

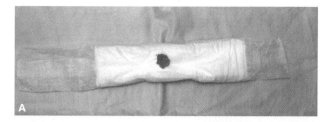

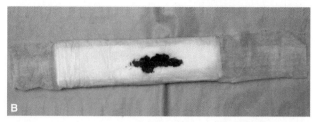

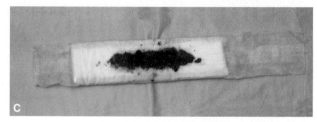

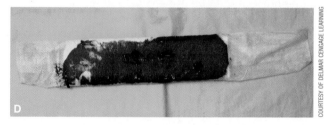

**FIGURE 4-11** An assessment of lochia is based on the amount of blood saturation on a peripad. *A*, Scant: 2-inch stain (10 mL); *B*, Small: 4-inch stain (10-25 mL); *C*, Moderate: 6-inch stain (25-50 mL); *D*, Large: >6-inch stain (50-80 mL).

COURTESY OF DELMAR CENGAGE LEARNING

a vaginal birth. The lochia also usually changes from rubra to serosa sooner because the inside of the uterus is wiped with sponges during a cesarean birth, removing some of the endometrium.

**Odor** Lochia has a nonoffensive odor. If the lochia has a foul odor, an infection is present and the certified nurse-midwife (CNM)/physician must be notified at once.

**Presence of Clots** A few small clots, which occur when blood pools in the vagina, are normal. Passing many or large clots is not normal and requires further investigation. Any clot that is larger than the size of an egg should be cause for further investigation and assessment by the nurse.

## Episiotomy

Assess the episiotomy with the mother in Sims' position (Figure 4-12). This can be done when the mother is on her side for lochia assessment. With a gloved hand, very gently raise the upper buttock just enough to see the episiotomy. Changes in the episiotomy should be noted. See Memory Trick for episiotomy assessment.

With the client in the same position, gently touch the external labia and note whether this causes pain. The labia should also be inspected for ecchymosis and edema. The anus can be inspected for hemorrhoids.

# MEMORY**TRICK**
## Episiotomy Assessment

When assessing a client's episiotomy, remember to assess the 5 items that are recalled by the **REEDA** mnemonic:

**R** = Redness—inflammation

**E** = Ecchymosis—bruising

**E** = Edema—swelling

**D** = Discharge—from incision

**A** = Approximation of suture line (Davidson, 1974).

# CLIENT**TEACHING**
## Techniques to Decrease Episiotomy Discomfort

Instruct mother to:

- Tighten her buttocks and perineum before sitting to prevent pulling on the episiotomy and perineal area, and to release the tightening after being seated.
- Rest several times a day with feet elevated.
- Practice the Kegel exercise many times a day to increase circulation to the perineal area and to strengthen the perineal muscles.
- Use peri-bottle when urinating to relieve pain and ease in lochia cleansing.

## Vital Signs

Assess vital signs every 15 minutes for the first 1 to 2 hours after birth. If no problems are identified, vital signs may then be checked every 8 hours.

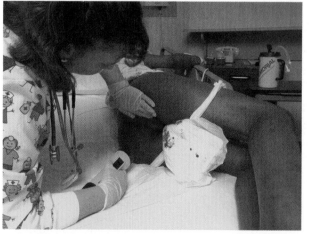

COURTESY OF DELMAR CENGAGE LEARNING

**FIGURE 4-12** The episiotomy is assessed with the mother lying on her side. The upper buttock is raised gently, just enough to see the episotomy. The anal area can be assessed for hemorrhoids at the same time.

**Temperature** Temperature may increase to 100.4°F (38°C) during the first 24 hours. After the first 24 hours, a temperature over 100.4°F suggests an infection.

**Pulse** After the first hour after the birth, the mother's pulse rate may decrease to 50 to 70 beats/minute for 6 to 8 days. An elevated pulse may indicate excessive blood loss, infection, anxiety, or pain.

**Blood Pressure** Blood pressure should remain consistent with the baseline during pregnancy. An increase suggests PIH, whereas a decrease may indicate excessive bleeding.

## Lower Extremities and Homans' Sign

Examine the mother's legs for signs of thrombophlebitis such as redness, heat, edema, and tenderness. Palpate the pedal pulses. Perform the assessment for Homans' sign.

To assess for Homans' sign, support the client's leg under the knee while sharply dorsiflexing the foot (Figure 4-13). Homans' sign is positive if the client experiences calf discomfort when the foot is dorsiflexed and negative if the client does not experience discomfort in the calf. When Homans' sign is positive, it must be reported at once to the CNM/physician because it may indicate thrombophlebitis.

## Bonding/Attachment

Assess the interaction of the mother with her infant for the expected behaviors of bonding and beginning attachment. The manner in which the mother holds, examines, and speaks to the infant is important. For instance, the mother who cradles her infant, gazes at her infant's face, and speaks in a pleasant manner to the infant is exhibiting signs of bonding and attachment.

## Parenting

Assess the skill with which the mother cares for her infant. For example, observe feeding, diapering, bathing, and consoling skills to determine whether additional teaching is required.

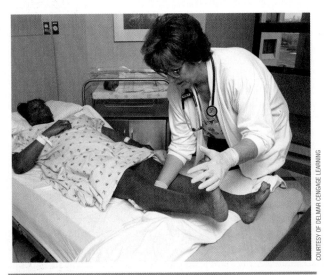

COURTESY OF DELMAR CENGAGE LEARNING

**FIGURE 4-13** **Homans' Sign Assessment. Discomfort experienced in the calf when the foot is sharply dorsiflexed is considered positive and may indicate thrombophlebitis.**

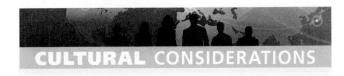

## CULTURAL CONSIDERATIONS

### Rest

Expectations of maternal activity during the postpartum period may be influenced by cultural norms. For example:

- Korean women rest an average of 21 days following birth (Howard & Berbiglia, 1997).
- Southeast Asian, Vietnamese, Cambodian, and Laotian women stay in bed without a pillow and keep warm for 2 days (Mattson, 1995).

## ▼ SAFETY ▼

### First Ambulation

The first time a new mother gets out of bed, the nurse should be at her side and ready to assist in case the mother becomes lightheaded, weak, or dizzy. Encourage client to sit at the side of the bed for a few moments before ambulating. Leave bathroom door slightly ajar and stay within close proximity to client in case she begins to feel faint.

## Activity

Determine that the mother is ambulating, that is, getting up to go to the bathroom and frequently walking around. Many complications such as thromboses, emboli, and hypostatic pneumonia occur when the mother is in bed for extended periods.

Rest is just as important as activity. The mother expended a great deal of energy during labor and birth. Care should be planned so the mother has some uninterrupted periods of rest.

## Comfort

Comfort is essential to rest. Many new mothers never say anything about discomforts because they are so excited and pleased with their new infant. Be alert to any behavioral signs of discomfort. Most discomfort is related to perineal pain or afterpains.

## Self-Care

Assessment of self-care includes the mother's knowledge of how to care for herself and also whether she actually performs the care. Self-care includes showering, perineal care, checking the fundus, breast care, and rest. Support the client's recovery by encouraging her to bathe, toilet, and feed herself independently.

**Nursing diagnoses for a postpartum mother include the following:**

| NURSING DIAGNOSES | PLANNING/OUTCOMES | NURSING INTERVENTIONS |
|---|---|---|
| *Urinary Retention* related to sensory motor impairment from bladder trauma during labor and birth as evidenced by client being unable to urinate after delivery | The client will have appropriate urinary elimination (no bladder distention). | Monitor intake for adequate amount.<br><br>Assess for bladder distention every 2 to 4 hours.<br><br>Assist client to bathroom for elimination.<br><br>Pour warm water over vulvar area or run water in the sink to stimulate urination.<br><br>Catheterize, if necessary, as ordered. |
| *Risk for Infection* related to episiotomy | The client will have no signs of infection. | Assess episiotomy for redness and swelling.<br><br>Teach mother pericare: wash hands, remove peripad from front to back, pour warm water over perineum, pat dry from front to back, apply clean peripad front first then toward the back, wash hands.<br><br>Advise client to change peripad every 2 to 4 hours and every time she goes to the bathroom. |
| *Acute Pain* related to episiotomy, engorged breasts, or involution of the uterus | The client will state that discomfort has decreased. | *Episiotomy*<br><br>Assess perineum for edema.<br><br>Apply ice pack for 20 minutes; remove for at least 10 minutes before reapplying.<br><br>Assist mother with Sitz bath as ordered, and watch for dizziness, floating feeling, or difficulty hearing (signs of possible fainting).<br><br>Apply Dermoplast spray or Americain spray (topical anesthetics) to perineum after a sitz bath or pericare, as ordered.<br><br>Emphasize the need to wash hands before and after any care of the episiotomy.<br><br>Teach mother to squeeze buttocks together before sitting, release after sitting.<br><br>Encourage mother to practice Kegel exercise 4 or 5 times a day.<br><br>Administer analgesic as ordered.<br><br>Avoid using rectal suppositories for clients with 3rd- or 4th-degree episiotomy.<br><br>*Engorged Breasts* (not breastfeeding)<br><br>Encourage mother to wear a well-fitting supportive bra, removing it only for showers, to suppress lactation.<br><br>Provide ice pack to axillary area and side of breast for 20 minutes 4 times a day to suppress lactation.<br><br>Advise mother to avoid any stimulation to breast; stand with back to shower so warm water does not hit breasts.<br><br>Administer analgesic as ordered.<br><br>*Engorged Breasts* (breastfeeding)<br><br>Encourage the mother to feed her infant approximately every 2 hours; empty (until soft) one breast; then feed from second breast or pump to soften.<br><br>Administer antiinflammatory pain medication as ordered.<br><br>Apply ice pack between feedings for 15 minutes on and 45 minutes off as ordered.<br><br>*Involution of Uterus* (afterpains)<br><br>Assess fundus for firmness and position. |

*(Continues)*

| **Nursing diagnoses for a postpartum mother include the following: (Continued)** | | |
| --- | --- | --- |
| **NURSING DIAGNOSES** | **PLANNING/OUTCOMES** | **NURSING INTERVENTIONS** |
| | | Determine when mother has pain. |
| | | Explain, if mother is breastfeeding, that the oxytocin released in response to breastfeeding causes the uterus to contract. The discomfort lasts only a few minutes at the beginning of each breastfeeding session for the first 4 to 6 days. |
| | | Administer analgesic as ordered. |

**Evaluation:** Evaluate each outcome to determine how it has been met by the client.

# HEALTH PROMOTION

The mother's record must be checked to determine the mother's need for Rh immune globulin (RhoGAM) and rubella immunization. When required, these two items protect the fetuses of future pregnancies.

## RH IMMUNE GLOBULIN

Rh immune globulin (RhoGAM) is given within 72 hours after birth to prevent sensitization of Rh-negative mothers who gave birth to Rh-positive infants. The RhoGAM promotes lysis of fetal Rh-positive red blood cells before the mother's body is able to form antibodies against them.

## RUBELLA IMMUNIZATION

It is recommended that all women who have not had rubella or who have a 1:8 rubella titer be given rubella vaccine in the immediate postpartum period. This will prevent fetal anomalies in future pregnancies if the mother is exposed to rubella. Breastfeeding is not a contraindication to receiving the immunization. Because the vaccine may be teratogenic, pregnancy must be avoided for 2 to 3 months

# CESAREAN BIRTH

All of the assessments just discussed are also performed on a mother who has had a cesarean birth. In addition, postoperative assessments are performed, including incision, respirations and breath sounds, abdomen and bowel sounds, fluid intake, urine output, and the degree of pain.

## INCISION

Inspect the dressing for intactness and any bleeding or discharge. After the dressing is removed, assess the incision for

### PROFESSIONAL TIP

#### Rh Immune Globulin (RhoGAM) Administration

Rho-GAM is considered a blood product. Some patients with cultural aversions to blood products might refuse administration. Since this is a blood product, two nurses must check labs and orders before administration.

signs of infection such as redness, heat, pain, or edema and the suture line for approximation.

## RESPIRATIONS AND BREATH SOUNDS

If the mother received narcotics either epidurally or with patient-controlled analgesia (PCA), assess respirations frequently because narcotics depress the respiratory center. Assess respiratory rate and depth every 15 minutes for the first hour, every 30 minutes for the next 4 to 5 hours, and every hour for the remainder of the first 24 hours. Some institutions may use an apnea monitor. Auscultate breath sounds at each respiratory check to identify whether secretions are beginning to pool in the bronchioles. Assess the client's efforts of turning (changing position), coughing, deep breathing, and use of the incentive spirometer.

## ABDOMEN AND BOWEL SOUNDS

In addition to the incision, assess the abdomen for softness or distention. Auscultate bowel sounds until peristalsis is noted in all four quadrants. Ask the mother whether she has been able to pass any flatus (gas) rectally.

## FLUID INTAKE

Frequently assess the flow rate of intravenous fluids as well as the site. Record the amount of intravenous fluid and any oral fluid intake.

## URINE OUTPUT

A Foley catheter is generally inserted into the bladder before the cesarean birth. Assess and record the amount of urine output as well as the clarity and color. Make sure that client is eliminating at least 30 mL/hour. If urine output is less than 30 mL, notify the attending physician.

## PAIN

Most new mothers who have a vaginal birth are eager to interact with their newborn infant. This is no different following a cesarean birth; however, these mothers will need to be taught how to hold and carry the infant in a way that will not disturb or irritate their incisions. The mothers may not want pain medication because they want to stay awake with and enjoy their infants.

Breastfeeding mothers who have had a cesarean birth may also not admit to having pain because they are concerned that pain medication will be present in the breast milk. Pain medication is generally required for 24 to 48 hours following a cesarean birth. These mothers are taught to support the baby with a pillow to avoid incisional pain while nursing.

## SAMPLE NURSING CARE PLAN

## The Postpartum Client

S.V. and her husband, J.V, have just participated in the birth of their first child, a daughter, weighing 6 lbs, 8 oz, and measuring 21 inches long. A small episiotomy was made. J.V. has "always wanted a son" and is "disappointed about having a daughter." He looks at the infant but does not touch her or speak to her.

S.V. is exhausted from the labor and birth, says she is too tired to hold the baby and wants only to sleep. Her vital signs are within normal range, and the uterus tends to relax. Within 1-1/2 hours, she has saturated three peripads. A bulge is noted above the symphysis. S.V. is unable to urinate at this time.

**NURSING DIAGNOSIS 1** *Risk for Deficient Fluid Volume* related to early postpartum hemorrhage as evidenced by saturating three peripads in 1-1/2 hours

**Nursing Outcomes Classification (NOC)**
*Fluid Balance*

**Nursing Interventions Classification (NIC)**
*Fluid Monitoring*

| PLANNING/OUTCOMES | NURSING INTERVENTIONS | RATIONALE |
|---|---|---|
| S.V.'s fluid volume will be maintained by reducing the amount of lochia discharge. | Palpate and monitor fundal height, location, and consistency. | Determines status of uterus (firm or boggy) and height and location relative to umbilicus. |
| | For boggy uterus, gently massage and assess muscle tone. | Promotes uterine contraction and increases uterine tone. |
| | Monitor lochia (amount and color), time peripad changed, and degree of peripad saturation. | Evaluates the amount of lochia. |
| | Assess for bladder fullness and encourage voiding. | A full bladder interferes with contracting of the uterus. |
| | Monitor intake and output. | Identifies potential need to urinate. |
| | Monitor vital signs, skin temperature, and color. | Detects signs of shock. |
| | Administer oxytocic agent as ordered. | Promotes uterine contraction. |
| | Explain involution process to S.V. and teach her to check and gently massage her uterus. | Involves S.V. in self-care. |

## EVALUATION

S.V.'s fluid volume is maintained. S.V. is voiding adequately, allowing the uterus to contract and the amount of lochia to decrease.

**NURSING DIAGNOSIS 2** *Risk for Impaired Parenting* related to not gender desired as evidenced by J.V. expressing a desire for a son, showing seeming disappointment with a daughter, not touching or speaking to the infant, and S.V. saying she is too tired to hold the baby

**Nursing Outcomes Classification (NOC)**
*Parent–Infant Attachment*

**Nursing Interventions Classification (NIC)**
*Parenting Promotion*

*(Continues)*

## SAMPLE NURSING CARE PLAN (Continued)

| PLANNING/OUTCOMES | NURSING INTERVENTIONS | RATIONALE |
|---|---|---|
| S.V. and J.V. will demonstrate bonding and attachment behaviors with their daughter. | Assist S.V. in holding her daughter. | Emphasizes holding infant as important. |
| | Point out unique characteristics about the infant (e.g., dimple in right cheek, long fingers). | Helps S.V. and J.V. get acquainted with their daughter. |
| | Ask S.V. and J.V. who the infant looks like. | Assists S.V. and J.V. in identifying family characteristics. |
| | Model bonding and attachment behaviors for S.V. and J.V. such as talking to infant, finger-tipping, and examining infant. | Shows S.V. and J.V. how to interact with their daughter. |
| | Describe infant's behavior and explain that the infant can see and hear her parents. | Enables S.V. and J.V. to understand their infant and her abilities. |

### EVALUATION
S.V. follows nurse's example and strokes the infant's head and face with her fingertips and talks to her. J.V. touches the infant's fingers but does not watch her intently or for longer than a few seconds.

**NURSING DIAGNOSIS 3** *Urinary Retention* related to sensory motor function impairment as evidenced by client's inability to urinate after delivery, as well as a bulge above the pubic symphysis, indicating bladder distention

**Nursing Outcomes Classification (NOC)**
*Urinary Elimination*

**Nursing Interventions Classification (NIC)**
*Urinary Elimination Management*
*Urinary Catheterization*

| PLANNING/OUTCOMES | NURSING INTERVENTIONS | RATIONALE |
|---|---|---|
| S.V. will have regular urinary elimination with no bladder distention. | Palpate bulge above symphysis while asking S.V. whether bladder feels full. | Confirms that bulge is a full bladder. |
| | Assist S.V. to the bathroom or onto bedpan if she is unable to ambulate. | Allows S.V. to empty her bladder. |
| | Run water in sink, place S.V.'s hands in warm water, or pour water over her perineum. | Stimulates urination. |
| | Administer analgesic as ordered if S.V. has vulvar/perineal discomfort and is afraid to void. | Relieves discomfort; may help S.V. relax and void. |
| | Catheterize if necessary, as ordered. | Empties bladder, allowing uterus to contract and promoting comfort. |

## SAMPLE NURSING CARE PLAN (Continued)

### EVALUATION

S.V. empties her bladder when assisted to the bathroom.

**NURSING DIAGNOSIS 4** *Risk for Infection* related to tissue destruction at episiotomy site and increased environmental exposure to pathogens as evidenced by inflammation and drainage at episiotomy site

**Nursing Outcomes Classification (NOC)**
*Infection Status*
*Primary Intention*

**Nursing Interventions Classification (NIC)**
*Infection Protection*
*Incision Site Care*
*Health Education*

| PLANNING/OUTCOMES | NURSING INTERVENTIONS | RATIONALE |
|---|---|---|
| S.V. will have no evidence of infection. | Follow Standard Precautions, especially good hand hygiene before and after providing care, and wear gloves when contact with lochia or urine is possible. | Prevents spread of infection. |
| | Use strict aseptic technique when inserting a catheter or starting an intravenous infusion. | Reduces the risk of a nosocomial infection. |
| | Monitor vital signs. | If elevated, may indicate an infection. |
| | Monitor for loss of appetite, malaise, and chills. | May indicate infection. |
| | Assess episiotomy for redness, edema, drainage, and pain; and lochia for a foul odor. | Indicates infection. |
| | Teach S.V. proper perineal care. | Keeps perineum clean and prevents contamination of episiotomy by anal organisms. |

### EVALUATION

S.V. has no signs of infection.

## COMPLICATIONS

The most common complications of childbirth are postpartum hemorrhage, infection, thromboembolic conditions, and disseminated intravascular coagulation.

### ■ POSTPARTUM HEMORRHAGE

Postpartum hemorrhage is defined as a blood loss of more than 500 mL after the third stage of labor or 1,000 mL after a cesarean birth. The hemorrhage is identified as either early, within the first 24 hours, or late, generally occurring 1 to 2 weeks after the birth, but may occur up to 6 weeks after the birth.

A postpartum hemorrhage can occur rapidly and may not be recognized until the client is in moderate to severe shock (Table 4-1).

## EARLY POSTPARTUM HEMORRHAGE

Early postpartum hemorrhage has several possible causes: uterine atony, retained placental fragments, lacerations of the birth canal, and hematomas. Predisposing factors for postpartum hemorrhage include the following:

- Overdistention of the uterus (large infant, multiple gestation, or hydramnios)
- Grandmultiparity (more than 5)
- Precipitate labor or birth

**TABLE 4-1  Hemorrhagic Shock**

|  | BP | PULSE | RESP | SKIN | URINE OUTPUT | BLOOD LOSS | LEVEL OF CONSCIOUSNESS |
|---|---|---|---|---|---|---|---|
| Mild | Normal or increased | Increased becoming weaker | Increased deep | Cool, pale | Normal 30 mL/hr | 500–900 mL | Alert, oriented, anxious |
| Moderate | Systolic 60–90 | Tachycardia becoming irregular | Tachypnea becoming shallow | Cool, pale, moist | Decreased 10–22 mL/hr | 1,200–1,500 mL | Oriented, increasing anxiety, restless |
| Severe | Systolic <60 | 120–160 irregular | 30–50 shallow | Cool, clammy | Oliguric <10 mL/hr | 1,800–2,100 mL | Lethargic |
| Very Severe | May not be detected | May be absent | >50 | Cyanotic | Oliguria to anuria | >2,400 mL | Slipping into unconsciousness |

COURTESY OF DELMAR CENGAGE LEARNING

- Prolonged labor
- Use of forceps or vacuum extractor
- Use of tocolytic drugs
- Use of oxytocin to augment or induce labor
- Cesarean birth
- Manual removal of the placenta
- Clotting disorders

## UTERINE ATONY

Uterine atony is a lack of muscle tone in the uterus. The uterus feels soft and boggy. Hemorrhage from uterine atony is usually a steady flow. Blood pressure and pulse changes may not occur until the blood loss is severe because during pregnancy there is an increase in blood volume.

## RETAINED PLACENTAL FRAGMENTS

Occasionally, small pieces of the placenta may not be expelled. These pieces prevent the uterus from contracting effectively, and bleeding continues.

## LACERATIONS OF THE BIRTH CANAL

Factors predisposing a woman to lacerations of the birth canal include the following:

- Nulliparity
- Forceps-assisted or vacuum-assisted birth
- Precipitous birth
- Macrosomia
- Epidural anesthesia

Lacerations may occur in the perineum, vagina, cervix, or around the urethral meatus. Most lacerations are identified and repaired by the CNM/physician immediately following the birth. Occasionally, a laceration is overlooked and bright red bleeding persists when the uterus is firmly contracted. It is at this point that the nurse should suspect a laceration and notify the attending CNM/physician.

## HEMATOMA

A hematoma forms when there is bleeding into the tissues; there is no external laceration. Spontaneous or forceps-assisted births may result in hematoma formation. The most common sites are the vulva, vagina, and retroperitoneal area (Figure 4-14). A hematoma is a bluish-purple mass that produces deep, severe, unrelenting pain and a feeling of great pressure. When the uterus is firmly contracted, the amount of lochia is within normal limits, and the mother has a falling blood pressure or tachycardia and persistently describes severe pain, suspect a hematoma.

## LATE POSTPARTUM HEMORRHAGE

A late postpartum hemorrhage usually occurs 1 to 2 weeks after the birth because of **subinvolution** (incomplete return of the uterus to its prepregnant size and consistency) or retained placental fragments. Clots may form around the retained placental

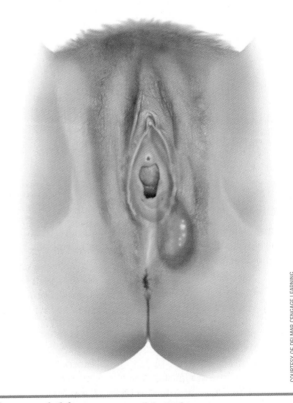

COURTESY OF DELMAR CENGAGE LEARNING

**FIGURE 4-14  Hematoma of the Vulva**

fragments immediately postpartum, thus keeping lochia within normal limits. Several days later, when the clots slough, excessive bleeding occurs. There is usually no warning of a late postpartum hemorrhage. This should be viewed as a medical emergency. The nurse teaches clients prior to discharge the signs and symptoms of a late postpartum hemorrhage.

## MEDICAL–SURGICAL MANAGEMENT

### Medical

The CNM/physician carefully palpates the uterus to make sure it is contracting after the birth. A thorough examination of the birth canal for lacerations or hematomas is also undertaken. A sonogram may be used to determine the presence of retained placental fragments.

### Surgical

Cunningham et al. (2005) report that curettage, formerly the usual treatment, is now believed to cause more bleeding because of trauma to the placental site. It now is performed when other methods have failed to control the bleeding.

Surgical evacuation of a large hematoma or one increasing in size may be necessary to attain hemostasis. The bleeding vessel is identified and ligated (tied).

### Pharmacological

Oxytocin (Pitocin), methylergonovine maleate (Methergine), misoprostol (Cytotec), or prostaglandins may be given to contract the uterus. Methylergonovine maleate (Methergine) should not be given to a client with an elevated blood pressure. The strong contractions produced by these medications often loosen the retained placental fragments, which are then discharged with the lochia. Antibiotics are often used prophylactically to prevent infection. Blood transfusion or replacement of coagulation factors may be necessary depending on the amount of blood lost.

### CRITICAL THINKING

#### Contracted Uterus and Heavy Lochia

A client with a well-contracted uterus is having an extremely heavy lochia discharge. What assessments does the nurse make? What nursing care should be provided?

### PROFESSIONAL TIP

#### Factors That Predispose a Postpartum Client to Hemorrhage:

If the postpartum client has any of these predisposing factors, carefully assess for hemorrhage.

- Low platelets count
- A history of bleeding
- A history of alcohol abuse
- Taking any herbal or homeopathic remedies
- Taking any aspirin or NSAIDs
- Obese or suffering from poor nutrition

Catastrophic Intraoperative Hemorrhage, by D. Gallup, 2005, June, *OBG Management*, 54--61.

### Activity

The mother is usually kept in bed until the bleeding is under control.

## NURSING MANAGEMENT

Monitor vital signs; urine output; uterine height, firmness, and position; blood loss; and level of consciousness. Assess bladder for distension. Save all peripads, linen, and linen savers for estimate of blood loss.

For a hematoma, apply ice, assess pain using pain scale, and continue assessing the hematoma size.

## NURSING PROCESS

### ASSESSMENT

#### Subjective Data

The mother may either describe feeling like a lot of blood is coming from her vagina or a severe pain in the vulvar or perineal area.

#### Objective Data

Palpate the fundus for size, consistency, and position. Check how long the peripad has been in place, how much lochia is present, and whether the bladder is distended. Vital signs will probably be within the normal range.

**Nursing diagnoses for a client with a postpartum hemorrhage include the following:**

| NURSING DIAGNOSES | PLANNING/OUTCOMES | NURSING INTERVENTIONS |
|---|---|---|
| Risk for *Imbalanced Fluid Volume* related to significant blood loss from uterine atony, as evidenced by client's fundus displaced from | The client will maintain adequate fluid volume. | Assess vital signs and the bladder for distension. |
| | | Assess fundal height, firmness, and location as per agency protocol. If client has predisposing factors for postpartum hemorrhage, assess more frequently. |
| | | Assess lochia amount and color and relate to firmness of fundus. Notify CNM/physician about excessive bleeding. |

*(Continues)*

**Nursing diagnoses for a client with a postpartum hemorrhage include the following: (Continued)**

| NURSING DIAGNOSES | PLANNING/OUTCOMES | NURSING INTERVENTIONS |
|---|---|---|
| midline and unable to maintain a firm fundus on palpation | | Maintain mother on bed rest. |
| | | Call for assistance; one nurse to monitor vital signs while a second nurse monitors fundus and lochia. |
| | | Save all peripads, linen, and linen savers for more accurate estimate of blood loss. |
| | | Document all assessments, interventions, and each time CNM/physician is notified. |
| | | Administer medications as ordered. |
| *Acute **Pain*** related to tissue damage from hematoma formation, as evidenced by client crying during peri care when RN was assessing the hematoma area | The client will describe having less pain. | Apply ice pack to hematoma. |
| | | Continue assessment of hematoma size. |
| | | Assess client's pain using 0 to 10 pain scale (0 = no pain, 10 = most pain). |
| | | Notify CNM/physician of hematoma and pain assessment. |
| | | Administer medications as ordered. |
| | | Document all assessments, interventions, and each time CNM/physician is notified. |

**Evaluation:** Evaluate each outcome to determine how it has been met by the client.

## ■ INFECTIONS

**P**uerperal (postpartum) infection is an infection after childbirth occurring between the birth and 6 weeks postpartum. It is defined as a temperature of 38°C (100.4°F) or more on two separate occasions, after the first 24 hours, on any two of the first 10 postpartum days (Bowes, 1996).

Because all parts of the reproductive tract are connected to each other, it is easy for organisms to move from the vagina through the cervix, to the uterus, through the fallopian tubes, and out to the ovaries and peritoneal cavity. The increased blood supply to the reproductive tract during pregnancy provides more avenues for invading bacteria to be spread throughout the body with the possibility of causing a life-threatening septicemia.

Amniotic fluid and lochia are alkaline, so during labor and in the postpartum period, the normal acidity of the vagina is reduced, which encourages bacterial growth. Predisposing factors include the frequency of vaginal examinations during labor, the length of time membranes had been ruptured, and the length of labor. The growing rates of cesarean sections in the United States have been a major concern and risk factor for postpartum infection. Research has shown that women who underwent labor before having a cesarean birth were at greater risk for postpartum infection (Tharpe, 2008)

It is currently recommended that a prophylactic antibiotic be given to the mother having a cesarean birth after the cord is clamped. This prevents masking or partial treatment of any neonatal infections (Normand & Damato, 2001). The use of prophylactic antibiotics after a caesarean delivery has been noted to reduce postpartum infection by up to 75% (Tharpe, 2008).

It is seldom necessary to keep the baby separated from the mother during maternal infection because they generally share the same organisms. Someone should be available to care for the infant because the mother is usually tired and does not have the energy to fully care for her infant.

Common postpartum infections are wound infection, metritis, mastitis, and urinary tract infection. Predisposing factors for puerperal infection are listed in Table 4-2.

## WOUND INFECTION

The break in the skin from lacerations, episiotomies, and surgical incisions from cesarean birth provides an easy portal of entry for bacteria. Localized signs of infection (redness, warmth, edema, and tenderness) are assessed at the skin break, which, if untreated, will develop into generalized signs of infection, including an elevated temperature and malaise. Wound edges may separate and drainage may be evident.

## METRITIS

**Metritis**, inflammation of the uterus, includes both endometritis (inflammation of the inside of the uterus, or endometrium) and parametritis (inflammation of the outside of the uterus, or parametrium, including the connective tissue of the broad ligaments). The usual causes are the organisms that normally inhabit the vagina and cervix. This infection easily spreads through the fallopian tubes (**salpingitis**) to the

## TABLE 4-2 Predisposing Factors for Postpartum Infection

| PREDISPOSING FACTORS | DESCRIPTION/ EXPLANATION |
|---|---|
| **Antepartum** **Medical conditions** | |
| • Diabetes <br> • Alcoholism <br> • Drug abuse <br> • Anemia <br> • Poor nutrition/ malnutrition <br> • Immunosuppression | Ability to defend against any infection is decreased |
| History of previous infections | Possibly more vulnerable to infections |
| **Intrapartum** | |
| Prolonged rupture of membranes | Provides direct access to interior of uterus |
| Chorioamnionitis | Organisms already in uterus |
| Prolonged labor | More time for bacteria to multiply |
| Excessive number of vaginal examinations | Increases opportunity for organisms from outside source or vagina to be introduced into the uterus |
| Internal fetal monitoring | Provides opportunity for introduction of organisms |
| Bladder catheterization | Possible introduction of organisms into bladder |
| Episiotomy, lacerations, and cesarean birth | Provide portals of entry for organisms |
| **Postpartum** | |
| Retained placental fragments | Good medium for bacterial growth |
| Hematoma | Makes tissues more susceptible |
| Hemorrhage | Infection-fighting components of blood are lost |

COURTESY OF DELMAR CENGAGE LEARNING

ovaries (**oophoritis**). The client may not appear ill except for chills and fever spikes (Ernest & Mead, 1998).

# MASTITIS

**Mastitis** is inflammation of the breast, generally during breastfeeding. The usual cause is *Staphylococcus aureus* but may also be *Candida albicans*. Symptoms appear between 2 and 4 weeks after birth. There is usually a crack or fissure in the nipple for the portal of entry. Nipple soreness may result in shorter breastfeeding times, allowing milk stasis, which is a good medium for bacterial growth.

# URINARY TRACT INFECTION

Approximately 2% to 4% of new mothers will have a urinary tract infection (UTI) (Murray et al., 2005). Trauma to the bladder and urethra during labor and birth, urinary stasis after the birth, and catheterization all contribute to the development of a UTI.

## MEDICAL–SURGICAL MANAGEMENT

### Medical

The goal of treatment is to confine the infection and prevent it from spreading systemically.

A culture of drainage from a wound, the uterine cavity, or urine is performed to identify the causative agent of the infection. Breastfeeding should continue during an infection unless the antibiotic used is contraindicated during lactation. Even with mastitis, breastfeeding should continue; emptying the breast at regular intervals is beneficial. If an abscess forms and ruptures into the breast ducts, the breast should be pumped and the milk discarded. Breastfeeding should continue with the unaffected breast.

### Surgical

Some sutures may be removed from the episiotomy, laceration repair, or abdominal incision to allow for drainage. If an abscess forms in mastitis, it may require an incision to allow drainage.

### Pharmacological

As soon as a culture is taken, a broad-spectrum antibiotic is usually administered pending the results of the culture.

• *Wound infection*: Iodoform gauze may be placed in the open incision. An analgesic may be necessary.
• *Metritis*: Intravenous administration of antibiotics may be required initially. An antipyretic is given to reduce fever, and methylergonovine maleate (Methergine) is given to increase lochia drainage and promote involution.
• *Mastitis*: Early antibiotic therapy usually prevents abscess formation. An analgesic may be necessary.

### Diet

A diet high in protein and vitamin C is needed for wound healing. Fluid intake should be increased to 3,000 mL/day for mothers with a urinary tract infection. Maintaining the increased fluid intake necessary for breastfeeding is essential even when the mother has mastitis.

### Activity

Extra rest periods are necessary for all new mothers with an infection. This is especially important for mothers with metritis and mastitis, who should ambulate only enough for their own self-care initially. While in bed, the mother with metritis should be in Fowler's position to aid in lochial drainage from the uterus.

## Health Promotion

Strict aseptic technique during labor and birth as well as frequent hand hygiene by those providing care to the mother are major factors in preventing postpartum infections.

## NURSING MANAGEMENT

Monitor vital signs and assess pain level. Perform a BUBBLE assessment at least every shift. Administer medications as ordered. Encourage client to stay in bed to rest and to increase fluid intake. Maintain client with metritis in the Fowler's position. Assist client to feed and interact with her infant.

## NURSING PROCESS

### ASSESSMENT

### Subjective Data

The mother may describe nausea, fatigue, malaise, pelvic pain or heaviness, leg tenderness, or breast tenderness.

### Objective Data

The objective data may include fever; chills; foul-smelling lochia; redness, edema, drainage, or wound separation; dysuria, frequency, or urgency; cracked nipple; and redness and edema of the breast.

| Nursing diagnoses for a client with a postpartum infection include the following: | | |
|---|---|---|
| **NURSING DIAGNOSES** | **PLANNING/OUTCOMES** | **NURSING INTERVENTIONS** |
| *Deficient Knowledge* related to unfamiliarity with information resources about the etiology, management, as well as the prevention of postpartum infection as evidenced by client's inaccurate follow through of instruction given by RN. | The client will follow the management plan for her infection. | Teach client how changes after birth predispose to infection. Explain the specific management for client's infection. Answer client's questions. |
| *Acute Pain* related to wound infection, metritis, mastitis, or urinary tract infection, as evidenced by client reporting her pain as greater than 2/10 on the pain scale on assessment. | The client will describe less discomfort. | Administer analgesics and antibiotics as ordered. Continue assessing degree of pain using 0 to 10 pain scale (0 = no pain, 10 = worst pain). |
| *Interrupted Family Processes* related to shift in health status of family member (mother) | The family will make adjustments for the mother's infection. | Assist family in understanding mother's limitations. Help family identify resources, people that assist with care, until the mother is well. |

**Evaluation:** Evaluate each outcome to determine how it has been met by the client.

## ■ THROMBOEMBOLIC CONDITIONS

Thrombophlebitis refers to the formation of a clot in an inflamed vein. Superficial thrombophlebitis is more common when the mother had preexisting varicose veins. Deep vein thrombosis (DVT) may or may not be related to vein inflammation and is seen more in women with a history of thromboses. Pulmonary embolism may be a complication of DVT. Septic pelvic thrombophlebitis is more commonly found in a mother with metritis as the inflammation spreads to the pelvic veins.

The incidence of thromboembolic conditions has decreased since early ambulation has become a standard practice after childbirth (Lowdermilk & Perry, 2007). Venous stasis and hypercoagulation, which are present during pregnancy, are the major causes. Other risk factors include maternal age older than 35, cesarean birth, prolonged time in stirrups during second stage of labor, obesity, smoking, and a history of varicosities or venous thromboses.

### MEDICAL–SURGICAL MANAGEMENT

#### Medical

Thrombophlebitis is usually managed with rest, elevation of the affected leg, and local application of heat. Elastic stockings are fitted for use when the mother is able to ambulate. Doppler ultrasound is an accurate diagnostic test for DVT. The mother who is receiving a broad-spectrum antibiotic for metritis and whose symptoms are not diminishing should be suspected of having septic pelvic thrombophlebitis.

#### 🔲 Pharmacological

An analgesic is given to relieve discomfort. Antibiotics are often given if the mother has a fever. DVT and septic pelvic thrombophlebitis are usually treated with intravenous heparin for 5 to 7 days. During this time, warfarin sodium (Coumadin) is begun and is usually continued for several months.

## Activity

Follow the CNM/physicians orders for all thromboembolic conditions. When the mother is allowed to ambulate, she must wear elastic stockings. In thrombophlebitis and DVT, the affected leg is elevated until symptoms decrease.

## Health Promotion

Instruct the client to avoid prolonged standing or sitting. Legs are not to be crossed when sitting. Encourage walking to increase venous return. Pad stirrups and properly adjust for correct support and to prevent pressure on the legs.

## NURSING MANAGEMENT

Maintain client in postion ordered by CNM/physician. Elevate the affected leg. Measure legs for elastic stockings for client to wear when able to ambulate. Administer medications as ordered. Teach client to avoid prolonged sitting or standing and to never cross her legs.

## NURSING PROCESS

### ASSESSMENT

Subjective Data The mother may describe discomfort or pain in the leg affected with superficial thrombophlebitis or DVT and a fullness/heaviness or pain in the pelvis if septic pelvic thrombosis occurs.

### Objective Data

Signs of superficial thrombophlebitis include redness, warmth, and swelling where the vein is inflamed. Deep vein thrombosis may manifest as edema and calf pain. A positive Homans' sign may be present, but may also be caused by a strained muscle or improper use of stirrups during the birth. The classic sign of septic pelvic thrombophlebitis is fever of unknown origin. When it is untreated, tachycardia, ileus, and an elevated white count develop.

### A nursing diagnosis for clients with thromboembolic conditions may be:

| NURSING DIAGNOSIS | PLANNING/OUTCOME | NURSING INTERVENTIONS |
|---|---|---|
| *Ineffective Peripheral Tissue Perfusion* related to mechanical reduction of venous blood flow as evidenced by positive Homans' Sign and pain on palpation of client's calf | The client will maintain adequate tissue perfusion. | Ensure affected leg is properly elevated. Apply heat to affected leg, as ordered. Measure client for antiembolic stockings and teach proper application when able to ambulate. Encourage fluid intake to prevent dehydration. Administer analgesics, antibiotics, heparin, and Coumadin as ordered. Assess for signs of pulmonary embolism (chest pain and dyspnea) and evidence of bleeding (i.e., petechiae, bruising, nosebleed, hematoma) related to heparin therapy. Emphasize importance of having prothrombin time checked while taking warfarin sodium (Coumadin). Keep protamine sulfate, the heparin antagonist, readily available. |

**Evaluation:** Evaluate each outcome to determine how it has been met by the client.

## ■ DISSEMINATED INTRAVASCULAR COAGULATION

Disseminated intravascular coagulation (DIC) is an abnormal stimulation of the clotting mechanism, which consumes clotting factors, causing small clots throughout the vascular system and widespread bleeding internally, externally, or both. This results in platelet and clotting factor depletion. DIC may result from a missed abortion, abruptio placenta, amniotic fluid embolism, severe preeclampsia, hemorrhage, and a dead fetus. It is a complication of a preexisting problem.

Correction of the underlying cause is the main aspect of medical management. Blood replacement products including whole blood, packed red cells, or cryoprecipitate may be administered. Nursing care includes continued assessment for signs of bleeding and of complications from the blood products. Intake and output is recorded; urinary output must be maintained at more than 30 mL/hour.

## CASE STUDY

R.L. and his wife, M.L, had a second son yesterday, their third child. The baby weighed 8 lbs, 10 oz, the largest of their three children. The labor lasted 5 hours. An episiotomy was performed this time but had not been for the previous births.

M.L. is having problems walking to the bathroom and says she feels faint and dizzy when she stands up. She talks constantly about the pain from the episiotomy. A bruised, edematous area is noted beside the episiotomy. Analgesics provide little relief. Plans were to breastfeed this infant as she had the first two. Today she does not want to feed the baby because she "hurts too much."

The following questions will guide your development of a nursing care plan for this case study.
1. What assessments should be made?
2. Identify three nursing diagnoses for M.L.
3. Identify planning/goals for M.L.
4. List nursing interventions to help M.L. meet the goals.
5. How can the effectiveness of this plan be evaluated?

## SUMMARY

- The first 6 weeks after the birth of an infant is called the puerperium or postpartum period.
- Mothers, fathers, siblings, and grandparents all make special adaptations for the neonate.
- During the postpartum period, most of the physiologic changes of pregnancy are reversed and the mother's body returns to its prepregnant state.
- Immediate weight loss of the mother is 13 lbs with an additional 8- to 9-lb loss during the first 6 weeks postpartum.

- Rubin describes three phases of maternal restoration/adaptation—taking in, taking hold, and letting go.
- Unexpected emotional/behavioral changes include postpartum depression, postpartum psychosis, and reaction to an infant with problems.
- Specific assessments for the first few days postpartum include BUBBLE (breasts, uterus, bladder, bowel, lochia, and episiotomy), vital signs, Homans' sign, bonding/attachment, parenting, activity, comfort, and self-care.

## REVIEW QUESTIONS

1. Client R.H. is 3 days postpartum and needs RhoGam. Before administering the injection, what should the nurse do?
   1. Check the orders and lab result to make sure that the Coomb's test was negative.
   2. Make sure the infant is Rh negative.
   3. Prepare a sub-q injection for the shot.
   4. Prepare to give the injection to the infant.
2. The nurse is checking a client after a scheduled cesarean delivery. On palpation of the fundus, the RN notices that the fundus is deviated to the right, firm, and with moderate lochial flow. What would be the nurse's first response to the situation?
   1. Administer 20 units of pitocin IM.
   2. Call the CNM/physician.
   3. Palpate the bladder and ask the client when she last voided.
   4. Insert a straight catheter into the client.
3. What is the best position to assess a postpartum woman's fundus?
   1. On her right side.
   2. Semi-Fowler position.
   3. Supine with knees slightly flexed.
   4. In a chair, with feet elevated.

4. A nurse is working triage in a busy labor and delivery unit when a patient calls, stating that "she is alone in her house and wants to harm herself and her new baby." The nurse's first response should be?
   1. "Let me help you schedule an appointment to see the doctor."
   2. Keep the client on the phone and call for police assistance to her house.
   3. Reassure the patient that she will be okay if she just gets some sleep.
   4. Have the patient drive herself to the emergency room.
5. The nurse is teaching a non-breastfeeding mother about breast care. The nurse knows that more teaching is needed when the client responds with the following statement:
   1. "I will make sure I wear a tight-fitting bra when my breast milk comes in."
   2. "I will express my milk to help it dry up."
   3. "I will avoid hot water on my breasts until my breast milk dries up."
   4. "I will use ice packs to help relieve the pain of engorgement."

6. The nurse observes passive and dependent behaviors displayed by a postpartum client. According to Reva Rubin, the client is in the:
   1. taking-in phase.
   2. letting-go phase.
   3. taking-hold phase.
   4. transitional phase.

7. A client has excessive vaginal bleeding after delivery. The assessment reveals a soft, boggy uterus located above the level of the umbilicus and displaced to the right side. The first action of the nurse should be to:
   1. notify the CNM/physician.
   2. massage the fundus and take vital signs.
   3. initiate measures that encourage voiding.
   4. put the client flat, take vital signs, and notify the CNM/physician.

8. A new mother tells the nurse that she is afraid of her baby and that she doubts she will be able to love the baby. The most appropriate action for the nurse would be to:
   1. tell the client she will learn fast.
   2. tell the client what a beautiful baby she has.
   3. encourage the client to talk about her feelings.
   4. have a psychiatrist visit the client immediately.

9. A client has excessive vaginal bleeding following the birth. The nurse should suspect a cervical or vaginal tear if the client assessment reveals:
   1. acute pelvic pain.
   2. a hard, contracted uterus.
   3. an elevation of blood pressure.
   4. a firmly contracted uterus with blood spurting from the vagina.

10. A client wants to know when she can begin breast-feeding and is anxious for her milk to start. The best response of the nurse would be:
    1. "Ask your CNM/physician."
    2. "Your baby will be brought to you at the next feeding time. Your milk will start right after that."
    3. "We encourage you to breastfeed as soon as you wish. Your milk will probably "come in" in about 3 days."
    4. "The baby can breastfeed anytime after birth. After your colostrum is gone (3 to 4 days), your milk will come in (5 to 6 days)."

## REFERENCES/SUGGESTED READINGS

Albright, A. (1993). Postpartum depression: An overview. *Journal of Counseling Development* 71(3), 316.

Ament, L. (1990). Maternal tasks of the puerperium reidentified. *JOGNN, 19*(4), 330.

American Academy of Pediatrics (AP) & American College of Obstetricians and Gynecologists (ACOG). (1977). *Guidelines for perinatal care* (3rd ed.). Elk Grove Village, IL: American Academy of Pediatrics.

Bandyopadhyay, M. (2009). Impact of ritual pollution on lactation and breastfeeding practices in rural West Bengal, India. *International Breastfeeding Journal, 4*(10), 1186/1746-4358-4-2.

Beck, C., & Gable, R. (2001). Further validation of the Postpartum Depression Screening Scale. *Nursing Research, 50*(3), 155.

Beeber, L. (2002). The pinks and the blues. *AJN, 102*(11), 91–97.

Berger, D., & Loveland-Cook, C. (1998). Postpartum teaching priorities: The viewpoints of nurses and mothers. *JOGNN, 27*(2), 161–168.

Bowes, W. (2001). Postpartum care. In S. Gabbe, J. Niebyl, & J. Simpson (Eds.), *Obstetrics: Normal and problem pregnancies* (4th ed.). New York: Churchill Livingstone.

Brown, S., & Johnson, B. (1998). Enhancing early discharge with home follow-up. A pilot project. *JOGNN, 27*(1), 33–38.

Bulechek, G., Butcher, H., McCloskey, J., & Dochterman, J., eds. (2008). *Nursing Interventions Classification (NIC)* (5th ed.). St. Louis, MO: Mosby/Elsevier.

Burroughs, A., & Leifer, G. (2007). *Maternity nursing* (10th ed.). Philadelphia: W. B. Saunders.

Callister, L., & Vega, R. (1998). Giving birth: Guatemalan women's voices. *JOGNN, 27*(3), 289–295.

Cesario, S. (2001). Care of the Native American woman: Strategies for practice, education, and research. *JOGNN, 30*(1), 13–19.

Cheng, C., Fowles, E., & Walker, L. (2006). Postpartum Maternal Health Care in the United States. *The Journal of Perinatal Education, 15* (3), 34-42.

Cunningham, F., Grant, N., Leveno, K., Gilstrap, L., & Cox, S. (2005). *William's obstetrics* (22nd ed.). Norwalk, CT: Appleton & Lange.

Davis, R. (2001). The postpartum experience for Southeast Asian women in the United States. *MCN, 26*(4), 208–213.

Davidson, N. (1974). REEDA: Evaluating postpartum healing. *Journal of Nurse Midwifery, 19*(2), 6-8.

Ernest, J., & Mead, P. (1998). Postpartum endometritis. *Contemporary OB/GYN, 43*(1), 33–38.

Ferguson, S., & Engelhard, C. (1996). Maternity length of stay and public policy: Issues and implications. *Journal of Pediatric Nursing, 11*(6), 392.

Ferketich, S., & Mercer, R. (1995). Paternal–infant attachment of experienced and inexperienced fathers during infancy. *Nursing Research, 44*(1), 31–37.

Gallup, D. (2005, June). Catastrophic Intraoperative Hemorrhage. *OBG Management, 54–61.*

Gennaro, S., Kamwendo, L., Mbweza, E., & Kershbaumer, R. (1998). Childbearing in Malawi, Africa. *JOGNN, 27*(2), 191–196.

Green, S., & Adams, W. (1993). Chronic psychiatric illness and pregnancy: Nursing implications. *Journal of Perinatal, Neonatal Nursing, 7*(3), 7–18.

Ha, L. (1994, December). *Culturally sensitive caregiving for Vietnamese women.* Lecture presented at the Medical College of Virginia Hospitals, Richmond, VA.

Harvard's Women's Health Page. (2008, June). Retrieved July 2, 2009, from Harvard Health: https://www.health.harvard.edu/newsweek/Hemorrhoids_and_what_to_do_about_them.htm

Havens, D., & Hannan, C. (1996). Legislation to mandate maternal and newborn length of stay. *Journal of Pediatric Health Care, 10*(3), 141.

Health Care Financing Administration (2002). The Newborns' and Mothers' Health Protection Act of 1996. [Online]. Retrieved from http://www.hcfa.gov/medicaid/hipaa/content/nmhpa.asp

Higgins, P. (2000). Postpartum complications. In S. Mattson & J. E. Smith (Eds.). *Core curriculum for maternal-newborn nursing* (2nd ed.). Philadelphia: W. B. Saunders.

Howard, J., & Berbiglia, V. (1997). Caring for childbearing women. *JOGNN, 26*(6), 665–671.

Hutchinson, M., & Baqi-Aziz, M. (1994). Nursing care of the childbearing Muslim family. *JOGNN, 23*(9), 767–771.

Johnson & Johnson (1996). *Compendium of postpartum care.* Skillman, NJ: Johnson & Johnson Consumer Products.

Kim-Godwin, Y. (2003). Postpartum beliefs & practices among non-western cultures. *MCN, 28*(2), 74–78.

Ladewig, P., Moberly, S., Olds, S., & London, M. (2009). *Contemporary maternal-newborn nursing care* (7th ed.). Menlo Park, CA: Addison-Wesley.

Leifer, G. (2007). *Maternity nursing: An introductory text (Burroughs)* (10th ed). Philadelphia: W.B. Saunders.

Littleton, L., & Engebretson, J. (2002). *Maternal, neonatal, and women's health nursing.* Clifton Park, NY: Delmar Cengage Learning.

Lowdermilk, D., & Perry, S. (2007). *Maternity and women's health care* (9th ed.). St. Louis, Missouri: Mosby Elsever.

Luegenbiehl, D., Brophy, G., Artigue, G., Phillips, K., & Flack, R. (1990). Standardized assessment of blood loss. *MCN, 15*(4), 241–244.

Martell, L. (1996). Is Rubin's "taking-in" and "taking-hold" a useful paradigm? *Health Care Women International 17*(1), 1.

Mattson, S. (1995). Culturally sensitive perinatal care for Southeast Asians. *JOGNN, 24*(4), 335–341.

Montigny, F., & Lacharité, C. (2005). Father's perceptions of the imediate postpartal period. *JOGNN, 33* (3), 328–339.

Moorhead, S., Johnson, M., Maas, M., & Swanson, E. (2007). *Nursing Outcomes Classifications (NOC)* (4th ed). St. Louis, MO: Elsevier–Health Sciences Division.

Murray, S., McKinney, E., & Gorrie, T. (2005). *Foundations of maternal–newborn nursing* (4th ed.). Philadelphia: W. B. Saunders.

Neal, J. (2001). RhD isoimmunization and current management modalities. *JOGNN, 309*(6), 589–606.

Normand, M., & Damato, E. (2001). Postcesarean infection. *JOGNN, 30*(6), 642–647.

North American Nursing Diagnosis Association International. (2010). *NANDA-I nursing diagnoses: Definitions and classification 2009-2011.* Ames, IA: Wiley-Blackwell.

Oyeku, S. (2003). *A Closer Look at Racial/Ethnic Disparities in Breastfeeding.* Boston: Harvard Pediatric Health Services.

Placksin, S. (2000). *Mothering the new mother: Women's feelings and needs after childbirth. A support and resource guide.* New York: Newmark Press.

Rubin, R. (1961). Puerperal change. *Nursing Outlook, 9*(12), 743–755.

Ruchala, P., & Halstead, L. (1994). The postpartum experience of low-risk women: A time of adjustment and change. *MCN, 22*(3), 83.

Savoia, M.. (1999). Bacterial, fungal, and parasitic disease during pregnancy. In G. Burrow, T. Duffy, & R. Kersey (Eds.). *Medical complications during pregnancy* (5th ed.). Philadelphia: W. B. Saunders.

Schneiderman, J. (1996). Postpartum nursing for Korean mothers. *MCN, 21*(3), 155–158.

Sharts-Hopko, N. (1995). Birth in the Japanese context. *JOGNN, 24*(4), 343–351.

Simpson, K., & Creehan, P. (2007). *AWHONN perinatal nursing* (3rd ed.). Philadelphia, Lippincott Williams & Wilkins.

Sit, D., Rothschild, A., & Wisner, K. (2006). A Review of Postpartum Psychosis. *Journal of Women's Health, 15* (4), 352–368.

Smith-Hanrahan, C., & Deblois, D. (1995). Postpartum early discharge. *Clinical Nursing Research, 4*(1), 50.

Spratto, G., & Woods, A. (2008). *PDR nurse's drug handbook.* Clifton Park, NY: Delmar Cengage Learning.

Squires, A. (2003). Documenting surgical incision site care. *Nursing2003, 33*(1), 74.

Staff, M. (2008, January). Infant and toddler health. Retrieved July 2, 2009, from Mayo Clinic: http://www.mayoclinic.com/health/infant-development/PR00061/NSECTIONGROUP=2

Tharpe, N. (2008). Postpregnancy Genital tract and Wound Infections. *Journal of Midwifery and Women's Health, 53*(3), 236–246.

Troy, N. (2003). Is the significance of postpartum fatigue being overlooked in the lives of women? *MCN, 28*(4), 252–257.

Visness, C., Kennedy, K., & Ramos, R. (1997). The duration and character of postpartum bleeding among breast-feeding women. *Obstetrics and Gynecology, 89*(2), 159.

Wilkerson, N. (1996). Appraisal of early discharge programs. *Journal of Perinatal Education, 5*(2), 1.

Wrasper, C. (1996). Discharge and timing and Rubin's concept of puerperal change. *Journal of Perinatal Education, 5*(2), 13.

Zlatnik, F. (1999). The normal and abnormal puerperlium. In J.R. Scott, P.J. Di Saia, C.B. Hammond, & W.N. Spellacy (Eds.), *Danforths' obstetrics and gynecology* (8th ed.). Philadelphia: Lippincott Williams & Wilkins.

# RESOURCES

**Association of Women's Health, Obstetric and Neonatal Nurses (AWHONN),** http://www.awhonn.org

**Depression After Delivery (DAD), Inc.,** http://www.depressionafterdelivery.com

**Health Science Consortium,** http://www.healthsciencesconsortium.com/

**Hollister, Inc.,** http://www.hollister.com

**International Lactation Consultant Association (ILCA),** http://www.ilca.org

**Johnson & Johnson Consumer Products, Inc.,** http://www.JNJ.com

**Postpartum Support International,** http://www.postpartum.net

# CHAPTER 5
## Newborn Care

## MAKING THE CONNECTION

*Refer to the following chapters to increase your understanding of newborn care:*

*Maternal & Pediatric Nursing*

- *Complications of Pregnancy*
- *The Birth Process*
- *Postpartum Care*

- *Basics of Pediatric Care*
- *Infants with Special Needs: Birth to 12 Months*

## LEARNING OBJECTIVES

- Define key terms.
- Describe the immediate needs of the newborn.
- Discuss what initiates breathing in the newborn.
- Describe the newborn's methods of heat production and heat retention.
- Identify the four ways heat is lost and nursing interventions to prevent heat loss.
- Describe the immediate care of the newborn.
- Discuss the Apgar score and how it is used.
- Describe the physical characteristics of the newborn.
- Identify the common variations in the newborn.
- Elicit the newborn's reflexes.
- Determine the gestational age of a newborn.
- Discuss the newborn's nutritional needs and how they can be met by breastfeeding and bottle feeding.
- Identify common problems the newborn may encounter and nursing interventions for each.
- Plan the care and then care for a newborn.

## KEY TERMS

| | | |
|---|---|---|
| acrocyanosis | hindmilk | nevus vascularis |
| appropriate for gestational age | hydrocele | nonshivering thermogenesis |
| caput succedaneum | hyperbilirubinemia | ophthalmia neonatorum |
| cephalhematoma | hypospadias | phimosis |
| circumcision | kernicterus | polydactyly |
| cold stress | lanugo | pseudomenstruation |
| conduction | large for gestational age | radiation |
| convection | meconium | small for gestational age |
| cryptorchidism | meningocele | spina bifida occulta |
| Down syndrome | milia | syndactyly |
| epispadias | molding | talipes equinovarus (clubfoot) |
| Epstein's pearls | mongolian spots | telangiectactic nevi |
| erythema toxicum neonatorum | myelomeningocele | thermogenesis |
| evaporation | neonatal transition | thermoregulation |
| foremilk | neutral thermal environment | vernix caseosa |
| hallux varus | nevus flammeus | witch's milk |

## INTRODUCTION

At the time of birth, the newborn must quickly make changes in the respiratory system to allow gas exchange to take place in the lungs and also make changes in the circulatory system to support the change to respiratory gas exchange. These profound, vital changes are critical to maintaining extrauterine life. The first few hours after birth wherein the newborn makes these changes and stabilizes respiratory and circulatory functions is called the **neonatal transition** period (Figure 5-1). Other body systems also make changes in their functioning over a longer period, although they are not crucial to the immediate survival of the infant.

Nurses are instrumental in assisting the newborn and mother through the neonatal transition period.

## IMMEDIATE NEEDS OF THE NEWBORN

The immediate needs of the newborn are airway, breathing, circulation, and warmth.

### AIRWAY

A clear airway is necessary for adequate gas exchange.

### BREATHING

In utero, the fetus relied on the placenta and the mother's respirations for gas exchange; however, fetal breathing movements, from approximately 11 weeks' gestation, help develop the chest wall muscles and the diaphragm (Ladewig, Moberly, Olds, & London, 2005). By approximately 35 weeks' gestation, the surfactant produced by the alveoli is sufficient in

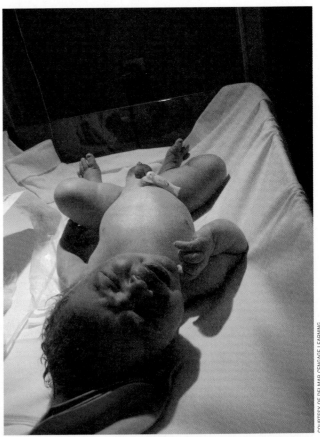

COURTESY OF DELMAR CENGAGE LEARNING

**FIGURE 5-1** The first few hours after birth are called the neonatal transition period, during which the infant experiences profound changes.

## PROFESSIONAL TIP

### Healthy People 2010

Healthy People 2010 includes initiatives to help people have good health and live longer lives. The following are the initiatives geared toward healthy mothers and their children:

- Increase the percentage of healthy full-term infants who are put down to sleep on their backs.
- Increase the proportion of mothers who breastfeed their babies.
- Ensure appropriate newborn bloodspot screening, follow up testing, and referral to services. (Healthy People 2010, 2009)

amount (L/S ratio 2:1) to allow the alveoli to remain partially expanded when the newborn begins to breathe at birth.

For the lungs to function, two changes must happen:

- Pulmonary ventilation must be established with lung expansion at the first breath.
- Pulmonary circulation must greatly increase.

The initiation of breathing is influenced by four factors—physical, chemical, thermal, and sensory—which work together.

## Physical Factors

The physical (sometimes called mechanical) factors include the compression of the fetal chest as it moves through the birth canal, which squeezes fluid from the lungs and increases intrathoracic pressure; and the chest wall recoil, which occurs as the newborn's trunk emerges. The chest recoil creates negative intrathoracic pressure, which causes a small amount of air to replace the fluid that was squeezed out of the lungs and some of the lung fluid to move across the alveolar membranes into the interstitial tissue of the lungs. Each breath allows more air into the alveoli and more fluid into the interstitial tissue. Because the protein concentration is higher in the capillaries, the interstitial fluid is drawn into them. All of the alveolar fluid is absorbed within the first day after birth.

## Chemical Factors

When the cord is clamped, placental gas exchange ceases, causing an increase in $PaCO_2$ and a decrease in $PaO_2$ and pH (a transitory asphyxia). These changes stimulate the carotid and aortic chemoreceptors, which send impulses to the respiratory center in the medulla, which in turn stimulates respirations. A brief period of asphyxia stimulates respirations, whereas prolonged asphyxia is a central nervous system (CNS) respiratory depressant.

## Thermal Factors

The change in temperature from the intrauterine environment to the extrauterine environment, a decrease of more than 20°F, is also a stimulus to breathing. The colder temperature stimulates the skin nerve endings and the newborn breathes as a response. Cold stress and respiratory depression result from excessive cooling of the newborn.

## Sensory Factors

The comfortable, relatively quiet uterine environment is left behind for an environment full of sensory stimuli. The auditory and visual stimuli associated with birth, along with the tactile stimulation of being handled, assist in the initiation of respirations.

## CIRCULATION

Several circulatory changes are necessary for the successful change from fetal circulation to neonatal circulation. These changes involve the pulmonary blood vessels, ductus arteriosus, foramen ovale, and ductus venosus.

### Pulmonary Blood Vessels

The dilation of these blood vessels begins with the first breath taken by the newborn. This results in lower pulmonary resistance, which allows the blood to freely circulate through the lungs to be oxygenated.

### Ductus Arteriosus

Within minutes after birth, the ductus arteriosus has a reversal of blood flow caused by the increased pressure in the aorta and the increase of oxygen in the blood. This results in more blood flowing through the pulmonary arteries for oxygenation. Closure of the ductus arteriosus is complete within 24 hours and is permanent in 3 to 4 weeks.

### Foramen Ovale

The foramen ovale closes within minutes after birth because of the higher pressure in the left atrium than in the right atrium. The increased blood flow in the lungs decreases pressure in the right atrium, and the return of blood from the lungs increases the pressure in the left atrium. Closure of the foramen ovale is permanent in approximately 3 months.

### Ductus Venosus

When the cord is clamped, the blood ceases flowing through the umbilical vein to the ductus venosus and into the inferior vena cava. Blood now flows through the liver and is filtered as in adult circulation.

## WARMTH

At birth the newborn must begin **thermoregulation**, maintenance of body temperature. Three factors are instrumental in thermoregulation: heat production, heat retention, and heat loss.

### Heat Production

The newborn produces heat (**thermogenesis**) through general metabolism, muscular activity, and nonshivering thermogenesis (unique to the newborn). Newborns rarely shiver as adults do to increase heat production. Shivering seen in a newborn indicates that the metabolic rate has already doubled (Ladewig et al., 2005).

When the infant is in a cool environment and requires more heat, the metabolic rate increases, producing more heat. The newborn may cry and have muscular activity when cold, but there is no voluntary control of muscular activity.

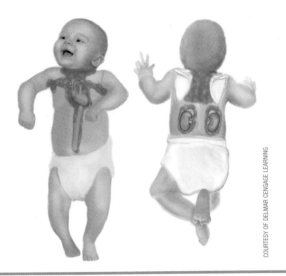

COURTESY OF DELMAR CENGAGE LEARNING

**FIGURE 5-2** **Brown fat distribution in the newborn.**

If the infant's temperature is not adequately raised through increased metabolism, **nonshivering thermogenesis**, the metabolism of brown fat, begins. Brown fat is a special fat found only in newborns. It appears at about 26 to 30 weeks of gestation and increases until 2 to 5 weeks of age (unless depleted by cold stress). The fat is highly vascularized, which gives it the brown color. The brown fat is located at the back of the neck, between the scapula, around the kidneys and adrenals, in the axilla, and around the heart and abdominal aorta (Figure 5-2). Once the brown fat has been metabolized, the infant no longer has this method of heat production available.

## Heat Retention

Newborns retain heat by staying in a flexed position. This reduces the area of skin exposed to the environmental temperature, thus decreasing heat loss. They also use the mechanism of peripheral vasoconstriction to retain heat.

## Heat Loss

The newborn has thin skin with blood vessels close to the surface and little subcutaneous fat to prevent heat loss. Heat moves from the warm internal areas to the cooler skin surface and then to the surrounding environment. Excessive heat loss is called **cold stress**. An increase in metabolism leads to a significant increase in the need for oxygen. When oxygen is used for metabolism (heat production), the infant may experience hypoxia. There may not be enough oxygen for the metabolic rate to increase, and the newborn will not be able to maintain body temperature. Prolonged cold stress causes respiratory difficulties and a decrease in surfactant production. Less surfactant hinders lung expansion, which in turn leads to more respiratory distress. Decreased blood oxygen may cause vasoconstriction of the pulmonary vessels with a return to fetal circulation patterns, which further increases respiratory distress.

The glucose necessary for increased metabolism is made available when glycogen stores are converted to glucose. If the glycogen is depleted, hypoglycemia results.

Brown fat metabolism results in the release of fatty acids. Continuous brown fat metabolism, when the newborn is in a cold stress situation for a considerable time, results in metabolic acidosis, which can be life-threatening. Excess fatty acids in the blood interfere with bilirubin transportation to the liver, which increases the risk of jaundice.

There are four methods by which the newborn loses heat: conduction, convection, evaporation, and radiation.

**Conduction** **Conduction** is the loss of heat by direct contact with a cooler object. When a newborn is touched by cold hands or a cold stethoscope or is placed on a cold surface such as a scale, heat is lost. Heat loss can be prevented by warming objects touching the newborn. If a newborn is wrapped in a warmed blanket or placed against the mother's warm skin, heat will be lost by the blanket or mother's skin to the cooler newborn and the newborn is warmed.

**Convection** **Convection** is the loss of heat by the movement of air. When air moves (air currents), heat is transferred to the air. Air currents from an open door or window, air conditioning, or from people moving around increase heat loss. A radiant warmer is often used for the newborn immediately after birth to prevent heat loss by convection (Figure 5-3).

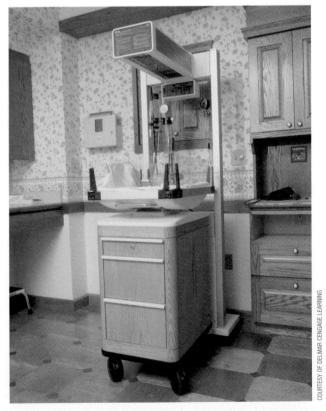

COURTESY OF DELMAR CENGAGE LEARNING

**FIGURE 5-3** **A radiant warmer keeps the air surrounding the newborn warm, preventing heat loss by convection.**

## ▼ SAFETY ▼

### Newborns and Standard Precautions

Penny-MacGillivray (1996) explains that blood and amniotic fluid, once believed to be sterile, are now considered contaminated with blood-borne pathogens. All newborns are now also considered contaminated until the first bath has removed all blood and amniotic fluid from the infant's body. The nurse performing the assessment and giving the first bath *must wear gloves*.

Heat loss in the newborn can be prevented by wrapping the infant in a blanket and placing a stocking cap on the head and by keeping the newborn out of any drafts.

**Evaporation** Evaporation is the loss of heat when water is changed to a vapor. When a wet body dries, heat is lost, such as a newborn wet with amniotic fluid or during a bath. The insensible water loss from the skin and respiratory tract also results in heat loss. Heat loss can be prevented by immediately drying the newborn at birth and after receiving a bath, and by changing wet clothing and diapers promptly.

**Radiation** Radiation is the loss of heat by transfer to cooler objects nearby, but not through direct contact. An infant placed near a cold window loses heat by radiation to the sides of the crib and the window. If the walls of an incubator are cold, the infant loses heat. Heat loss can be prevented by keeping cribs and incubators away from cold windows.

## IMMEDIATE CARE OF THE NEWBORN

The immediate care of the newborn includes obtaining the Apgar score, resuscitation (if needed), providing a neutral thermal environment, proper identification of the infant, parent/infant bonding, and prophylactic care.

### APGAR SCORE

The Apgar score, which assesses the infant's cardiopulmonary adaptations to extrauterine life, is given immediately after the delivery. The Apgar scores are assigned by the nurse caring for the infant. More information on Apgar scoring can be found in the Birth Process chapter.

### RESUSCITATION

Resuscitation is begun if no respirations are initiated by the infant. The LP/VN may be asked to use a bulb syringe to suction mucus from the infant's oropharynx, gently rub the infant's back for stimulation, or provide oxygen. More intense resuscitation would typically be performed by an RN or physician who have gone through a Neonatal Resuscitation Program (NRP).

## NEUTRAL THERMAL ENVIRONMENT

A **neutral thermal environment** is an environment in which the newborn can maintain internal body temperature with minimal oxygen consumption and metabolism. In this environment, the newborn's body does not have to focus on temperature maintenance but can focus on growth and development.

## IDENTIFICATION

Proper identification of the newborn is vital. The identification bands must be checked and compared to the mother's band each time the baby is brought into the mother's room. No infant should ever leave the hospital without having their bands checked against the mother's bands. One band will usually be kept in the infant's hospital records when the infant is discharged. The process of applying the identification bands is discussed in the Birth Process chapter.

## PARENT/INFANT BONDING

Interaction between the parents and infant should be promoted as soon as the infant is stable. The nurse assists the parents in holding their baby or to give them permission to examine the infant. This is a good time for the nurse to answer any questions that the parents might have.

## PROPHYLACTIC CARE

Prophylactic care includes the administration of vitamin K and hepatitis B vaccine, instillation of an antibiotic ophthalmic ointment, and umbilical cord care.

### Vitamin K

At birth, newborns lack vitamin K, which is necessary for the clotting process. Vitamin K is synthesized in the intestine and requires food and normal intestinal flora for the process. Because the intestines are sterile at birth, no vitamin K can be produced for several days. An intramuscular (IM) injection of vitamin K, phytonadione (aquaMEPHYTON), is generally given within the first hour after birth to prevent hemorrhagic disorders. A normal newborn is able to produce vitamin K by the eighth day (Lowdermilk & Perry, 2007).

### Hepatitis B Vaccination

The Centers for Disease Control and Prevention (CDC), along with the Advisory Committee on Immunization Practices (ACIP), the American Academy of Pediatrics (AAP), and the American Academy of Family Physicians (AAFP), recommend giving the first dose of hepatitis B (Hep B) vaccine within 12 hours of birth. Infants whose mothers have hepatitis B should also receive hepatitis B immune globulin (HBIG) at the same time, but at a different site than the vaccine. The HBIG provides passive immunity until the newborn develops antibodies. In many agencies, the parents must give written permission for the infant to receive the hepatitis B vaccine. Parents who do not wish to vaccinate their infant should sign a refusal of treatment after the infant is born. Many parents will opt to have their pediatrician vaccinate the infant at their one week visit.

## Eye Prophylaxis

In the United States, it is mandatory to instill a prophylactic agent in the eyes of all neonates to prevent **ophthalmia neonatorum**. This is an inflammation of the newborn's eyes that results from passing through the birth canal when a gonorrheal or chlamydial infection is present. The medication used for prophylaxis varies with agency protocol but is generally erythromycin (Ilotycin Ophthalmic Ointment) or tetracycline (Achromycin Ophthalmic Ointment) (Lowdermilk & Perry, 2007). Silver nitrate 1% is now seldom used because it protects only against gonorrheal infection and not chlamydial infection. To promote parent/infant eye contact, bonding, and attachment, some agencies delay the eye prophylaxis for an hour or so.

## Umbilical Cord Care

Umbilical cord care is similar to caring for an open sore or wound. In the past, agencies used triple blue dye, alcohol, or an erythromycin solution to clean the cord. Keeping the cord dry and clean is the best way to promote healing and prevent infection of the cord. Early signs of infection to inspect for at the cord and the skin at the base include purulent drainage, pus, active bleeding from the site, infant showing signs of pain, and redness and irritation at site. Make sure parents are informed that the infant should not be fully bathed until the cord falls off. The prevention of or early identification of any hemorrhage or infection is the goal of care.

**▼ SAFETY ▼**

**Cord Hemorrhage**

- When bleeding from the cord is noted, check the clamp and apply a second clamp on the body side of the first one.
- If the bleeding does not stop immediately, notify the health care provider.

# PHYSICAL CHARACTERISTICS OF THE NEWBORN

The newborn infant is not just a miniature adult. Identification of the physical characteristics and common variations of the newborn found in the infant are documented. This provides a basis for nursing diagnoses and care. Agencies generally have a form to follow such as the one shown in Figure 5-4. This form incorporates data about the mother, the delivery, Apgar score, and gestational age along with the physical assessment of the infant.

## WEIGHT AND LENGTH

Most full-term newborns weigh between 2,500 g and 4,000 g or approximately 5 lb, 8 oz to 8 lb, 13 oz. Newborns lose 5% to

**Initial Newborn Profile**
Hollister Maternal/Newborn Record System
To order call: 1.800.323.4060 Re-order No. 5720

**Admit Data** Date __/__/__ Date ____
ID/Band No. ____ Name ____
Admitted By ____
Medications ☐ None ☐ See Delivery Data
Date Time Medication Dose Route Site Inits
Eye Prophylaxis Erythromycin
Vitamin K

**Newborn Data** ☐ male ☐ Female ☐ Breast ☐ Bottle
Birthdate __/__/__ Time ____
Place of Birth ☐ Hospital ☐ ____
☐ Vertex ☐ Breech ☐ Vaginal ☐ Cesarean
Delivered by ____
Apgar ____ 1min ____ 5min ____ 10min
Cord Blood pH ____ Type/Rh ____ Coombs ____
Intrapartum Problems Identified ☐ None
1. ____
2. ____
3. ____

**Maternal Data** G T Pt A L
Name ____ Age ____
Record No. ____ Room No. ____
Blood Type/Rh ____ Antibody + -
Screens Neg Pos Comments
STD ☐ ☐
Urine Tox ☐ ☐
Hepatitis B ☐ ☐

**Measurements/Gestational Age Assessment**
See Delivery Data
☐ Weight ____ lbs ____ gms
☐ Length ____ cms ____ ins
☐ Head Circ ____ cms ____ ins
☐ Chest Circ ____ cms ____ ins
☐ Abd Cric ____ cms ____ ins
Gest Age by Dates ____ Wks
Gest Age by Exam ____ Wks
☐ Preterm ☐ Term ☐ Postterm
☐ SGA ☐ AGA ☐ LGA

**Physical Assessment**
Date __/__/__ Time ____ Age ____ hrs
Temp ____ Pulse Rate/Rhythm ____ Resp ____ BP ☐ Not done ☐ ____
Head/Neck — Detail Abnormal Findings
1. Fontanels Level Bulging Depressed
Anterior ☐ ☐ ☐
Posterior ☐ ☐ ☐
2. Sutures ☐ Open ☐ Closed ☐ Overriding
3. Variations ☐ None ☐ Molding ☐ Caput ☐ Cephalhematoma
4. Lacerations ☐ No ☐ Yes

Normal / Abnormal
5. Face ☐ ☐
6. Eyes ☐ ☐
7. Ears ☐ ☐
8. Nose ☐ ☐
9. Mouth ☐ ☐
10. Neck ☐ ☐
Chest
11. Breath sounds ☐ ☐
12. Thorax ☐ ☐
13. Clavicles ☐ ☐
Cardiovascular
14. Heart sounds ☐ ☐
15. Pulses ☐ ☐
Abdomen
16. Structure ☐ ☐
17. Bowel sounds ☐ ☐
18. Cord ☐ ☐
19. Liver ☐ ☐
20. Spleen ☐ ☐
21. Kidneys ☐ ☐
Genitalia
22. Female ☐ ☐
23. Male ☐ ☐

Musculoskeletal — Normal / Abnormal — Detail Abnormal Findings
24. Tone ☐ ☐
25. Extremities ☐ ☐
26. Hips ☐ ☐
27. Spine ☐ ☐
Neurologic
28. Reflexes ☐ ☐
29. Cry ☐ ☐
Skin
30. Condition ☐ Smooth ☐ Dry ☐ Peeling ☐ Vernix ☐ Mec Stain
31. Color ☐ Pink ☐ Ruddy ☐ Pale ☐ Mottled ☐ Cyanotic ☐ Jaundice (time noted ____ )
32. Variations (i.e. rash, lesion, birthmark) ____
Elimination
33. Bowel Anus Patent ☐ Yes ☐ No ____
First Meconium (date, time) ____
34. Urine First Void (date, time) ____

Problems identified ☐ None
1. ____
2. ____
3. ____
Comments/Plan

Hollister Incorporated, 2000 Hollister Drive, Libertyville, Illinois 60048

Newborn Risk Indicators

**Observable at birth**

☐ **No risk factors noted**
☐ Abnormal presentation
☐ Multiple birth
☐ Low birth rate
☐ Resuscitation at birth
☐ 1 min. Apgar <5
☐ 5 min. Apgar <7
☐ Placental Abnormalities
☐ Two cord vessels
☐ Difficult catheterization
☐ > 20 ml. of gastric aspirate
☐ Small mandible with cleft palate
☐ Grunting
☐ Deep retractions
☐ Imperforate anus
☐ Pallor
☐ Jaundice
☐ Plethora
☐ Convulsions
☐ Decreased tone
☐ Congenial malformations
☐ ____
☐ ____
☐ ____

**Within 24 hrs. postpartum**

☐ **No risk factors noted**
☐ Abdominal presentation
☐ Vomiting
☐ Failure to pass meconium (if skin not stained)
☐ Melena
☐ Apneic episodes (>20 seconds)
☐ Tachypnea (transient)
☐ See-saw breathing
☐ Cyanosis
☐ Petechiae/Ecchymoses
☐ Jaundice
☐ Pallor
☐ Plethora
☐ Fever
☐ Hypothermia
☐ Arrhythmias
☐ Murmur
☐ Lethargy
☐ Tremors (jitters)
☐ Convulsions
☐ ____
☐ ____
☐ ____

____
Signature

**FIGURE 5-4** **Initial Newborn Profile with Newborn Risk Indicators** (*Permission to use this copyright material has been granted by the owner, Hollister Incorporated.*)

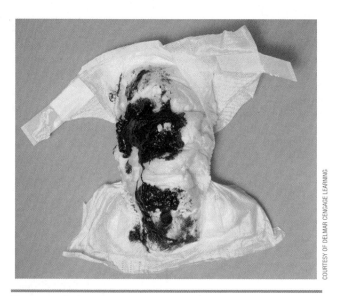

FIGURE 5-5 **Meconium Stool**

10% of their body weight in the first 3 to 4 days. This is a result of small fluid intake, volume of **meconium** (first bowel movements of newborn, black and tarry) (Figure 5-5), and urination. Birth weight is generally regained by 10 days of age.

Their head-to-heel length is 48 cm to 53 cm (approximately 19 in. to 21 in.), and crown-to-rump length is 31 cm to 35 cm (approximately 12 in. to 14 in.) or approximately equal to the head circumference.

## VITAL SIGNS

The axillary temperature should be between 36.5°C and 37.2°C (97.6°F and 98.9°F). A continuous skin probe is best for small newborns or those in a radiant warmer. Normal skin temperature is 36°C to 36.5°C (96.8°F to 97.6°F). Crying may slightly increase temperature.

The apical heart rate is 120 to 160 beats per minute. When the newborn is sleeping, the heart rate decreases, and when crying, the heart rate increases.

Respirations are 30 to 60 breaths per minute. As with the heart rate, sleep decreases respirations and crying increases respirations.

Blood pressure ranges between 60 and 80 mm Hg systolic and 40 and 45 mm Hg diastolic. By 10 days of age, it is 100/50 mm Hg. Activity and crying will increase the newborn's blood pressure.

## GENERAL APPEARANCE

Full-term newborns have a flexed posture. The head is flexed, the arms are flexed on the chest, and the legs are flexed on the abdomen.

### Skin

At birth, the skin is red, puffy, and smooth. Some **vernix caseosa** (a white, creamy substance) may thinly cover the skin, with large amounts found in body creases. **Lanugo** (fine, downy hair) may still be seen on the forehead and shoulders, or it may all have disappeared. **Acrocyanosis**, blue coloring of the hands and feet, is generally present for several hours until the cardiopulmonary changes have stabilized and fully oxygenated blood has reached the hands and feet. Edema may

be present around the eyes, face, dorsa of hands, legs, feet, and labia or scrotum.

### Head

The head circumference, measured over the most prominent part of the occiput and just above the eyebrows, is between 33 cm and 35 cm (approximately 13 in. to 14 in.). There are two fontanelles, one anterior and one posterior. The anterior fontanelle is largest, diamond shaped, and closes by 18 months of age. The posterior fontanelle is triangular in shape and closes about 2 months after birth. The fontanelles should be soft and flat.

### Eyes

Eye color varies, being either slate gray, blue, or brown. Permanent eye color is usually established by 3 months of age. The eyelids are usually edematous, and there are no tears.

### Ears

The ears are soft, pliable, and recoil swiftly when bent and released. Ear placement should be so the top of the ear is in line with the outer canthus of the eye (Figure 5-6).

### Neck

The neck is short, thick, and usually has several skin folds.

### Chest

Chest circumference is 30.5 cm to 33 cm (approximately 12 in. to 13 in.). It is measured directly over the nipple line and lower edge of the scapulas. The chest circumference is 2 cm to 3 cm smaller than the head circumference. The diameters front to back and side to side are equal (Figure 5-7).

### Abdomen

The abdomen is cylindrical in shape. The bluish-white umbilical cord protrudes from the center.

### Genitalia

The labia are usually edematous with vernix caseosa between the labia.

If the testes are descended, the scrotum is large, pendulous, and edematous; if the testes are not descended, the scrotum is small. In either case, the scrotum is covered with rugae. The newborn with dark skin has a deeply pigmented scrotum. The newborn should urinate within 24 hours.

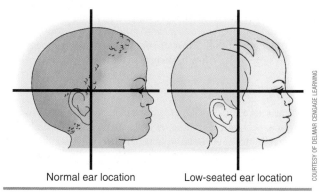

Normal ear location          Low-seated ear location

FIGURE 5-6 **Ear Placement. Top of ear should be in line with the outer canthus of the eye.**

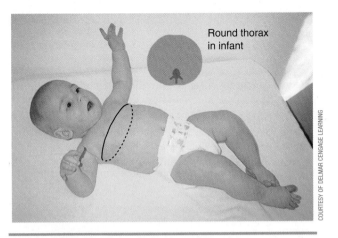

Round thorax in infant

COURTESY OF DELMAR CENGAGE LEARNING

**FIGURE 5-7** Newborn chest is round, having the same diameter front to back and side to side.

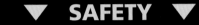
## ▼ SAFETY ▼

### Disposable Paper Tape Measure

When a measurement has been completed, either roll the infant off the paper tape measure or lift the newborn and remove the paper tape measure. Never pull the tape measure out from under the newborn; a paper cut on the newborn's body may result.

## Back

The spine is intact with no openings, masses, or prominent curves. Tufts of hair on the spinal area should be reported for evaluation.

## Extremities

The extremities are usually flexed, have a full range of motion, and are symmetrical. Ten fingers and ten toes are present, with creases visible on the anterior two-thirds of the sole of the foot.

# COMMON VARIATIONS IN THE NEWBORN

Many variations seen in the newborn are perfectly normal and cause no trouble. Any one newborn may have some of these variations but not all. Most of these variations disappear in a few days or weeks, a few in several years.

## SKIN

Several colorations or skin eruptions may be present, including jaundice, ecchymoses, milia, erythema toxicum neonatorum, telangiectatic nevi, nevus flammeus, nevus vascularis, and mongolian spots.

## Jaundice

Jaundice occurring *after* the first 24 hours of life is related to the normal destruction of the excess red blood cells (RBCs) in

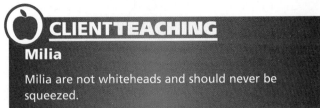
## CLIENTTEACHING
### Milia

Milia are not whiteheads and should never be squeezed.

the newborn. With direct oxygenation of the blood in the newborn's lungs, the extra RBCs of the fetus are no longer needed. The infant's immature liver is often unable to conjugate all of the bilirubin released by the destroyed RBCs, and this is evident as jaundice. The jaundice usually peaks at 72 hours and then disappears in a couple of weeks. Jaundice appearing *within* the first 24 hours of life is discussed later in this chapter.

## Ecchymosis

Areas of ecchymosis (bruising) may be evident after a difficult delivery. Petechiae may also be present.

## Milia

Milia are white, pinhead-size, distended sebaceous glands on the cheeks, nose, chin, and occasionally on the trunk. After a few weeks of bathing, they usually disappear.

## Erythema Toxicum Neonatorum

Erythema toxicum neonatorum is a pink rash with firm, yellow-white papules or pustules found on the chest, abdomen, back, and buttocks of some newborns. It only appears in the neonatal period and the pathophysiology is unknown. It may appear 24 to 48 hours after birth and dissapears in a few days without any treatment.

## Telangiectactic Nevi

Telangiectactic nevi ("stork-bites") are birthmarks of dilated capillaries that blanch with pressure. They may appear on the eyelids, nose, occipital area, or nape of the neck and fade between 1 and 2 years of age.

## Nevus Flammeus

Nevus flammeus (port-wine stain) is a large reddish-purple birthmark usually found on the face or neck that does not blanch with pressure. It is not raised above the skin. This does not spontaneously disappear but may be lightened with special laser treatments.

## Nevus Vascularis

Nevus vascularis (strawberry mark) is a birthmark of enlarged superficial blood vessels. They are elevated, red, and of variable

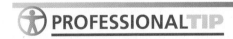
## PROFESSIONALTIP

### Mongolian Spots

Carefully document the presence of mongolian spots on the newborn's record. This may prevent charges of child abuse being filed later against the parents or caregivers.

size and shape. They are most often found on the head, face, neck, and arms. By school age, they have generally disappeared.

## Mongolian Spots

Mongolian spots are deep blue areas of coloration, usually in the sacral region, at birth. They are seen mainly in infants of African, Asian, American Indian, Hispanic, and Southern European descent.

# HEAD

Three common variations in newborns involve the head: molding, caput succedaneum, and cephalhematoma.

## Molding

Molding is the shaping of the fetal head to adapt to the mother's pelvis during labor. In 2 to 3 days the cranial bones typically return to their proper placement (Figure 5-8).

## Caput Succedaneum

Caput succedaneum, edema of the newborn's scalp that is present at birth, may cross suture lines and is caused by head compression against the cervix (Figure 5-9A). The edema disappears in 2 to 3 days. No treatment is needed.

## Cephalhematoma

Cephalhematoma is a collection of blood between the periosteum and the skull of a newborn. It appears several hours to a day after birth, does not cross suture lines, and is caused by the rupturing of the periosteal bridging veins

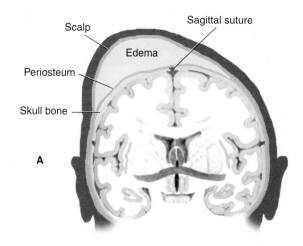

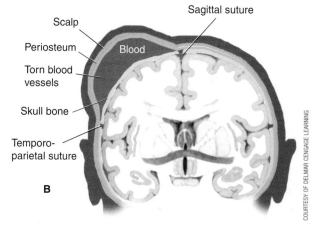

FIGURE 5-9 *A*, Caput Succedaneum; *B*, Cephalhematoma

because of friction and pressure during labor and delivery (Figure 5-9B). It is usually the largest on the second or third day and spontaneously reabsorbs in 3 to 6 weeks. Table 5-1 compares caput succedaneum and cephalhematoma.

# EYES

The newborn's eyes may show signs of strabismus, which is caused by poor neuromuscular control. This usually disappears in 3 to 4 months. Subconjunctival hemorrhages are present in approximately 10% of newborns (Ladewig et al., 2005). Change in vascular tension or ocular pressure during birth

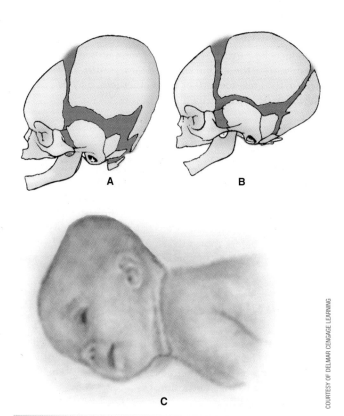

FIGURE 5-8 **Molding;** *A,* **Movement of the Cranial Bones during Labor;** *B,* **Cranial Bones Return to their Proper Placement in 2 to 3 days;** *C,* **Infant Exhibiting Molding**

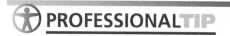

**PROFESSIONALTIP**

### Newborn Skin Variations

Many of the newborn skin variations can be surprising and upsetting to new parents. The nurse should educate the parents and help them understand that several of these skin variations are common and that often they will disappear over time without any interventions.

**TABLE 5-1  Comparison of Caput Succedaneum and Cephalhematoma**

| CHARACTERISTIC | CAPUT SUCCEDANEUM | CEPHALHEMATOMA |
| --- | --- | --- |
| Fluid | Edema | Blood |
| Layer involved | Scalp | Between periosteum and skull |
| Relationship to suture lines | May cross suture lines | Does not cross suture lines |
| Appears | Present at birth | First or second day |
| Disappears | 2 to 3 days | 3 to 6 weeks |

causes these hemorrhages. They last for a few weeks and do not impair vision.

## EARS

The ears may be of irregular shape and size. The pinna may be flat against the head.

## MOUTH

Precocious teeth may be present at birth in the center of the lower gum. If loose, they should be removed to prevent aspiration. **Epstein's pearls**, small, whitish-yellow epithelial cysts, are found on the hard palate. They disappear within a few weeks.

## CHEST

Many newborns, both male and female, have engorged breasts as a result of maternal hormones. This occurs by the third day and may last 2 weeks. The nipples may secrete a whitish fluid, often called "**witch's milk**." Witch's milk is a term for any milk that comes from the breast of someone who is not lactating. This phenomena is only seen in full term infants.

## GENITALIA

There are several variations in the female and male genitalia.

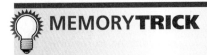

## MEMORY TRICK

**Caput Succedaneum**

| R | U |
| O | T |
| S | U |
| S | R |
| E | E |
| S | S |

If you can remember that this collection of fluids crosses the suture lines you will automatically know that the Cephalhematoma does not.

## Female

**Pseudomenstruation**, a blood-tinged mucous discharge from the vagina, may be evident in the first week after birth. It is caused by the withdrawal of maternal hormones. A vaginal tag or hymenal tag may be present but will disappear in a few weeks.

## Male

**Hypospadias**, placement of the urinary meatus on the underside of the penis, may be present. **Phimosis**, when the opening in the foreskin is so small that it cannot be pulled back over the glans, may interfere with urination. **Cryptorchidism**, failure of one or both testes to descend, may be evident. **Hydrocele**, fluid around the testes in the scrotum, usually disappears without any treatment. **Epispadias** is the placement of the urinary meatus on the top of the penis.

## EXTREMITIES

There may be partial **syndactyly** (fusion of two or more fingers or toes) of the second and third toes. **Hallux varus**, placement of the great toe farther from other toes, may be present. The infant born with extra fingers or toes has **polydactyly**.

## REFLEXES

Many of the newborn's movements are reflexive in nature. Some reflexes, such as sneezing, coughing, swallowing, blinking, yawning, and hiccupping, are present throughout life. Others disappear at various times throughout the first 2 years of life; these are discussed next. These neonatal reflexes must be lost before motor development can proceed (Estes, 2010). The presence of the reflexes indicates neurological integrity.

## ROOTING REFLEX

The rooting reflex is elicited by stroking the skin at one corner of the infant's mouth. The infant will turn the head toward the side stroked (Figure 5-10). This reflex is present up until 3 or 4 months of age. Absence of the reflex during this time frame may indicate a frontal lobe lesion.

## SUCKING REFLEX

Touching the newborn's lips elicits the sucking reflex (Figure 5-11). This reflex occurs until approximately 10 months of

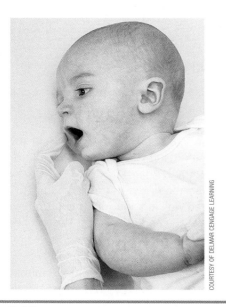

FIGURE 5-10    Rooting Reflex

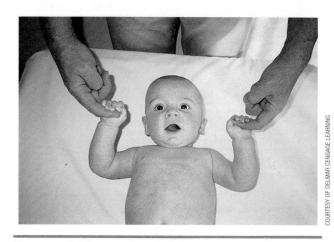

FIGURE 5-12    Palmar Grasp Reflex

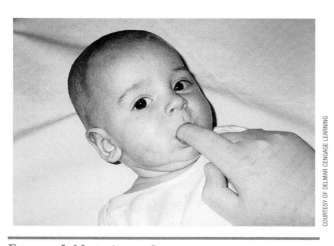

FIGURE 5-11    Sucking Reflex

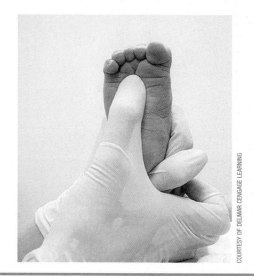

FIGURE 5-13    Plantar Grasp Reflex

age. Preterm infants or an infant who is breastfed by a mother taking barbiturates will not exhibit the sucking reflex because of central nervous system depression.

## EXTRUSION REFLEX

When the tip of the tongue is touched or depressed, the infant will force the tongue outward. This reflex disappears at approximately 4 months of age. Feeding an infant food with a spoon before 4 months of age is difficult because of the extrusion reflex.

## PALMAR GRASP REFLEX

When a finger is placed across the palm, the infant's fingers flex and grasp the examiner's finger (Figure 5-12). If the palmar grasp reflex is present after 4 months of age, frontal lobe lesions are suspected.

## PLANTAR GRASP REFLEX

When the infant's leg is held in one hand, and the plantar surface of the foot is touched below the toes with the other hand, the infant's toes will curl downward (Figure 5-13). This reflex

lasts until 8 months of age. If the plantar grasp reflex is absent on one foot, an obstructive lesion is suspected. Absence of the reflex in both feet is seen with neurological alterations such as cerebral palsy.

## TONIC NECK REFLEX

The tonic neck reflex is sometimes referred to as the "fencing" reflex because of the position assumed by the infant. This reflex is elicited by placing the infant supine and rotating the head to one side. The arm and leg on the side to which the jaw is turned will extend and the opposite arm and leg will flex (Figure 5-14). Sometimes, this reflex may not be displayed until 6 to 8 weeks of age. If it is still seen after 6 months of age, cerebral damage is suspected.

## MORO REFLEX

The Moro reflex is sometimes called the startle reflex. It is elicited either by holding the newborn in a semisitting position and then allowing the head to fall backward to an angle of 30°, or having the infant lying on a flat surface and then hitting the surface to startle the infant. The response by the infant less than 4 months of age is to quickly extend and abduct the arms with the fingers fanning out. The thumb and forefinger form a "C" followed by adduction of the arms in an embracing motion. A slight tremor may be noted. The legs may also

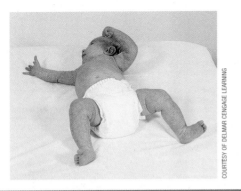

**FIGURE 5-14** Tonic Neck Reflex

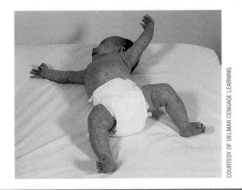

**FIGURE 5-15** Moro (Startle) Reflex

extend and then flex (Figure 5-15). The Moro reflex is present at birth and disappears between 4 and 6 months of age. Possible brain damage is indicated if the response persists after 6 months of age. An asymmetrical response may be caused by an injury to the clavicle, humerus, or brachial plexus.

## GALLANT REFLEX

The Gallant reflex is elicited with the infant lying prone with the hands under the abdomen. The infant's skin is stroked along one side of the spine; the infant's shoulders and pelvis turn toward the stimulated side (Figure 5-16). A spinal cord lesion is suspected if there is no response from an infant younger than 2 months of age. This reflex is present from birth to age 2 months.

## STEPPING REFLEX

To elicit the stepping reflex, the newborn is held under the arms with the feet placed on a firm surface. The infant will lift

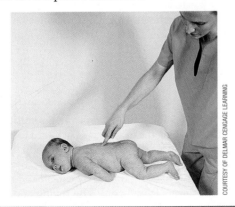

**FIGURE 5-16** Gallant Reflex

alternate feet as if walking (Figure 5-17). This reflex disappears at about 3 months of age.

## BABINSKI'S REFLEX

To elicit Babinski's reflex, the plantar surface of the infant's foot is stroked from the lateral heel area upward and across under the toes. The great toe should dorsiflex and the other toes fan out (Figure 5-18). The presence of Babinski's reflex after the infant has mastered walking (12 to 18 months of age) is abnormal.

## CROSSED EXTENSION REFLEX

The crossed extension reflex is elicited with the infant supine by holding one leg extended with the knee pressed down and stimulating the bottom of that foot. The other leg should flex, adduct, and then extend as if trying to push away the stimulus. This reflex should be present during the first 4 weeks of life.

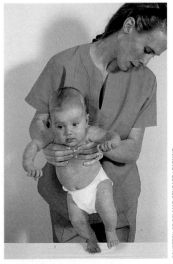

**FIGURE 5-17** Stepping Reflex

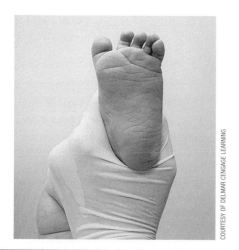

FIGURE 5-18  Babinski's Reflex

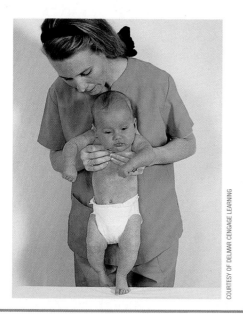

FIGURE 5-19  Placing Reflex

## PLACING REFLEX

To elicit the placing reflex, the infant is held under the arms from behind then brought to a standing position, touching the dorsum of one foot on the edge of the table. The tested leg will flex and lift onto the table (Figure 5-19). It is abnormal for there to be no response. An infant born in a breech presentation or one with paralysis or cerebral cortex difficulties may not respond to this stimulus.

# BEHAVIORAL CHARACTERISTICS

During the first 6 to 10 hours after birth, the infant has a fairly predictable pattern of behavior called the periods of reactivity. Following that, the infant will exhibit various behavioral states, divided into sleeping and waking phases.

## PERIODS OF REACTIVITY

Two periods of reactivity occur during the first few hours of life, separated by a period of sleep.

## First Period of Reactivity

During the first period of reactivity, the first 30 minutes after birth, the newborn is awake, alert, and active. It is a prime time for parent/infant interaction. The newborn may act hungry, with a strong sucking reflex evident. If the mother plans to breastfeed, this is the ideal time for her to begin. During this period, the newborn's heart rate and respirations are rapid, and bowel sounds are seldom heard.

## Sleep Period

The newborn enters a sleep period that usually lasts from 2 to 4 hours. This is a time of deep sleep, from which it is difficult to awaken the newborn. The heart and respiratory rates return to baseline and bowel sounds become audible.

## Second Period of Reactivity

The second period of reactivity lasts from 4 to 6 hours. The newborn is once again awake and alert. Physiologic responses vary. The heart and respiratory rates increase, yet there may be periods of apnea, which may cause the heart rate to decrease. During these fluctuations, the newborn may become mottled or slightly cyanotic.

The newborn may gag, spit up, or choke as gastric and respiratory mucus increases. Close observation is a must during this period of activity so that appropriate interventions may be taken to maintain a clear airway for the infant.

The first meconium stool is often passed as the gastrointestinal tract becomes more active. The first voiding may now occur. The newborn may begin rooting, sucking, and swallowing, indicating a readiness for feeding.

## BEHAVIORAL STATES

Brazelton (1995) identified that newborns have different states of being. He categorized them as sleep states and alert states.

## Sleep States

Two sleep states have been identified for the newborn: quiet sleep and active sleep. At term, a newborn changes from one sleep state to the other approximately every 45 to 50 minutes during sleep. Of the total amount of sleep, 45% to 50% is active sleep, 35% to 45% is quiet sleep, and 10% is shifting between the two sleep states (Ladewig et al., 2005).

**Quiet Sleep State** In quiet sleep, the eyes are closed and there are no eye movements. Respirations are regular, quiet, and slower than in any other state. The heart rate is 100 to 120 beats per minute. There are startles or jerky movements at regular intervals. Stimuli in the environment are not likely to cause a change in the newborn's state.

**Active Sleep State** During active sleep, respirations are rapid and irregular and sucking movements may be observed.

The infant stretches, moves extremities, makes faces, and may fuss briefly. Rapid eye movements (REM) occur. Environmental stimuli may startle the infant, who may then go back to sleep or awaken.

## Alert States

There are four alert states: drowsy, quiet alert, active alert, and crying.

**Drowsy State** The transition between sleep and awake is called the drowsy state. The eyes open and then slowly close, as if unable to stay open. When open, the eyes appear glazed and unfocused. From this state, the infant may go back to sleep or awaken.

**Quiet Alert State** In the quiet alert state, the infant focuses on people or objects, responds with intense gazing, and seems very interested in the immediate environment. Body movements are minimal. When the infant is in the quiet alert state, it is a good time to enhance bonding. Parents should be made aware of this so they can take advantage of this opportunity.

**Active Alert State** The infant is often fussy and restless in the active alert state, with more rapid and irregular respirations. The awareness of discomfort from hunger or cold is more intense. Motor activity is quite frequent. The infant is less focused on visual stimuli than in the quiet alert state.

**Crying State** Crying is generally accompanied by jerky motor activity. Crying serves as a distraction from disturbing stimuli, allows a discharge of energy, and is a method of communication to elicit appropriate responses from parents or caregivers.

## GESTATIONAL AGE

According to Alexander and Allen (1996), gestational age must be determined in the first 4 hours after birth so that age-related problems can be identified and appropriate care initiated.

The New Ballard Score is the most commonly used tool (Figure 5-20). It has two elements: external physical characteristics and neuromuscular maturity. If the findings of neuromuscular maturity are not in line with the findings of the external physical characteristics, a second assessment should be performed within 24 hours.

### ASSESSMENT OF EXTERNAL PHYSICAL CHARACTERISTICS

The nurse should begin with resting posture, then skin, lanugo, plantar creases, breast, eye/ear, and then genitals.

### Resting Posture

Although resting posture is a characteristic of neuromuscular maturity, it should be assessed first. The posture the newborn assumes when lying undisturbed is to be assessed. The very preterm infant has no flexion of the extremities, while the full-term infant is fully flexed.

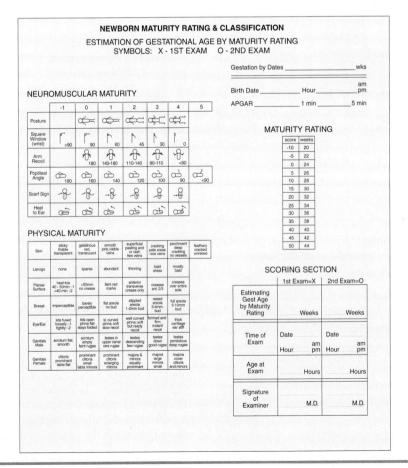

**FIGURE 5-20** New Ballard Score (*Courtesy of Mead Johnson Nutritionals.*)

## Skin

The skin of a preterm infant is very transparent and thin. As gestation progresses, the veins disappear from view as subcutaneous fat is deposited. Vernix caseosa disappears near term but may remain in the creases. There may be some cracking and peeling of the skin, especially around the ankles and feet. As the skin loses moisture after birth, peeling is more apparent.

## Lanugo

Lanugo is most abundant between 28 and 30 weeks' gestation. It disappears as the gestational age increases, first disappearing from the face, then the extremities and trunk. A small amount may remain on the shoulders, ears, and sides of the forehead at full term.

## Plantar Creases

During the first 12 hours of life, the plantar creases are reliable signs of gestational age. Sole creases develop from the top (under toes) beginning about 32 weeks of gestation. The creases cover two-thirds of the sole by 37 weeks and cover the sole at 40 weeks' gestation.

## Breast

The size of the breast bud tissue is measured by placing the forefinger and middle finger on each side of the breast tissue and measuring between the fingers. At term, the breast bud tissue should be 1 cm. This procedure should be performed gently to prevent tissue damage.

## Eye/Ear

The eyelids are fused until 26 to 28 weeks of gestation. The upper pinna begins to curve over at about 33 to 34 weeks of gestation. The curving over continues until it is complete at 39 to 40 weeks of gestation.

The infant at less than 32 weeks of gestation has almost no ear cartilage. When folded, the ear remains folded. By 36 weeks, there is enough cartilage for the ear to slowly return to its original state when folded. The ear of a full-term infant springs back quickly when folded.

## Male Genitals

The male genitals are evaluated for descent of the testes, presence of rugae on the scrotum, and scrotal size. The testes are formed in the abdomen, move into the inguinal canal at 30 weeks of gestation, then into the upper scrotum by 37 weeks of gestation, and are fully descended by full term. Before 36 weeks, there are few rugae on the scrotum. By 38 weeks, rugae have formed on the anterior part of the scrotum and

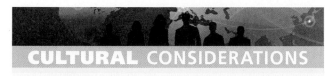

### Lanugo

There may be more lanugo on infants with dark skin coloring than on fair-skinned infants with light-colored hair.

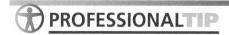

### Ears

When caring for an infant of 32 weeks' gestation or less, be sure the infant's ears are flat to the head and not bent over. Lying on a bent ear can impair circulation to the ear.

cover the scrotum by 40 weeks of gestation. The scrotum is large and pendulous by 40 weeks.

## Female Genitals

Deposits of subcutaneous fat related to nutritional status as well as gestational age determine the appearance of the female genitals. The clitoris and labia minora seem large in comparison to the labia majora, which are small and widely separated at 30 to 32 weeks of gestation. By 36 to 38 weeks of gestation, the clitoris is mostly covered by the labia majora. By 40 weeks of gestation, the labia majora covers the labia minora and clitoris.

## NEUROMUSCULAR MATURITY

The five remaining neuromuscular characteristics to be evaluated are square window, arm recoil, popliteal angle, scarf sign, and heel to ear.

## Square Window

The square window sign is elicited by bending the wrist so the palm is as flat against the arm as possible. If the angle between the palm and arm is 90 degrees and looks like a square window, the gestational age is 32 weeks or less and receives a score of 0. If the angle is greater than 90 degrees, the score is $-1$. The angle becomes smaller the more mature the infant is, until the palm can fold flat against the arm in a full-term newborn.

## Arm Recoil

The infant's arms are held with the elbows fully flexed for 5 seconds. Then the arms are pulled straight down at the infant's sides and quickly released. The elbows of a full-term newborn, when released, rapidly recoil and have an angle less than 90 degrees. That infant is given a score of 4. Very preterm infants may not move their arms (no recoil) and receive a score of 0.

## Popliteal Angle

The popliteal angle is measured when the thigh is flexed on the abdomen, the hips remain flat on the table, and the lower leg is straightened just until met by resistance. Then the angle behind the knee is scored. When the leg can be fully extended, a score of $-1$ is given, but if the popliteal angle is less than 90 degrees, a score of 5 is given.

## Scarf Sign

The newborn's arm is drawn across the body toward the opposite shoulder until resistance is felt. The shoulder of the arm being tested should remain on the table. The relation of the elbow to the infant's midline is noted for scoring. If the elbow does not reach near the midline, it is a score of 4. When the elbow goes across and beyond the infant's body, a score of −1 is given.

## Heel to Ear

With the hips remaining on the surface of the table, the newborn's foot is moved toward the ear on the same side. When resistance is felt, foot position relative to the ear and the degree of knee extension is noted. The preterm infant's leg will remain straight and the foot will be near the ear. The more mature the infant, the more resistance will be felt and more flexion will be noted.

## GESTATIONAL AGE RELATIONSHIP TO INTRAUTERINE GROWTH

There is a normal range of birth weight for each week of gestation as well as for length, head circumference, and intrauterine weight–length ratio (Figure 5-21). Birth weight is classified as follows:

- **Large for gestational age (LGA)**: Infant's weight falls above the 90th percentile for gestational age.

- **Appropriate for gestational age (AGA)**: Infant's weight falls between the 90th and 10th percentile for gestational age.
- **Small for gestational age (SGA)**: Infant's weight falls below the 10th percentile for gestational age.

The correlation of the infant's measurements for length and head circumference also documents the infant's level of maturity and appropriate classification of LGA, AGA, or SGA.

All of these determinations assist caregivers to expect possible physiologic complications, and together with the results of a physical assessment are the basis for preparing an appropriate care plan for the infant.

## SLEEPING POSITION

In 1992, the American Academy of Pediatrics (AAP) recommended that babies be put to sleep on their back to prevent sudden infant death syndrome (SIDS). Since the AAP started their program "back to sleep" and suggested that parents allow infants to use a pacifier when sleeping, the incidence of SIDS has greatly decreased. Another easily prevented and treated condition, positional plagiocephaly, has increased. The recommendation for back sleeping still stands. Both conditions

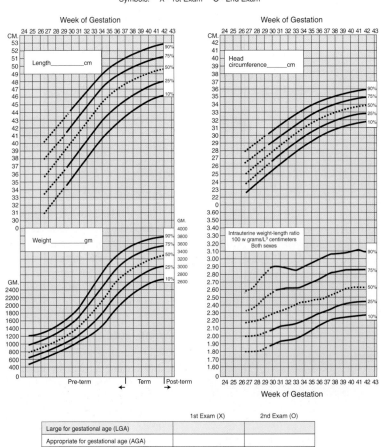

**FIGURE 5-21** Intrauterine Growth Grids (*Courtesy of Mead Johnson Nutritionals.*)

are discussed in the chapter on Infant with Special Needs: Birth to 12 Months.

# FIRST BATH AND CORD CARE

The infant's first bath, and the type of bath for the next 10 days to 2 weeks, is a sponge bath. Newborns are not generally given a tub bath until after the cord has fallen off and healing is complete. Placing the infant under a radiant warmer during the bath helps prevent heat loss. Follow agency protocol for the order of the bath.

Nurses giving the first bath to newborns must wear gloves to comply with Standard Precautions regarding contact with blood or body fluids. A study by Varda and Behnke (2000) found that bathing could be done safely as soon as 1 hour after birth if the newborn's condition is stable and appropriate care is provided. Bathing newborns at 1 hour could decrease exposure of the family and health care providers to blood-borne pathogens (Varda & Behnke, 2000).

Wipe each eye with either a separate cotton ball or a separate place on a washcloth. The eyes are wiped from the inner to outer canthus. The entire face is washed. All of the creases of the ears are cleaned with a corner of a washcloth; a cotton-tipped applicator should never be used in the ears.

Using gauze squares and the approved soap, firmly wash the head to remove all blood and body fluids. Infants with a large amount of hair may require the use of a comb to remove all traces of substances in the hair. A second washing and rinsing of the head may be necessary. The head must be well dried when finished.

Soap or a cleansing agent is used on the rest of the body according to agency protocol. Creases must have special attention to be sure that all traces of blood and the majority of vernix caseosa are removed. The skin should be well rinsed to reduce the drying or potential irritating effect of the soap or cleansing agent (Lund et al., 1999). When completely washed and rinsed, the infant is dried and wrapped in a dry, warm blanket.

The infant may remain in the radiant warmer on dry linens or may be dressed, wrapped in a blanket with a hat on the head, and placed in a regular crib and covered with another blanket. Within 30 minutes to 1 hour, the infant's temperature should be checked. Some infants maintain body temperature better than others. It is important to check the infant's temperature often and according to agency protocol so that when the infant is at an appropriate temperature he can leave the radiant warmer and be taken to his mother to feed.

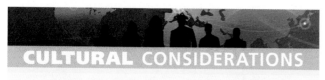

## CULTURAL CONSIDERATIONS

### Umbilical Cord

In Malawi, Africa, infants are kept indoors and are not named until the umbilical cord falls off, typically within the first 2 weeks (Gennaro, Kamwendo, Mbweza, & Kershbaumer, 1998).

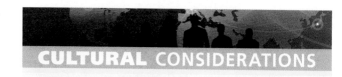

## CULTURAL CONSIDERATIONS

### Infant Care

Nurses must be aware of different cultural practices in order to provide sensitive care. A few examples include:

- Korean tradition is to consider a newborn 1 year old at the time of birth.
- Korean parents will often tightly wrap a newborn in a blanket to prevent possible harm from the wind (Howard & Berbiglia, 1997).
- Japanese parents often choose to immerse the infant for a bath before the cord is healed (Sharts-Hopko, 1995).
- Muslim fathers traditionally call praise to Allah in the newborn's right ear before cleansing the infant.
- Most infants of Muslim parents are not named until they are 7 days old (Hutchinson & Baqi-Aziz, 1994).
- Babies of Southeast Asian parents are kept swaddled for the first few days (Mattson, 1995).
- Jewish male infants are not to be named until the eigth day of life when they have their circumcision.

The cord should be cleaned, at least daily, with alcohol. The diaper should be folded under to allow the cord to dry and prevent urine from getting on the cord.

# CIRCUMCISION

**Circumcision** is the surgical removal of the prepuce (foreskin), which covers the glans penis. In 1999, the American Academy of Pediatrics made a policy statement on circumcision that "data are not sufficient to recommend routine neonatal circumcision. . . . If a decision for circumcision is made, procedural analgesia should be provided" (AAP, 1999). Circumcision is considered an elective procedure for which parents must give written consent. Only full-term, healthy newborns should be circumcised.

## PROCEDURE

The infant is placed on a circumcision board just before the procedure begins (Figure 5-22). Because infants prefer a flexed position, being placed on a circumcision board is frustrating to the newborn. Crying often begins at this point, before the procedure is started.

The best pain relief is provided by a penile nerve root block (Lenhart, Lenhart, Reid, & Chong, 1997; Pasero, 2001). A pacifier with 20% sucrose provides comfort and has been shown to be analgesic (Pasero, 2001). The physician

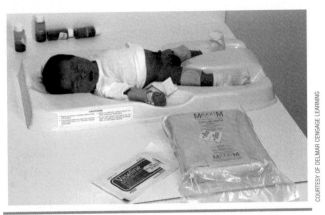

FIGURE 5-22  Circumcision Board. The infant is restrained just before the procedure begins.

then makes a slit in the prepuce and then uses either a Gomco (Yellen) clamp (Figure 5-23) or Plastibell (Figure 5-24) to control bleeding when the prepuce is cut off. After a circumcision with the Gomco clamp, A+D ointment or petroleum jelly is put on the penis to prevent the diaper from sticking to the site. At each diaper change, new ointment is applied for at least 24 to 48 hours.

## NURSING MANAGEMENT

The nurse ensures that the circumcision permit has been signed by a parent. Equipment and supplies are set up, and the infant is placed on the circumcision board with diaper removed. Most infants are not fed for 2 to 4 hours before the procedure to prevent regurgitation. The nurse administers

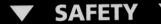

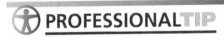

### ▼ SAFETY ▼

#### Gomco (Yellen) Clamp

Inspect the clamp before use for inadequate closure or corrosion. Check the marks on component parts to make sure they match.

### PROFESSIONALTIP

#### Reasons for and against Circumcision

*For:*
- Religious rite.
- Prevent need for procedure later in life.
- May reduce urinary tract infections, penile cancer, and sexually transmitted diseases.

*Against:*
- Procedure is painful.
- Possibility of hemorrhage, infection, or adhesions.

(*Kaufman, Clark & Castro, 2001*)

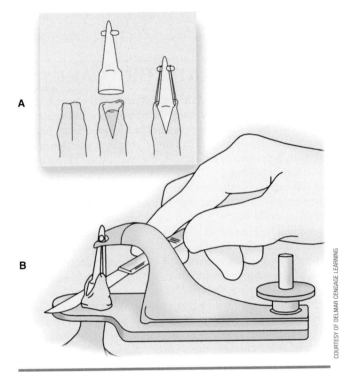

FIGURE 5-23  Gomgo (Yellen) Clamp Used for Circumcision; *A,* After slit is made in prepuce, the cone is placed over the glans and the prepuce is pulled up around the cone; *B,* The cone is placed in the clamp, which is tightened to obliterate the blood vessels. This prevents bleeding. The prepuce is cut away and the clamp is removed in 3 to 5 minutes.

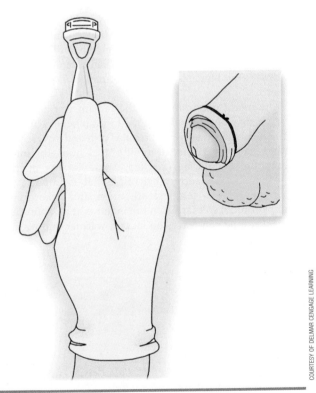

FIGURE 5-24  Plastibell Used for Circumcision. The plastibell is placed over the glans after a slit is made in the prepuce. A suture is tied around the ring. This prevents bleeding when the prepuce is cut away. The handle is removed, leaving the ring to fall off in 5 to 8 days, after healing.

ordered pain medication for the infant 20 to 30 minutes before the procedure.

During the procedure, comfort the infant by talking to the infant, playing a tape of soft music or intrauterine sounds, or lightly stroking the infant. The infant should be kept warm during the circumcision procedure with a well-placed heat lamp. After the procedure, hold the infant to provide comfort. Care following a circumcision includes checking hourly for 12 hours to see if any bleeding is occurring and that the infant is voiding.

If the infant goes home within the first 12 hours after circumcision, bleeding must be minimal and the infant must have voided. Ensure that the parents know how to care for the circumcision and that they have the physician's telephone number.

# NUTRITION

Feeding the newborn is an important aspect of parenting. Nurses assisting in the choice of a feeding method must have knowledge of the newborn's nutritional needs. The American Academy of Pediatrics recommends breast milk for at least 12 months (AAP, 1997).

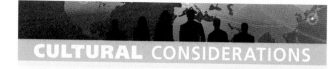

# NUTRITIONAL NEEDS OF NEWBORN

The full-term newborn needs a sufficient intake of calories to meet energy and growth requirements. There should be adequate carbohydrates and fats for energy so that proteins can be used for growth. A newborn requires 110 to 120 kcal/kg (50 to 55 kcal/lb) each day to meet these needs.

This equates to approximately 20 oz of breast milk or formula each day. Newborns lose weight the first few days of life partly because their intake of calories is less than their requirement. One reason is that the newborn's stomach capacity is only 20 mL (30 mL = 1 oz). This capacity increases rapidly, so that by 7 days of age the infant may consume 2 to 3 oz at each feeding. The infant regains birth weight by age 10 days.

# BREAST MILK AND INFANT FORMULA COMPOSITION

The compositions of breast milk and infant formula are different.

## Breast Milk

Breast milk is biologically designed to meet the needs of human infants. Its composition changes to meet the changing nutritional and immunologic needs of the infant. Breast milk is easily digested.

The colostrum (first few days) is rich in immunoglobulins to protect the newborn's gastrointestinal tract from infection. Colostrum helps establish normal intestinal flora and has a laxative effect that assists in the passage of meconium.

In 2 weeks, mature milk is being produced. It contains sufficient nutrients to meet the infant's needs and has 20 kcal/oz. Breast stimulation and removal of milk from the breast stimulates the secretion of prolactin by the anterior pituitary of the mother. Prolactin increases milk production. As the demand becomes greater (infant feeding longer and more frequently), the milk supply increases.

The mother's diet makes little difference in the proportions of carbohydrates, protein, and most minerals in her breast milk, but fat content and the amount of vitamins are affected. The breastfeeding mother must eat a well-balanced diet to provide the most nutritious milk for her infant and to maintain her own health and energy level. An extra 500 calories per day is needed to support breastfeeding.

## Infant Formula

Many infant formulas are modified to match the components in breast milk as nearly as possible. Most formulas are modified cow's milk. Protein is reduced, saturated fat is removed and replaced with vegetable fats, and vitamins and some minerals are added. Soy formulas are used for infants with allergies or who do not tolerate cow's milk–based formula. Nutramigen is a protein hydrolysate formula made from cow's milk but treated to be hypoallergenic. Nutramigen typically is used only when all other formulas have failed as it can be very costly for the parents.

Special formulas are made to meet special needs of some infants. Preterm infants need more calories but less quantity; these formulas provide 24 kcal/oz. Other formulas are modified to be low in the amino acid phenylalanine for infants with phenylketonuria (PKU), who cannot digest phenylalanine.

## FEEDING METHOD

Nutrition is provided for the newborn either through breastfeeding or bottle feeding. Whichever method the parents choose, nurses must support and assist the parents to make the experience meaningful. Some of the advantages and disadvantages of breastfeeding and bottle feeding are identified in Table 5-2.

Other factors besides the advantages and disadvantages of breastfeeding and bottle feeding enter into the decision of how to feed the newborn. These factors include support offered by the infant's father; support by other family members; the need to work outside the home by the mother; and age, educational level, and income level of the parents.

When the mother is breastfeeding (8 to 12 times a day at first), she is focused on the infant. Various tasks around the home may need to be left undone or the father will need to do them. Support from other family members may be based on how other family members have chosen to feed their infants.

**TABLE 5-2 Breastfeeding/Bottle Feeding, Advantages and Disadvantages**

| | BREASTFEEDING | BOTTLE FEEDING |
|---|---|---|
| Advantages | Nonallergenic | Father or others may feed infant day or night |
| | Meets infant's specific nutritional needs | Feed less frequently (3 to 4 hours) |
| | Immunologic properties help prevent infections | Amount of milk taken at each feeding known |
| | Easily digested | Easier to go back to work |
| | Constipation unlikely (Figure 5-25) | Caregiver determines amount |
| | Overfeeding less likely | |
| | Convenient, always available | |
| | No formula or bottles to buy | |
| | No formula and bottles to prepare | |
| | Oxytocin release helps involution | |
| | Mother more likely to eat well-balanced diet | |
| | May help with mother's weight loss | |
| | Enhances mother/infant attachment through skin-to-skin contact | |
| | Infant determines amount | |
| Disadvantages | Feed more frequently (2 to 3 hours) | Expense of formula, bottles ($50 to $200 per month) |
| | More frequent diaper changes | Washing bottles |
| | Amount of milk taken at each feeding unknown | Fixing and refrigerating formula |
| | Medications taken by mother present in milk | Carrying bottles on outings |
| | Discomfort of some mothers to nurse in public | May cause constipation |
| | Expense of pumping and storing milk for periods when mother is unavailable (such as work hours) | |

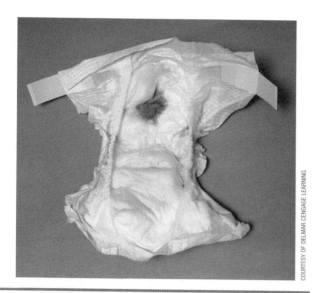

COURTESY OF DELMAR CENGAGE LEARNING

**FIGURE 5-25** Stool of a Breastfed Infant

# BREASTFEEDING

Many factors influence breastfeeding, including positions for feeding, latching on, and length of feeding.

## Positions for Feeding

The infant should be held with the head slightly higher than the rest of the body. The cradle hold, with the infant's head in the bend of the mother's elbow and the arm supporting the infant's body, is probably the most common. It can be used whether breastfeeding or bottle feeding. Other positions that are particularly adaptable to breastfeeding are the football hold, side-lying position, and across-the-lap position (Figure 5-26). The mother's free hand should be in a "C" position, supporting the underside of her breast with the fingers.

## Latching On

The mother should use the infant's rooting reflex to allow proper positioning of the nipple in the infant's mouth. Brushing the nipple against the infant's lower lip will cause the infant to open the mouth. When the mouth is wide open and the tongue is down, the mother quickly brings the infant closer to the breast so the infant can latch on to the nipple and areola. When properly positioned, the tongue is on top of the lower gum and

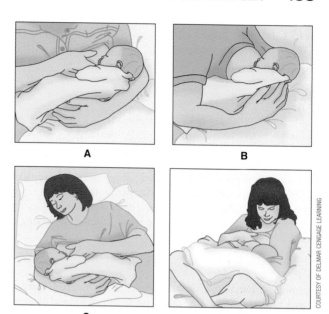

COURTESY OF DELMAR CENGAGE LEARNING

**FIGURE 5-26** Positions for Feeding Infant; *A*, Cradling, used for Breast and Bottle Feeding; *B*, Football Hold; *C*, Lying Down; *D*, Across Lap.

under the breast, with the lips flared outward. When the infant is properly latched on, the suction is strong. To remove the infant from the breast, the mother should insert a finger into the corner of the infant's mouth between the gums to break the suction and quickly remove the breast. The nipple should never be simply pulled out from the infant's mouth because this will cause the mother pain and may also result in tissue damage to the nipple.

## Length of Feeding

Feeding length varies with each mother/infant unit; however, the feeding should be long enough to remove all of the **fore-milk**, the watery first milk from the breast, which is high in lactose, like skim milk, and is effective in quenching thirst. This allows the infant to receive the **hindmilk**, which is higher in fat content, leads to weight gain, and is more satisfying.

The average time for a feeding session is approximately 30 minutes. It is more important to know when the infant is finished feeding than to go by the clock. When an infant is satisfied, the sucking and swallowing will be much slower and the breast will be soft. The infant may fall asleep and release the nipple.

The first breast should be emptied (very soft) before moving the infant to the other breast. At the next feeding, the breast used last at the previous feeding should be used first. This ensures that each breast is emptied at least at every other feeding. As the infant grows and requires more milk, both breasts may be emptied at each feeding.

**CLIENTTEACHING**

### Timing of Feedings

Feedings should be given when the infant is hungry (demand feeding) rather than on a fixed schedule. The infant is ready to eat when wide awake, sucking on hands, rooting, and slightly fussy. New mothers are encouraged to feed on demand as this will help their milk supply build. Some breastfeeding mothers fear that they will overfeed or spoil their infant if they are fed on demand. Teach the mother that this is acceptable and that they should continue to observe the infant for hunger clues and then feed them.

**CRITICAL THINKING**

### Breastfeeding

Your client is trying to breastfeed her second child. With her first child, she gave up in three weeks because of cracked, sore nipples. What factors may affect her success or failure? What nursing interventions should be planned and implemented?

## BOTTLE FEEDING

Factors related to bottle feeding include bottles, formula preparation, and amount of feeding.

### Bottles

Babies will generally feed well from any bottle and nipple, although many babies will eventually develop a preference and may refuse a new type of nipple. Whatever choice the parents make will be fine. Washing the bottles and nipples with a bottle and nipple brush in warm, soapy water is necessary for thorough cleaning. Rinsing thoroughly removes all traces of soap. Only if there is a question regarding the safety of the water supply (e.g., well water on a farm or ranch) is boiling of the bottles and nipples necessary.

### Formula Preparation

Formulas are available in three forms: ready to feed, concentrated, and powdered. The latter two require addition of water. The choice of formula is generally left up to the parents. There is a great difference in price, so the choice may be made based on finances. Mixing of formula must be accurate to provide the 20 kcal/oz.

### Amount of Feeding

Most newborns begin by drinking 7.5 mL to 15 mL (1/4 to 1/2 oz) at a feeding but gradually increase to approximately 90 mL to 120 mL (3 to 4 oz) at each feeding in 2 weeks. The infant's appetite will generally increase during growth spurts at 2 weeks, 6 to 9 weeks, and 3 to 6 months, so the amount of formula should be increased by 30 mL (1 oz) in each bottle to meet this need.

## BURPING

All infants require burping, whether breastfed or bottle fed. Burping is needed to expel the air swallowed when the infant sucks. Some infants swallow more air than others and require more frequent burping.

To facilitate burping, the infant can be held upright on the feeder's shoulder, in a sitting position on the feeder's lap with the head and chest supported with one hand, or prone across the feeder's lap (Figure 5-27). The other hand is used to gently pat or rub the infant's back.

Burping should be done generally about halfway through the feeding for bottle feeding and when changing breasts for breastfeeding. Parents soon learn the infant's cues regarding the need to be burped.

### Pacifiers

Many parents are anxious to comfort their new baby. This usually means offering the infant a pacifier to help sooth them. The best practice is to wait at least 4 to 6 weeks to prevent nipple confusion and ensure that the infant has a solid feeding relationship with either breast or bottle.

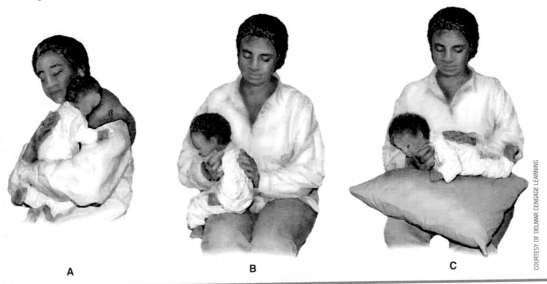

FIGURE 5-27  Burping positions: *A*, Supported on the shoulder; *B*, Upright on the lap; *C*, Face down across the lap.

## SAMPLE NURSING CARE PLAN

## Newborn Infant

S.S., born at 36 weeks' gestation, weighs 6 pounds 3 ounces and is 19 inches long. Her Apgar score was 8 at 1 minute and 9 at 5 minutes. Axillary temperature is 96.5°F (35.8°C), respirations 56, and apical pulse 148. The parents are very excited about S.S., their first child. S.S. is very sleepy and is not breastfeeding well.

**NURSING DIAGNOSIS 1** *Ineffective Thermoregulation* related to immaturity as evidenced by birth at 36 weeks' gestation

## SAMPLE NURSING CARE PLAN (Continued)

**Nursing Outcomes Classification (NOC)**
*Thermoregulation: Neonate*

**Nursing Interventions Classification (NIC)**
*Temperature Regulation*

| PLANNING/OUTCOMES | NURSING INTERVENTIONS | RATIONALE |
|---|---|---|
| S.S.'s temperature will be between 97.5°F (36.4°C) and 98.9°F (37.2°C). | Keep S.S. adequately clothed and covered. | Maintains her temperature. |
| | Maintain ambient room temperature between 77.2°F (25.1°C) and 78.1°F (25.6°C). | Is optimum environmental temperature. |
| | Keep S.S. away from air conditioning vents, drafts, and fans. | Prevents heat loss by convection. |
| | Use warm water when bathing S.S., wrap her in a towel, and dry her quickly. Dry her head thoroughly and put a cap on her head. | Prevents heat loss by evaporation. |
| | Cover scales and examination area before S.S. is laid down. | Prevents heat loss by conduction. |
| | Keep S.S.'s crib away from outside windows. | Prevents heat loss by radiation. |
| | Teach S.S.'s parents how to maintain a neutral thermal environment for S.S. | Prevents S.S. from using her brown fat too fast. |

## EVALUATION

S.S.'s temperature is 97.8°F.

**NURSING DIAGNOSIS 2** *Risk for Infection* related to risk factor of inadequate primary defenses as evidenced by cut umbilical cord and immature immune system

**Nursing Outcomes Classification (NOC)**
*Infection Status, Wound Healing, Immune Status*

**Nursing Interventions Classification (NIC)**
*Infection Control, Wound Care*

| PLANNING/OUTCOMES | NURSING INTERVENTIONS | RATIONALE |
|---|---|---|
| S.S. will have no signs of infection of the eyes, diaper area, or umbilical cord. | Use good hand hygiene technique (caregivers and parents) before and after caring for S.S. | Prevents spread of infection. |
| | Provide prescribed eye prophylaxis and keep eyes clean. | Prevents infection. |
| | Keep diaper area clean and dry. | Prevents skin irritation and infection. |
| | Place diaper below the umbilical cord. | Allows cord to dry and heal. |

## EVALUATION

S.S. shows no signs of infection.

*(Continues)*

## SAMPLE NURSING CARE PLAN (Continued)

**NURSING DIAGNOSIS 3** *Imbalanced Nutrition, less than body requirements* related to infants prematurity and limited nutritional intake as evidenced by infant remaining sleepy and not breastfeeding well during feedings

**Nursing Outcomes Classification (NOC)**
*Nutritional Status*

**Nursing Interventions Classification (NIC)**
*Nutrition Management, Nutrition Monitoring*

| PLANNING/OUTCOMES | NURSING INTERVENTIONS | RATIONALE |
|---|---|---|
| S.S. will lose only 5 to 10 ounces of weight during the first 3 days. | Assist mother in breastfeeding S.S. | Provides support for first time breastfeeding. |
| | Demonstrate use of rooting reflex to ensure proper latch on. | Uses natural response of infant for proper position of mouth and tongue. |
| | Explain that S.S. will suck in spurts. | Assists mother in knowing that S.S. has not finished breastfeeding when she rests. |
| | Explain that the breast has foremilk and hindmilk (needed for growth), so breasts must be emptied. | Ensures that mother will allow S.S. to empty one breast before changing to the other breast. |

**EVALUATION**
S.S. lost 7 ounces during the first 3 days.

# PROBLEMS OF THE NEWBORN

Problems of the newborn identified either at birth or before discharge include hyperbilirubinemia, respiratory distress, cleft lip/palate, hydrocephalus, spina bifida, Down syndrome, and talipes equinovarus. Newborn problems may also occur when the mother is diabetic, HIV positive, or a substance abuser. Phenylketonuria must be tested for as soon as possible so treatment can begin immediately.

## HYPERBILIRUBINEMIA

Hyperbilirubinemia, an excess of bilirubin in the blood, may be related to physiologic jaundice or pathologic jaundice. Physiologic jaundice does not appear until after 24 hours of age and is more commonly seen after the infant has gone home. It is discussed in the Infants with Special Needs: Birth to 12 Months chapter.

Pathologic jaundice appears in the first 24 hours and may lead to **kernicterus** (deposits of bilirubin causing yellow staining in the brain, especially the basal ganglia, cerebellum, and hippocampus). The exact level of total bilirubin when kernicterus occurs is not known but may occur at 20 mg/dL in full-term infants and at a lower level in preterm neonates. Kernicterus is a chronic and clinically permanent result of bilirubin toxcity. Preterm infants are at a greater risk of developing kernicterus, and the most common cause is Rh incompatibility and severe dehydration (AAP, 2004)

## MEDICAL–SURGICAL MANAGEMENT
### Medical

Phototherapy is the most common treatment for jaundice. The "bili" lights are special flourescent lamps (in the blue-light spectrum) placed over the infant. Only a diaper and an eye covering are on the infant to expose the most skin surface to the light. A fiber-optic phototherapy blanket and the BiliBed® with the Bilicombi™ blanket (Figure 5-28) have been designed to provide phototherapy without the eyes needing to be covered. Because the infant is covered, thermal regulation is no longer a problem, and interaction with the parents can take place. The infant may experience frequent, green, loose stools as the bilirubin is excreted.

### Surgical

If the bilirubin level cannot be reduced quickly or maintained below 12 mg/dL with phototherapy treatment, exchange transfusion is necessary. Blood type O, Rh-negative blood is used. During this procedure, 5 mL to 10 mL of blood are removed from the infant and replaced with a like amount of donor blood. This is a very slow process. Complications of hypervolemia, hypovolemia, infection, cardiac arrhythmias, and air embolism may occur.

This procedure is seldom necessary today because of the widespread use of RhoGAM to prevent Rh incompatibility.

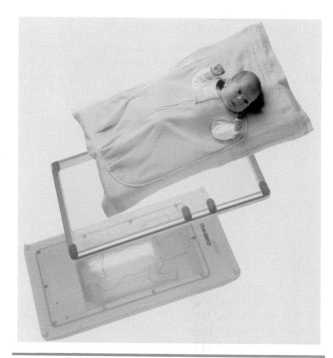

FIGURE 5-28  Bilibed® with Bilicombi™ Blanket (*Photo courtesy of Medela, Inc.*)

## Diet

Fluid intake is increased to assist in elimination of the bilirubin through the urine.

## NURSING MANAGEMENT

Review record to identify factors predisposing the infant to jaundice. Assess infant for jaundice every 4 hours. Encourage adequate amount taken at each feeding. Breastfeeding mothers should feed their infants at least 8 to 12 times a day for the first several days after delivery. Make sure to keep diaper area clean and protected. The American Academy of Pediatrics (2004), recommends against supplementations with extra fluids such as water or dextrose with water, as they will not prevent or lower the bilirubin levels.

## NURSING PROCESS

### ASSESSMENT

#### Subjective Data

None.

#### Objective Data

Prenatal and perinatal records are reviewed to identify factors predisposing to jaundice. Jaundice in light-skinned infants is assessed by blanching the skin (pressing firmly with the thumb) over a bony prominence such as the forehead, nose, or sternum. When the thumb is removed, the area has a yellowish appearance before normal color returns if jaundice is present. In darker-skinned infants, the infant's oral mucosa, posterior aspect of the hard palate, or conjunctival sacs will have a yellow coloring when jaundice is present.

**Nursing diagnoses for an infant with hyperbilirubinemia include the following:**

| NURSING DIAGNOSES | PLANNING/OUTCOMES | NURSING INTERVENTIONS |
|---|---|---|
| *Risk for Deficient **F**luid Volume* related to increased insensible water loss and frequent loose stools secondary to phototherapy | The infant's intake will be at least 100 to 150 mL/kg/day. | Encourage adequate feedings of infant by mother. |
| *Risk for **N**eonatal Jaundice* related to abnormal weight loss (>7% to 8% in breastfeeding newborn; 15% in term infant) as evidenced by infant experiencing difficulty in establishing a consistent breastfeeding pattern | The infant will maintain a 2% to 3% in weight prior to discharge. | Assist in proper latch on technique. Instruct parents on weighing wet diapers to help ensure appropriate intake. |
| *Risk for Impaired **S**kin Integrity* related to frequent loose stools secondary to phototherapy | The infant's diaper area will maintain skin integrity. | Check diaper frequently and change as soon as soiled. Apply A+D ointment or petroleum jelly to diaper area after cleansing. |

**Evaluation:** Evaluate each outcome to determine how it has been met by the client.

## RESPIRATORY DISTRESS

Two types of respiratory distress may occur in a newborn: respiratory distress syndrome (RDS) and transient tachypnea of the newborn (TTN).

Respiratory distress syndrome is associated with preterm infants and surfactant deficiency. Verma (1995) describes

respiratory distress syndrome as caused by alterations in surfactant quantity, composition, function, or production. These infants have hypoxia, respiratory acidosis, and metabolic acidosis.

Transient tachypnea of the newborn is found mainly in AGA and near-term infants (Ladewig et al., 2005). Either intrauterine or intrapartum asphyxia has been experienced by these infants. This results in the newborn's failure to clear the airway of lung fluid and mucus or aspiration of amniotic fluid. No respiratory difficulties are experienced at birth, but shortly after birth, the newborn may have flaring of the nares and expiratory grunting. By 6 hours of age, tachypnea is noted, with respirations as high as 100 to 140 breaths per minute.

## MEDICAL–SURGICAL MANAGEMENT
### Medical

The goal is to determine which type of respiratory distress is affecting the newborn and begin treatment. For RDS, the goals of treatment are maintenance of adequate oxygenation and ventilation and correction of the respiratory and metabolic acidosis. Mild RDS is often treated only with increased, humidified oxygen concentration. Infants with moderate RDS may require continuous positive airway pressure (CPAP). Mechanical ventilation is required for severe RDS. The oxygen needs of infants with RDS increase over the first 48 hours.

Infants with TTN generally require ambient oxygen of 30% to 50% initially. This need for increased oxygen generally decreases over the first 48 hours. Treatment is usually required only for 4 days.

## NURSING MANAGEMENT

Monitor respirations and pulse oximetry at least hourly. Use the Silverman-Anderson index to rate respiratory effort. Provide oxygen as ordered. Monitor oxygen concentration. Use strict aseptic technique when caring for the infant.

## NURSING PROCESS

### ASSESSMENT
#### Subjective Data

None.

#### Objective Data

There will be cyanosis pallor or mottling of the skin, tachypnea, grunting respirations, retractions, and nasal flaring. To rate the infant's respiratory effort, the Silverman-Anderson index is often used (Figure 5-29). The heart rate is generally within the expected range.

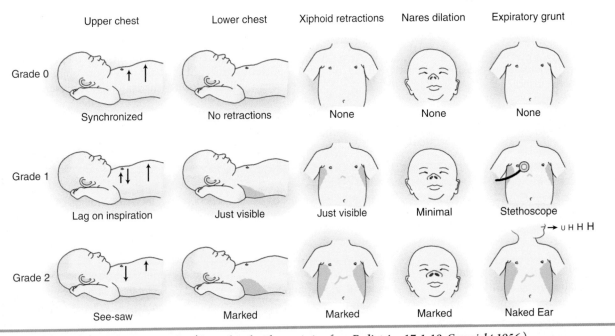

**FIGURE 5-29** Silverman-Anderson Index (*Reproduced with permission from* Pediatrics *17:1-10. Copyright 1956.*)

### Nursing diagnoses for an infant with respiratory distress include the following:

| NURSING DIAGNOSES | PLANNING/OUTCOMES | NURSING INTERVENTIONS |
|---|---|---|
| *Respiratory Distress* related to premature infant lung maturity | The infant will maintain optimum lung function as evidenced by pulse oximetry within normal limits 98% or higher. | Monitor arterial blood gases.<br>Administer oxygen as ordered.<br>Assess infant for periods of apnea.<br>Monitor infant's skin and reposition as needed.<br>Monitor for nasal flaring. |
| *Risk for Infection* related to invasive procedures | The infant will show no signs or symptoms of infection at the procedure site. | Assess procedure site for signs of infection (redness, swelling, color, size, and odor). |

**Nursing diagnoses for an infant with respiratory distress include the following: (Continued)**

| NURSING DIAGNOSES | PLANNING/OUTCOMES | NURSING INTERVENTIONS |
|---|---|---|
| | | Monitor infant's temperature hourly. |
| | | Maintain strict aseptic technique when caring for infant. |
| | | Review all lab work and report status changes. |

**Evaluation:** Evaluate each outcome to determine how it has been met by the client.

## CLEFT LIP/PALATE

The immediate concern with cleft lip/palate (Figure 5-30) is the problem of feeding the infant. The size of the cleft and whether the palate is also involved determine the difficulty of feeding. Special nipples and feeding devices are available. Hold the infant in an upright sitting position when feeding. Burp frequently because these infants swallow more air than usual. When sleeping, keep the infant in a side-lying position.

Parents of an infant with any congenital anomaly need support from the nurse as they learn to care for an infant with special needs. The nurse must role model interacting with the infant. Complete coverage is found in the Infants with Special Needs: Birth to 12 Months chapter.

## HYDROCEPHALUS

Hydrocephalus, excess cerebrospinal fluid in the cerebral ventricles, causes the infant's head to be enlarged. Head circumference is measured daily, fontanelles checked to see whether they are flat or bulging, and the infant's position changed frequently. The infant usually cannot move the head. Complete coverage is found in the Infant with Special Needs: Birth to 12 Months chapter.

## SPINA BIFIDA

There are three types of spina bifida (neural tube defects): spina bifida occulta, meningocele, and myelomeningocele (Figure 5-31). **Spina bifida occulta** is a failure of the vertebral arch to close. There is a dimple on the back, which may have a tuft of hair in it. No care is required.

A **meningocele** is a saclike protrusion along the vertebral column filled with cerebrospinal fluid and meninges. Surgery is required to repair the defect, but there are no long-term effects.

A **myelomeningocele** is a saclike protrusion along the vertebral column filled with spinal fluid, meninges, nerve roots, and spinal cord. Because of the nerve root and spinal cord involvement, there will be paralysis at some level after surgical repair.

The saclike protrusions must be kept covered with sterile saline dressings, and the infant handled carefully when changing position from side to side. The sac must be kept free from contamination by urine and stool. Head circumference is measured and fontanelles checked for bulging on each shift because hydrocephalus often develops. Complete coverage of myelomeningocele is found in the Infant with Special Needs: Birth to 12 Months chapter.

## DOWN SYNDROME

**Down syndrome** is caused by a chromosomal abnormality, also called trisomy 21. Routine care is provided in the newborn period. Complete coverage is found in the Infant with Special Needs: Birth to 12 Months chapter.

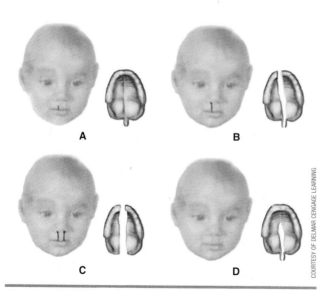

COURTESY OF DELMAR CENGAGE LEARNING

**FIGURE 5-30** Types of Cleft Lip/Palate; *A*, Small Notch in Lip, Palate Normal; *B*, Cleft Lip and Cleft Palate; *C*, Bilateral Cleft Lip and Cleft Palate; *D*, Lip Normal, Cleft Palate

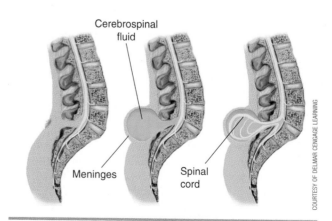

Cerebrospinal fluid

Meninges

Spinal cord

COURTESY OF DELMAR CENGAGE LEARNING

**FIGURE 5-31** Types of Spina Bifida; *A*, Spina Bifida Occulta; *B*, Meningocele; *C*, Myelomeningocele

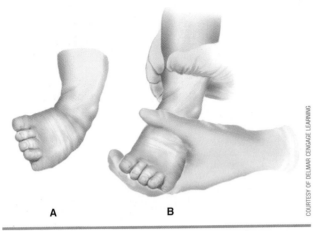

FIGURE 5-32 *A,* Talipes Equinovarus (clubfoot); *B,* Foot Moves to Midline; Positional, not Clubfoot

## ■ TALIPES EQUINOVARUS

**T**alipes equinovarus, also called clubfoot, is a congenital deformity in which the foot and ankle are twisted inward and cannot be moved to a midline position (Figure 5-32). The foot or feet of some infants appear to turn inward, but if they can be moved to the midline, the cause is intrauterine position. Range-of-motion exercises will often correct this problem.

Infants with true clubfoot may have a cast on before going home. Complete coverage is found in the Infant with Special Needs: Birth to 12 Months chapter.

## ■ INFANT OF A DIABETIC MOTHER

**T**he infant of a diabetic mother (IDM) requires close observation the first few hours to several days after birth. If the mother has vascular complications with the diabetes, the infant is generally SGA. If the mother has gestational diabetes or diabetes without vascular changes, the infant is generally LGA, especially if the diabetes has not been well-controlled. The large size is the result of fat deposits and increased size of all organs except the brain. The IDM has less total body water, especially in the extra-cellular spaces. The following are complications seen most often in the IDM:

- *Hypoglycemia*: The loss of maternal glucose at birth and the high level of insulin produced by the infant decrease the infant's blood glucose within hours after birth. It takes a period of time for insulin production to be reduced in the newborn.
- *Respiratory distress*: Insulin is antagonistic to the cortisol-induced stimulation of lecithin (phospholipid necessary for lung maturation) synthesis. This results in less-mature lungs than would be expected for the gestational age. This does not seem to be a problem if the mother has vascular complications with her diabetes.
- *Hyperbilirubinemia*: Hepatic immaturity and a decreased extracellular fluid volume, which increases hematocrit, may be the cause of the hyperbilirubinemia seen 48 to

72 hours after birth (Ladewig et al., 2005). Any bruises from a difficult delivery may also be a cause.

- *Birth trauma*: The large size of many IDMs predisposes them to trauma during labor and delivery.
- *Congenital birth defects*: Birth defects may include patent ductus arteriosus, ventricular septal defect, transposition of the great vessels, small left colon syndrome, and sacral agenesis.

## MEDICAL–SURGICAL MANAGEMENT

### Medical

Blood glucose monitoring is performed hourly during the first 4 to 6 hours of life and then every 4 hours for 24 hours, or per agency protocol. Blood is generally obtained by heelstick (Figure 5-33).

### 🔖 Pharmacological

An intravenous infusion of glucose may be necessary if early feeding does not keep the blood glucose at 45 mg/dL or above.

### Diet

A feeding of 5% glucose water may be given soon after birth, followed in 1 hour by a breast or formula feeding, which is continued on a regular basis.

## NURSING MANAGEMENT

Monitor blood glucose level as ordered. Ensure timely feedings. Administer glucose orally or IV as ordered. Prevent cold stress. Hold and comfort the infant after heelsticks.

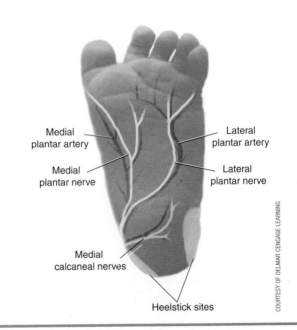

FIGURE 5-33 Shaded areas shown are heelstick sites.

# NURSING PROCESS

## ASSESSMENT

### Subjective Data

None.

### Objective Data

Blood glucose screening of less than 45 mg/dL should be verified by laboratory analysis. The infant may show signs of jitteriness or tremors. Diaphoresis, although uncommon for a newborn, may occur with hypoglycemia. Poor muscle tone, low temperature, and rapid respirations may also be noted.

### Nursing diagnoses for an infant with hypoglycemia include the following:

| NURSING DIAGNOSES | PLANNING/OUTCOMES | NURSING INTERVENTIONS |
| --- | --- | --- |
| *Imbalanced **N**utrition: Less Than Body Requirements* related to increased glucose use secondary to being IDM | The infant will maintain an adequate glucose level. | Initiate feedings as soon as possible. |
| | | Prepare dextrose solution IV if infant is unable to take PO fluids. |
| | | Weigh infant every day at the same time for adequate weight checks. |
| | | Monitor infant's temperature and the temperature in the isolette to maintain warm environment and to prevent cold stress, which could increase the glucose levels. |
| | | Monitor lab work and report any changes. |
| | | Ensure timely infant feedings. |
| | | Monitor blood glucose level according to protocol. |
| | | Prevent cold stress and identify other stressors (hypoxia, sepsis, RDS) that increase glucose use. |
| *Acute **P**ain* related to physical injury of heelsticks for glucose monitoring | The infant will decrease crying after each heelstick. | Warm infant's heel before heelstick to increase blood flow to the area. |
| | | Properly perform heelstick to avoid nerves and arteries. |
| | | Hold and comfort infant after heelstick procedure. |

**Evaluation:** Evaluate each outcome to determine how it has been met by the client.

## ■ INFANT OF AN HIV-POSITIVE MOTHER

The transmission rate of HIV infection from mother to infant is 28% to 35% (Merenstein, Adams, & Weisman, 2006). This transmission may occur through the placenta at various gestational ages, through maternal blood and secretions during labor and birth, and through breast milk after the birth (Fanaroff & Martin, 2005).

Every infant born to an HIV-seropositive mother will have HIV antibodies that have crossed the placenta from the mother. By 8 to 15 months of age, uninfected infants have lost the maternal antibodies; but the infected infants have begun to develop their own antibodies and remain HIV seropositive (Fanaroff & Martin, 2005).

At birth, the HIV-infected infant typically has no symptoms. The appearance of an opportunistic disease between 3 and 6 months of age may alert caregivers to the presence of HIV infection. Lymphoid interstitial pneumonitis is considered a criterion for diagnosis (Fanaroff & Martin, 2005). As a basis for care, all infants of HIV-positive mothers must be presumed to be HIV positive.

Breastfeeding is not recommended. HIV-positive women that breastfeed their infants increase the risk of trasmission by 15% to 40%. HIV transmission occurs most often in the first few months of the infants life. In the United States, the rate of transmission has been significantly reduced due to medications and formula that are available for HIV-positive mothers (Amman, 2009).

## ■ INFANT OF A SUBSTANCE-ABUSING MOTHER

The infant of a substance-abusing mother (ISAM) is a substance abuser at birth. When the umbilical cord is cut at birth, the newborn experiences withdrawal. The severity of withdrawal symptoms depends on the substance(s) abused by the mother and the time and amount of the last dose. The symptoms may occur within the first 24 to 48 hours after birth or not until 4 or 5 days of age. Alcohol withdrawal symptoms often appear within 6 to 12 hours after birth or at least within the first 3 days. Infant alcohol dependence is physiologic. It may be very difficult for the substance-abusing mother to care for her infant initially and/or long term.

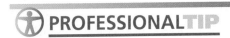

### Narcotic Antagonists

The use of naloxone (Narcan) is contraindicated for infants born to narcotic abusers. It may cause severe signs and symptoms of narcotic withdrawal, especially seizures.

Complications commonly found in an ISAM include withdrawal, respiratory distress, jaundice, behavior problems, congenital anomalies, and growth retardation. Infants of alcohol-dependent mothers may also have fetal alcohol syndrome (FAS). Narcon (Naxalone), an opiod antagonist, is pulled for delivery whenever the client has tested positive for drugs on admission. Narcan is used when a mother has had a narcotic during delivery for pain relief.

## MEDICAL–SURGICAL MANAGEMENT

### Medical

Treatment is focused on management of the previously mentioned complications that may be present. Approximately 50% of these infants experience withdrawal symptoms severe enough to require treatment.

### Pharmacological

Phenobarbital or tincture of opium may be used to control drug withdrawal symptoms. Phenobarbital or diazepam (Valium) may be used to control seizures in the alcohol-dependent infant.

### Diet

Formula supplying 24 kcal/oz is recommended for the infant who experiences vomiting and diarrhea or who is excessively active.

## NURSING MANAGEMENT

Monitor the infant's temperature, weight, skin turgor, and fontanells. Maintain strict intake and output. Provide small, frequent feedings. Provide a quiet environment and keep stimulation at a minimum. Administer medications as ordered. Role model interacting with the infant and encourage the mother to do so. Make referrals as necessary to social agencies and infant development programs.

## NURSING PROCESS

### ASSESSMENT

#### Subjective Data

None.

#### Objective Data

The drug-dependent infant may experience hyperactivity, persistent high-pitched shrill cry, tremors, seizures, tachypnea, fever, disorganized sucking and swallowing, vomiting, diarrhea, stuffy nose, yawning, sneezing, and sweating. The alcohol-dependent infant may or may not have FAS, which includes mental retardation, hyperactivity, growth deficiency, distinctive facial abnormalities, and other congenital anomalies. This infant may also experience tremors, seizures, inconsolable crying, abdominal distention, great activity, and exaggerated rooting and sucking.

**Nursing diagnoses for an infant experiencing withdrawal include the following:**

| NURSING DIAGNOSES | PLANNING/OUTCOMES | NURSING INTERVENTIONS |
|---|---|---|
| *Imbalanced Nutrition: Less Than Body Requirements* related to disorganized sucking and swallowing, vomiting, diarrhea, and hyperactivity | The infant will not lose excessive weight (more than 10% of birth weight). | Monitor infant's temperature so environment can be adjusted to maintain normal infant temperature. Provide small frequent feedings. Administer medications as ordered. Position infant on the side to avoid possible aspiration. Maintain strict intake and output. Weigh infant every 8 hours. Monitor for signs of dehydration (sunken fontanel, dry mucous membranes, poor skin turgor, weight loss). |
| *Risk for Injury* related to effects of substancewithdrawal (seizures, hyperactivity) | The infant will not exhibit signs of seizures. | Administer medications as ordered. Decrease environmental activity. Plan care to necessitate minimum stimulation. Wrap infant snugly. Monitor activity level. |

| **Nursing diagnoses for an infant experiencing withdrawal include the following: (Continued)** | | |
|---|---|---|
| **NURSING DIAGNOSES** | **PLANNING/OUTCOMES** | **NURSING INTERVENTIONS** |
| *Risk for Impaired **P**arenting* related to substance abuse and difficult temperament of the infant | The parent will show signs of bonding/attachment and an interest in infant care. | Explain effects of maternal substance abuse on infant and the process of withdrawal. |
| | | Role model interacting with the infant. |
| | | Encourage mother to interact with her infant. |
| | | Explain and demonstrate infant care procedures, especially how to avoid excess stimulation of the infant. |
| | | Make referrals to social agencies and infant development programs. |

**Evaluation:** Evaluate each outcome to determine how it has been met by the client.

## PHENYLKETONURIA

Most states require neonatal screening for the genetic disease phenylketonuria (PKU), an inborn error of metabolism in which the infant has a deficiency of the enzyme required to digest the amino acid phenylalanine. The infant must ingest an ample amount of phenylalanine, found in both breast milk and regular infant formulas, for the PKU test to be reliable. The test is performed at least 24 hours after the initial breast or formula feeding.

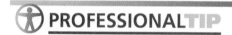

## PROFESSIONALTIP

### PKU

The time of the first breast or formula feeding is to be documented so at least 24 hours passes before the heelstick for the PKU test is performed.

An infant with PKU must be put on a diet low in phenylalanine, preferably by 1 month of age. Infant formulas that are very low in phenylalanine are available. Without screening and diet modification, severe mental retardation results. Even with neonatal PKU screening, many affected children have some intellectual impairment (Lowdermilk & Perry, 2007).

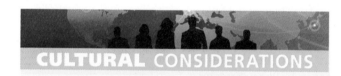

## CULTURAL CONSIDERATIONS

### Phenylketonuria

The highest incidence of PKU is found in the white populations of Northern Europe and the United States; it is less common in populations of African, Chinese, and Japanese descent (Hardelid & Etal, 2008).

## CASE STUDY

Baby boy H.R., a full-term newborn, is 36 hours old. He has type B, Rh-positive blood and his mother has type O, Rh-positive blood. There is a small cephalhematoma on the right parietal bone. Routine assessment identified the appearance of jaundice when the skin was blanched on his forehead. His bilirubin level was 2 mg/dL on the cord blood and 4 mg/dL at 24 hours of age.

The following questions will guide your development of a nursing care plan for the case study.

1. What factors may be causing the jaundice?
2. What orders would you anticipate the physician would write?
3. What are the critical levels of bilirubin?
4. Phototherapy is begun using "bili" lights. What assessments and precautions must be taken when these lights are used?
5. Identify two possible nursing diagnoses and a goal for each for baby boy H.R.
6. Describe nursing interventions for meeting the goals.
7. How can the goals be evaluated?

## SUMMARY

- The immediate needs of the newborn are airway, breathing, circulation, and warmth.
- The initiation of breathing is related to physical, chemical, thermal, and sensory factors.
- Circulatory changes include the closing of the three fetal structures: the ductus arteriosus, foramen ovale, and the ductus venosus.
- Nonshivering thermogenesis, metabolism of brown fat, is the newborn's unique method of heat production.
- Infants lose heat through conduction, convection, evaporation, and radiation.
- The immediate care of the newborn includes obtaining the Apgar score, resuscitation (if required), providing a neutral thermal environment, identification, parent/infant bonding, and prophylactic care.
- Common variations of the newborn must be carefully documented, especially mongolian spots, to possibly prevent parents from being charged with child abuse.
- Neurologic integrity can be assessed through the many reflexes of the newborn. Most of these reflexes disappear during the first 2 years of life.
- Six states of being have been identified for the newborn: quiet sleep, active sleep, drowsy, quiet alert, active alert, and crying.
- Gestational age can be determined by assessing six physical characteristics and six neuromuscular maturity characteristics.
- Infants are considered contaminated with blood-borne pathogens until after the first bath.
- Problems of the newborn include hyperbilirubinemia, respiratory distress, cleft lip/palate, hydrocephalus, spina bifida, Down syndrome, talipes equinovarus, and phenylketonuria.
- Infants need special care when the mother is a diabetic, HIV positive, or a substance abuser.

## REVIEW QUESTIONS

1. Which of the following is the result of a metabolic error in the newborn?
   1. Leukemia.
   2. Patent ductus arteriosus.
   3. Phenylketonuria.
   4. Pyloric stenosis.

2. A nurse working in the special care nursery admits a 35 4/7 newborn. Given the infants prematurity, the nurse would want to monitor for which of the following conditions?
   1. Hypothermia.
   2. Hyperthermia.
   3. Hyperglycemia.
   4. Tachycardia.

3. A nurse is teaching new parents safety positions for their new baby to sleep in. The nurse knows that the parents understand the teaching when they make which of following statements.
   1. "We will place our baby on her stomach to sleep."
   2. "We will place our baby on her back to sleep."
   3. "We will place our baby on her pillow to sleep."
   4. "We will place our baby under the covers to sleep."

4. A new mother calls the nurse and states, "My baby has been sleeping for the past 3 hours and does not want to wake up to feed, I am so worried" The mother has just given birth 5 hours ago. Which explanation by the nurse would be the most appropriate to put the new mother at ease?
   1. "I would be worried too. How about we wake the baby up together."
   2. "Let me go get a bottle warmed up and see what I can do."

3. "Do not worry; your baby is going through a sleep period. You should try to get some rest."
4. "I will call the pediatrician's office right away to see what they can do."

5. A newborn male is scheduled for a circumcision. Which of the following is essential for the nurse to teach the parents after the procedure is over?
   1. Apply Emla cream to the penis for pain relief.
   2. Give Tylenol every 4 to 6 hours round the clock.
   3. Apply A+D ointment and gauze to the penis with every diaper change for the first 24 hours.
   4. Withhold feedings for 4 hours after the procedure.

6. The nurse is aware that survival of a newborn infant depends primarily on:
   1. the infant's regulation of body temperature.
   2. prompt expansion of the lungs and the establishment of gaseous exchange.
   3. the infant's energy provided from materials obtained from the environment.
   4. the rise in the infant's arterial oxygen tension and a rapid fall in carbon dioxide tension.

7. When assisting the establishment of respirations in a newborn, which of these actions should the nurse do first?
   1. Tie the cord.
   2. Provide continuous oxygen.
   3. Use a resuscitation machine.
   4. Remove mucus from the mouth, throat, and nose.

8. The nurse dries a newborn infant as soon after birth as possible, primarily to help:
   1. stimulate the infant's circulatory system.
   2. avoid excess heat loss from the infant's body.
   3. remove organisms from the infant's skin acquired during birth.
   4. remove the amniotic fluid so the infant is not so slippery.

9. A new mother asks the nurse about the bluish area on her infant's buttocks. The nurse's response is based on knowledge that this discoloration:
   1. is called mongolian spots.
   2. may need to be removed surgically.
   3. is a birthmark that the infant will have for life.
   4. should be checked about twice a year for precancerous cells.

10. The nurse is aware that the most generally accepted theory of the cause of physiologic jaundice is that it results from:
    1. dehydration fever.
    2. congenital obliteration of the bile ducts.
    3. rapid destruction of excess red blood cells.
    4. antibodies caused by the Rh negative factor in the maternal blood.

# REFERENCES/SUGGESTED READINGS

Alexander, G. & Allen, M. (1996). Conceptualization, measurement, and use of gestational age: I. clinical and public health practice. *Journal of Perinatology, 16*(1), 53.

Alexander, I., & Reuters, T. (2009). *PDR nurse's drug handbook 2010.* Montvale, NJ: Physicians' Desk Reference.

Allard-Hendren, R. (2000). Alcohol use and adolescent pregnancy. *MCN, 25*(3), 159–162.

American Academy of Pediatrics (AAP). Committee on Pediatrics and Committee on Genetics (1996). Newborn screening fact sheets. *Pediatrics, 98*(3), 473.

American Academy of Pediatrics (AAP). Work Group on Breastfeeding (1997). Breastfeeding and the use of human milk. *Pediatrics, 100*(6), 1035.

American Academy of Pediatrics. (1999). Task force on circumcision. Circumcision policy statement. *Pediatrics, 103*(3), 686–693.

American Academy of Pediatrics. (2004). Management of hyperbilirubinemia in the newborn infant 35 or more weeks of gestation. *Pediatrics , 114*, 297–316.

Ammann, A. (2009). Global stratagies for HIV prevention. Retrieved July 2, 2009, from http://www.globalstrategies.org/new_documents/resources/PMTCToverviewweb06.pdf.

Armentrout, D., & Huseby, V. (2003). Polycythemia in the newborn. *MCN, 28*(4), 234–240.

Ballard, J. Khoury, J. Wedig, K., Wang, L., Eilers-Walsman, B. & Lipp, R. (1991). New Ballard Score, expanded to include extremely premature infants. *Journal of Pediatrics, 19*(3), 417–423.

Behrman, R. Kliegman, R. & Jenson, H. (Eds.). (2007). *Nelson's textbook of pediatrics* (18th ed.). Philadelphia: W. B. Saunders.

Blackwell, W. (2009). In H. Herdman, Ed., *Nursing Diagnosis 2009–2011.* Iowa: Blackwell.

Blecher, M. (2001). Cutting to the point on circumcision. Retrieved from: http://www.webmd.com/content/article/3609.220.

Brazelton, T. & Nagent, J. (1995). *Neonatal behavioral assessment scale* (3rd ed.). London: Cambridge University Press.

Bulechek, G., Butcher, H., McCloskey, J., & Dochterman, J., eds. (2008). *Nursing Interventions Classification (NIC)* (5th ed.). St. Louis, MO: Mosby/Elsevier.

Burroughs, A., & Leifer, G. (2001). *Maternity nursing* (8th ed.). Philadelphia: W.B. Saunders.

Callister, L., & Vega, R. (1998). Giving birth: Guatemalan women's voices. *JOGNN, 27*(3), 289–295.

Choudhry, U. (1997). Traditional practices of women from India: Pregnancy, childbirth, and newborn care. *JOGNN, 26*(5), 533–539.

Clinical Rounds. (2002). Why circumcision helps protect against infection. *Nursing2002, 32*(10), 33–34.

Estes, M. (2010). *Health assessment & physical examination* (4th ed.). Clifton Park, NY: Delmar Cengage Learning.

Fanaroff, A., & Martin, R. (2005). *Neonatal-perinatal medicine: Diseases of the fetus and infant* (7th ed.). St. Louis, MO: Mosby–Year Book.

Gennaro, S., Kamwendo, L., Mbweza, E., & Kershbaumer, R. (1998). Childbearing in Malawi, Africa. *JOGNN, 27*(2), 191–196.

Hardelid, P., Cortina-Borja, M., Munro, A., Jones, H., Cleary, M., Champion, M., et al. (2008). The birth prevalence of PKU in populations of European, South Asian and Sub-Saharan African Ancestry. *Annals of Human Genetics, 72*, 65–71.

Healthy People 2010. (2009, July). Retrieved July 2, 2009, from http://www.healthypeople.gov/Document/HTML/Volume2/16MICH.htm#_Toc494699664.

Howard, J., & Berbiglia, V. (1997). Caring for childbearing Korean women. *JOGNN, 26*(6), 665–671.

Hutchinson, M., & Baqi-Aziz, M. (1994). Nursing care of the childbearing Muslim family. *JOGNN, 23*(9), 767–771.

Kaufman, M., Clark, J., & Castro, C. (2001). Neonatal circumcision: Benefits, risks, and family teaching. *MCN, 26*(4), 197–201.

Ladewig, P., Moberly, S., Olds, S., & London, M. (2005). *Contemporary maternal–newborn nursing care* (6th ed.). Menlo Park: CA: Addison-Wesley.

Lenhart, J. Lenhart, N. Reid, A., & Chong, B. (1997). Local anesthesia for circumcision: Which techniques are more effective? *Journal of the American Board of Family Practice, 10*(1), 13–19.

Letko, M. (1996). Understanding the Apgar score. *JOGNN, 25*(4), 299.

Littleton, L., & Engebretson, J. (2002). *Maternal, neonatal, and women's health nursing.* Clifton Park, NY: Delmar Cengage Learning.

Lowdermilk, D., & Perry, S. (2007). *Maternity and women's health care* (9th ed.). St. Louis, Missouri: Mosby Elsever.

Lund, C., Kuller, J., Lane, A., Lott, J., & Raines, D. (1999). Neonatal skin care: The scientific basis for practice. *JOGNN, 28*(3), 241–254.

Matsuura, T., Callister, L., & Schwartz, R. (2003). First-time mothers' views of breastfeeding support from nurses. *MCN, 28*(1), 10–15.

Mattson, S. (1995). Culturally sensitive perinatal care for Southeast Asians. *JOGNN, 24*(4), 335–341.

McCaffery, M. (2002). Circumcision: Is a local anesthetic appropriate? *Nursing2002, 32*(4), 24.

Merenstein, G., Adams, K., & Weisman, L. (2006). Infections in the neonate. In G. Merenstein & S. Gardner (Eds.), *Handbook of neonatal intensive care* (6th ed.). St. Louis, MO: Mosby–Year Book.

Moorhead, S., Johnson, M., Maas, M., & Swanson, E. (2007). *Nursing Outcomes Classification* (NOC) (4th ed.). St. Louis, MO: Elsevier-Health Sciences Division.

Murray, S., McKinney, E., & Gorrie, T. (2002). *Foundations of maternal–newborn nursing* (3rd ed.). Philadelphia: W. B. Saunders.

North American Nursing Diagnosis Association International. (2010). *NANDA-I nursing diagnoses: Definitions and classification 2009–2011.* Ames, IA: Wiley-Blackwell.

Pasero, C. (2001). Circumcision requires anesthesia and analgesia. *American Journal of Nursing, 101*(9), 22–23.

Penny-MacGillivray, T. (1996). A newborn's first bath: When. *JOGNN, 25*(6), 481.

Queenan, J. (2001). Positional plagiocephaly (flattened head). Retrieved from: http://kidshealth.org/parent/general/ sleep/positional_plagiocephaly.html.

Reifsnider, E., & Gill, S. (2000). Nutrition for the childbearing years. *JOGNN, 29*(1), 43–55.

Schneiderman, J. (1996). Postpartum nursing for Korean mothers. *MCN, 21*(3), 155–158.

Sharts-Hopko, N. (1995). Birth in the Japanese context. *JOGNN, 24*(4), 343–351.

Simpson, K., & Creehan, P. (2007). *AWHONN perinatal nursing* (3rd ed.). Philadelphia: Lippincott Williams & Wilkins.

Swayze, S. (1999). Clamping down on circumcision. *Nursing99, 29*(9), 73.

Task Force on Sudden Infant Death Syndrome. (2005). *Pediatrics, 116*(5), 1245–1255.

Thoyre, S. (2003). Technique for feeding preterm infants. *AJN, 103*(9), 69–73.

Tiedje, L., Schiffman, R., Omar, M., Wright, J., Buzzitta, C., McCann, A., & Metzger, S. (2002). An ecological approach to breastfeeding. *MCN, 27*(3), 154–161.

Varda, K., & Behnke, R. (2000). The effect of timing of initial bath on newborn's temperature. *JOGNN, 29*(1), 27–32.

Verma, R. (1995). Respiratory distress syndrome of the newborn infant. *Obstetric Gynecologic Survey, 50*(7), 542.

Workman, E. (2001). Guiding parents through the death of their infant. *JOGNN, 30*(6), 569–573.

York, R., Bhuttarowas, P., & Brown, L. (1999). The development of nursing in Thailand. *MCN, 24*(3), 145–150.

## RESOURCES

**Association of Women's Health, Obstetric and Neonatal Nurses AWHONN,** http://www.awhonn.org
**International Lactation Consultant Association (ILCA),** http://www.ilca.org

**LaLeche League International,** http://www.llli.org
**Women, Infants, and Children (WIC),** http://www.fns.usda.gov/wic

# UNIT 2 | Nursing Care of the Client: Childrearing

# CHAPTER 6
## Basics of Pediatric Care

## MAKING THE CONNECTION

*Refer to the following chapters to increase your understanding of pediatric care:*

*Maternal & Pediatric Nursing*
- *Infants with Special Needs: Birth to 12 Months*
- *Common Problems: 1 to 18 Years*

## LEARNING OBJECTIVES

Upon completion of this chapter, you should be able to:
- Define key terms.
- Discuss the role of the nurse in preparing a child and family for hospitalization.
- Explain the role of the nurse in admission and discharge of the pediatric client.
- Prepare children at different developmental stages for procedures.
- Discuss various methods for assessing basic needs and planning daily care.
- Safely perform supportive pediatric procedures.
- Identify the child's concept of death at various developmental stages.
- Describe common responses (child, family, siblings, nurses) to a dying child.
- Discuss sources of support for the dying child.

## KEY TERMS

assent
child life specialist

emancipated minor
family-centered care

rooming-in

# INTRODUCTION

Nursing care of children centers on promoting, maintaining, and restoring the health of the child and family. While families are very important to all clients in the health-care area, caregivers are essential to the care and nurturing of the pediatric client. For this reason, when providing care to children, inclusion of the family is essential. **Family-centered care** recognizes the family as the constant in a child's life. Family-centered care describes a philosophy of care recognizing the centrality of the family in the child's life and including the family's contribution and involvement in the plan of care and its delivery. An additional factor that impacts the health care of children is their rapidly evolving growth and development.

Children differ from adults in their physical, emotional, and cognitive responses. Physical, emotional, and cognitive immaturity affects the child's response to comprehension of and reaction to illness or injury. For that reason, a child's developmental level always is assessed and care plans based on that level. Nursing care of children covers the neonatal period (birth to 28 days), infancy (1 month to 1 year), toddlerhood (12 months to 3 years), preschool age (3 to 6 years), school age (6 to 10 years), preadolescence (10 to 12 years), and adolescence (13 to 20 years). For more detailed information on physical, emotional, cognitive, and moral development, refer to the lifespan development chapter.

Trends in health care, leading to shorter hospital stays, provision of care in the home, outpatient surgery, and managed care, have changed the settings in which children and their caregivers receive care. These settings include the home, school-based and outpatient clinics, 24-hour observation and outpatient surgery areas, emergency rooms, rehabilitative care, hospitals, and intensive care units. Nurses must be able to rapidly assess, plan, implement, and evaluate care in these diverse settings.

Although any illness of a child is a major stressor for a family, it can also result in a positive experience. Nurses can maximize the client/family/nurse contact by fostering parent–child relationships, providing educational opportunities, promoting self-mastery, and providing socialization.

This chapter discusses preparing the child and family for hospitalization, pediatric procedures, and dealing with the dying child.

# PREPARING THE CHILD AND FAMILY FOR HOSPITALIZATION

Foremost in the preparation of children for hospitalization on any unit is preparing the family. If the family is well informed about and understands the child's illness, confidence in their medical recommendations, and the support of understanding nurses, then they are more likely to be able to assist in preparing the child for the hospital experience. Hospitalization may be planned or unexpected. When the hospitalization is planned, the caregivers and child have time to prepare for the event. Many hospitals and agencies concerned with the care of the young child provide age-appropriate materials to assist caregivers and children to prepare for the experience of hospitalization. These materials include tours of the hospital with dress-up in surgical attire and playing with equipment, photographs and videotapes, health fairs to explain procedures, and books and films to explain in age-appropriate terms of what to expect. Adolescents require different approaches in preparation for hospitalization; they not only learn from written materials, models, and films but also benefit from peers who have experienced the same procedures. Allowing them to ask questions of health-care workers without their caregivers being present is also beneficial.

When hospitalization is unexpected, it is of utmost importance that children be given opportunities to explore their new surroundings and encouraged to view hospitalization as an adventure that they can handle. The nurse treats all children and their caregivers with respect, listening attentively, with an open-mind, in a nonjudgmental way.

Many hospitals have **child life specialists**, who are health-care professionals with extensive knowledge of psychology and early childhood development, trained to prepare the child and caregivers for hospitalization, surgery, and procedures. Their goals include maintaining normalcy, minimizing psychological trauma, and promoting optimal development of the child and family. A collaborative effort between the nurse, the child life specialist, and other health-care providers ensures the best possible hospital experience for the child and family.

Many hospitals provide various educational programs such as an open house for well children and preadmission orientation. These programs are designed to orient the child and family to the environment and procedures and may incorporate such learning activities as audiovisuals, art, puppets, tours, and role-play.

The preparation of the child and family should be guided by consideration of the child's developmental level. Caregivers of infants and toddlers must be reassured of their important role as primary care providers, even during hospitalization (Figure 6-1). Caregivers are encouraged to make the necessary arrangements that will allow them to room-in with the hospitalized child. **Rooming-in** is the practice of staying with a hospitalized client (child) 24 hours a day to provide care and comfort to that child. It may also be the method of choice when caregivers need to learn and practice specialized treatments that they will be performing at home for the child.

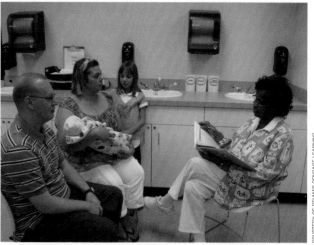

COURTESY OF DELMAR CENGAGE LEARNING

**FIGURE 6-1** The nurse helps prepare the caregivers for an infant's hospitalization.

## ADMISSION

In the past, most care provided to ill children was in the hospital setting. The current trend is to use community-based areas such as clinics, free-standing surgical units, schools, and the home. Children admitted to the hospital are more acutely ill, yet the time spent in the facility often is shorter. Nursing's role in the care of pediatric clients is changing and expanding. In planning care for children, prevention is a key component as well as teaching for the child and family. The nurse is frequently the first person who sees the child and family when they enter the health-care system. The nurse's ability to assess the child and family for physical, psychosocial, cultural, spiritual, and growth and developmental factors sets the stage for the plan of care.

The plan of care begins with admission to the health care facility. The completion of admission information includes previous data regarding the child and family as well as information regarding peers and play patterns, eating patterns, sleeping patterns, school history, normal activity patterns, fears, comfort measures, habits, primary language spoken, language development and level of understanding, usual reaction to pain, special routines, and perception of caregivers regarding prior or present hospitalizations. In addition, an assessment of basic needs and daily care planning information is obtained. Most healthcare facilities have policies and procedures for admission. Many institutions have a form for caregivers to complete regarding the child's routines, previous illnesses, current medications, and specific adaptations needed for the child and family. This form is usually signed by the parent and kept in the medical record. Although the

agency may have a set policy for admission, the routine may need to be altered based on the needs of the child and family. For example, a fearful child in pain may need to have pain medication and support before being interviewed. Always focus on the needs of the client and family in order to support and assist in mobilizing coping mechanisms rather than data gathering.

The initial assessment determines the need for immediate care. After the family and child are made comfortable or stabilized, a more thorough physical assessment and health history is obtained. The standard data collected are history of the client, allergies, nutritional intake, sleep, elimination, psychosocial information, spiritual and cultural factors, and the initial physical assessment. Data collected at the time of admission are used to identify nursing diagnoses and to establish a plan of care; these are placed in the child's medical record. Figure 6-2 shows an example of a pediatric admission form.

Many agencies have standardized care plans based on the most common problems identified by the assessment. These care plans are also placed on the medical records and are the basis of care. In addition to standardized care plans, many agencies are developing clinical paths or care paths for specific disease states. These tools assist the health care providers in giving care based on protocols that result in more rapid recovery, prevention of complications, reduction of length of stay, and cost-containing care for the client and family.

## PROTECTION/SAFETY

Situations may arise during hospitalization that may jeopardize the safety and well-being of the child. Be ever mindful of who has custody of the child, and screen visitors if there are threats to the child's safety. Issues of custody, disputes among family members, and kidnapping of children are no longer remote problems for hospital personnel. Security measures have been put in place on pediatric units with visible identification of caregivers, approved visitors, and personnel. Many units utilize electronic surveillance for visitors and monitoring devices for hospitalized children.

Informed consent of the legal guardian is obtained at the time of admission for general treatment, including procedures such as IV insertions, specimen collection, and medication and oxygen administration. Separate informed consents of the legal guardian must be obtained for procedures such as lumbar punctures, chest tube insertion, and bone marrow aspirations. Federal guidelines state that children older than 7 years of age have the right to give **assent** (the child's voluntary agreement to participate in a research project or to accept treatment) for treatment and research procedures. In most states, clients older than 18 years of age can legally give informed consent. In addition, most states allow some exceptions for parental consent in cases involving emancipated minors. An **emancipated minor** is a child who has the legal competency of an adult because of circumstances involving marriage, divorce, parenting a child, living independently without caregivers, or enlistment in the armed services.

Choking and falls are also areas of concern with hospitalized children. To avoid choking, the environment must be free of objects that could be placed in the mouth and possibly occlude the airway (e.g., broken balloons, syringe caps, toys, food). An adult should always be present when a young child

**ADMISSION FORM PART 1 OF 2**
**PARENT / PATIENT INFORMATION**

Dear Parent,
We want to work with you to individually plan the care which your child will receive. You can help us by completing this form. The information will help us learn about your child's illness or condition and about his/her general health. If you have any questions or if you do not want to answer any or all of the questions, please return the form to the nurse. Your nurse will review your answers and together we will develop a plan for your child's care.
Thank you for your cooperation.

The DCH Nursing Staff

Primary language _____ Interpreter _____

**GENERAL INFORMATION**

Where will you be staying during your child's hospitalization? _____ RELATIONSHIP: _____
Whom should we call in case of emergency, NAME: _____ Phone, days _____
in case you are not available: Phone, days _____ Phone, nights _____
What do you expect to happen during this hospitalization? _____
What childhood disease has your child had? ☐ measles; ☐ chicken pox; ☐ mumps; ☐ rubella;
Has your child been exposed to any of these within the past two weeks? ☐ Yes ☐ No
Do you have child's Immunization card? ☐ Yes ☐ No
Are your child's Immunizations current? ☐ Yes ☐ No   Check those which your child has had.
DPT ☐ 2 mo. ☐ 4 mo. ☐ 6 mo. ☐ 15 mo. ☐ 4-6 yrs.   OPV ☐ 2 mo. ☐ 4 mo. ☐ 15-18 mo. ☐ 4-6 yrs
HIB ☐ 2 mo. ☐ 4 mo. ☐ 6 mo. ☐ 12-15 mo.   MMR ☐ 15 mo. ☐ 11-12 yrs
Td ☐ 14-16 yrs.   Hepatitis ☐ Birth ☐ 1-2 mo. ☐ 6-18 mo.
What is your child's grade in school? _____ TB Skin Test _____ Boosters _____
(Patient only) Do you...smoke? ☐ No ☐ Yes _____ use alcohol? ☐ No ☐ Yes _____
Previous hospitalization _____
Where? _____ Why? _____

**DISCHARGE PLANNING INFORMATION**

Parent/Guardian: present ☐ Not available ☐ Telephone interview ☐
Have you been receiving help from any agencies? ☐ Yes ☐ No
☐ Home Health ☐ Visiting Nurse ☐ WIC ☐ AFDC ☐ CIDCS ☐ Early Childhood Intervention
If you need help with your child at home, who can assist you? _____
Does your child require any special equipment or supplies in his/her daily home care? ☐ Yes ☐ No
(apnea monitor, oxygen, suction, etc...)
What information do you need regarding your child's illness and/or hospitalization? _____

**IF YOU NEED HELP ARRANGING FOR POSTHOSPITAL SERVICES INFORM YOUR PHYSICIAN OR NURSE THAT YOU WOULD LIKE TO TALK TO A PROFESSIONAL STAFF MEMBER WHO HANDLES DISCHARGE PLANNING.**

**MEDICATION HISTORY**

In this section, please list for each medication your child takes, the dose, how often taken, the time of the last dose, and you/your child's understanding of the reason the drug has been prescribed. If there are problems taking the drug, please describe those also. While your child is in the hospital, ALL medications will be provided. If you have brought medications with you, please do not leave them. Please take them home. Thank you.

| Medication | Dose | Frequency | Last Taken | Purpose/Problems Taking |
|---|---|---|---|---|
| | | | | |
| | | | | |
| | | | | |

Allergies: Not known ☐ Medications _____ Foods _____ Other: _____

DRISCOLL CHILDREN'S HOSPITAL
CHILDREN'S MEDICAL CENTER OF SOUTH TEXAS

**ADMISSION ASSESSMENT**

---

For the following questions, please check your answer – yes or no – and use the space provided to describe or provide more information.

**NUTRITIONAL METABOLIC**

YES NO
☐ ☐ Use a pacifier, bottle, cup, special nipple, feeding tube? _____
☐ ☐ Type of diet? _____
☐ ☐ Take formula? Type _____ Amount? _____ How often? _____
☐ ☐ Has your child had any recent weight change? Loss _____ Gain _____
☐ ☐ Any changes in appetite or thirst? _____
☐ ☐ Any difficulties with eating, or swallowing food? _____
☐ ☐ When did child last eat or drink? _____

**ELIMINATION**

☐ ☐ Is child potty trained? Special words _____
☐ ☐ Diapers? Type _____ Size _____
☐ ☐ Has your child experienced any changes or difficulties with urination? _____
☐ ☐ Does your child have a history of bed wetting? _____
☐ ☐ Does your child often have diarrhea or constipation? _____
☐ ☐ Are laxatives or other aids used for regularity? _____

**ACTIVITY EXERCISE**

☐ ☐ Does your child have preferred play activities? _____
☐ ☐ Does your child tire easily with play? _____
☐ ☐ Does your child have appliances or need assistance for walking or mobility? (walker, wheelchair) _____
Briefly describe your child's usual daily routine: _____

**COGNITIVE-PERCEPTUAL**

YES NO
☐ ☐ Does your child have any difficulty hearing? Use a hearing aid? _____
☐ ☐ Does your child have any difficulty seeing? When were the eyes last checked? _____ Type: _____ Wear glasses? _____
☐ ☐ Does your child sometimes have difficulty learning? _____
What is the easiest way for him/her to learn? (books, film watching, demonstrations) _____
What do you do special to comfort your child when having pain/discomfort? _____

**COPING-STRESS**

☐ Are there any recent changes in family life that may affect this hospitalization? _____
☐ How have your child/you and your family responded to these changes? _____
☐ Are there other children in family? _____ Ages. _____
☐ Do you have family or friends in the Corpus Christi area? _____
☐ Whom do you define as your family or support system? _____
☐ Being in the hospital is stressful for many people. Is there anything we can do to make it easier for you or for your child? _____

**ORIENTED TO**
☐ Phone; ☐ Bed; ☐ Call light/intercom; ☐ Parent bed/regulations (Recliners up by 8 a.m.) ☐ Patient Rights & Responsibilities
☐ Playroom; ☐ Mealtimes; ☐ Smoking policy; ☐ IV, VS routine, a.m. wts. ☐ Visitation Limits/hrs. ☐ Intake & Output Monitored
☐ Care of valuables; ☐ Side rails; ☐ TV; ☐ Isolation; ☐ ID Band ☐ Car seat for discharge ☐ Save diapers
☐ Bear Questionaires ☐ No electrical appliances
Oriented by: _____

Parent Signature: _____ Date: _____ Time: _____

(Continues)

FIGURE 6-2  Pediatric Admission Form  (Courtesy of Driscoll Children's Hospital, Corpus Christi, TX.)

ADMISSION FORM PART 2 OF 2

**TO BE COMPLETED BY ADMITTING NURSE.**       Attn. Physician/Time Notified _____ by _____
Arrival to RM _____ Date _____ Time _____ Resident _____ by _____
Brief History _____

**GENERAL APPEARANCE:** _____
_____

**NEUROLOGICAL:** Responds to: ☐ Verbal ☐ Pain ☐ Nonresponsive
Gait: ☐ N/A ☐ Walks ☐ Unable to stand ☐ Uncoordinated   LOC: ☐ Lethargic ☐ Semi-Comatose   ☐ Comatose ☐ Alert
Movement: ☐ Coordinated ☐ Voluntary ☐ Involuntary; Speech _____ Head Circ _____
Anterior Fontanel _____
Seizures _____
Developmental level: _____

Pupil Scale: (mm)    1  2  3  4  5  6  7  8    · • ● ● ● ● ⬤ ⬤

**CARDIO VASCULAR:**                                          HR _____
Apical pulse: rhythm _____ Peripheral pulses:  RA _____ RL _____ LA _____ LL _____    BP _____
Clubbing: _____ Nailbed Color _____ Capillary Refill _____
Comments: _____
                                                              Temp. _____
**RESPIRATORY:**
Breath Sounds: ☐ Clear ☐ Crackles ☐ Wheezing ☐ Coarse ☐ Diminished _____ RR _____
Retractions: ☐ None ☐ Substernal ☐ Intercostal ☐ Subcostal _____ Chest Circ _____
Effort: ☐ Shallow ☐ Deep ☐ Labored ☐ Unlabored; Cough _____ Sputum _____
Chest Symmetry _____ Comments: _____

**GASTRO-INTESTINAL:**
Abdomen: ☐ Soft ☐ Tender ☐ Nontender ☐ Rigid ☐ Distended; Last B.M. _____   Wt _____
Bowel Sounds: ☐ Active ☐ Hyperactive ☐ Hypoactive; Appetite _____   Ht _____
Tubes: ☐ OG ☐ NG ☐ GT ☐ JT _____   Abd girth _____
Comments: _____
**GYNECOLOGICAL:** ☐ No abnormalities reported ☐ Sexually active; LMP _____
Discharge _____ Lesions _____ Comments: _____

**GENITOURINARY:** Urine color _____ Amt. _____ Odor _____ Discharge _____
Incontinent _____ Last void _____
Comments: _____
**MUSCULO-SKELETAL:**
☐ Moves all extremities ☐ Limited ROM; Swelling _____
Contractures _____ Edema _____ Prosthetic devices _____
Comments: _____
**INTEGUMENTARY:** (on figure in box, note location of any items with the appropriate letter and check the box by the letter)
☐ Skin intact ☐ Warm ☐ Cool ☐ Cold ☐ Moist ☐ Dry; Color: ☐ Pale ☐ Pink ☐ Jaundiced ☐ Cyanotic ☐ Mottled
Turgor _____ Masses/Size _____ IV site, condition, fluids _____
Wounds/Dressings _____
Comments: _____

☐ B - Bruise
☐ D - Decubitus
☐ L - Laceration
☐ R - Rash
☐ S - Scar

Nursing Process/Plan of care inititated _____ Nurse initials _____
**Allergies:** Not Known _____ Medications _____
                Foods _____ Environmental _____
R.N. _____ Date/Time _____

**FIGURE 6-2** *Continued*

is eating. Other safety concerns in the hospital setting include machinery (e.g., IV pumps and equipment, needles). Doors to treatment rooms, staircases, supply closets, and rooms containing extra equipment need to be equipped with locks preventing access by children.

Side rails on cribs must be up at all times. If a toddler is able to climb over the rails, a safety cover is placed over the crib, or a regular bed is used. Never turn your back to a child or reach for materials when the side rail is down if the child is not properly secured.

## PEDIATRIC CLIENTS EXPERIENCING SURGERY

The child and family experience with surgery may be an elective procedure, planned in advance, or the result of an emergency with little time for planning. When possible, pre-admission visits are an excellent way to prepare the child and family for surgery. Sessions are scheduled within the week

before admission. Table 6-1 contains suggestions for hospital preparation and surgery that are appropriate for planned procedures. As with any preparation, a multidisciplinary approach that includes caregivers, nursing staff, child life

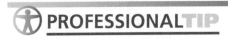
**PROFESSIONALTIP**

### ID Bands

It is very important for all clients to have a hospital identification (ID) band on at all times (Figure 6-3). It is equally important that all health-care providers check the band for proper client identification before performing any procedure. The nurse replaces an ID band on any child that does not have a band before performing treatments.

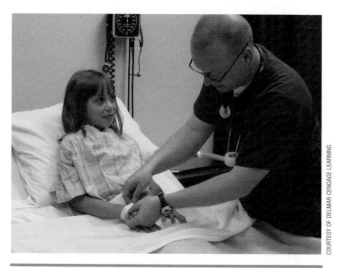

COURTESY OF DELMAR CENGAGE LEARNING

**FIGURE 6-3** All hospitalized children will have an ID band.

specialists, medical staff, and other involved professionals is best.

Preparation for surgery includes both psychosocial and physical preparation. The purpose of preoperative preparation is to reduce fear and anxiety associated with the surgical procedure and the surrounding environment. Play can facilitate preparation for hospitalization. Visits to units before the experience can familiarize the child and family with sights, sounds, smells, and equipment. Anatomically correct dolls and puppets, drawings, and models can be used to teach the child and family about the procedures. Through play, the child experiences the use of equipment to take vital signs and become familiar with other health-care interventions.

The nurse reassures the child that she will be transported to the operating room accompanied by caregivers and that her caregivers will be there when she wakes up. Inform caregivers of the expected length of the surgery and inform them of the child's status throughout the procedure. The child and caregivers feel more secure if one nurse is designated to be the contact before, during, and after surgery.

Many hospitals and surgical units allow and encourage caregivers to be present during anesthesia induction. The presence of caregivers and familiar objects such as blankets and toys in the presurgical area decreases the child's and caregivers' anxiety. Decreased anxiety lessens the need for premedication for the child. Some common induction techniques for young children include concealing the breathing circuit in a play phone, behind a pacifier, or within a stuffed animal, and providing a choice of flavored gases (e.g., watermelon, grape, chocolate).

**TABLE 6-1 Nursing Responsibilities to the Child Having Surgery**

| PREPARATION FOR SURGERY | AGE CONSIDERATIONS |
|---|---|
| **Psychological** | |
| Explain surgery. | *Infant:* Allow infant to remain on caregiver's lap as long as possible. |
| Prepare for separation from family. | *Toddler:* Use dolls, puppets, play hospital. |
| Conduct preadmission visit. | *Preschooler:* Use books, videos, art. Assure toddlers and preschoolers that the surgery is not their fault and is not a punishment. |
| | *School-age Child:* Offer brief explanations with supporting visuals. |
| | *Adolescent:* Involve in the procedure planning and decision making. |
| **Physical** | |
| Discontinue food and drink after specified time. | *Infant:* Explain to caregivers only. |
| Monitor fluid level (child has less fluid within body and can become dehydrated quickly). | *Toddler:* Explain 3 days in advance. |
| Perform specific preparation for procedure. | *Preschooler:* Prepare formally no more than 1 week in advance. |
| Ensure that consent form is signed by guardian. | *School-age Child:* Videos and tours. |
| Administer preoperative medication. | *Adolescent:* Provide detailed information and encourage questioning. |
| **Postoperative Care** | |
| Make preparations for return of child. | *Infant:* Maintain body warmth. Monitor intake and output. |
| Obtain vital signs. | *Toddler and Preschooler:* Give favorite animal or try to provide comfort. |
| Assess pain level. | *School-age Child:* Ask about comfort and preferred distraction activities. |
| Inspect operative site. | |
| Check dressings for bleeding or other drainage. | *All children:* Presence of caregivers on return to postoperative area and in child's room is important. Know the manifestations of pain and medicate as needed. |
| Check bowel and bladder function. | |
| Observe for signs of shock, dehydration, infection. | *Adolescent:* Provide privacy |

COURTESY OF DELMAR CENGAGE LEARNING

During the postoperative period, the child is monitored for bleeding, pain level, and pulmonary and circulatory status. When the child awakens, it is important that the caregivers be present to calm and comfort the child. Comfort objects from home such as favorite toys may assist the child in feeling at ease. Use pain medication as necessary. Most health-care facilities have instructions to follow for general and specific surgical procedures.

The child may be discharged home or admitted to an inpatient unit for further care. Because children recuperate more quickly in a familiar environment, they are discharged as soon as is safely possible following surgery. Discharge planning ideally is initiated at admission. The ability of the caregivers to provide adequate care at home determines the extent of education provided before discharge and the involvement of a home health agency after discharge.

## DISCHARGE/DISCHARGE PLANNING

Use a multidisciplinary approach that includes the social service department, home care agencies, rehabilitation therapists, and the family to plan for equipment, procedures, and other home care needs. Discharge plans begin with admission of the child. Many agencies have a discharge planning nurse who coordinates the plans for home care. The nurse working with the client and family takes part in the planning and communicates frequently with the discharge nurse regarding information about the client and family.

Make the caregivers aware that behavioral changes often occur after hospitalization. These changes are most evident in children 6 months to 6 years of age. The changes may include fear or anxiety about sleeping and separation, regression, withdrawal, aggression, and demanding behavior.

Assessment of the family's ability to manage the child's care and the ability of the home environment to support the care needed by the child is important. Early planning gives the health-care providers and family time to investigate financial support by agencies such as Medicaid and private insurance. If the child is school-aged, involve the school district to plan for continued education. This may require special assessment by the school system and a plan of educational care developed to include home tutors, specialized services such as speech therapists and occupational therapists, and/or transportation to school with specialized medical care delivered at the school.

Caregivers may need to learn special or rehabilitative procedures for the child's care. Demonstrate, explain, and observe as the caregivers assume the care they will be responsible for at home. The education provided and the caregivers' ability to perform care are discussed with the public health nurse, home health nurse, or individual who will be managing the home care program. Assist caregivers in exploring options for relief from the child's care, such as respite care, relatives, church groups, or lists of caregivers with ability to give specialized care.

The family is the most important advocate and spokesperson for the child. When a child needs long-term care, the family will need the services of many agencies and numerous health-care personnel. To coordinate health care and to prevent gaps and overlaps, one person is identified as the case manager. The parent may decide to act as the child's case manager with support and education from discharge planners.

Discharge documentation includes the condition and behavior at discharge, instructions given to caretaker, the mode of transportation, time of discharge, and who accompanied the child.

## PEDIATRIC PROCEDURES

In preparing the child and family for procedures performed either at home or in an agency, consider the child's growth and development, cognitive abilities, and physical and psychosocial factors. The nurse performs the procedures effectively and efficiently with the least amount of discomfort to the client and family. The following procedures are common to the care of children. While they are similar to procedures performed on adults, they also may differ in several ways. Be knowledgeable about variations in preparation, equipment, positioning, and specific steps when performing procedures on children.

### PHYSICAL ASSESSMENT

Physical assessments for the child are similar to those for the adult with a few differences. Measurements of physical size are significant in evaluating a child's health status. Deviation from the established norms may indicate a significant health problem.

### Growth Measurements

Growth measurements for children are recorded at each well-child visit as well as visits for disease episodes. Take measurements correctly and accurately. Values for growth parameters are placed on percentile charts and evaluated with those of the general population. In general, percentiles from 5% to 95% are considered within normal ranges. All growth evaluations take into consideration a child's genetic predisposition. As well as genetic concerns, ethnic and socioeconomic background may influence growth norms. It is unknown whether the differences within the ethnic and socioeconomic backgrounds are from the cultural norms or the result of nutritional differences.

The growth charts most commonly used in the United States are those from the National Center for Health Statistics (NCHS) and are available for boys and girls of different ages. There are growth charts available for children 2 to 3 based on whether their height is measured in a lying or standing position. Lying position is referred to as recumbent, and height while standing is referred to as stature. Most children younger than age 2 are measured in a recumbent position, and children older than 2 are measured in a standing position.

**Children Younger Than Two Years of Age** Growth measurements for children younger than 2 differ in the procedure and types of measurements taken. Typical measurements taken for the child younger than 2 are length; weight; and head, chest, and abdominal circumferences.

*Length* Measurement of length is taken with the child in a supine position. The method for children younger than 2 is as follows:

1. Use a paper sheet to lay the infant in a recumbent (lying down) position. Extend the infant's body.
2. Ensure that the infant's head is in midline and legs are extended. Gently grasp knees and push toward table to fully extend legs (Figure 6-4).
3. Place a mark on the paper at the crown of the infant's head.
4. Extend the leg and place a mark on the paper at the base of the heel (toes pointing upward).
5. If a measuring board is used, place the infant's head against the board and extend the legs, placing the heels of the feet on the footboard.
6. Measure the distance between the two marks or on the measuring board.
7. Record the length.

*Weight* Infants are weighed on a platform scale. They may be placed in either a sitting or supine position, depending on their ability to sit unsupported. Before weighing the infant, make sure the scale is cleaned, a paper cover is placed on the

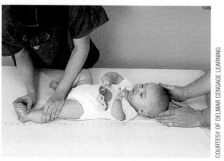

COURTESY OF DELMAR CENGAGE LEARNING

FIGURE 6-4 **Measuring Recumbent Length of an Infant**

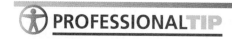

## PROFESSIONALTIP

### General Instructions for All Pediatric Procedures

**Preprocedure**
Check physician's orders.
Review procedure in agency procedure manual.
Gather equipment and assistance if necessary.
Introduce yourself and assistants to child and caregivers.
Identify child by name band or approved identification method.
Give instructions and explanation to the child and parent and ask if there are any questions.
If parent is going to hold child, demonstrate exactly what you want done. Make sure the parent feels secure about assisting with the procedure. Make sure you know the agency policy regarding caregivers assisting with procedures by holding the child.
Wash your hands.
Don protective clothing if necessary.

**During the Procedure**
Maintain privacy.
Tell the child exactly what is expected of her, never threaten or tell a child you will have to "hold him/her down."
Have someone assist you if necessary and if it will facilitate the procedure being completed more quickly.
Maintain a conversation with parent and child, explaining what you are doing, in a calm soothing voice.
Keep the child and parent informed of the procedure's progress.
Tell the child when the procedure is nearly complete.

**Support of Child and Family**
Offer ways of coping with pain or discomfort (imagery, music). Give permission to cry.
Use developmentally appropriate words.
Give child as much choice over the procedure as possible.

## PROFESSIONALTIP

### Growth

Growth is a continuous and uneven process, and the most important point for monitoring the growth of children is comparison over time.

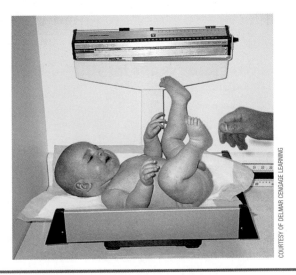

FIGURE 6-5   Measuring Weight of an Infant

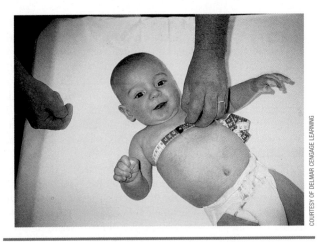

FIGURE 6-6   Measuring Chest Circumference of an Infant

scale, and the room is warm. The nurse balances the scale before weighing the infant. The method for weighing is as follows:

1. Place the nude child on the scale, making sure never to turn your back to the child on the scale. Hold your hand over the infant but do not touch the infant while obtaining the weight (Figure 6-5).
2. Measure to the nearest 10 grams or 2 ounces and record the weight.

**Head Circumference**   During the first year or two of life, head circumference is measured as an important indication of brain growth. The method for obtaining head circumference is as follows:

1. Measure the head at its greatest circumference.
2. Wrap a measuring tape around the infant's head, placing it above the brows, the pinna of the ears, and around the occipital prominence. Make sure the tape is flat against the skin.
3. Record the circumference.

**Chest Circumference**   The chest circumference is often measured during the first year of life as an indicator of adequate growth. During the first year, head circumference is greater than chest circumference; after age 1, chest circumference exceeds head circumference. The method for obtaining chest circumference is as follows:

1. Measure the chest at its greatest circumference.
2. Wrap a measuring tape around the infant's chest, placing it under the axilla and over the nipple line (Figure 6-6).
3. Measure between inspiration and expiration.
4. Record the circumference.

**Abdominal Circumference**   The abdominal circumference is obtained on very young or preterm infants to detect abdominal distention. The method for measuring abdominal circumference is as follows:

1. Measure the abdomen at its point of greatest girth.
2. Place a paper tape around the infant's abdomen at the umbilicus.
3. Record the circumference.

**Children Older Than Two Years of Age**   Typical measurements taken on children older than 2 years of age include height and weight.

**Height**   After the age of 2 or 3, height is measured with the child standing upright. Remove the child's shoes before the measurement is taken, and have the child stand upright, with the back to the wall or scale. Ask the child to stand very straight with head in midline and shoulders, buttocks, and heels touching the wall or the attachment to a balance scale. The method for measuring height is as follows:

1. On the balance scale, lower the ruler device until it touches the top of the child's head (Figure 6-7). Take the measurement.
2. If measuring the child against a wall, place a flat edge such as a ruler on top of the child's head. Make a mark on the wall; measure from the floor to the mark.
3. Record the height.

**Weight**   After a child can stand and balance well, weight is taken on a standing scale. Standing scales are digital or balance. Remove shoes for all children. Toddlers are weighed in their underclothes, older children are weighed in street clothes with heavy jackets removed. The method for weighing is as follows:

1. Keep the room warm and ensure privacy.
2. Balance the scale before asking the child to step on it.
3. Place child in center of scale and, with a balance scale, move the weights until the scale is balanced.
4. On digital scale, have child stand in center of scale and take reading.
5. Measure to the nearest 100 grams or 1/4 pound and record the weight.

▼ **SAFETY** ▼

**Paper Tape Measures**

Use care when placing paper tape measures. Place under the infant and wrap around carefully. Do not slide the tape around an infant because this may result in paper cuts on the baby.

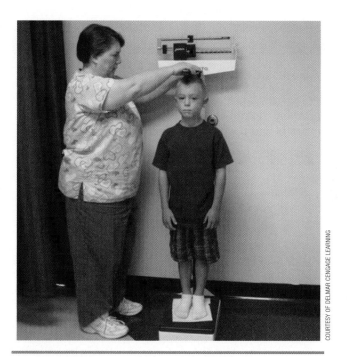

COURTESY OF DELMAR CENGAGE LEARNING

FIGURE 6-7 **Measuring Height of a Child**

## Vital Signs

Assessment of vital signs (temperature, pulse, respiratory rate, and blood pressure) is an important method for measuring and monitoring vital body functioning. In children, vital signs may change quickly and will provide the basis for decisions regarding care. Table 6-2 describes normal vital signs by age.

Body Temperature Temperature assessment is a simple, objective, inexpensive, and reliable indicator of illness and is part of the pediatric assessment. Currently, there are three types of thermometers utilized in pediatric agencies: electronic, digital, and tympanic membrane. The electronic and tympanic

membrane thermometers are the most common types utilized in acute care agencies. Another type of thermometer known as a thermograph (plastic strips or dots) is used for screening only. Each agency will have guidelines to follow in taking temperatures.

Four routes are utilized for obtaining temperatures: axillary, oral, rectal, and tympanic. Axillary temperatures are usually taken on newborns, preterm infants, and infants and children younger than 3 years of age. The thermometer is placed in the axilla and the child's arm pressed close to the body for a minimum of 5 minutes if it is a mercury device or until the electronic thermometer registers.

An oral temperature may be taken in most children 6 years of age or older, including adolescents; the procedure is the same as for adults.

Because of the risk of complications, rectal temperatures are taken only when no other route is available (Betz & Sowden, 2008). The child is positioned supine, prone, or side-lying, and a well-lubricated thermometer is inserted no more than a maximum of 2.5 cm for 3 to 5 minutes. Rectal temperatures are contraindicated on preterm infants, immunosuppressed children, and children with rectal surgery or gastrointestinal disorders (i.e., diarrhea and any bleeding disorder).

Tympanic temperature measurement is more quickly and easily obtained. The procedure appears to be less upsetting to children and is easy to learn by caregivers for home care. Tympanic temperatures and rectal temperatures appear to strongly correlate. Technique is very important in using the tympanic thermometer. Position of the thermometer enhances the accuracy of the reading. The ear canal must be straightened as when using an otoscope. With the ear tugged correctly and the probe tip pointing at the midpoint between the eyebrow and the sideburn on the opposite side of the face, more accurate temperature readings are obtained. Size of the probe also influences temperature. Using appropriately sized ear probes for children increases the accuracy of the reading.

TABLE 6-2 **Normal Vital Signs by Age**

| AGE | TEMPERATURE | PULSE RATE | RESPIRATORY RATE | BLOOD PRESSURE |
| --- | --- | --- | --- | --- |
| Newborn | 98.8–99°F | 100–170 | 30–50 | Systolic: 65–95<br>Diastolic: 30–60 |
| 6 months–1 year | 97.5–98.6°F | 80–130 | 20–40 | Systolic: 65–115<br>Diastolic: 42–80 |
| 3 years | 97.5–98.6°F | 80–120 | 20–30 | Systolic: 72–122<br>Diastolic: 46–84 |
| 6 years | 97.5–98.6°F | 70–115 | 16–22 | Systolic: 85–115<br>Diastolic: 48–64 |
| 10–14 years | 97.5–98.6°F | 60–110 | 14–20 | Systolic: 93–137<br>Diastolic: 46–71 |
| 14–19 years | 97.5–98.6°F | 60–100 | 12–20 | Systolic: 99–140<br>Diastolic: 51–80 |

COURTESY OF DELMAR CENGAGE LEARNING

### Measuring Temperature

Regardless of the type of thermometer used, the child's temperature should be measured at the same site and with the same type of device to maintain consistency and allow for reliable comparison and tracking of temperatures over time.

The method for taking a temperature is as follows:

1. Prepare the child and family for the procedure and assure them that little discomfort will arise from the procedure.
2. Select the appropriate method for obtaining the temperature measurement based on the child's age and condition.
3. Provide an explanation of the procedure to the child and family.
4. Assist the child into a position of comfort. The child may remain on the parent's lap if preferred.
5. Wash hands.
6. Don gloves and use Standard Precautions.
7. Obtain the child's temperature using method chosen.
8. Offer praise to the child for cooperating.
9. Document and report core temperatures of less than 36°C (96.8°F) or greater than 38.5°C (101.4°F) or specified parameters for individual child.
10. Reassess the child's temperature every one-half to 1 hour, or per instructions.
11. Document method of temperature assessment, measurement obtained, and any resulting action.

**Heart Rate or Pulse** For children younger than age 2 and those having irregular heart rhythms or congenital heart disease, apical pulse is the preferred site. Radial pulse is taken for children older than 3 years of age unless contraindicated. The method for taking a heart rate/pulse is as follows:

1. To count the pulse rate, place the stethoscope on the anterior chest at the fifth intercostal space in a mid-clavicular position (Figure 6-8).
2. Count the rate for 1 full minute.

3. Note whether the rhythm is regular or irregular.
4. Note whether the pulse is normal, bounding, or thready.
5. Compare the distal and proximal pulses for strength.
6. Pulse rates may be checked at sites other than the apex of the heart, for example, the carotid, brachial, radial, femoral, and dorsal pedis sites.
7. Record rate, quality, and rhythm.

**Respiratory Rate** The rate, depth, and ease of respiration are observed in the child. Respiratory rate will vary by age of the child. Therefore, the nurse counts the respiratory rate for 1 full minute because it is irregular. It is best if the child is unaware that respirations are being counted. The method for obtaining a respiratory rate is as follows:

1. Children's respirations are diaphragmatic, so observe abdominal movement to count respirations.
2. Count respirations before obtaining temperature or pulse rates (expect abdominal respirations to be irregular).
3. Count for 1 full minute.
4. Record rate, quality, and rhythm.

**Blood Pressure** Blood pressure measurement for the child is basically the same as for an adult. The size of the cuff is determined by the size of the child's arm or leg. To obtain an accurate blood pressure, the bladder of the cuff encircles 80% of the limb in which the BP is measured. If the bladder is too small, the pressure will be falsely high; if it is too large, the pressure will be falsely low. Blood pressure may be taken on the upper or lower extremities. General instructions for BP measurement are as follows:

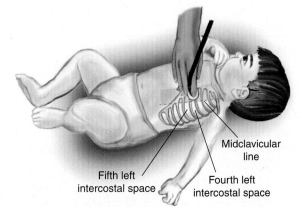

**FIGURE 6-8** Apical Pulse Position for Infant and Child

Midclavicular line

Fifth left intercostal space

Fourth left intercostal space

COURTESY OF DELMAR CENGAGE LEARNING

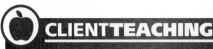

## CLIENTTEACHING
### Measuring Pulse Rate

Teach caregivers that have children taking medication, such as digoxin, how to take a pulse rate on their child before administering the drug. The nurse demonstrates the method of taking the pulse and observes the caregivers as they take the pulse on their child. Teach the caregivers the acceptable pulse range for their child as well as the method of obtaining the pulse.

*Electronic Monitoring:*

1. Place the cuff around the desired extremity.
2. Activate the equipment according to the manufacturer's recommendations.
3. Stabilize limb during inflation and deflation because movement sometimes interferes with the device's ability to measure the blood pressure accurately.
4. For some devices, the first reading is a priming reading and the second reading is considered the true blood pressure reading. Refer to manual.
5. Record the reading.

*Manual Cuff:*

1. Position limb at level of heart.
2. Rapidly inflate cuff to about 20 mm Hg above point at which radial pulse disappears.
3. Release cuff pressure at a rate of about 2 to 3 mm Hg per second during auscultation of artery.
4. Record systolic value as onset of a clear tapping sound.
5. Record diastolic pressure as disappearance of all sounds. Record systolic, diastolic pressures, limb used, position, cuff size, and method.

## DEVELOPMENTAL ASSESSMENT

Developmental assessment for the growing child is an important measure. A tool that is frequently used for the child younger than 6 years of age is the Denver Developmental Screening Test II (DDST-2). The test is composed of four sections: personal–social, fine motor-adaptive, language, and gross motor. Of the 125 items on the test, responses can be obtained by observing the child, asking the parent, and having the child perform a task.

Inform the parent that the DDST-2 is not an I.Q. (intelligence quotient) test but a helpful measure of the child's growth and development. The parent and child are made comfortable in the testing environment. Age-appropriate communication and approaches are directed toward the child (e.g., very young children may prefer to sit on parent's lap). The child is then evaluated on a series of tasks, and rated on each with a "P" for pass, "F" for refuse, and "NO" for no opportunity. A caution is given when the child fails to perform an item that has been achieved by 75% to 90% of children of the same age. A delay indicates the child's inability to perform a task that would be expected to be mastered by children in the developmental stage just before the child's current developmental stage. A suspect test is one with one or more delays and/or two or more cautions.

Current illness, lack of sleep, anxiety, chronic disability, or sensory deficits can affect a child's performance. If these factors can explain a child's failure to successfully complete the DDST-2, then the test may be readministered in 1 month, providing resolution of the problem has occurred. If a developmental delay exists, early detection can lead to intervention and possible resolution.

## CHILD SAFETY DEVICES

Restraints are rarely used in the pediatric unit. Some alternatives are having a person sit with the child, using diversion with the child, and using some behavior modification techniques. IVs, dressings, or other equipment is hidden from the child's view by taping a washcloth over an IV site or covering a dressing with a gown. If the child does not see the IV, dressing, or other equipment; he may forget about the item of interest.

The Joint Commission provides guidelines for the use of restraints that provide for the self-respect and safety of the client (The Joint Commission, 2009). The use of a restraint requires a physician's order stating the reason the restraint is needed and how long it will be left in place.

## SPECIMEN COLLECTION

Specimens are collected from children the same as adults with a few modifications. Children require more specific explanations and directions in an age-appropriate format. Explain any sensation that may be felt. Regardless of the type of specimen collected, the nurse follows Standard Precautions.

### Urine

A urine sample is obtained to assess for infection and to determine levels of blood, protein, glucose, acetone, bilirubin, drugs, hormones, metals, and electrolytes excreted by the kidneys. Urine also is assessed for concentration/specific gravity, pH, and other substances.

A collection bag is used to obtain a clean-catch urine sample from an infant and non-toilet-trained children. Intermittent catheterization is used when obtaining a specimen for culture to decrease the risk of contamination (Bekeris et al., 2008). Older children, after being given clear instructions, are usually capable of collecting their own urine. Usually, 5–10 mL of urine is adequate.

The method of obtaining a urine sample for the infant is as follows:

1. Remove the diaper and clean the skin around the meatus; allow to dry thoroughly.
2. Attach the bag with the adhesive tabs, for girls, around the labia, and for boys, around the scrotum (Figure 6-9).
3. Make sure the seal is tight to prevent leakage.
4. Check the bag frequently for urine.
5. To remove the bag, pull away gently from the skin using moistened cotton balls to assist in releasing the adhesive.
6. Pour into container and cap tightly.
7. Double bag the specimen and then send it to the lab immediately.
8. Document color, amount, clarity, and lab tests requested.

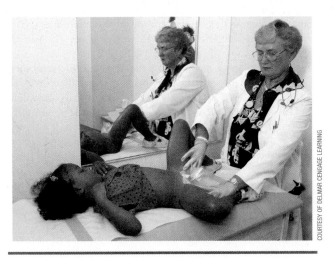

**FIGURE 6-9** Applying a Urine Collection Bag to a Child

A clean-catch sample for a male older child is collected in the following manner:

1. Instruct the older child to clean the head of his penis (after retracting the foreskin, if not circumcised) three times, each time using a different towelette, moving from the urethral meatus outward.
2. Have the child urinate into the toilet and, while urinating, collect urine in the sterile container. Have the child remove the container before stopping the flow of urine.
3. Proceed as above.

A clean-catch sample for a female older child is collected in the following manner:

1. Instruct the child to sit back on the toilet as far as possible with her legs apart. Have her spread her labia with her fingers and wipe each side with a separate towelette using a front-to-back stroke. Tell the child to use a third wipe to clean the meatus, repeating the front-to-back motion.
2. Have the child urinate into the toilet and, while urinating, collect urine in the sterile container. Have the child remove the container before stopping the flow of urine.
3. Proceed as above.

## Stool

Stool specimens are used in pediatric clients to check for the presence of fat, blood, bacteria, parasites, or reducing substances. If the stool specimen is needed from an infant or incontinent child, scrape it from the diaper and place in the appropriate container. If the child is potty-trained, use a bedpan or container to collect the specimen. Record the time the specimen is obtained, color, consistency, any odor, and disposition.

## Blood

Blood specimens are obtained from children by accessing veins of the hand or antecubital space, heelsticks, and femoral and jugular venipunctures. Collection of blood is very distressing to young children because of their lack of discrete body boundaries and the pain involved. The use of EMLA, a topical anesthetic cream, can reduce the discomfort of the needle penetrating the skin. EMLA contains lidocaine-prilocaine

5% and can be used to decrease pain associated with selected procedures: venipuncture, lumbar puncture, suture removal, immunizations, bone marrow aspiration, and removal of foreign bodies. EMLA is not approved for infants because of lack of testing and is not placed on skin that is broken. The cream is applied to the site liberally with an occlusive dressing and left in place 60 minutes before the procedure. The duration of the anesthesia is at least 2 and not more than 5 hours. Permission to use EMLA varies by institution; some may require a physician's order, and others allow the nurse to use it without an order. Children still may fear the needlestick; however, when the stick is not painful, they are more content. Venipunctures that are the same as those in adults are not covered in this section.

**Jugular Venipuncture** Jugular and femoral venipunctures are performed by a physician, with the nurse assisting and monitoring the child. The blood specimen is obtained from the large superficial external jugular vein. The nurse assists the physician by doing the following:

1. Place child in mummy restraint (possibly just hold child's arms).
2. Position child with head and shoulders extended over the edge of a table or small pillow with neck area hyperextended (Figure 6-10).
3. Take care that circulation and breathing during the procedure are not impaired.
4. Make sure that the nose and mouth are not covered by the restrainer's hand.
5. Document in the chart the amount of blood drawn, the site, condition of the site, and the type of dressing applied.

**Femoral Venipuncture** The nurse assists the physician by doing the following:

1. Place child in modified mummy restraint with legs exposed.
2. Position child's legs in a froglike position to provide extensive exposure of the groin area (Figure 6-11).
3. Restrain legs in frog position with hands while controlling the child's arm and body movements with downward and inward pressure of forearms.

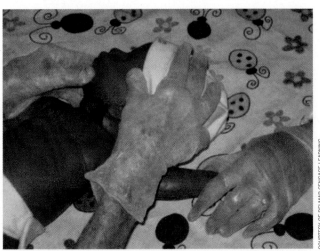

**FIGURE 6-10** Positioning for Jugular Venipuncture

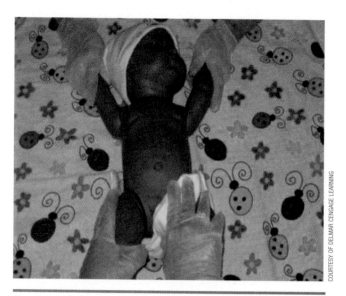

FIGURE 6-11  Positioning for Femoral Venipuncture

4. Cover genitalia to avoid contamination if the child urinates.
5. Document in chart amount of blood drawn, site, condition of the site, and type of dressing applied.

## Lumbar Puncture

Lumbar puncture (spinal tap) requires the infant or child to be held perfectly still. It is desirable to have an experienced staff member hold the child for the procedure. Lumbar puncture is performed as follows:

1. Place infant in sitting or side-lying position (neonates) with modified head extension to decrease respiratory distress during procedure.
2. Immobilize arms and legs with nurse's hands.
3. Observe child for difficulty in breathing.
4. Place child on side with back close to or extended over the edge of examining table, head flexed, and knees drawn up toward the chest.
5. Reach over the top of the child and place one arm behind child's neck and the other behind the knees (Figure 6-12).

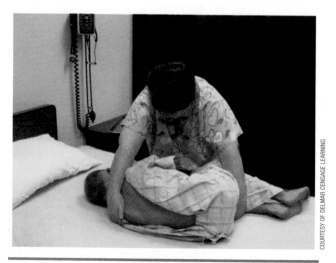

FIGURE 6-12  Positioning for Lumbar Puncture

6. Stabilize this position by clasping own hands in front of the child's abdomen.
7. Observe carefully for compromise in circulatory or respiratory systems. The restrainer's body should not cover the nose and mouth of the child.
8. Document number of attempts to obtain spinal fluid, number of cc's to lab, lab tests requested, color and consistency of spinal fluid, and response of child to procedure.

## INTAKE AND OUTPUT

Most children in acute care agencies will be on intake and output, which is critical for children with the following conditions:

- Anyone receiving IV fluids or TPN
- Major surgery
- Prematurity
- Renal disease or dysfunction
- Congestive heart failure
- Heart disease or anomalies
- Endocrine disorders
- Gastrointestinal disorders
- Shock
- Burns
- Taking medications such as digoxin (Lanoxin), furosemide (Lasix), or corticosteriods
- Neurological conditions

To measure output for infants, the nurse should:

1. Weigh the diaper before placing it on the infant and then again when wet. For each mg the diaper weighs, record 1 mL of urine. *Caution:* For those diapers that protect against wetness, the accuracy may be distorted because of the absorbent material embedded in the diaper.
2. A urine bag with adhesive may be placed on the child and the urine collected measured in this way. This is not usually done because of the irritation of the adhesive over time.

For toddlers and older children, measure urine and stool output in a bedpan or other container. All intake is measured and recorded on the intake and output sheet. If caregivers are present, instruct them to measure and record fluids taken in and those eliminated. Record all fluids from IVs and other sources. Measure drainage from stomas, colostomies, fistulas, and emesis and record.

## ADMINISTRATION OF MEDICATIONS

Administration of medications to infants and children presents a number of adaptations. The medication dosage is determined by the physician; however, the nurse observes the five rights of medication administration. Explain all procedures or treatments to the child and caregivers based on the child's developmental stage and the level of understanding of both parties. The nurse gives explanations truthfully, using nonthreatening words. All questions posed by the caregivers and child are answered before giving the medication.

## Approaches to Pediatric Clients

Children's reactions to medication administration are affected by developmental characteristics such as physical skills and

## Medication Administration in Children

Suggestions to facilitate successful medication administration in infants and children:

- Be honest with the child.
- Allow the child choices when possible.
- Provide distraction when appropriate.
- Praise the child for doing her best.
- Expect success; use a positive approach.
- Allow the child opportunity to express feelings.
- Involve the child in order to gain cooperation.
- Provide a developmentally appropriate explanation.
- Do not use basic foods such as milk to disguise medication.
- Spend some time with the child after administering the medication.

cognitive understanding, environmental influences, past experiences, cultural influences, parental responses, current relationship with the nurse, and perception of the present situation.

## Calculating Dosages for Children

Standardized doses of medication for children do not exist. The most common method of determining medication amounts is based on the child's weight. This method of determining the medication amount is more reliable because it allows for a more precise dose based on weight (see example in Professional Tip box). Medication doses also may be calculated by body surface area (BSA, mg/m²). The formula to calculate dosage using surface area is:

$$\text{Approximate dose} = \frac{\text{BSA of child (m}^2)}{1.7} \times \text{Adult dose}$$

## Oral Medications

The oral route of medication is the preferred method of administering medication to a child. Oral medications may come in liquids, pills, tablets, and caplets. Pediatric medications are frequently in a liquid suspension that tastes "good" and is colorful. Many medications have an unpleasant after-taste. Become aware of medications that are bitter or unpleasant and methods to decrease the unpleasant taste such as numbing the tongue before administration by giving a flavored ice popsicle or small ice cube. The method for administering oral medication to a child is as follows:

1. Select appropriate vehicle (e.g., calibrated cup, syringe, dropper, measuring spoon, nipple)
2. Prepare medication
3. Measure into appropriate vehicle

4. Avoid mixing medications with essential food items such as milk, formula, etc. (The child may later refuse the essential food item because of the association with medication.)
5. Administer the medication, employing safety precautions in identification and administration

Specific instructions for administering oral medications to infants are as follows:

1. Hold infant in semi-reclining position
2. Place syringe, measuring spoon, or dropper with medication in mouth well back on the tongue or to the side of the tongue
3. Administer slowly and wait for the child to swallow to reduce likelihood of choking or aspiration
4. Allow infant to suck medication placed in nipple

Specific instructions for administering oral medications to the older infant or toddler are as follows:

1. Explain in developmentally appropriate terms what you are going to do
2. Allow the child to sit on your lap or the parent's lap in a sitting or modified supine position
3. Use mild or partial restraint
4. Administer the medication slowly with a syringe or small medicine cup
5. Never force actively resistive children because of the danger of aspiration; postpone 20 to 30 minutes and offer medication again

Specific instructions for administering oral medications to a preschool child are as follows:

1. Use a straightforward approach
2. For a reluctant child, use the following:

   - Simple persuasion (e.g., "When you take your medicine, we can go to the playroom.")
   - Reinforcement, such as stickers or other rewards for compliance

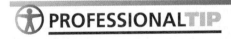

## PROFESSIONALTIP

### Dosage Calculations for Children

The recommended dose of ampicillin is 50–100 mg/kg/day in equally divided doses every 6 hours. For a child weighing 5 kg, the dose would be 250–500 mg divided by 4, or 63–125 mg every 6 hours.

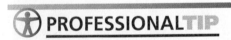

## PROFESSIONALTIP

### Resistant Child

If the nurse holds the small child on his/her lap with the child's right arm behind the nurse, and the left hand firmly grasped by the nurse's hand, the medication can be slowly poured into the mouth of a resisting child (Figure 6-13).

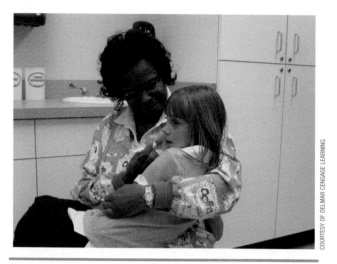

FIGURE 6-13 **Administering Oral Medication to a Child**

## CRITICAL THINKING

### Needle Threats

A child who has received multiple intramuscular injections has a real fear of the "needle." The caregivers threaten the child that if he does not do what they say, the nurse will come and give him a "needle." How would you approach the caregivers? What interventions would assist the child to lessen his fear and regain control?

## Intramuscular Injections

Intramuscular injections are used for pediatric clients but avoided when possible because of physical discomfort and psychological distress (Potts & Mandleco, 2007). Medications given by the intramuscular route include immunizations, antibiotics, and other drugs. Preparation of the child is important as injections can be painful and a source of stress to children (Carter-Templeton & McCoy, 2008). The task for nurses is to support the child while administering the medication quickly, safely, and with the least amount of pain and stress to the child. Pain perception is lessened with a distraction such as the child blowing bubbles or the skin being stroked around the injection site before and during the injection (Sparks, 2001).

## Otic Medications

Otic medication is used frequently in children who have ear infections. Because of pain associated with cold coming in contact with the tympanic membrane, warm all otic medications to room temperature before administering. The child should receive an age-appropriate explanation regarding what will be felt and heard and what can be done to help. Assistance in restraining a young child may be needed.

Position the child on the side with the affected ear up, and clean any discharge with a clean gauze pad. Brace the administering hand above the ear on the head. To instill the solution in a child younger than 3 years of age, pull the pinna of the ear back and down; for an older child, the pinna is pulled back and up. After instillation, the tragus of the ear is massaged to ensure the drops reach the tympanic membrane. If ordered, place cotton loosely into the ear canal to allow for drainage.

## Intravenous Medications

Children in acute care settings frequently receive intravenous (IV) medications. Children who have poor absorption as a result of dehydration, malabsorption syndromes, shock, and those in need of a high concentration of the drug quickly would receive IV fluids and medication. Children needing continuous pain relief benefit from IV medication administration. Advantages of IV medications are the immediate effect and the ability to control blood levels of the drugs used. Disadvantages are the same: side effects occur very quickly, and the drug may be very harmful to the veins. Once the drug is administered into the bloodstream, further control is limited.

All drugs given by IV route require a specified minimum dilution and specific rate of flow. It is difficult to control the IV flow rate in children by gravity. Children are at risk for fluid overload when IV rates are not controlled; therefore, all children receiving IV fluids or medications should receive those fluids through a volumetric infusion pump. IV medication may be delivered as a continuous infusion or intermittently. Syringe pumps are used in many agencies to deliver small amounts of medication.

Nursing care of the client receiving IV fluids and/or medication includes site assessment every hour for signs and symptoms of infiltration. Site assessment includes color of the site, tension of the skin, and skin temperature. When administering IV fluids and medications to the pediatric client, know the following:

- Type of fluid.
- Compatibility of medication and IV solutions.
- Recommended dilution of the drug.
- Recommended time frame for administration.
- Amount of flush needed.
- Any precautions to observe before administration (e.g., for aminophylline [Aminophyllin], take apical pulse before administering).
- Side effects of the drug.

## THE DYING CHILD

Care of the dying child presents one of the greatest challenges to nurses. It involves sensitive, gentle physical care and comfort measures for the child as well as continuing emotional support for the family and caregivers.

## CHILD

Children's understanding of death parallels their cognitive and psychosocial development. Preverbal infants and toddlers have no clear concept of death. Children between the ages of 3 and 5 may view death as a kind of sleep that is interchangeable with life. Because of their concrete thinking, school-age children begin developing the concept of death as final. Adolescents have a maturing understanding of death. In addition to their developmental level, children are greatly influenced by their life experiences and the attitudes of those around them.

Children can sense when they are seriously ill. They may realize they are dying because of the effects of disease and treatments on their body. The child usually experiences fear of death, of dying alone, and of pain. Nursing interventions include promoting socialization with family and peers, providing avenues for self-expression (i.e., drawings, fantasy play, storytelling), dealing directly with the child's questions, and allowing the death to occur in peace and with dignity.

## CAREGIVERS

When death is expected, the family begins a mourning process called anticipatory grieving. Manifestations of this process include denial, anger, and depression. It is important to acknowledge the caregivers' feelings, encourage expression, and guide them through the gradual process to reorganization. Spouses may need additional support when they are at different levels of grieving to prevent a sense of loneliness and isolation.

Explore options with the family concerning the child's care. The child and family have a right to request termination of treatment and to determine the care setting.

Caregivers who are caring for their dying child usually fear what the death will be like, not being present at the death, and pain the child will experience. The family needs to be encouraged to talk to the child about dying. Families need help to focus on the time that remains with the child. Openness and honesty allow the health-care providers and the family to provide effective care, to avoid misunderstandings, to see that the child and the family resolve problems, and to share their love.

## SIBLINGS

The nurse must recognize that each family member will handle the grief process in a different and personal way. Like their caregivers, siblings may experience anticipatory grief in the form of anger, denial, or fear. They may resent the attention given to the dying child. Siblings may fear that they caused their brother or sister to become ill or that the same thing will happen to them. They may need help in adapting to their caregivers' distraction, grief, and increased protectiveness. The death of a sibling can affect a child's ability to make and maintain friendships (Hinds, Schum, Baker, & Wolfe, 2005). Encourage caregivers to include siblings in the care of the dying child, in discussions about dying, and in the funeral. Like the dying child and the grieving caregivers, siblings need acknowledgment of their feelings and opportunities for expression.

## NURSE

Caring for the dying is usually a team effort, but often the nurse is the coordinator of the care. Working effectively with dying children and their families requires confidence, empathy, and competence in addition to attention to managing personal stress. Nurses who are comfortable with their own mortality can help make the remainder of the child's life more meaningful and the family's mourning experience more healing.

Nurses experience reactions to caring for dying children including denial, anger, depression, guilt, and ambivalent feelings. Nurses may even cry in the presence of the child and the family. Learning to care for the dying involves talking with other professionals, sharing concerns, comforting each other in stressful times, maintaining good general health, using distancing techniques, and focusing on the positive aspects of the caregiver role.

## SOURCES OF SUPPORT

Hospice care may be an option for the dying child. Hospice services provide palliative care for the dying to live life to the fullest without pain, with choices of dignity, and with family support including follow-up care after death. Self-help groups such as Compassionate Friends, an international organization for bereaved caregivers and siblings, are available in many communities.

---

### CASE STUDY

T.C., a 5-year-old client with an inoperable abdominal tumor, lives with her caregivers and a 7-year-old sister, M.C. The decision has been made to discontinue chemotherapy. T.C. has been involved in decisions about her care throughout her illness. When asked about her condition, she states, "I'm very sick and I'm not getting better." T.C. spends much of her time curled in a fetal position with her favorite toy, a tattered rag doll named Dolly. T.C. refuses physical exams and pills and gets little sleep because of her pain.

The following questions will guide your development of a nursing care plan for the case study.

1. List subjective and objective data a nurse would want to know about T.C. and her family.
2. List three nursing diagnoses and goals for T.C.
3. What would you expect a 5-year-old client to understand about death?
4. List affective nursing interventions for T.C. and her family?
5. List three successful outcomes for T.C. and her family.

## SUMMARY

- Even though hospitalization places great stress on children and their families, it can be a positive growth experience for the child.
- Teaching children and their families what to expect and explaining what is going to happen before, during, and after procedures helps reduce anxiety.

- Children's developmental stage and cognitive ability influence the preparation for treatments and procedures.
- Children must be protected from hazards that can cause harm to them.
- The child's stage of development, cognitive ability, and life experiences contribute to the child's understanding of death.

## REVIEW QUESTIONS

1. The major stressor of hospitalization for infants and young children is:
   1. pain.
   2. bodily injury.
   3. loss of control.
   4. separation anxiety.

2. Because of their stage of development, preschoolers may view hospitalization as:
   1. abuse.
   2. rejection.
   3. punishment.
   4. abandonment.

3. Before drawing blood on a 9-year-old client, the nurse tells the child:
   1. a Band-Aid will not be necessary.
   2. the procedure will not be painful.
   3. not to worry about the tight tourniquet.
   4. the body will produce more blood to replace what is being taken.

4. An appropriate method for administering oral medication to a small child is to mix it with:
   1. milk.
   2. food from the child's plate.
   3. a large amount of water.
   4. sweet-tasting food or syrup.

5. The physician orders Demerol 10 mg for pain after an infant has surgery. The stock medication is 50 mg/mL. The nurse would administer:
   1. 5.0 mL
   2. 0.5 mL
   3. 2.0 mL
   4. 0.2 mL

6. The nurse would expect the normal pulse range of a school age child to be:
   1. 70–115
   2. 90–120
   3. 60–110
   4. 80–130

7. When administering medications to children, what strategies does the nurse include to facilitate the process? (Select all that apply.)
   1. Give the child choices when possible.
   2. Do not use foods such as milk to disguise medications.
   3. Praise the child when possible.
   4. Do not let the child know that they are taking medication.
   5. Leave the medication with the parent to decrease anxiety.
   6. Explain medication procedure according to child's developmental stage.

8. Additional assessments done with the pediatric client that differ from an adult client include: (Select all that apply.)
   1. blood pressure.
   2. pulse.
   3. weight.
   4. head circumference.
   5. abdominal circumference.
   6. height.

9. The sibling of a terminally ill child may experience all of the following except:
   1. fear.
   2. anxiety.
   3. denial.
   4. acceptance.

10. The nurse understands that which of the following affects a child's ability to understand death: (Select all that apply.)
    1. developmental stage.
    2. cognitive ability.
    3. pain.
    4. life experiences.
    5. ability to express feelings.
    6. age-appropriate explanations.

# REFERENCES/SUGGESTED READINGS

Alam, M., Coulter, J., Pacheco, J., Correia, J., Ribeiro, M., Coelho, M., et al. (2005). Comparison of urine contamination rates using three different methods of collection: Clean-catch, cotton wool pad and urine bag. *Annals of Tropical Paediatrics, 25*(1), 29–34.

Allen, L. (2008). Dosage form design and development. *Clinical Therapeutics, 30*(11), 2102–2111.

Ball, J., & Bindler, R. (2000). *Pediatric nursing* (2nd ed.). Norwalk, CT: Appleton & Lange.

Ball, J., & Bindler, R. (2007). *Pediatric Nursing,* (4th ed.). Upper Saddle River, NJ: Pearson.

Bekeris, L., Jones, B., Walsh, M., & Wagar, E. (2008). Urine culture contamination: A college of American pathologists Q-probes study of 127 labora. *Archives of Pathology & Laboratory Medicine, 132*(6), 913–917.

Betz, C., & Sowden, L. (2008). *Mosby's Pediatric Nursing Reference* (6th ed.). St. Louis, MO: Mosby.

Carter-Templeton, H., & McCoy, T. (2008). Are we on the same page?: A comparison of intramuscular injection Explanations in Nursing Fundamental Texts. *MEDSURG Nursing, 17*(4), 237–240.

Cooper, L., Gooding, J., Gallagher, J., Sternesky, L., Ledsky, R., & Berns, S. (2007). Impact of a family-centered care initiative on NICU care, staff and families. *Journal of Perinatology, 27,* 32–37.

Eland, J., & Anderson, J. (1977). The experience of pain in children. In A. Jacox (Ed.), *Pain: A sourcebook for nurses and other health professionals.* Philadelphia: Lippincott Williams & Wilkins.

Estes, M. (2010). *Health assessment & physical examination* (4th ed.). Clifton Park, NY: Delmar Cengage Learning.

Gedaly-Duff, V., & Burns, C. (1992). Reducing children's pain-distress associated with injection using cold: A pilot study. *Journal of the American Academy of Nurse Practitioners, 4*(3), 95–99.

Hinds, P., Schum, L., Baker, J., & Wolfe, J. (2005). Key factors affecting dying children and their families. *Journal of Palliative Medicine, 8,* 70–78.

Hockenberry, M., & Wilson, D. (2008). *Wong's essentials of pediatric care* (8th ed.). St. Louis, MO: Mosby.

Hockenberry, M., Wilson, D., & Barrera, P. (2006). Implementing evidence-based nursing practice in a pediatric hospital. *Pediatric Nursing, 32*(4), 371–377.

Hughes, R., & Edgerton, E. (2005). First, do no harm: Reducing pediatric medication errors. *American Journal of Nursing, 105*(5), 79–92.

James, S., Ashwill, J., & Droske, S. (2002). *Nursing care of children: Principles and practice* (2nd ed.). Philadelphia: W. B. Saunders.

Johnston, A., Bullock, C., Graham, J., Reilly, M., Rocha, C., Hoopes, J., et al. (2006). Implementation and case-study results of potentially better practices for family-centered care: The family-centered care map. *Pediatrics, 118,* 108–114.

Jones, H., Kleber, C., Eckert, G., & Mahon, B. (2003). Comparison of rectal temperature measured by digital vs. mercury glass thermometer in infants under two months old. *Clinical Pediatrics, 42*(4), 357.

Kliegman, R., Jenson, H., & Behrman, R. (2000). *Nelson textbook of pediatrics* (16th ed.). Philadelphia: W. B. Saunders.

Leifer, G. (2006). *Introduction to maternity and pediatric nursing* (5th ed.). Philadelphia: W.B. Saunders.

Moldow, D., & Martinson, I. *Home care for seriously ill children: A manual for caregivers.* Children's Hospice International, 901 N. Washington Street, 7th Floor, Alexandria, VA 22314, (800) 24-CHILD.

Morgan, D. (2009). Caring for dying children: Assessing the needs of the pediatric palliative care nurse. *Pediatric Nursing, 35*(2), 86–90.

Newton, M. (2000). Family-centered care: Current realities in parent-participation. *Pediatric Nursing, 26*(2), 164–168.

North American Nursing Diagnosis Association International. (2010). *NANDA-I nursing diagnoses: Definitions and classification 2009–2011.* Ames, IA: Wiley-Blackwell.

Parson, A., & White, J. (2008). Learning from reflection on intramuscular injections. *Nursing Standard, 22*(17), 35–40.

Potts, N., & Mandleco, B. (2007). *Pediatric nursing: Caring for children and their families* (2nd ed.). Clifton Park, NY: Delmar Cengage Learning.

Timby, B., & Harrison, L. (2005). *Fundamental Skills and Concepts in Patient Care* (8th ed.). Philadelphia: Lippincott.

The Joint Commission. (2009). The Joint Commission 2009 requirements that support effective communication, cultural competence, and patient-centered care hospital accreditation program (HAP) (Standard PC.03.02.03, Standard PC.03.02.05, & Standard PC.03.02.07). Retrieved November 25, 2009 from http://www.jointcommission.org/NR/rdonlyres/B48B39E3-107D-495A-9032-24C3EBD96176/0/PDF32009HAPSupportingStds.pdf

# RESOURCES

**Association for the Care of Children's Health,**
http://www.acch.org

**Children's Hospice International,**
http://www.chionline.org

**Compassionate Friends, Inc.,**
http://www.compassionatefriends.org/index.html

**National Father's Network,**
http://www.fathersnetwork.org

**Sibling Support Project,**
http://www.chmc.org/departmt/sibsupp

# CHAPTER 7
## Infants with Special Needs: Birth to 12 Months

## MAKING THE CONNECTION

*Refer to the following chapters to increase your understanding of infants with special needs:*

*Maternal & Pediatric Nursing*
- *Basics of Pediatric Care*

## LEARNING OBJECTIVES

Upon completion of this chapter, you should be able to:
- Define key terms.
- Differentiate the most common respiratory conditions affecting infants.
- Describe nursing care for infants with circulatory conditions.
- Discuss nursing considerations for infants with digestive conditions.
- Explain the evaluative techniques used for infants suspected of having musculoskeletal alterations.
- Differentiate among the skin disorders most commonly seen in infants.
- Explain the causes and effects of nervous system disorders seen in infants.
- Describe nursing care for infants with genitourinary conditions.
- Outline teaching strategies for caregivers of infants with visual and hearing impairments and cognitive disorders.
- Implement nursing interventions for infants who have been abused.
- Describe teaching guidelines for families of infants who have unsafe environments.

## KEY TERMS

| | | |
|---|---|---|
| abduction | erythematous | milia |
| antipyretic | hypotonia | mongolian spots |
| atresia | intussusception | multifactorial inheritance |
| child abuse | jaundice | myelomeningocele |
| circumoral cyanosis | kernicterus | myringotomy |
| colic | lecithin | projectile vomiting |
| dislocation | meconium ileus | pruritus |
| dysplasia | meningitis | stridor |

# INTRODUCTION

The immaturity of all body systems leaves infants vulnerable to numerous illnesses and disorders. Most health problems during infancy are caused by respiratory and gastrointestinal infections or congenital anomalies. Although infants can become ill rapidly, they usually recover quickly. This chapter describes common conditions and illnesses affecting all systems of the infant, typical medical and surgical management, and nursing care of infants.

## RESPIRATORY SYSTEM

In the normal infant, breathing is quiet and shallow with variations in rate and rhythm. Respiratory movement is primarily abdominal. Respirations should be counted for 1 full minute while watching the rise and fall of the abdomen. The normal rate ranges from 30 to 50 breaths per minute. A persistent rate greater than 60 breaths per minute is an important sign of respiratory distress.

The child's respiratory tract is constantly changing and growing during the first 12 years of life. Differences between the respiratory tract of the adult and the infant contribute to the greater potential for obstruction, aspiration, infection, and airway resistance in the child (Table 7-1). In the infant, the most common respiratory disorders include otitis media, laryngotracheobronchitis, pneumonia, respiratory distress syndrome, cystic fibrosis, and sudden infant death syndrome.

## ■ OTITIS MEDIA

Otitis media, an inflammation of the middle ear, can occur unilaterally or bilaterally. The eustachian tubes, which allow for drainage from the middle ear to the nasopharynx, are shorter, wider, and more horizontal in infants than in adults (Figure 7-1). As a result, drainage is frequently impaired, resulting in retention of secretions and air in the middle ear. This positioning also facilitates

## TABLE 7-1 Respiratory Tract Characteristics in Infants

| FINDINGS IN CHILDREN | SIGNIFICANCE |
|---|---|
| Small nares, oral cavity, and nasopharynx; large tongue | Increases risk for obstruction |
| Obligatory nose breathers (<6 months) due to immature neurological function | Increases risk for obstruction |
| Rapid growth of lymph tissue | Increases risk for obstruction with infection |
| Larynx and glottis high in neck | Increases risk for aspiration |
| Large amount of soft tissues and loose, poorly anchored mucous membranes; long floppy epiglottis | Increases risk for obstruction with infection |
| Fewer functional airway muscles | Increases risk for aspiration |
| Immature cartilages that may collapse when neck is flexed | Increases risk for obstruction |
| Short neck resulting in structures being closer together | Increases risk for infection |
| Short, narrow airway | Increases risk for obstruction and aspiration; increases airway resistance/respiratory effort |
| Bifurcation of trachea at the third thoracic space | Increases risk for infection and aspiration |
| Immature intercostal muscles and cartilaginous ribs; primarily diaphragmatic breathers | Increases respiratory effort |
| Eustachian tube shorter, wider, and straighter | Increases risk for infection |

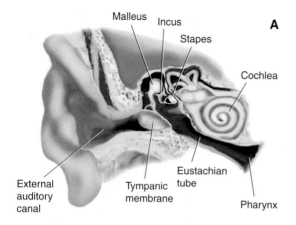

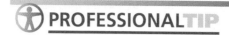

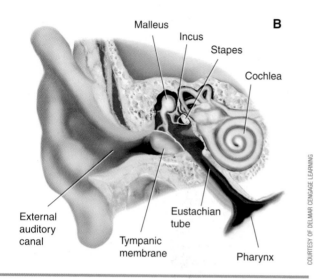

FIGURE 7-1 Eustachian Tubes; *A,* Infant; *B,* Adult

## PROFESSIONAL TIP

### Pertussis

*Incidence*

Bacterial infection of the respiratory tract

Caused by *Bordatella pertussis*

Transmitted through aerosolized droplets of respiratory secretions

5,000 to 7,000 cases reported each year

### Clinical Manifestations

Nasal congestion

Runny nose

Mild sore throat

Minimal or no fever

Mild dry, intermittent cough (initially)

Paroxysmal spasms of severe coughing, whooping

Posttussive vomiting

### Treatment

Erythromycin, clarithromycin, and azithromycin are the preferred antibiotics for infants ≥1 month

For infants <1 month, azithomycin is preferred.

### Nursing considerations

Vaccinate with diphtheria, tetanus, and acellular pertussis (DTaP) vaccine at ages 2, 4, 6, 15 to 18 months, and 4 to 6 years.

Protect children that are too young to have completed the primary vaccination series.

---

the movement of bacteria up the eustachian tube from the pharynx into the middle ear. An upper respiratory infection often precedes the development of otitis media in infants. *Streptococcus pneumoniae, Haemophilus influenzae,* and *Moxarella catarrhalis* are the most common causative agents of otitis media in infants (AAP 2004; Ramakrishnan et al., 2007).

The onset of signs and symptoms in otitis media is usually rapid and abrupt (AAP, 2004; Ramakrishnan et al., 2007). Infants with otitis media may be irritable, pull at the infected ear, or have diarrhea, vomiting, fever, and hearing loss. Upon inspection, the ear drum will be red, bulging, and nonmobile. Prolonged otitis media may result in sensorineural and/or conductive hearing loss, which is further discussed in the hearing impairment section of this chapter.

## MEDICAL–SURGICAL MANAGEMENT

### Medical

Medical treatment focuses on elimination of the infection and follow-up evaluation to determine the extent of hearing loss, if any.

### Surgical

If infections recur, **myringotomy** (surgical incision of the eardrum) may be performed and tympanoplasty tubes inserted to drain the fluid from the middle ear.

### Pharmacological

Treatment usually includes antibiotics, **antipyretics** (drug used to reduce an abnormally high temperature), and analgesics. Considerations when deciding which antibiotic to administer include compliance of caregivers in giving the medication, the child's willingness to take oral medications, and the pain involved with injections. The most common used antibiotic is amoxicillin (Amoxil) at 80 to 90 mg/kg/day for 10 days. Amoxicillin (Amoxil) is a safe, low-cost antibiotic, that when used in sufficient doses kills susceptible bacteria and has an acceptable taste to the child (AAP, 2004; Ramakrishnan et al., 2007). Another commonly used antibiotic is cefaclor (Ceclor), and newer antibiotics such as cefixime (Suprax) and loracarbef (Lorabid) also are used (Spratto & Woods, 2009). Another option for managing otitis media is observation without the use of antibiotics. This option is for select children based on their age (> 6 months), illness severity, and assurance of follow-up. This option involves treating the child only for pain and waiting 48 to 72 hours to reassess for improvement. If there is no improvement then antibiotic therapy is initiated (AAP, 2004; Spiro et al., 2006).

## NURSING MANAGEMENT

The primary nursing concerns are relieving fever and pain and teaching the caregivers about signs and symptoms, management, and prevention of otitis media. Acetaminophen (Tylenol) or ibuprofen (Motrin) may be used to reduce fever. In addition to analgesic administration, pain may be minimized by applying a heating pad on the low setting or an ice pack compress to the affected ear. Lying on the affected side will facilitate drainage, if the eardrum has ruptured or myringotomy has been performed. Providing liquids and soft foods may minimize pain caused by chewing.

Teach caregivers to have the infant examined at the first sign of a possible ear infection. Early possible signs of infection include hearing difficulties, pulling or rubbing of the ears, and irritability.

If antibiotics are prescribed, it is imperative that the child be given all of the medication. Failure to adhere to prescribed treatment may lead to the need for additional antibiotics, hearing loss, potential speech and language problems, and antibiotic resistance.

Prevention of otitis media involves ensuring proper positioning during feeding. Infants who are bottle-fed should be held with the head slightly elevated to prevent formula from draining into the middle ear through the wide eustachian tube. Breastfed infants receive immunoglobulin A contained in the breast milk. Immunizations are also preventive (Burns et al., 2008).

Providing a smoke-free environment is another important element of prevention. Inform parents of the relationship between environmental tobacco smoke and otitis media in young children. Passive smoking has been associated with an increase in blocked eustachian tubes, which can lead to nasopharyngeal congestion and upper respiratory infections (Burns et al., 2008).

## LARYNGOTRACHEOBRONCHITIS

Laryngotracheobronchitis (LTB), the most common type of croup, is a viral illness that causes swelling (narrowing) of the upper airway (Figure 7-2).

Initial symptoms include inspiratory **stridor** (a high-pitched, harsh sound), a "barking" cough, and hoarseness. The child may have a persistent, low-grade fever and a history of profuse nasal drainage with increased respiratory effort for several days.

## MEDICAL–SURGICAL MANAGEMENT
### Medical

Treatment is focused on maintaining a patent airway and improving respiratory effort by creating a highly humid, cool-mist environment.

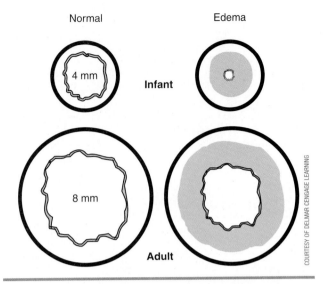

**FIGURE 7-2** Effect of edema on airway resistance in the infant versus the adult: Whereas 1 mm of circumferential edema (on right) can cause a 75% decrease in the cross-sectional area of an infant's airway, it only causes a 44% decrease in the adult's.

## Pharmacological

Use of medications such as bronchodilators, corticosteroids, and sedatives is controversial because of potential side effects. In severe cases caused by respiratory syncytial virus (RSV), ribavirin (Virazole), an aerosoled antiviral agent, may be used.

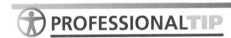

### PROFESSIONAL TIP

**Throat Procedures**

Procedures involving the throat (e.g., cultures and visual inspection) can cause laryngospasm and airway obstruction and should therefore be avoided when children present with symptoms such as inspiratory stridor, a barking cough, or hoarseness.

### COMMUNITY/HOME HEALTH CARE

**Managing LTB at Home**

- Observe for early signs of respiratory distress, such as stridor at rest; lower rib retractions; difficulty swallowing; absence of cough; agitation; respiration >50; flaring nares
- Maintain high humidity with cool-air vaporizer, 10 to 15 minutes in the bathroom with steam from a hot shower, cool air through a window
- Hydrate with cool, noncarbonated, nonacidic beverages of choice; ice pops; gelatin; small pieces of ice
- Provide rest by holding, rocking, soothing, and staying calm

# NURSING MANAGEMENT

Children with mild croup (no stridor at rest, mild retractions, no cyanosis, and restlessness only when disturbed) are managed at home. Teach caregivers how to monitor for signs of respiratory distress and ways to maintain high humidity and hydration. Instruct caregivers to not give the child red-colored drinks because it may be difficult to differentiate between the food coloring and blood in the client's vomit or stool.

Care for the hospitalized infant includes a mist hood or tent with oxygen and, if the child is refusing oral fluids or respirations are greater than 60 breaths per minute, intravenous (IV) therapy. Infants may be held with the mist blowing in the face if being in the tent causes distress. Caregivers should remain with the child and provide routine care throughout hospitalization in an effort to keep the infant calm, quiet, and in the tent. The presence of favorite toys and items from home can also be comforting to the infant. It is important to keep linens and clothes dry and the child in a comfortable position (usually semireclined in an infant seat placed under the tent). If oxygen is administered, the concentration delivered is regulated to maintain arterial saturation > 95% (according to pulse oximetry).

As with home care, monitoring for early signs of impending airway obstruction is paramount. Intubation equipment should be readily available at all times.

# PNEUMONIA

An inflammation of the bronchioles and alveolar spaces of the lungs, pneumonia is most commonly caused by RSV in infants. Pneumonia is often preceded by an upper respiratory infection. Viral infections render the infant more susceptible to secondary bacterial invasion. Pneumococcal pneumonia is the most common form of bacterial pneumonia found in infants.

Onset is usually abrupt, with rapidly increasing fever, flaring nostrils, **circumoral cyanosis** (bluish discoloration surrounding the mouth), chest retractions, pulse rate of 140 to 180 beats per minute, respiratory rate of 60 to 80 breaths per minute, and nonproductive cough. Chest x-rays and secretion cultures are used to confirm the diagnosis.

# MEDICAL–SURGICAL MANAGEMENT

## Medical

Treatment involves oxygen and cool-mist administration, chest physiotherapy, postural drainage, hydration, caregiver support, antipyretics, and antibiotics (if causative agent is bacterial) such as penicillin and macrolides (erythromycin, azithromycin, and clarithromycin) (Klugman & Lonks, 2005).

# NURSING MANAGEMENT

Assess lung sounds, monitor respiratory status, prevent further infection, and promote safety. Monitor hydration by accurate intake and output (I&O) measurement and assessment of skin turgor and anterior fontanel. Use a bulb syringe to suction the nose and nasopharynx as needed and before feeding. Saline nose drops may aid in clearing passages. Change the infant's position frequently to prevent both stasis of secretions in the lungs and secretion drainage into the eustachian tubes. Encourage caregivers to be active participants in their infant's routine daily care.

# RESPIRATORY DISTRESS SYNDROME

Preterm infants often have respiratory distress syndrome (RDS) because the lungs are deficient in surfactant, a substance that reduces surface tension inside the air sacs. The lungs collapse after each breath, greatly reducing the infant's supply of oxygen. This, in turn, damages the lung cells, contributing to the formation of hyaline membrane. This membrane blocks gas exchange in the alveoli. Infants born at 28 weeks' gestation or less are most at risk for developing respiratory distress syndrome (Hermansen & Lorah, 2007).

Clinical manifestations include tachypnea (70 to 120 breaths per minute in children), retractions, grunting, crackles, pallor, cyanosis, slow capillary refill, hypothermia, peripheral edema, flaccid muscle tone, gastrointestinal (GI) shutdown, jaundice, and acidosis. Chest radiographs confirm the diagnosis.

The first 96 hours are critical to the recovery of infants with RDS. Complications of RDS include complications of oxygen administration; intraventricular hemorrhage; bronchopulmonary dysplasia (BPD); and necrotizing enterocolitis.

# MEDICAL–SURGICAL MANAGEMENT

## Medical

Treatment includes administration of surfactant through the endotracheal tube immediately at or soon after birth. In addition, continuous positive airway pressure (CPAP) helps keep the lungs partially expanded until they begin producing surfactant (approximately 5 days).

## Health Promotion

Attempts may be made to prevent the occurrence of RDS. Surfactant may be administered to at-risk infants before the development of RDS. If preterm delivery is expected, **lecithin**, the major component of surfactant, may be measured to determine lung maturity. If insufficient lecithin is present, the mother may be given a glucocorticosteroid (betamethasone) that crosses the placenta and causes the infant's lungs to produce surfactant within 72 hours.

# NURSING MANAGEMENT

Closely monitor respirations, eliminate unnecessary physical stimulation and metabolic demands, and establish a positive relationship with the caregivers. Place the infant in a warmer under an oxygen hood or with mechanical ventilation.

# CYSTIC FIBROSIS

Cystic fibrosis (CF), a major dysfunction of all exocrine glands, primarily affects the lungs, pancreas, liver, and reproductive organs. Characteristics of this disease include increased viscosity of mucous gland secretions, elevated sweat electrolytes, increased organic and enzymatic constituents of saliva, and abnormalities in autonomic nervous system function. This disease is transmitted as an autosomal-recessive trait, meaning that both parents must be carriers (Table 7-2). Therefore, it is common that infants with CF also have siblings with CF.

Most children show evidence of the disease by 1 year of age. The earliest manifestation of CF is **meconium ileus** (impacted feces in the newborn, causing bowel obstruction).

**TABLE 7-2 Autosomal-Recessive Inheritance**

| | | MOTHER (CARRIER: HAS TRAIT) | |
|---|---|---|---|
| GAMETES | | A | a |
| Father (Carrier: Has Trait) | A | AA (no disease/trait) | Aa (has trait) |
| | a | Aa (has trait) | aa (has disease) |

COURTESY OF DELMAR CENGAGE LEARNING

**Intussusception** (telescoping of the bowel) may be another sign of the disorder. Rectal prolapse is a common problem resulting from difficulty passing the sticky, thick, fatty stools. These GI problems result from the lack of pancreatic enzymes. Most children have difficulty gaining and maintaining weight, despite a voracious appetite. Failure to thrive is common in these infants. Pulmonary complications, such as chronic moist, productive cough and frequent infections, are present in most children with CF due to their inability to clear mucoid secretions. Many children develop barrel chests and clubbed fingers because of the chronic lack of oxygen. Fertility is low in females and males are usually sterile (Burns et al., 2008).

Caregivers frequently report that their infants taste like salt when they kiss them. This common manifestation is a result of the elevated sweat electrolytes. Diagnosis is confirmed with the sweat chloride test. Results greater than 60 mEq/L of chloride are considered positive for CF (Burns et al., 2008).

Although CF is a life-threatening illness, families must be encouraged to focus on positive outcomes. The life expectancy continues to rise, and the search for improved treatments continues. In 2008, the median predicted age of survival for children affected with CF rose to 37.4 years, up from 32 in 2000.

## MEDICAL–SURGICAL MANAGEMENT

### Medical

Treatment focuses on managing pulmonary complications, ensuring adequate nutrition, and assisting the child and family in adapting to a chronic disorder. Chest physiotherapy (CPT, postural drainage) is usually performed one to three times per day to maintain patent airways.

## Pharmacological

Aerosol treatments and antibiotic therapy may be used as indicated. Commercially prepared pancreatic enzymes are given with meals and snacks to aid digestion and absorption of fats and proteins.

VX (a chemical derivative of existing lead compounds) is a new protein repair therapy that may interact directly with the cystic fibrosis transmembrane regulator (CFTR) protein, the product of the CF gene. It appears to repair the faulty protein, thereby curing the basic CF defect. Clinical studies of this new drug began in August 1998. Researchers are evaluating the safety and pharmacodynamics of oral doses of VX during phase 3 clinical trials starting in 2009 (Cystic Fibrosis Foundation, 2009).

### Diet

Well-balanced, high-caloric diets should be maintained because children with CF often absorb only 50% of ingested foods.

## NURSING MANAGEMENT

Monitor respiratory status, adventitious lung sounds, cough, stools, abdominal distension, and weight. Assess growth and development, hydration, and nutrition. Administer oxygen and medications as ordered. Encourage physical activity. Teach family skills needed to follow the prescribed therapeutic plan.

## NURSING PROCESS

### ASSESSMENT

#### Subjective Data

Assess the child and caregivers for indications of anxiety and fear. Interview the caregiver about activities or events leading up to the crisis, effects of illness on day-to-day functioning, previous hospitalizations, and knowledge about the condition.

#### Objective Data

Physical assessment focuses on respiratory status, growth and development, hydration, and nutrition. Observe for adventitious lung sounds, cough, finger clubbing, barrel chest, frequency and nature of stools, abdominal distension, weight loss, fatigue, and pallor. Routinely plot height and weight on a growth chart, and assess developmental level using the Denver II test.

**Nursing diagnoses for the infant with CF include the following:**

| NURSING DIAGNOSES | PLANNING/OUTCOMES | NURSING INTERVENTIONS |
|---|---|---|
| *Ineffective Airway Clearance* related to thick, tenacious secretions | The client will maintain a clear airway. | Initiate aerosol therapy, CPT, and breathing exercises as prescribed; schedule at least 1 hour before or after meals. |
| | | Administer oxygen as prescribed and monitor closely for level of consciousness. |
| | | Calculate and maintain required fluid intake. |
| | | Observe for signs of infection. |
| | | Assess respiratory status frequently. |
| | | Administer antibiotics as prescribed. |

**Nursing diagnoses for the infant with CF include the following: (Continued)**

| NURSING DIAGNOSES | PLANNING/OUTCOMES | NURSING INTERVENTIONS |
|---|---|---|
| *Delayed **G**rowth and Development* related to inability to digest nutrients and possible loss of appetite | The client will exhibit signs of adequate growth and development. | Ensure high-caloric intake. Administer prescribed pancreatic enzymes with meals and snacks. Offer small, frequent feedings if appetite poor. Monitor weight and height (plot on growth chart). Assess developmental level (e.g., with the Denver II test). Encourage physical activity limited only by the child's endurance. |
| *Fear (family)* related to long-term care and prognosis | The family will verbalize knowledge of disease and demonstrate proper techniques for care. The family will verbalize lessened fears and anxiety. The family will utilize available support systems and community resources. | Teach the family the importance of carrying out prescribed therapeutic plan. Teach the family skills for carrying out prescribed therapeutic plan. Provide numbers for CF Foundation and community resources. Encourage expression of feelings and concerns. Refer the family for genetic counseling. |

**Evaluation:** Evaluate each outcome to determine how it has been met by the client.

## ■ SUDDEN INFANT DEATH SYNDROME

Sudden infant death syndrome (SIDS), commonly called "crib death," is the sudden, unexpected death of an apparently healthy infant in whom the postmortem fails to reveal an adequate cause. It is the leading cause of death in infants older than 1 month of age, peaking between 2 and 30 months of age (AAP, 2005). Although numerous theories have been proposed regarding the cause of SIDS (including airway obstruction, abnormal cardiorespiratory control, and hyperactive airway reflexes), no single cause has been identified.

In 1994 the American Academy of Pediatrics (AAP) implemented the "Back to Sleep" campaign, recommending that infants be laid down for sleep in a supine position (AAP, 2005). Since then, the incidence of SIDS has dramatically decreased. Other modifiable risk factors to focus on are sleeping on a soft surface, maternal smoking, bed sharing, and overheating (AAP, 2005). Hersheberger (Dowshen, Hersheberger & Rutherford, 2001) states: "Parents need to know that SIDS is not caused by vomiting and choking or other minor illnesses. It is not caused by vaccines or other immunizations."

Typically, the infant is found huddled in the corner of a disheveled bed, with blankets over the head. Frothy, blood-tinged fluid fills the mouth and nose, and the infant may be lying face down in the secretions. The diaper is wet and full of stool. The hands may be clenched.

## NURSING MANAGEMENT

Provide empathic support to the family. Ask caregivers only factual questions, with no suggestion of responsibility. It is vital to reassure them that death caused by SIDS is not predictable or completely preventable. Inform the caregiver that an autopsy must be performed to confirm the diagnosis of SIDS. Encourage them to hold their child and say "good-bye." If the mother was breastfeeding, provide information about abrupt discontinuation of lactation. Refer to the SIDS Foundation.

Ideally, the family will receive a visit from a competent, qualified professional as soon after the death as possible. Areas needing to be discussed include expression of feelings, coping mechanisms, siblings' reactions, and birth of a subsequent child.

## CARDIOVASCULAR SYSTEM

Indications that the heart is functioning normally include warm skin, pink mucous membranes, easily palpated pulses, symmetrical chest, normal growth and development, and high activity tolerance. Upon auscultation of a healthy heart at the point of maximum intensity (PMI), two sounds (S1 ["lub"] and S2 ["dub"]) are heard. Heart sounds should be clear and distinct, regular and even. The rate should be the same as the radial pulse. In many children, a *sinus arrhythmia*, wherein the heart rate increases on inspiration and decreases on expiration, is considered normal.

During fetal life, the lungs are inactive and require only a small amount of blood to nourish their tissues. Blood is circulated through the umbilical arteries to the placenta, where waste products and carbon dioxide are exchanged for oxygen and nutrients. The blood is then returned to the fetus through the umbilical vein.

At birth, the umbilical cord is cut, and the infant's own independent system is established. The ductus arteriosus, the foramen ovale, and the ductus venosus are no longer needed. They normally close and atrophy during the first several weeks after birth. Figure 7-3 illustrates the circulatory patterns of the healthy prenatal and postnatal heart.

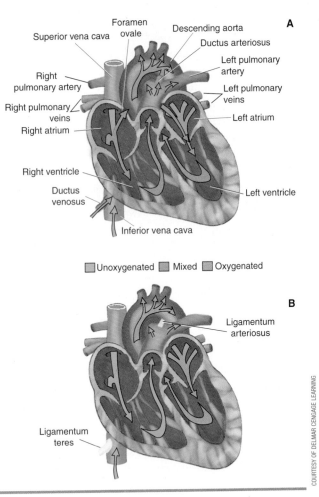

Unoxygenated ☐ Mixed ☐ Oxygenated

COURTESY OF DELMAR CENGAGE LEARNING

**FIGURE 7-3** Circulation of the Heart; *A,* Prenatal; *B,* Postnatal

Congenital cardiovascular defects range from mild to severe. They may be detected immediately at birth or may not be detected for several months.

# CONGENITAL CARDIOVASCULAR DEFECTS

Congenital cardiovascular defects are among the leading causes of death during the first year of life (American Heart Association, 2009). Errors in formation of the heart or great vessels can occur prenatally, and persistence of fetal circulation can occur postnatally. Cardiovascular defects are best categorized according to blood flow patterns: (1) increased pulmonary blood flow, (2) decreased pulmonary blood flow, (3) obstructed blood flow out of the heart, or (4) mixed blood flow. Four of the most common cardiovascular defects in infants are listed in Table 7-3. Congenital heart disease is considered to be of **multifactorial inheritance**, a combination of genetic and environmental factors.

Rubella in the mother during the first trimester of pregnancy is a common cause of heart defects in infants. Other possible maternal causes include alcoholism, irradiation, ingestion of drugs, diabetes, malnutrition, and being more than 40 years of age. Heredity is seldom a contributing factor.

Infants with severe cardiovascular defects may be born with obvious distress caused by hypoxia. Those with less serious defects may compensate and appear to be healthy at birth. Heart murmurs and delayed growth and development observed later may call attention to problems. Infants with severe defects will often manifest signs and symptoms of CHF, such as fatigability; orthopnea; failure to thrive;

## TABLE 7-3 Common Cardiovascular Defects in Infants

| | VENTRICULAR SEPTAL DEFECT (VSD) | ATRIAL SEPTAL DEFECT (ASD) | PATENT DUCTUS ARTERIOSUS (PDA) | TETRALOGY OF FALLOT (TOF) |
|---|---|---|---|---|
| **Description** | Opening between ventricles | Opening between atria; incompetent foramen ovale | Failure of fetal ductus arteriosus to close postnatally | Four defects: (VSD), pulmonic stenosis, overriding aorta, and right ventricular hypertrophy |
| **Blood Flow Pattern** | ↑Pulmonary flow, left-to-right shunting | ↑Pulmonary flow; left-to-right shunting | ↑Pulmonary flow, left-to-right shunting | ↓Pulmonary flow; right-to-left shunting |
| **Manifestations** | ↑Respiratory infections; normal growth and development; congestive heart failure (CHF), if defect large | Usually asymptomatic, possible dysrhythmias, CHF if defect large | Usually asymptomatic, CHF possible, machinery-like murmur | Hypoxia, murmur, delayed growth and development |
| **Treatment** | Surgical correction by 2 years of age; prognosis dependent on extent of defect | Surgical correction by 6 years of age; excellent prognosis | Possiblity indomethacin (Indocin) administration to premature babies; surgical correction by 2 years; excellent prognosis | Surgical correction by 1 year of age |

COURTESY OF DELMAR CENGAGE LEARNING

pale, mottled, or cyanotic skin; hoarse or weak cry; tachycardia; and signs of respiratory distress, such as rate > 60 breaths per minute, costal retractions, orthopnea, wheezing, and coughing.

## MEDICAL–SURGICAL MANAGEMENT

### Surgical

Surgical intervention to repair a defect may be postponed until the child develops CHF. Generally, the older the infant, the better the surgical outcome. Refer to Table 7-3 for treatments of common heart defects.

### Pharmacological

Digoxin (Lanoxin) is the drug most often used to improve the heart's contractility and increase its output. Furosemide (Lasix) is the most commonly used diuretic. Because most diuretics cause potassium loss, serum potassium level is monitored, and potassium supplements may be ordered. Oxygen therapy and fluid management are also part of the treatment plan.

### Diet

When infants experience significant dyspnea while feeding, special feeding techniques are needed, such as providing small, frequent feedings and softer nipples. Some infants need higher caloric formulas and diets to meet nutritional needs. Gavage feedings may be required if the infant becomes fatigued before taking an adequate amount of formula.

## NURSING MANAGEMENT

Assess cardiac and respiratory function. Monitor behavioral patterns and growth and development. Administer oxygen and medications as ordered. Accurately record I&O. Weigh daily. Provide high-calorie feedings. If infant tires easily when eating, implement gavage feedings.

## NURSING PROCESS

### ASSESSMENT

#### Subjective Data

Take a history of the child's previous hospitalizations and assess the caregiver's knowledge about the condition. Note the caregiver anxiety level, coping strategies, and economic status.

#### Objective Data

Assess the child's behavioral patterns, cardiac and respiratory function, fluid status, and growth and development. Obtain a detailed history of onset of symptoms and a typical day's activity schedule.

### Nursing diagnoses for the infant with a heart defect include the following:

| NURSING DIAGNOSES | PLANNING/OUTCOMES | NURSING INTERVENTIONS |
|---|---|---|
| Decreased **Cardiac Output** related to structural defect | The client will demonstrate sufficient cardiac output to meet metabolic demands. | Administer digoxin as prescribed. Monitor vital signs (including apical pulse for 1 minute), potassium level, urine output, cardiac rhythm, activity tolerance. Assess for signs of digoxin toxicity (vomiting, anorexia, dysrhythmias, bradycardia [pulse rate < 90 to 110]), peripheral perfusion. Provide periods of rest each hour. |
| Ineffective **Breathing Pattern** related to pulmonary congestion | The client will breathe effortlessly at rest. | Keep the client in semi-Fowler's position (i.e., use infant seat). Administer humidified oxygen as prescribed, assess respiratory rate and effort, color, and oxygen saturation. Employ comfort measures (e.g., holding, rocking, presence of caregivers). Respond quickly to crying. |
| Excess **Fluid Volume** related to fluid accumulation | The client will experience decreased edema. | Administer diuretics as prescribed. Measure I&O. Weigh daily (same time and scale). Assess skin for edema, breakdown. Turn every 2 hours and elevate edematous extremities. Monitor electrolytes. |

*(Continues)*

**Nursing diagnoses for the infant with a heart defect include the following: (Continued)**

| NURSING DIAGNOSES | PLANNING/OUTCOMES | NURSING INTERVENTIONS |
|---|---|---|
| *Imbalanced **N**utrition: Less than Body Requirements* related to fatigue and dyspnea | The client will demonstrate normal weight gain for age. | Give small, frequent, high-caloric feedings.<br><br>Use soft nipple with large hole.<br><br>Implement gavage feeding, if the infant tires before taking prescribed amount of formula.<br><br>Make feeding time as stress free as possible.<br><br>Hold the infant when bottle-feeding (preferably by primary caregiver). |
| *Delayed **G**rowth and Development* related to low energy level | The client will meet developmental milestones for age. | Encourage age-appropriate activities, stimulation, and socialization.<br><br>Allow the child to set own pace. |
| *Interrupted **F**amily Processes* related to child with life-threatening illness/condition | The family will receive needed support. | Teach the family as needed about medication administration, signs and symptoms of CHF and when to report, feeding techniques, and appropriate activities for the child.<br><br>Refer the family to appropriate community resources. |

**Evaluation:** Evaluate each outcome to determine how it has been met by the client.

## HEMATOLOGIC AND LYMPHATIC SYSTEMS

The hematologic system regulates, directly or indirectly, the functions of all body tissues and organs. Some of the most common disorders occurring in infants include hyperbilirubinemia, iron-deficiency anemia, and sickle-cell anemia (SCA).

## HYPERBILIRUBINEMIA

Hyperbilirubinemia, often referred to as jaundice, is a common occurrence in neonates. Jaundice is the yellow discoloration of the skin, sclera, mucous membranes, and body fluids resulting from excess bilirubin and deposition of bile pigments. Physiologically, hemoglobin is broken down by the liver into iron, protein, and bilirubin. The bilirubin binds to albumin and is transported to the liver, where it is conjugated. Conjugated bilirubin is then eliminated through the intestines. Neonates have an intestinal enzyme that can convert the conjugated bilirubin back to unconjugated bilirubin, which can be reabsorbed into the bloodstream. This process can contribute significantly to the amount of bilirubin that the immature liver must break down. As the bilirubin level rises, some of the excess bilirubin is deposited in body tissues, resulting in a temporary yellow discoloration of the skin and sclera. A high level of bilirubin can penetrate and damage brain cells, causing severe neural symptoms (kernicterus). Hyperbilirubinemia develops during the first few days of life, with a greater incidence in preterm infants.

### MEDICAL–SURGICAL MANAGEMENT

#### Medical

The main objective of treatment is to reduce the amount of unconjugated bilirubin and aid in the conversion of bilirubin to a form that can be excreted by the body (urobilinogen). Full-term infants with jaundice may benefit from early and frequent breastfeeding (every 2 hours) (Moerschel et al., 2008). Otherwise, treatment usually begins with a phototherapy light, called a bililight, or a fiber-optic blanket. This light causes a chemical reaction in the skin and converts unconjugated bilirubin to a form that can be excreted by the body (lumirubin). Therapy is usually continual, with short breaks for feeding and holding. Phototherapy may be done at home because it is less expensive than treatment in the hospital and the caregivers will not have to be separated from their newborn.

### ⊕ PROFESSIONALTIP

#### Stress at Feeding Time

Ways to decrease stress at feeding time include the following:
- Decrease the noise level.
- Hold the infant while sitting in a rocker.
- Assess the infant's readiness to eat. (Infant is calm, demonstrates rooting, latches onto nipple eagerly, opens mouth voluntarily, looks at caregiver.)

## Pharmacological

If the bilirubin level responds slowly to phototherapy, pheno-barbital is sometimes given to enhance both the liver enzyme action and bilirubin excretion. Breastfed infants should continue nursing (8 to 12 times per day) whether or not phototherapy is required. Increasing the frequency of breastfeeding aids in the removal of bilirubin from the gastrointestinal tract. In cases where the mother's milk supply is inadequate, substituting formula for breastfeeding or incorporating it as a supplement may help decrease bilirubin levels. Ideally, breastfeeding should not be interrupted. (AAP, 2004; Moerschel et al., 2008).

## NURSING MANAGEMENT

Frequently assess for jaundice. Encourage frequent feedings. Maintain phototherapy as prescribed. Teach caregivers to do phototherapy at home.

## NURSING PROCESS

### ASSESSMENT

#### Subjective Data

Assess perinatal risk factors such as familial history of hyper-bilirubinemia and induced delivery.

#### Objective Data

Assess for jaundice by applying light pressure to the skin over either the tip of the nose or the sternum in natural daylight. For dark-skinned infants, observe the sclera, conjunctiva, and oral mucosa for a yellow color. Bruising, petechiae, and pallor are also suggestive of hyperbiliru-benemia.

### Nursing diagnoses for the infant with hyperbilirubinemia include the following:

| NURSING DIAGNOSES | PLANNING/OUTCOMES | NURSING INTERVENTIONS |
|---|---|---|
| *Risk for Deficient **F**luid Volume* related to insensible losses | The client will maintain fluid balance. | Assess skin for signs of dehydration (i.e., dry mouth, sleepiness, decreased urine output). Calculate needed fluid intake to compensate for losses. Monitor I&O. |
| *Risk for Impaired **S**kin Integrity* related to use of phototherapy | The client's skin will remain intact. | Assess skin for breakdown. Monitor temperature every 2 to 4 hours. Keep skin clean and dry, do not apply any oils or lotions. |
| *Interrupted **F**amily Processes* related to situational crisis | The family will receive needed support. | Encourage bonding by removing eye shields and allowing the caregivers to hold/feed the infant. Teach the importance of eye shields under light. Support the breastfeeding mother. Encourage pumping the breasts if feeding must be stopped temporarily. Keep the caregivers informed. |

**Evaluation**: Evaluate each outcome to determine how it has been met by the client.

## ■ IRON-DEFICIENCY ANEMIA

The incidence of iron-deficiency anemia is usually related to the infant's consuming large amounts of milk and foods that do not contain supplemental iron. These babies are often overweight because of excessive intake of cow's milk, which is a poor source of iron. In addition, cow's milk can cause loss of blood in the stool.

Because full-term infants have iron stores from fetal circulation that usually last for 5 to 6 months, iron-deficiency anemia usually surfaces between 9 and 24 months of age. Clinical manifestations may include extreme pallor (porcelain-like in fair-skinned infants), tachycardia, lethargy, irritability, and below-normal hemoglobin, hematocrit, and iron levels.

## MEDICAL–SURGICAL MANAGEMENT

### Pharmacological

Iron therapy is usually prescribed and continued for 3 months after hemoglobin and hematocrit levels return to normal. An increase in hemoglobin level can be expected within 4 to 30 days. Ascorbic acid may also be prescribed in an attempt to facilitate iron absorption. Intramuscular (IM) or IV injections may be necessary if the level does not improve after 1 month of oral iron. Transfusions are indicated only for the most severe cases.

### Diet

Long-term therapy is directed at increasing the dietary intake of iron and continuing the use of iron-fortified formula until

## PROFESSIONALTIP

### WIC

The federal supplemental food program called Women, Infants, and Children (WIC) is an excellent resource for nutritious food for low-income families with pregnant, postpartum, or lactating women and children up to 5 years of age. In addition to food, this program provides nutritional education and screening.

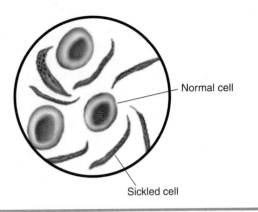

**FIGURE 7-4** Sickling Cells

12 months of age. At 4 to 6 months of age, iron-fortified cereal can be used (Burns et al., 2008).

## NURSING MANAGEMENT

Prevent anemia by educating the caregivers about administration of iron. It is important to explore any misconceptions caregivers may have, such as "milk is a perfect food" and "excessive weight gain equates to a healthy child and good mothering."

Encourage foods rich in iron, such as dried beans, iron-fortified cereals, apricots, prunes, egg yolks, and dark-green, leafy vegetables. Infants should remain on iron-fortified formulas until 12 months of age.

Instruct caregivers in the proper administration of oral iron. When administering IM preparations, no more than 1 mL should be given deep into the muscle using the Z-track method to prevent staining of tissues and to minimize irritation.

## ■ SICKLE-CELL ANEMIA

Sickle-cell anemia is a genetic disorder characterized by the production of abnormal hemoglobin and resulting in red blood cells (RBCs) taking on a "sickle" shape (Figure 7-4). Because of the presence of fetal hemoglobin, clinical symptoms usually do not appear until 6 months of age. Episodes of sickling may be triggered by infection, dehydration, hypoxia, trauma, or general physical or emotional stress resulting in impaired circulation and increased RBC destruction.

The most common symptoms of SCA include abdominal pain (caused by sludging in the spleen and leading to its enlargement), fever, severe leg pain, and hot, swollen joints. In addition, growth retardation, chronic anemia, and increased susceptibility to infection may be experienced. This disease occurs primarily among African Americans and is transmitted as an autosomal-recessive trait wherein both parents are carriers (refer back to Table 7-2).

## MEDICAL–SURGICAL MANAGEMENT

### Medical

Between episodes, the goal is to prevent crises with adequate hydration (1,500 to 3,000 mL per day). During crises, treatment may include bed rest, oxygen, analgesics (morphine), and fluids.

### Pharmacological

Children with this disease must be immunized with influenza, pneumococcal, meningococcal, and hepatitis B vaccines because of increased susceptibility to infection and the likelihood of transfusion therapy. Prophylactic oral penicillin is often prescribed twice a day until age 5 or 6, and a daily supplement of folic acid is taken (Mayo Clinic, 2009).

## CLIENTTEACHING

### Administration of Iron to Infants

When instructing caregivers in the administration of iron to infants, teach to:

- Administer with citrus fruit or juice in order to increase its absorption.
- Administer through a straw or medicine dropper placed at the back of the mouth, to decrease staining of the teeth.
- Brush or wipe the infant's teeth after administration.
- Expect dark, black stools.

## MEMORYTRICK

### Sickle-Cell Anemia

When a client is experiencing a sickle-cell crisis, remember the 5 "**A**s:"

**A** = Administer analgesics

**A** = Administer antibiotics

**A** = Administer oxygen

**A** = Administer fluids

**A** = Apply heat to affected area

## Health Promotion

Avoid high altitudes, poorly pressurized airplanes, and exposure to extreme heat or cold. Maintaining hydration is of paramount importance. Neonatal screening, early intervention, prophylactic antibiotics, and parent education have allowed children with SCA to live into adulthood.

## NURSING MANAGEMENT

Encourage continuous adequate hydration and immunizations. Prevent exposure to extreme heat or cold. Provide caregiver education. Monitor growth and development. When in crisis, administer analgesics, antibiotics, oxygen, and fluids as ordered. Apply heat to affected area.

## NURSING PROCESS

### ASSESSMENT

#### Subjective Data

Interview the caregivers about activities or events leading up to the crisis, a history of child's health, and previous episodes. Evaluate the caregivers level of knowledge about the condition.

#### Objective Data

Assess all areas and systems that can be affected by circulatory obstruction, such as vital signs, vision, hearing, growth and development, and the respiratory, GI, renal, neurological, and musculoskeletal systems.

### Nursing diagnoses for the infant with sickle-cell anemia include the following:

| NURSING DIAGNOSES | PLANNING/OUTCOMES | NURSING INTERVENTIONS |
|---|---|---|
| *Ineffective **T**issue Perfusion* related to vaso-occlusion and anemia | The client will maintain oxygen saturation levels at 95% or greater. | Administer oxygen as prescribed. Monitor oxygen saturation, capillary refill, and respiratory status. Maintain the client in a position of comfort (semi- to high-Fowler's). Administer packed RBCs as prescribed. |
| *Acute **P**ain* related to vaso-occlusion and tissue ischemia | The client will be pain free. | Apply heat to affected area; avoid cold compresses. Administer analgesics as prescribed (preferably morphine) and assess effectiveness by assessing behavior and vital signs. Reassure the caregivers that opioids are appropriate, high doses may be needed, and addiction is rare. Position the client carefully and handle gently. |
| *Risk for **I**nfection* related to splenic malfunction | The client will be infection-free. | Provide one to one and one-half daily fluid requirement as determined by body weight. Provide daily food requirements as determined by body weight and length. Administer antibiotics as prescribed. Ensure that the infant avoids contact with known sources of infection. Ensure that immunizations are up-to-date. |
| *Deficient **K**nowledge (family)* related to cause and treatment of disease | The family will verbalize an understanding of the risk factors and ways to minimize them. | Teach need for one to one and one-half times daily fluid requirement. Teach importance of hand hygiene and avoiding known sources of infection. Reinforce importance of up-to-date immunizations for the infant. Teach to shield the infant from overexertion, emotional stress, and low-oxygen environments. Teach early intervention for any sign of infection (e.g., temperature of 101.5°F or greater) or dehydration (weight loss, dry skin and mucous membranes, sunken fontanel). Teach medication administration as ordered. |

*(Continues)*

**Nursing diagnoses for the infant with sickle-cell anemia include the following: (Continued)**

| NURSING DIAGNOSES | PLANNING/OUTCOMES | NURSING INTERVENTIONS |
|---|---|---|
| *Interrupted Family Processes* related to child with chronic condition | The family will adjust to lifelong, potentially fatal hereditary disease. | Explain procedures and planned treatments. |
| | | Allow the family to provide care in the hospital. |
| | | Provide information about appropriate developmental activities. |
| | | Encourage the family to talk about feelings and concerns. |
| | | Stress positive outcomes (e.g., that most of the time, children are asymptomatic and can participate in appropriate activities without restrictions). |
| | | Provide information regarding transmission of the condition; refer for genetic counseling. |
| | | Provide numbers for American Sickle Cell Anemia Association and available support groups. |

**Evaluation:** Evaluate each outcome to determine how it has been met by the client.

# GASTROINTESTINAL SYSTEM

Infants have minimal saliva, no voluntary control of swallowing, a small stomach, rapid intestinal motility, a relaxed cardiac sphincter, deficiency of enzymes in the duodenum, and immature liver function. This accounts for the numerous GI problems that occur during the first 12 months of life, such as vomiting, diarrhea, colic (sudden, recurrent bouts of abdominal pain), and failure to thrive. In addition, because the immune system is also immature, the infant is highly susceptible to infection. Congenital defects resulting in atresia (absence or closure of a body orifice), malposition, nonclosure, or other abnormalities can occur in any area of the GI tract. Any GI problem, whether a lack of nutrients, an infection, or a congenital disorder, can quickly affect other parts of the body and ultimately affect general health and growth and development. The GI disorders discussed following include thrush, acute gastroenteritis, colic, failure to thrive, cleft lip/palate, esophageal atresia with tracheoesophageal fistula, pyloric stenosis, Hirschsprung's disease, gastroesophageal reflux, and intussusception.

## ■ THRUSH

Thrush (moniliasis, candidiasis) is an oral fungal infection that is transmitted from the vaginal canal of an infected mother to the newborn. Other contributing factors include poor hand hygiene by care providers, inadequate washing of bottles and nipples, and antibiotic therapy. Thrush is characterized by painless, white patches that look like curdled milk on the oral mucosa (Figure 7-5). Bottle-fed infants are at greater risk of developing thrush than breastfed infants.

## MEDICAL–SURGICAL MANAGEMENT
### ◨ Pharmacological

Topical nystatin (Mycostatin) is the most commonly used treatment for thrush. It is applied to the oral mucosa four times per day with an applicator or a gloved finger and then swallowed (Su et al., 2008). Rinse the mouth before medicating. In addition, if infants are breastfed, apply the medication to the breasts.

## NURSING MANAGEMENT

Teach caregivers proper hand hygiene. Boiling bottles, pacifiers, and nipples for 20 minutes will kill the spores.

## ■ ACUTE GASTROENTERITIS

Acute gastroenteritis (AGE) is an inflammation of the stomach and intestines that may be accompanied by diarrhea and vomiting. This common condition may be caused by malnutrition, lactose intolerance, chronic conditions, or infections by viruses, bacteria, and parasites.

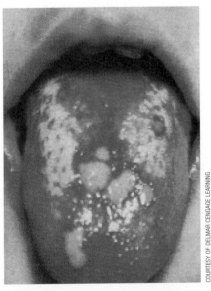

**FIGURE 7-5** Thrush

COURTESY OF DELMAR CENGAGE LEARNING

The infant with AGE will have an increased number of green, liquid stools tinged with mucus or blood. In addition, symptoms of fluid and electrolyte imbalance, cramping, extreme irritability, and vomiting may be exhibited. Depending on age and nutritional status and on the severity and duration of the diarrhea, the infant may become severely dehydrated and gravely ill.

# MEDICAL–SURGICAL MANAGEMENT
## Medical

Regaining and maintaining fluid balance is paramount. Use oral rehydrating fluids such as Pedialyte and Lytren for mild dehydration. For severe dehydration, IV solutions are needed to replace fluids and electrolytes. Antibiotics may be prescribed if bacterial infection is indicated from stool cultures.

## Diet

Once rehydration is attained, the usual diet is continued. Research has indicated that early reintroduction of normal nutrients is desirable, and delayed introduction of food may be harmful in terms of nutritional status and duration of illness. Breastfed infants should continue on supplemental oral rehydrating solutions throughout the illness. If formula feedings are not tolerated, suggest lactose-free formulas. Complex carbohydrates, lean meats, fruits, and vegetables are well tolerated. Foods high in simple sugars such as carbonated soft drinks, juice, and gelatin should be avoided (MMWR, 2003).

# NURSING MANAGEMENT

Assess for dehydration. Monitor I&O and electrolyte levels. Administer fluids and electrolytes as ordered. Provide clear fluids and oral rehydrating solutions every 30 minutes. Follow proper hand hygiene and teach to caregivers. Keep diaper area clean and apply a barrier ointment.

# NURSING PROCESS
## ASSESSMENT
### Subjective Data

Question caregivers regarding probable etiologic agents such as introduction of new food; exposure to infectious agents; travel to an area where the infectious agent is endemic; contact with foods that might be contaminated; crowded, dirty living conditions; and contact with pets that are known to be sources of enteric infections, such as pet turtles. Obtain allergy, drug, health, and diet histories.

## Objective Data

Assessing for dehydration is paramount for infants with AGE (Table 7-4). Assess the diaper area for skin breakdown resulting from repeated contact with diarrheal stools.

## INFECTION CONTROL

### Diaper Hygiene

- Change diapers as soon as they are soiled.
- Wear gloves when changing diapers.
- Fold the used diaper with soiled area to the inside and immediately place the diaper in a covered receptacle.
- Cleanse the skin and dispose of wipes along with the diaper.
- Remove gloves after disposal of wipes.
- Rediaper.
- Wash hands immediately after rediapering is complete.
- Store soiled clothing, cloth diapers, and washcloths in a covered receptacle.
- Cleanse surface of changing area.

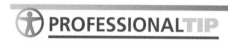

## PROFESSIONAL TIP

### Potassium Administration

Potassium is excreted by the kidneys. If kidney function is impaired, potassium can build up in the body and can lead to arrhythmias and become life-threatening. Therefore, urine output must be established prior to administering potassium.

**TABLE 7-4 Assessing Dehydration**

| SIGNS AND SYMPTOMS | MILD | MODERATE | SEVERE |
|---|---|---|---|
| Weight loss | <3% | 3–9% | >9% |
| Skin turgor | Taut | Tenting | Tenting |
| Skin color | Pale | Grey | Mottled |
| Mucous membranes | Slightly dry, pale | Very dry, grey | Parched |
| Urine output | Decreased | Absent | Absent |
| Blood pressure | Normal | Normal | Decreased |
| Pulse | Normal or increased | Increased | Increased/thready |
| Fontanelle | Flat | Depressed | Sunken |

**Nursing diagnoses for the infant with AGE include the following:**

| NURSING DIAGNOSES | PLANNING/OUTCOMES | NURSING INTERVENTIONS |
|---|---|---|
| *Deficient **F**luid Volume* related to excessive GI losses | The client will be adequately hydrated (specify). | Monitor I&O and notify physician if output <1 mL/kg/h. Assess weight daily and compare with previous weights. Assess for degree of hydration. Monitor electrolyte levels. Administer fluids and electrolytes as prescribed. Encourage clear liquids and oral rehydrating solutions (Pedialyte, Lytren) in small doses every 30 minutes until rehydrated; after rehydration, alternate with water, breast milk, or half-strength formula, as needed. |
| *Risk for **I**nfection* related to GI infection | The client and family will be infection free. | Teach proper hand hygiene and diaper hygiene to care providers. Wear gloves when handling diapers. |
| *Risk for Impaired **S**kin Integrity* related to frequent contact with diarrheal stools | The client's skin will remain intact. | Change diapers every 2 hours, as needed. Cleanse skin with mild soap (Dove) and water. Apply barrier (A&D Ointment). |

**Evaluation**: Evaluate each outcome to determine how it has been met by the client.

## ■ COLIC

Colic is a sudden, periodic attack of abdominal pain and cramping that is defined as "crying for more than three hours per day, for more than three days per week, and for longer than three weeks in an infant who is well-fed and otherwise healthy" (Roberts et al., 2004). It usually occurs between birth and 3 months of age and at approximately the same time each day (late afternoon, early evening hours). During these episodes, the infant is generally inconsolable, which may interfere with caregiver–child attachment and family relations.

The child is usually eager to eat and is growing appropriately. There is no known cause of colic; however, speculation points to overfeeding, overly rapid feeding, improper burping, the swallowing of large amounts of air, and emotional stress between parent and child (Hockenberry et al., 2006).

## MEDICAL–SURGICAL MANAGEMENT
### Medical

Sensitivity to formula, food allergies, peritoneal infection, and intestinal obstruction must be ruled out as specific causes of the distress. If sensitivity to formula is suspected, another brand

of formula may be substituted. In the case of breastfeeding mothers, avoid dairy products, onions, cabbage, and dry beans for several days in an attempt to relieve the infant's symptoms.

### 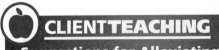 Pharmacological

Sedatives, antispasmodics, antihistamines, and antiflatulents are sometimes recommended in an attempt to relieve symptoms.

## NURSING MANAGEMENT

Assessing circumstances surrounding the colicky event, exploring techniques to relieve symptoms, and supporting

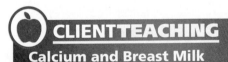

**CLIENTTEACHING**

**Calcium and Breast Milk**

If the breastfeeding mother maintains a milk-free diet for more than several days, she must take calcium supplements in order to maintain the calcium content of the breast milk.

**CLIENTTEACHING**

**Suggestions for Alleviating Colic**

- Provide rhythmic movement, such as rocking, swinging, and riding in the car.
- Alternate positions, such as placing the infant face down across the lap.
- Reduce environmental stimuli, especially during feedings.
- Provide a variety of tactile stimulation, such as rubbing the head or abdomen or placing prone on a warm heating pad.
- Provide small, frequent feedings.
- Burp during and after feedings.
- Respond immediately to crying.
- Provide background or "white" noise (vacuum cleaner, hair dryer) or play music.

caregivers during the colicky period are the primary nursing goals. Observe the feeding technique in order to assess the parent's sensitivity and response to the infant's cues of distress and evaluate the clarity of the infant's cues and the infant's responsiveness to the parent.

Reassure caregivers that colic usually resolves by 3 months of age and does not indicate poor or inadequate parenting. Encourage them to talk about their feelings toward the infant and any insecurities they may feel.

## ■ FAILURE TO THRIVE

Failure to thrive (FTT) is the label applied to infants who fail to gain weight and who show signs of delayed development. There are two categories of FTT: organic, which is caused by a physical defect or condition; and nonorganic, which is the result of psychosocial factors such as an impaired parent–child relationship. Manifestations of FTT include sustained growth failure (below the fifth percentile on the standardized growth chart), developmental delays in all areas, and poor feeding and sleeping patterns.

## MEDICAL–SURGICAL MANAGEMENT

### Medical

If FTT is the result of a physical defect or condition, the condition is treated. Regardless of the cause, the primary goals are to provide adequate nutrition, promote growth and development, and assist caregivers in developing the skills needed to nurture their infant.

### Health Promotion

In most cases of nonorganic FTT, a multidisciplinary health care team is needed to deal with the physical, psychosocial, mental, and emotional problems that may be occurring in the family. If the entire family is to become healthy, each member must be helped to change.

## NURSING MANAGEMENT

Monitor weight gain and development. Provide adequate nutrition. Assist caregivers to develop nurturing skills.

## NURSING PROCESS

### ASSESSMENT

#### Subjective Data

Focus on the infant's routine, respiratory status, and diet history. Assess the family for depression, substance abuse, mental retardation, and psychosis as well as socioeconomic level, education, social isolation, stress factors, and support systems.

#### Objective Data

Focus on signs of malnutrition (skin, hair, nails, mucous membranes, energy level, developmental milestones) and on parent–infant interactions (parent's cues, infant's cues, and synchrony).

### Nursing diagnoses for the infant with FTT include the following:

| NURSING DIAGNOSES | PLANNING/OUTCOMES | NURSING INTERVENTIONS |
|---|---|---|
| *Imbalanced Nutrition: Less than Body Requirements* related to insufficient intake of calories and/or impaired parent/child interaction | The client will demonstrate growth curve above the 5th percentile. | Provide consistent nursing staff and develop a structured routine. |
| | | Feed the infant on demand and increase intake as tolerated. |
| | | Monitor I&O. Weigh daily. |
| | | Encourage caregiver involvement in care, demonstrate and model appropriate care techniques, praise positive attempts at care, and provide for rooming-in. |
| | | Use a variety of methods to teach child care to the caregivers. |
| *Risk for Delayed Development* related to inadequate stimulation | The client will attain age-appropriate developmental milestones. | Begin a program of play that stimulates interest and responsiveness. |
| | | Teach the caregivers ways to play and interact with the infant and to cuddle the infant. |

**Evaluation:** Evaluate each outcome to determine how it has been met by the client.

## ■ CLEFT LIP/PALATE

The most common facial malformations are cleft lip and cleft palate. They may occur separately or together. Failure of the palates and/or lip to fuse is evident at birth. The defect may occur unilaterally on either side or bilaterally and with varying degrees of severity. The cause is unclear, but some genetic component seems likely.

Clinical manifestations include nasal, lip, and palate distortions. The child born with a cleft palate and intact lip does not manifest the external disfigurement so potentially distressing to caregivers, but the physical problems are more serious. The infant with a cleft palate is at risk for aspiration,

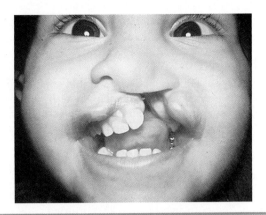

**FIGURE 7-6** **Older Child with Unrepaired Cleft Lip** (*Courtesy of Dr. Joseph Konzelman, School of Dentistry, Medical College of Georgia.*)

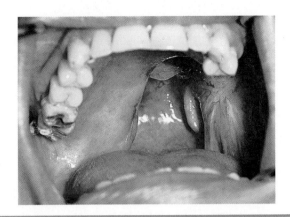

**FIGURE 7-7** **Older Child with Unrepaired Cleft Palate** (*Courtesy of Dr. Joseph Konzelman, School of Dentistry, Medical College of Georgia.*)

feeding difficulties, and respiratory infections (Figures 7-6 and 7-7).

# MEDICAL–SURGICAL MANAGEMENT

## Medical

Care is directed toward closing the defects, maintaining adequate nutrition, preventing complications, and fostering normal growth and development of the child. Total care may involve many specialists, including pediatricians, nurses, plastic surgeons, orthodontists, prosthodontists, otolaryngologists, speech therapists, and psychiatrists. The extent of multidisciplinary care depends on the severity of the defect. Infants with cleft lip and palate are prone to recurrent otitis media, which will likely be treated with antibiotics.

## Surgical

Closure of the lip precedes that of the palate, usually at 6 to 12 weeks of age. The palate is usually closed surgically at 12 to 18 months of age to facilitate speech development.

## Health Promotion

Maternal use of multivitamin supplements containing folic acid around the time of conception has been reported to reduce the risk of cleft malformations by up to 50% (Bailey & Berry, 2005).

# NURSING MANAGEMENT

Encourage caregivers to hold and interact with their infant and to participate in the care of the infant. Provide feedings as ordered using assistive devices. Keep infant in upright position for feeding. Burp frequently.

# NURSING PROCESS

## ASSESSMENT

### Subjective Data

Assess immediately the emotional impact of the birth of an infant with a facial deformity. Assess the caregivers acceptance of the child periodically, at various appointments and hospital admissions.

### Objective Data

Cleft lip and palate are observable at birth. A cleft palate is palpable with the finger. Document the degree of involvement. Evaluate the ability to suck, swallow, breathe, and handle secretions.

## Nursing diagnoses for the infant with cleft lip or palate include the following:

| NURSING DIAGNOSES | PLANNING/OUTCOMES | NURSING INTERVENTIONS |
|---|---|---|
| *Compromised Family Coping* related to birth of infant with visible and/or structural defect | The family will bond with the infant. | Encourage the caregivers to hold the infant. |
| | | Point out positive attributes of the infant (e.g., hair, eyes, alertness); convey attitude of acceptance of the infant and family. |
| | | Explain expected outcomes of surgical repair; show pictures of repaired children. |
| | | Allow expression of feelings. |
| | | Assess the caregivers' knowledge, degree of anxiety, level of discomfort, interpersonal relationships. |
| | | Explore reactions of extended family. |
| | | Encourage the caregivers to participate in care of the infant. |
| | | Refer to support groups and to other families in similar situations. |

**Nursing diagnoses for the infant with cleft lip or palate include the following: (Continued)**

| NURSING DIAGNOSES | PLANNING/OUTCOMES | NURSING INTERVENTIONS |
|---|---|---|
| *Imbalanced Nutrition: Less than Body Requirements* related to infant's inability to form an adequate seal when sucking on the nipple | The infant will maintain a growth curve above the 5th percentile. | Provide 100 to 150 cal/kg/d and 100 to 130 mL/kg/d. |
| | | Assess output daily. |
| | | Weigh daily. |
| | | Observe for respiratory impairment (i.e., for adventitious breath sounds, increased respiratory rate). |
| | | Facilitate breastfeeding; refer for ongoing support (e.g., to La Leche League). |
| | | Position the infant in an upright or semi-sitting position for feeding. |
| | | Use effective assistive devices (e.g., longer, softer nipples; feeders). |
| | | Feed small amounts slowly, allowing ample time for sucking and swallowing; burp after 15 to 30 mL. |
| | | Initiate nasogastric feeding if infant is unable to ingest sufficient calories by mouth. |
| | | Teach caregivers the proper placement and use of nasogastric tube. |
| *Impaired Tissue Integrity* related to surgical correction of cleft | The client's tissue will heal with minimal scarring. | Position the infant on side or back. |
| | | Use elbow restraints for 7 to 10 days as needed and teach proper application to caregivers. |
| | | Medicate for pain around-the-clock for at least 24 hours postoperatively. |
| | | Provide developmentally appropriate activities (e.g., music, mobiles, holding) to distract the infant's attention from the incision site. |
| | | Do not use pacifiers, spoons, or straws for 7 to 10 days postoperatively. |
| | | Progress to a soft diet appropriate for age and as ordered and tolerated within 48 hours. |
| *Risk for Infection* related to surgical procedure and accumulation of formula and secretions in oral cavity | The client's surgical site will be free of infection. | Assess vital signs and oral cavity every 2 hours. |
| | | Cleanse suture line with normal saline or sterile water, as ordered. |
| | | Give 5 to 15 mL water after each feeding to cleanse the mouth. |
| | | Apply antibiotic cream as ordered. |
| | | Ensure hand hygiene by all care providers. |
| | | Include caregivers in care and prepare for home care. |

**Evaluation:** Evaluate each outcome to determine how it has been met by the client.

## ESOPHAGEAL ATRESIA WITH TRACHEOESOPHAGEAL FISTULA

Esophageal atresia and tracheoesophageal fistula are rare malformations that may occur alone or in combination and represent a failure of the esophagus to develop as a continuous passage (atresia) to the stomach and/or an unnatural connection between the esophagus and the trachea (fistula) (Figure 7-8). The cause is unknown.

Manifestations include excessive salivation, drooling, coughing, choking when feeding, and cyanosis. A history of polyhydramnios (excessive production of amniotic fluid) during the prenatal period is common.

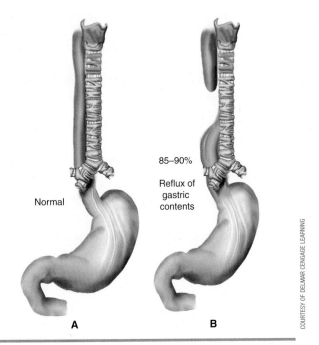

FIGURE 7-8 Esophagus; *A*, Normal; *B*, Atresia/Fistula

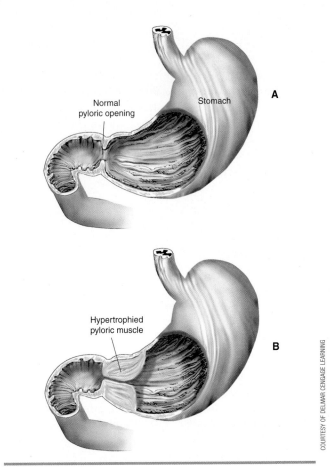

FIGURE 7-9 Stomach; *A*, Normal Opening; *B*, Pyloric Stenosis

## MEDICAL–SURGICAL MANAGEMENT

### Medical

The primary goal is prevention and treatment of aspiration pneumonia. The infant will be designated NPO and administered IV fluids. Removal of secretions from the mouth and esophagus requires frequent or continuous suctioning through a nasogastric tube (NGT). Antibiotics are prescribed for any developing pneumonia.

### Surgical

These defects represent a critical neonatal surgical emergency. Surgical correction may be accomplished in several stages depending on the size and condition of the infant and the extent of the defect. If closure of the gap requires staged repair, a gastrostomy tube will be placed for feeding. The prognosis is usually good with surgery.

## NURSING MANAGEMENT

Nursing responsibility for detection of this malformation begins immediately after birth. Assess the newborn for color, amount of saliva, ability to swallow, respiratory distress, and abdominal distention. A maternal history of polyhydramnios necessitates assessment for the defect with insertion of an NGT. Do not initiate feedings until the infant has been assessed. When the defect is diagnosed, prepare the infant and the family for immediate surgery. Postoperative care is the same as that provided to any high-risk newborn.

## ■ PYLORIC STENOSIS

Pyloric stenosis is a common disorder that occurs when the circular muscle surrounding the pylorus hypertrophies and blocks gastric emptying (Figure 7-9). It is rarely diagnosed before the third week of life. Manifestations include **projectile vomiting** (ejection of stomach contents up to 3 feet),

ravenous hunger, hyperactive bowel sounds, irritability, FTT, decreased number and volume of stools, an olive-shaped mass in the right upper quadrant, and visible peristaltic waves.

## MEDICAL–SURGICAL MANAGEMENT

### Medical

Diagnosis is usually made before malnutrition, dehydration, and alkalosis are severe. It is unusual for the infant to require IV fluid therapy before surgery.

### Surgical

The defect usually is discovered early and repaired immediately. Most infants recover rapidly and completely with surgery.

## NURSING MANAGEMENT

Recognize the signs and symptoms early. Pre- and postoperative care are the same as for any GI surgical client. Infants are allowed to resume feedings 4 to 6 hours postoperatively and may be discharged within 24 hours.

## ■ HIRSCHSPRUNG'S DISEASE/ MEGACOLON

Hirschsprung's disease is a congenital anomaly manifested as a partial or complete mechanical obstruction resulting from inadequate motility of part of the colon. There is an absence of parasympathetic ganglion cells and, thus, of peristalsis within the muscular wall of the distal colon and the rectum. As a result, the affected portion of the bowel narrows, and the portion directly above the affected area becomes greatly dilated and fills with feces and gas (Figure 7-10). Failure of the newborn to have a stool during the first 24 to 48 hours may indicate this defect. Older infants may have constipation or ribbonlike stools and an enlarged, distended abdomen.

## MEDICAL–SURGICAL MANAGEMENT
### Medical

For the child with a mild defect, management may involve dietary modification, stool softeners, and isotonic irrigations until the child is toilet trained. Most infants with Hirschsprung's require surgical intervention.

### Surgical

Surgical intervention involves removal of the aganglionic bowel and creation of a temporary colostomy. Resection and colostomy closure are performed after the child reaches 10 kg.

## NURSING MANAGEMENT

Assess the newborn for passage of stool during the first 24 to 48 hours and observe for signs of constipation and for malformed stools throughout infancy. Assess all infants with Hirschsprung's for weight gain, nutritional intake, and bowel

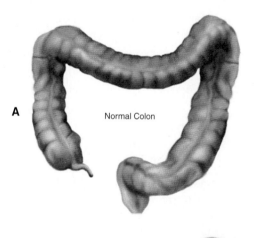

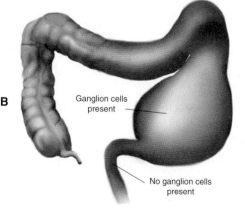

A  Normal Colon

B  Ganglion cells present

No ganglion cells present

FIGURE 7-10  Colon; *A*, Normal; *B*, Hirschsprung's Disease/Megacolon

habits. Teach caregivers both to ensure regular bowel habits with daily saline irrigations and a balanced diet and to observe for signs of fluid and electrolyte imbalances, such as dry mucous membranes and increased thirst.

Postoperative care may include reduction of anxiety and preparation for home care of the colostomy.

## ■ GASTROESOPHAGEAL REFLUX

Gastroesophageal reflux (GER) is the return of stomach contents into the esophagus caused by an immature sphincter. Manifestations such as hunger, irritability, FTT, vomiting, and frequent upper respiratory infections usually occur during the first 6 weeks of life.

Most infants have mild reflux and generally improve without surgical intervention by 1 year of age. Severe cases of GER that do not respond to therapy can result in esophageal strictures, respiratory distress, and FTT.

## MEDICAL–SURGICAL MANAGEMENT
### Medical

Gastroesophageal reflux often resolves with dietary modifications, medication, and positioning. Small, frequent feedings and frequent burping are measures for minimizing reflux. Thickening formula with cereal (1 to 3 teaspoons of cereal for each ounce of formula) may be recommended if FTT persists.

Placing the infant prone and with the head elevated 30 degrees is generally thought to be the most effective positioning for reducing the frequency of reflux (Orenstein, Izadnia & Khan, 1999). Positioning in an infant seat may cause increased intra-abdominal pressure and is not recommended.

### Surgical

Severe cases of GER that do not respond to medical interventions may be treated with a surgical procedure called fundoplication, which involves loosely wrapping the gastric fundus around the lower esophagus.

### Pharmacological

Medications such as cimetidine (Tagamet), ranitidine (Zantac), or famotidine (Pepcid) may be effective in reducing gastric acid content.

## NURSING MANAGEMENT

Recognize signs and symptoms of GER and educate caregivers regarding home care, including feeding, positioning, and medications. Pre- and postoperative care will be needed if the defect is surgically repaired.

## ■ INTUSSUSCEPTION

Intussusception is a disorder characterized by the telescoping of one portion of the bowel (usually the ileum) into a distal portion (usually the ascending colon). A previously healthy infant who develops intussusception will suddenly become pale, cry out sharply, and draw up the legs in a severe colicky spasm of pain. Such episodes last for several minutes and recur within 20 minutes. Vomiting and passage of "currant-jelly stools" (containing bloody mucus) also occur; however, these symptoms are present in fewer than 50% of infants with this condition (Kuppermann, O'Dea, Pincherry, & Hoecker, 2000). Symptoms of shock, such as increased heart rate and changes in level of consciousness, appear quickly. If the intussusception is detected and reduced within 24 hours, morbidity is minimal. Complications such as perforation, peritonitis, and sepsis can occur (Applegate, 2005).

## MEDICAL–SURGICAL MANAGEMENT

### Medical

Initial treatment involves hydrostatic reduction with barium or air enema at the time of diagnosis. Air enema is considered more successful at reduction and has significantly higher reduction rates when compared with liquid enemas; 82% versus 68% (Applegate, 2005).

### Surgical

If hydrostatic reduction fails or bowel damage is visualized during x-ray, surgical repair is done immediately. Surgery may consist of manual reduction of the telescoping, resection and anastomosis, or, possibly, colostomy, if the intestine is gangrenous.

## NURSING MANAGEMENT

Recognize early the signs and symptoms of intussusception (e.g., abrupt onset of colicky pain and vomiting with currant-jelly stools). Help caregivers visualize telescoping by pressing the finger of an inflated rubber glove into the glove; pressing on the glove will then demonstrate hydrostatic reduction as the finger is pushed back to its normal position.

## SAMPLE NURSING CARE PLAN

## The Infant Client with Abdominal Surgery

Eight-month-old N.W. was brought to the emergency room by his mother and father, who stated that he was perfectly fine until approximately 4 hours ago, when he refused to eat lunch or take his bottle. He wanted to be held and became increasingly irritable. He began alternating between inconsolable crying and being quiet and limp. Physical examination revealed a palpable abdominal mass and passage of currant-jelly stool. Barium enema confirmed the diagnosis of intussusception, but attempts to reduce the blockage were unsuccessful. N.W. was admitted and prepared for surgery. N.W. weighs 8.8 kg and is maintaining a normal growth curve at the 50th percentile. He has attained all appropriate developmental milestones. This is N.W.'s first illness and hospitalization. His mother begins to cry when she learns of the impending surgery and says, "What did I do wrong?" When the surgery is over, the doctor reports that N.W. has a temporary colostomy that will be closed in a few months. N.W. returns from surgery with a nasogastric tube and a urinary catheter in place and with dextrose 5% with normal saline being administered by IV at 40 mL per hour.

**NURSING DIAGNOSIS 1** *Risk for Injury* related to physical risk factors as evidenced by surgical procedure, loss of fluids, altered nutrition, and chemical risk factor of anesthesia

**Nursing Outcomes Classification (NOC)**
*Risk Control*

**Nursing Interventions Classification (NIC)**
*Surgical Precautions*
*Post-Anesthesia Care*

| PLANNING/OUTCOMES | NURSING INTERVENTIONS | RATIONALE |
|---|---|---|
| N.W. will be free of injury, infection, and complications. | Assess vital signs, skin, hydration, and respiratory status every 4 hours. | Facilitates early detection of signs of complications. |
| | Administer antibiotics as prescribed. | Prevents infection. |
| N.W. will demonstrate required fluid I&O. | Provide mouth care at least every 4 hours. | Mucous membranes become dry when clients are NPO. |
| | Maintain NPO and monitor IV as prescribed, and record I&O. | An empty stomach prevents aspiration, and fluids maintain hydration. |

## SAMPLE NURSING CARE PLAN (Continued)

| PLANNING/OUTCOMES | NURSING INTERVENTIONS | RATIONALE |
|---|---|---|
| N.W. will maintain growth curve at 50th percentile. | Assess bowel sounds every 2 hours. | Active bowel sounds indicate ability to tolerate food. |
| | When diet is ordered, offer small sips of water and advance as tolerated. | Small, frequent feedings decrease vomiting. |

### EVALUATION

Surgical site is infection free and shows signs of healing. Mucous membranes are moist. Fluid requirements are maintained. Client loses less than 5% of admission weight.

### NURSING DIAGNOSIS 2 _Acute **P**ain_ related to physical injury as evidenced by surgical procedure

**Nursing Outcomes Classification (NOC)**
_Pain Level_

**Nursing Interventions Classification (NIC)**
_Post-Anesthesia Care_
_Pain Management_

| PLANNING/OUTCOMES | NURSING INTERVENTIONS | RATIONALE |
|---|---|---|
| N.W. will be pain free. | Administer pain medications every 3 to 4 hours as prescribed and around-the-clock. | If child is able to sleep and rest, recovery is faster. |
| | Position for comfort; allow caregivers to hold and comfort. | |
| | Lubricate nostrils, if nasogatric tube present. | |
| | Perform procedures such as dressing changes and respiratory therapy after analgesia. | |

### EVALUATION

Child sleeps quietly and shows no signs of restlessness.

### NURSING DIAGNOSIS 3 _**A**nxiety (parental)_ related to hospitalization, colostomy, and home care as evidenced by parental reaction and questioning

**Nursing Outcomes Classification (NOC)**
_Coping_
_Acceptance: Health Status_

**Nursing Interventions Classification (NIC)**
_Coping Enhancement_
_Anticipatory Guidance_

| PLANNING/OUTCOMES | NURSING INTERVENTIONS | RATIONALE |
|---|---|---|
| N.W.'s parents will understand etiology, pathology, and treatment of illness. | Encourage expression of feelings. | Maintain positive family interaction during hospitalization. |
| | Explain procedures, keep informed of progress, and answer questions. | Facilitates development of rapport with the family. |

_(Continues)_

## SAMPLE NURSING CARE PLAN (Continued)

| PLANNING/OUTCOMES | NURSING INTERVENTIONS | RATIONALE |
|---|---|---|
| N.W.'s parents will provide comfort to their child. | Encourage parental presence and give positive reinforcement to client and family for cooperation and participation in care. | Active participation facilitates coping and decreases anxiety. |
| N.W.'s parents will demonstrate proper techniques for home care procedures. | Teach parents to provide colostomy care, dressing changes, fluids, nutrition, and growth-fostering activities. | Provides parents with skills required to care for N.W. at home. |
| | Refer to appropriate community resources. | Decreases parents' anxiety and ensures proper care is provided. |

### EVALUATION

Family care providers demonstrate skill and knowledge in caring for their child's needs. Parents verbalize decreased anxiety and return demonstrations of colostomy care and dressing changes.

# MUSCULOSKELETAL SYSTEM

The musculoskeletal system provides protection to vital organs, supports weight, stores minerals, and supplies RBCs. Disorders may be congenital or acquired and require short- or long-term care. Most alterations of the arms and legs are mild variations of normal posturing, but some are severe anomalies. The two most common congenital skeletal defects are clubfoot and dislocated hip.

## CONGENITAL TALIPES EQUINOVARUS (CLUB FOOT)

The equinovarus foot has a clublike appearance with the entire foot inverted, the heel drawn up, and the forefoot adducted (Figure 7-11). It can occur as a single anomaly or in connection with other defects such as **myelomeningocele** (a saclike protrusion situated along the vertebral column and filled with spinal fluid, meninges, nerve roots, and spinal cord). Club foot is apparent at birth and may be bilateral or unilateral. The degree of malformation and likelihood for complete correction varies. Even with correction, recurrence is common.

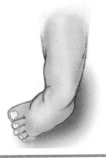

COURTESY OF DELMAR CENGAGE LEARNING

**FIGURE 7-11** **Club Foot**

## MEDICAL–SURGICAL MANAGEMENT

### Medical

Correction is usually started during the neonatal period with manipulation and casting of the foot. The long leg cast is changed every few days for the first few weeks and then every week or two for several months. Correction is confirmed by x-ray. Following casting, a splint with shoes attached is used for several months to maintain correction.

### Surgical

Children who do not respond to nonsurgical treatment within 3 to 6 months need surgical correction. Following surgery, a

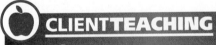

### CLIENT TEACHING

**Cast Care**

Instruct caregivers in the following regarding cast care:

- Casts must be changed as prescribed to maintain growth and comfort.
- Wet casts should be handled with the palms (to prevent indentations).
- Hair dryers should not be used to facilitate drying of the cast.
- Plaster of Paris casts should dry within 10 to 72 hours, depending on the size.
- Dry casts should be felt for "hot spots" and observed for visible stains due to drainage, which may indicate skin breakdown.
- Signs of swelling should be noted and reported immediately.
- Toes should be warm, pink, and moving.

cast is applied with the knee in a flexed position. After 6 to 12 weeks, casting is discontinued, and corrective shoes or bracing may be prescribed. Even with aggressive therapy, the foot is seldom entirely normal, and atrophy of the calf is common.

## NURSING MANAGEMENT

Assess and explore the caregivers' feelings about their less-than-perfect newborn, the caregivers knowledge about the defect, treatment, and need for long-term care. Nursing responsibilities include teaching the caregivers cast care, monitoring for complications, encouraging compliance with long-term follow-up, and facilitating normal development.

## ■ DEVELOPMENTAL DYSPLASIA OF THE HIP

Developmental **dysplasia** (abnormal development) of the hip (DDH) refers to a variety of conditions wherein the femoral head and the acetabulum are improperly aligned. These conditions include **dislocation** (displacement of the bone from its normal position in a joint), subluxation (partial dislocation), and acetabular dysplasia. These conditions can be congenital, but in some children, they develop after birth.

Manifestations include limited **abduction** (lateral movement away from body) of the affected hip, asymmetry of the gluteal and thigh fat folds, and telescoping or pistoning of the thigh. The walking infant may manifest minimal to pronounced variations in gait, with lurching toward the affected side. The longer the disorder goes untreated, the more pronounced the clinical manifestations become and the worse the prognosis.

## MEDICAL–SURGICAL MANAGEMENT

Early screening, detection, and treatment enable most affected children to attain normal hip function.

### Medical

For young infants, the Pavlik harness is used to maintain flexion, abduction, and external rotation (Figure 7-12). This harness is highly effective when used as prescribed. A hip spica cast may be necessary when the harness is ineffective. Older infants may require traction for weeks, either at home or in the hospital.

### Surgical

The older infant may require closed reduction under anesthesia and/or open reduction followed by a hip spica cast.

## NURSING MANAGEMENT

Teach caregivers how to use the Pavlik harness. If cast is necessary, teach caregivers cast care.

## NURSING PROCESS

### ASSESSMENT

#### Subjective Data

The nurse is alerted to the possibility of DDH when the infant has a history of being delivered by cesarean section or frank breech, is large for gestational age, or is a twin.

#### Objective Data

During the newborn assessment and routine nurturing activities, inspect the infant for limited abduction of the hip, a wide perineum, and unequal gluteal folds (Figure 7-13). The walking infant is assessed for a limp or an unusual gait.

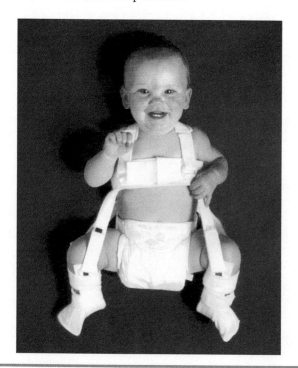

FIGURE 7-12 **A Pavlik harness is used to treat an infant with developmental dysplasia of the hip.** (*Courtesy Wheaton Brace Co., Carol Tream, IL.*)

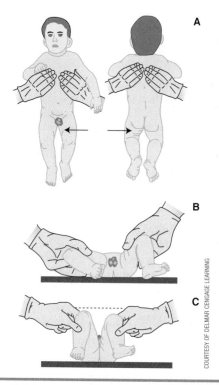

COURTESY OF DELMAR CENGAGE LEARNING

FIGURE 7-13 **Assessing for DDH; A, Thighs and gluteal folds will show asymmetry. B, Flexion will show limited hip abduction. C, Knee height will show uneven level caused by shortened femur.**

**Nursing diagnoses for the infant with DDH include the following:**

| NURSING DIAGNOSES | PLANNING/OUTCOMES | NURSING INTERVENTIONS |
|---|---|---|
| *Anxiety (parental)* related to having a less-than-perfect child and to the need to provide complex long-term care | The parents will verbalize feelings about their child and the condition.<br><br>The parents will carry out prescribed therapy and provide daily care with confidence. | Explore the parents' feelings about their less-than-perfect newborn and their knowledge about the defect, treatment, and need for long-term care.<br><br>Teach the parents about harness use (e.g., the hips should be flexed without being tight, the harness should be worn 23 hours per day).<br><br>Explore options for the safe transport of the infant (e.g., use of a special car seat, adaptation of stroller). |
| *Risk for Impaired **S**kin Integrity* related to devices | The client's skin will remain intact. | Teach the parents to assess the infant's skin for irritation and to change the infant's position every 2 to 4 hours.<br><br>Teach the parents ways of protecting the infant's skin from the brace (e.g., using a shirt that snaps at the crotch, long socks under the harness).<br><br>Teach the parents to change diapers without removing the harness.<br><br>Teach the parents to bathe the infant daily during the 1 hour that the harness is off. |
| *Delayed **G**rowth and Development* related to immobility and difficulty in positioning | The client will attain milestones appropriate for age and limitations. | Teach the parents to provide activities that stimulate the infant's upper extremities and all five senses (e.g., blocks, musical toys, balls, bright mobiles) and to interact with the infant.<br><br>Teach the parents methods of holding, nursing, feeding, and cuddling the infant when the harness is in use.<br><br>Instruct the parents to include the infant in family activities and outings. |

**Evaluation:** Evaluate each outcome to determine how it has been met by the client.

## ■ POSITIONAL PLAGIOCEPHALY

Positional plagiocephaly, also called flattened head syndrome, is a condition in which one side or the back of an infant's head is flattened. This can be caused when the infant is put to sleep in the same position repeatedly or by neck muscle problems. Queenan (2001) reports that the number of positional plagiocephaly cases increased six-fold from 1992 to 1994. These were the first two years following the American Academy of Pediatrics' (AAP) "Back to Sleep" promotion for infants to sleep on their backs to prevent sudden infant death syndrome (SIDS). SIDS has decreased, but positional plagiocephaly, which has an excellent corrective prognosis when treated early, has dramatically increased.

This head deformation is not self-correcting. Sometimes, after the infant's hair has grown, mild asymmetrical features may appear normal.

## MEDICAL–SURGICAL MANAGEMENT

Early identification and treatment allows time for reshaping of the head before sutures and fontanels close.

### Medical

When this positional deformity is detected, infants are generally placed in a light-weight plastic helmet or band, which redirects symmetrical growth of the infant's head (Figure 7-14).

## NURSING MANAGEMENT

Prevention is the key through caregiver teaching. Caregivers should be taught to alternate the infant's head position during sleep (one sleep period with the right side of the head touching the mattress and the next sleep period the left). The infant is supine to sleep. Infants should not be left in an infant carrier,

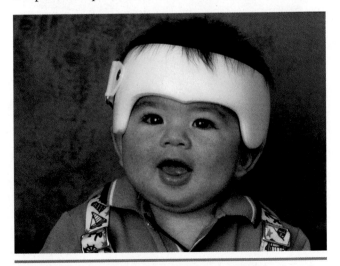

**FIGURE 7-14** **Child in DOC (Dynamic Orthotic Cranioplasy) Band for Positional Plagiocephaly** (*Courtesy of Cranial Technologies, Inc.*)

car seat, or swing for extended periods. Providing as much "tummy time" as possible when the infant is awake and supervised gives the back of the infant's head a rest and reduces the risk of developing positional plagiocephaly. This tummy position also strengthens neck muscles and arms and encourages learning and discovery of the world around.

# INTEGUMENTARY SYSTEM

Normally, infants have soft, smooth, dry, cool, taut, elastic skin. Color is evenly distributed but may display variations such as freckles, **mongolian spots** (large patches of bluish skin on the buttocks of dark-skinned infants), small hemangiomas called "stork bites" (on eyelids or back of the neck), and **milia** (pearly white cysts on the face). Most of these blemishes disappear within months and require no treatment.

The infant's skin is immature and, thus, susceptible to disorders. The most frequently seen skin disorders include milia rubra, diaper dermatitis, seborrheic dermatitis, and atopic dermatitis.

## ■ MILIA RUBRA

Milia rubra, also known as prickly heat, is most noticeable on the folds of the skin, chest, and neck. This rash appears as pinhead-sized **erythematous** (reddishness of the skin) papules. It commonly occurs when infants are febrile or overdressed in summer heat. Infants may be irritable because of itching.

### NURSING MANAGEMENT

Treatment is primarily preventive. Teach caregivers to avoid bundling infants in hot weather. Tepid baths may help alleviate itching.

## ■ DIAPER DERMATITIS

Diaper dermatitis, also called diaper rash, is characterized by erythema (redness), edema, vesicles, papules, and scaling on the perineum, genitals, buttocks, and skin folds. It is caused by repetitive exposure to an irritant such as urine, feces, soap, detergent, ointment, friction, or infection resulting from bacteria or yeast (*Candida albicans*) (Figure 7-15). The incidence is generally reported to be greater among bottle-fed than among breastfed infants (Hockenberry et al., 2006).

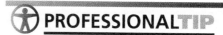

# PROFESSIONALTIP

### Mongolian Spots

It is important for nurses to be aware that blemishes such as mongolian spots are common in dark-skinned infants up to 24 months of age and, thus, should not be mistaken for signs of child abuse.

### NURSING MANAGEMENT

To prevent diaper rash, teach care providers to change diapers frequently and keep the infant's skin clean and dry. Use of disposable diapers and exposure of healthy skin to air, not heat, will help keep the skin dry. Ointments such as zinc oxide or petrolatum may be used to protect inflamed skin. Nystatin (Mycostatin) ointment or cream may be applied to treat *Candida*.

## ■ SEBORRHEIC DERMATITIS

Seborrheic dermatitis, also called cradle cap, is characterized by yellowish, scaly, or crusted patches on the scalp of infants up to 3 months of age (Figure 7-16). It typically results from excessive sebaceous gland activity.

### NURSING MANAGEMENT

Teach caregivers that cradle cap is not caused by poor hygiene but, rather, by increased sebum production by the scalp. It will eventually disappear, although children with dry skin may continue to have flakes on the scalp. A mild shampoo or mineral oil may be left on the scalp for a few minutes to help soften and loosen the crust. Then rinse and comb the hair with a fine-toothed comb to loosen and remove the crust. In most cases, no further treatment is needed. The crusting can usually be prevented by washing the infant's head with a washcloth and using a fine-toothed comb.

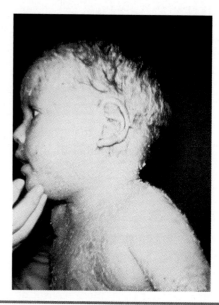

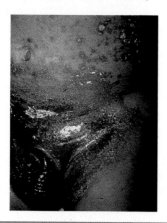

**FIGURE 7-15** Candidiasis (*Courtesy of the Centers for Disease Control and Prevention.*)

**FIGURE 7-16** Seborrheic Dermatitis (*Courtesy of the Center for Disease Control and Prevention.*)

## ATOPIC DERMATITIS

Atopic dermatitis, also called eczema, is a chronic, superficial inflammatory skin disorder characterized by intense **pruritus** (severe itching). It is considered to be at least in part an allergic reaction to irritants (wool, nylon, plastics, detergents, perspiration, cosmetics, and perfumed lotions and soaps) and allergens (dust, pollens, and foods). A strong family history of eczema, asthma, food allergies, or allergic rhinitis usually predisposes a child to eczema. The disorder is uncommon among breastfed infants before other foods are added to the diet.

Papules and vesicles usually begin forming on the cheeks and spread to the arms and legs and then to the trunk. Exudate and crust are often present.

Infantile eczema usually resolves by the age of 3 years; however, infants who have eczema tend to develop hay fever or asthma later in life.

## MEDICAL–SURGICAL MANAGEMENT
### Medical

Treatment is aimed at relieving pruritus, hydrating skin, reducing inflammation, and preventing secondary infections. Baths and compresses may provide temporary relief.

### Pharmacological

A variety of lotions, oral antihistamines, topical corticosteroids, and antibiotics may be prescribed.

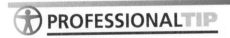

## PROFESSIONAL TIP

### Controlling Allergens

When teaching caregivers about the need to decrease allergens in the child's environment, the nurse should stress the following:

- "Smoking outside" rather than "not smoking"
- "Keeping pets outside" rather than "getting rid of pets"
- "Removing as much dust as possible from the child's room" rather than "removing as much dust as possible from the entire house"
- Consider using an air purifier or air-filtering machine

Providing alternatives to the ideal situation may empower caregivers to set more realistic goals for improving their child's environment.

### Diet

A diet including a milk substitute such as soy formula, a vitamin supplement, and foods known to be hypoallergenic may be instituted to rule out offending foods. If the child's skin improves, foods are added back into the diet one at a time at intervals of approximately 1 week. The effects are then noted and any allergenic foods eliminated from the child's diet.

### Health Promotion

Guidelines for preventing eczema include practicing breastfeeding; prohibiting cow's milk, eggs, fish, corn, citrus, peanuts, nuts, and chocolate for the first 12 months of life; and delaying introduction of solid foods until 6 months of age. Environmental control of dust, mold, animals, and cigarette smoke is also recommended.

## NURSING MANAGEMENT

The major nursing goals are to soothe and relieve pruritus, maintain skin integrity, provide adequate nutrition and fluids, offer sensory stimulation, and teach the family about the condition. Caregivers may feel apprehensive or repulsed by their infant's appearance. They need to be encouraged to express their feelings but be assured that eczema, while potentially distressing, is a temporary condition.

## NEUROLOGICAL SYSTEM

By the fourth week of gestation, the neural tube has closed, and the brain and the spinal cord have begun to form. By the second month of gestation, the brain is the most prominent part of the body. It grows rapidly and continues to grow through the fifth year of life. As myelinization of the peripheral nerves progresses, so do the child's coordination and fine motor abilities. The primitive reflexes (Moro, grasp, and rooting) disappear by 12 months of age. Alterations discussed following are spina bifida, hydrocephalus, febrile convulsions, **meningitis** (inflammation of the meninges), and cerebral palsy.

## SPINA BIFIDA

Spina bifida is a neural tube defect wherein incomplete closure of the vertebrae and neural tube results in an opening through which meninges and spinal cord may protrude. Although the cause remains undetermined, genetic predisposition, maternal folic acid deficiency during pregnancy, and environmental factors such as pollution may be implicated. The severity of the defect can vary, with manifestations ranging from a dimple or small tuft of hair (which may be overlooked at birth) to a large, saclike protrusion anywhere along the lumbar or sacral area (Figure 7-17). The most severe form is myelomeningocele. The degree of neurological impairment depends on the location of the defect on the spinal cord and the size of the defect. The child may be asymptomatic or display neurological impairments varying from mild sensory loss to complete paralysis below the lesion. Associated defects may include hydrocephalus (present in 90% of clients) and genitourinary and orthopedic defects. Although these children often require lifelong therapy and care, many ultimately go on to live independently and become productive adults.

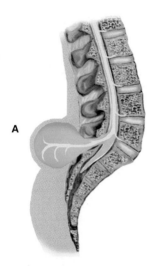

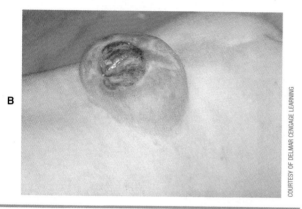

COURTESY OF DELMAR CENGAGE LEARNING

FIGURE 7-17  *A,* Illustration of Myelomeningocele; *B,* Myeleomeningocele

## MEDICAL–SURGICAL MANAGEMENT
### Medical

Specialists such as neurologists, neurosurgeons, orthopedic specialists, pediatricians, urologists, and physical therapists may be needed to provide surgical repair and follow-up treatment.

### Surgical

Surgery is required to close the defect but may not be performed immediately after birth. Waiting several days gives the family time to adjust to the initial shock and become involved in the decision-making process. Immediate closure reduces the risk of infection and allows for easier handling of the infant, which, in turn, facilitates earlier bonding.

## NURSING MANAGEMENT

Preoperatively, monitor vital signs, neurological status, and behavior. Maintain infant in a prone position. Keep sac covered with moist, warm, sterile dressings and change every 2 hours. Administer medications as ordered.

Postoperatively, monitor vital signs, I&O, and provide prescribed wound care. Teach caregivers intermittent catheterization to keep infant's bladder empty until incision heals. Teach caregivers how to elicit sucking and to feed and cuddle infant, signs of increased intracranial pressure, and signs of constipation. Refer to Spina Bifida Association.

## NURSING PROCESS

### ASSESSMENT
#### Subjective Data

Assess the caregivers' feelings about their less-than-perfect newborn and their knowledge about the defect, the treatment, and the need for long-term care.

#### Objective Data

At birth, assess the intactness of the membranous sac. Assess neurological impairment by noting movement of the extremities; reflexes; anal reflex; urinary output; vital signs; fontanelles; and head circumference.

### Nursing diagnoses for the infant with spina bifida include the following:

| NURSING DIAGNOSES | PLANNING/OUTCOMES | NURSING INTERVENTIONS |
|---|---|---|
| *Anxiety (parental)* related to having a less-than-perfect child and to the need to provide complex long-term care | The caregivers will verbalize their feelings about the child and condition.<br><br>The caregivers will carry out prescribed therapy and provide daily care with confidence. | Explore the caregivers' feelings about their less-than-perfect newborn and their knowledge about the defect, the treatment, and the need for long-term care.<br><br>Teach the caregivers ways to elicit sucking and to feed and cuddle the infant.<br><br>Teach the caregivers to assess for signs of constipation, such as abdominal distention, vomiting, and poor feeding.<br><br>Teach the caregivers to recognize signs of increased intracranial pressure, such as irritability, restlessness, and vomiting.<br><br>Explore options for mobility, such as splints, a walker, or a wheelchair.<br><br>Refer caregivers to the Spina Bifida Association and to local resources and support groups. |

*(Continues)*

**Nursing diagnoses for the infant with spina bifida include the following: (Continued)**

| NURSING DIAGNOSES | PLANNING/OUTCOMES | NURSING INTERVENTIONS |
|---|---|---|
| *Risk for Infection* related to vulnerability of the sac, the surgical procedure, and the lack of bowel and bladder control | The client will be infection free. | **Preoperative:**<br>Monitor the infant's vital signs, neurological status, and behavior.<br>Administer prophylactic antibiotics, as ordered.<br>Keep the sac covered with a moist, warm, sterile dressing and change every 2 hours.<br>Maintain the infant in the prone position.<br>Protect the sac from fecal contamination.<br>**Postoperative:**<br>Provide prescribed wound care.<br>Instruct the caregivers in the use of intermittent, clean catheterization to keep bladder empty. |
| *Delayed Growth and Development* related to immobility | The client will attain milestones appropriate for age and limitations. | Teach the caregivers to provide activities that stimulate the infant's upper extremities and all five senses and to interact with the infant.<br>Instruct the caregivers to include the infant in family activities and outings.<br>Explore options for education and vocational training as the child grows older. |

**Evaluation:** Evaluate each outcome to determine how it has been met by the client.

## ■ HYDROCEPHALUS

In hydrocephalus, the balance between the rate of cerebrospinal fluid (CSF) formation and absorption is disturbed. This disturbance may result from an obstruction in the circulation of CSF or from defective absorption. Hydrocephalus may be recognized at birth or weeks or months later. The condition may be congenital or occur as the result of a neoplasm, a head injury, or an infection.

Manifestations include an excessively large head at birth or rapid head growth along with widening cranial sutures. As pressure increases, the anterior fontanel becomes tense and bulges, and the eyes appear to be pushed downward, with the sclera visible above the iris ("sunset eyes"). Because of the increase in intracranial pressure, the infant may display irritability, restlessness, a high-pitched cry, vomiting, seizure, and change in level of consciousness.

### MEDICAL–SURGICAL MANAGEMENT

#### Surgical

Surgical intervention is the only effective means of relieving brain pressure and preventing further damage to the brain tissue. Surgery involves removing the obstruction or inserting a shunting device that bypasses the point of obstruction and drains the excess CSF into a body cavity, usually the peritoneum.

### NURSING MANAGEMENT

Monitor vital signs, head circumference, and neurological signs. Prevent infections, provide loving care to the child and

support to the caregivers, and increase the family's knowledge about the condition. Set realistic growth and development goals. Many infants with hydrocephalus are able to ultimately live independently and become productive adults despite associated neurological disabilities.

## ■ FEBRILE CONVULSIONS

A convulsion or seizure involves involuntary muscle contraction and relaxation. Seizures may be a symptom of a wide variety of disorders. In infants and children, febrile seizures usually accompany such infections as otitis media, upper respiratory infections, and meningitis. Clinical manifestations include sudden occurrence, body stiffening, and loss of consciousness followed by quick, jerking movements of the arms, legs, and facial muscles. Breathing may be irregular, and swallowing ability may be absent.

Febrile seizures usually occur early in the course of a high fever. Usually, only one seizure occurs, and it will last less than 3 minutes. Febrile seizures carry little risk of neurological damage.

### MEDICAL–SURGICAL MANAGEMENT

#### ■ Pharmacological

Most febrile seizures stop before the infant can be taken for medical attention. If the seizure continues, diazepam (Valium) is the drug of choice. Antipyretics such as acetaminophen (Tylenol) or ibuprofen (Motrin) may be used to reduce the infant's fever.

# NURSING MANAGEMENT

Focus on teaching caregivers about febrile seizures and treating a fever. caregivers are naturally extremely anxious when their child has experienced a seizure, especially the first time. Reassure the caregivers that febrile seizures are not life threatening, do not cause neurological damage, are common in children younger than 5 years of age who are experiencing infection, usually do not recur, and usually last less than 3 minutes.

## ■ MENINGITIS

The most common infection of the central nervous system (CNS) in infants is meningitis. The three main types of causative organisms are bacterial, tubercular, and viral. Meningitis may also occur as the result of complications of neurosurgery, trauma, systemic infection, or sinus or ear infection. Bacterial meningitis is the most common and serves as the focus of this discussion.

Clinical manifestations may occur suddenly or gradually and include neurological symptoms such as a high-pitched cry, fever, seizures, irritability, as well as vomiting, a bulging anterior fontanel, and poor feeding. Early diagnosis and treatment are essential for uncomplicated recovery.

## MEDICAL–SURGICAL MANAGEMENT

### Medical

Meningitis is a medical emergency. A spinal tap (lumbar puncture) is performed promptly whenever symptoms are present and before administration of antibiotics. The causative organism usually can be ascertained from stained smears of the spinal fluid. Appropriate IV antibiotics are prescribed for bacterial meningitis. The infant is isolated from other clients for at least 24 hours.

### Health Promotion

Current immunization schedules include the *Haemophilus influenzae* type b conjugate vaccine (HbCV). The incidence of *H. influenza* type B (Hib) has greatly decreased since the advent of this immunization.

### Nursing Management

After assisting with the spinal tap and starting the IV, complete the history and physical. It is important to note any food and fluid intake, nausea, vomiting, or loss of appetite, as well as recent immunizations, illnesses, surgery, and injuries and previous lumbar puncture.

Perform a complete neurological assessment and an evaluation of head circumference. Examine the fontanelles for bulging.

Maintain in isolation for at least 24 hours, administer antibiotics, monitor neurological status every 4 hours, maintain fluid balance, establish trust with the caregivers and infant, teach the caregivers about the disease and ways to care for their infant, and refer close contacts for possible prophylactic treatment.

## ■ CEREBRAL PALSY

Cerebral palsy (CP) is a nonprogressive motor disorder resulting from damage to the motor centers of the brain. This damage can occur during the prenatal, perinatal, or postnatal period.

Manifestations of CP vary in severity and may include delayed gross motor development (e.g., persistent head lag), alterations in muscle tone (e.g., body stiffness), abnormal motor performance (e.g., uncoordinated or involuntary movements), and reflex abnormalities (e.g., persistent tonic neck). In addition, the child may experience seizures, impaired vision and hearing, difficulty swallowing and speaking, and subnormal learning and reasoning. Less-severe cases of CP may not be diagnosed until 2 years of age.

## MEDICAL–SURGICAL MANAGEMENT

### Medical

A multidisciplinary team including the family, pediatricians, neurologists, surgeons, nurses, nutritionists, therapists, social workers, and special education teachers is necessary to assist the child in developing maximum potential.

### Surgical

Surgical intervention such as lengthening the Achilles' tendon and releasing the hamstrings may be necessary to improve ambulation.

## NURSING MANAGEMENT

Encourage caregivers to stimulate and interact with their infant and participate in an infant-stimulation program. Refer to nutritionist, occupational therapist, and speech therapist as needed.

# NURSING PROCESS

## ASSESSMENT

### Subjective Data

A history of conditions such as maternal diabetes, ABO or Rh incompatibilities, rubella in the first trimester, prematurity, prolonged labor, and postnatal infections or trauma may predispose an infant to brain damage and CP.

### Objective Data

Further observe the infant who feeds poorly and is rigid, tense, or hypotonic. Assess for developmental delays with an instrument such as the Denver II test.

---

### 🍎 CLIENT TEACHING

#### Tips for Treating a Fever

Teach caregivers to care for their febrile infant by:

- Administering acetaminophen or ibuprophen, but never aspirin
- Providing more clothing if the child is too cold and less clothing if the child is too warm, to prevent shivering
- Applying cool, moist compresses to the forehead 1 hour after administering an antipyretic
- Encouraging fluid intake (e.g., water, juice, ice, popsicles)

**Nursing diagnoses for the infant with CP include the following:**

| NURSING DIAGNOSES | PLANNING/OUTCOMES | NURSING INTERVENTIONS |
|---|---|---|
| *Imbalanced **N**utrition: Less than Body Requirements* related to difficulty chewing and swallowing and to increased muscle activity | The client will maintain a normal growth curve above the fifth percentile on the growth chart. | Encourage active swallowing by maintenance of a flexed sitting position, with the arms brought forward. Provide jaw stabilization from the front or side of the face. Provide a flexible feeding schedule with frequent, small feedings. Encourage use of adaptive utensils and foods to stimulate self-care (e.g., finger foods, foods that stick to utensils, spoon with padded handle). Refer to a nutritionist and an occupational therapist, as needed. |
| *Delayed **G**rowth and Development* related to neuromuscular impairment | The client will achieve maximum potential. | Teach the caregivers to stimulate the infant and to interact on the infant's functional level. Encourage early intervention and participation in infant-stimulation programs. |
| *Impaired Physical **M**obility* related to spasticity and muscle weakness | The client will attain mobility via assistive devices. | Refer to a physical therapist, as needed. Evaluate the need for special equipment. Ensure adequate rest. Perform prescribed range-of-motion and stretching exercises. Provide preoperative and postoperative care for the infant who requires corrective surgery. Select toys and activities that improve motor activity (e.g., place a desired toy such that the child must reach). |
| *Impaired Verbal **C**ommunication* related to neuromuscular impairment and difficulty with articulation | The client will develop methods of communication. | Refer to a speech therapist, as needed. Encourage the use of flash cards, articles, pictures, talking boards, a computer with a voice synthesizer. Encourage jaw-stabilization methods (as with feeding) to facilitate speech. |

**Evaluation**: Evaluate each outcome to determine how it has been met by the client.

# GENITOURINARY SYSTEM

During infancy, the kidneys are less able to concentrate urine, and output per kilogram of body weight is higher than that of an adult. Bladder capacity increases with age, from 20 to 50 mL at birth to 700 mL in adulthood, and the infant's urethra is shorter than the adult's. In addition, infants lack bladder control because of insufficient nerve development.

Most external defects of the genitourinary (GU) tract are not life threatening in the physical sense but may present social problems with lifelong implications for the child and family. More severe disorders such as exstrophy of the bladder and ambiguous genitalia lead to concerns about penis size, appearance of the genitalia, altered elimination, potential ability to procreate, and rejection by peers. These children and their caregivers need emotional support in order to adjust to these permanent alterations. Hypospadias, hydrocele, cryptorchidism, vesicoureteral reflux, and Wilms' tumor are the most common types of urinary alterations.

# HYPOSPADIAS

Hypospadias is a condition wherein the urethral opening is on the ventral (under) surface of the penis (Figure 7-18). It is often associated with undescended testes and inguinal hernia and is visible on inspection at birth.

## MEDICAL–SURGICAL MANAGEMENT
### Surgical

Hypospadias is surgically corrected during the first year of life. The infant is not circumcised at birth because the foreskin may be used to correct the defect.

## NURSING MANAGEMENT

Focus on preparing caregivers for the surgical procedure and for postoperative and home care. Assure caregivers that normal urination will be restored and that sexual function will

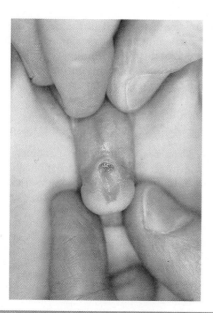

**FIGURE 7-18** Hypospadias (*Courtesy of Dr. James Mandell, Chief Surgeon, Urology, Albany Medical College, Albany, NY.*)

not be impeded. Tell them that the penis may never appear perfectly normal, even after the surgery. The infant may go home with a catheter in place until healing is complete. Teach caregivers proper catheterization technique and have them demonstrate catheter care before discharge.

## HYDROCELE

Hydrocele is the result of the processus vaginalis failing to close, which allows fluid to enter the scrotum. The scrotum contains a palpable, round, nontender mass. This defect is often associated with inguinal hernia.

## MEDICAL–SURGICAL MANAGEMENT

### Medical

Most hydroceles will close by 1 year of age without intervention.

### Surgical

If spontaneous closure does not occur by 1 year of age, surgical intervention may be done on an outpatient basis.

## NURSING MANAGEMENT

Preoperative preparation and postoperative care are the focus of the nurse. Postoperatively, focus on pain management, infection control, and activity restriction. Alert caregivers to the potential for temporary swelling and discoloration of the scrotum.

## CRYPTORCHIDISM

Cryptorchidism is a condition wherein one or both testes do not descend into the scrotal sac. One or both sides of the scrotum appear to be smaller than normal. When palpated, the scrotal sac is empty. This defect is often associated with inguinal hernia.

### COMMUNITY/HOME HEALTH CARE

**Infant with External GU Defect Repair**

*Pain Management*
- Medicate for pain as prescribed for 24 to 48 hours postoperatively.
- Protect the site by double diapering.

*Infection Control*
- Wash hands before and after diapering.
- Carefully and thoroughly cleanse any area soiled with stool or urine.
- Watch for signs of infection, such as fever, irritability, drainage, and redness.
- Increase fluid intake.

*Activity Restriction*
- Do not allow the infant to play on riding toys.
- Do not allow the infant to straddle the caregiver's hip when being carried.

## MEDICAL–SURGICAL MANAGEMENT

### Medical

The testes usually descend spontaneously by 1 year of age. If the testes have not descended after 1 year, hormone therapy may be prescribed.

### Surgical

Surgical correction, if required, is performed by 3 years of age to prevent sterility.

## NURSING MANAGEMENT

Preoperative preparation and postoperative care are the primary nursing concerns. Postoperative care focuses on pain management, infection control, and activity restriction.

## VESICOURETERAL REFLUX

Vesicoureteral reflux refers to the backflow of urine from the bladder into the ureters and, possibly, the kidneys. Reflux can result from abnormal insertion of the ureters into the bladder or from a urinary tract infection (UTI). The primary manifestation of vesicoureteral reflux is recurrent UTIs. Specific clues of a UTI in the infant include poor feeding; vomiting; and failure to gain weight. A UTI is confirmed by detection of bacteria in the urine. Early diagnosis with radiological studies is important to prevent renal injury.

## MEDICAL–SURGICAL MANAGEMENT

### Medical

The primary concern is preventing UTIs. Low-dose prophylactic antibiotic therapy is prescribed until the reflux is resolved. In addition, urine cultures, cystograms, and blood studies are necessary to monitor for UTI and kidney function. Less-severe refluxes will resolve spontaneously.

## Surgical

Surgical reimplantation of the ureter(s) into the bladder may be necessary if UTIs persist.

## NURSING MANAGEMENT

Nursing care includes treatment and prevention of UTIs (see the Urinary System chapter). Help caregivers understand that medical treatment may be needed for years and that compliance as well as follow-up is important. If surgery is required, provide pre- and postoperative care.

## ■ WILMS' TUMOR

Wilms' tumor (nephroblastoma) is found in the kidney region and is one of the most common early childhood cancers. The tumor arises from bits of embryonic tissue remaining after birth. The etiology is unknown, but Wilms' tumor is associated with other anomalies such as GU defects, microcephaly, and mental retardation. The most common manifestations are an abdominal mass located to one side of the midline, abdominal pain, malaise, anemia, and fever.

## MEDICAL–SURGICAL MANAGEMENT

### Surgical

Surgical removal of the involved kidney and lymph node is the treatment of choice. Chemotherapy and radiation may be used pre- and postoperatively, depending on the stage and size of the tumor.

## NURSING MANAGEMENT

If a mass is felt in a child's abdomen, stop palpation immediately because it is possible to dislodge cells and spread the tumor. Focus on pre- and postoperative care, chemotherapy administration, and caregiver support.

## COGNITIVE AND SENSORY SYSTEMS

Cognitive and sensory impairments result in a variety of lifelong challenges for infants and their families. Nurs-

### PROFESSIONALTIP

#### Wilms' Tumor

If a client has a Wilms' tumor, a sign stating, "Do not palpate the abdomen" should be posted at the head of the bed. Palpating the abdomen can dislodge cells and spread the tumor.

ing care focuses on assessment of the degree of impairment and on appropriate interventions for individual and caregiver adaptation. Some of the most common cognitive and sensory impairments occurring in infants include Down syndrome and visual and hearing impairments.

## ■ DOWN SYNDROME

Down syndrome is a chromosomal anomaly resulting in moderate to severe mental retardation. Evidence supports trisomy 21 (an extra chromosome); translocation of chromosomes 15, 21, and 22; and advanced parental age as possible causes of Down syndrome.

Manifestations include a variety of facial and body abnormalities and intellectual, language, and social alterations. Typically, the child with Down syndrome has upward- and outward-slanted (almond-shaped) eyes; a depressed nasal bridge; a protruding tongue; small, short, low-set ears; a short, broad neck; transverse palmar crease; broad, short hands with stubby fingers; a protruding abdomen; hypotonia (lax muscle tone); and a blunted affect (Figure 7-19). Numerous medical conditions may be associated with Down syndrome, including cardiac anomalies, GI defects, endocrine disorders, and leukemia.

### CLIENTTEACHING

#### Feeding the Infant with Down Syndrome

- The tongue thrust represents a physiologic response rather than a refusal to eat.
- Use a long, straight-handled spoon to place food to the back and side of the mouth.
- Refeed food that is thrust out of the mouth.
- Increase fluids and fiber to prevent constipation.
- Monitor height and weight by plotting on a growth chart each month.

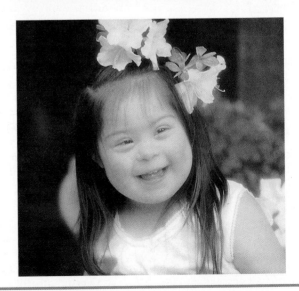

FIGURE 7-19 Young Girl with Down Syndrome (*Courtesy of Down Right Beautiful 1996 Calendar, Marijane Scott, Marijane's Designer Portraits.*)

## MEDICAL–SURGICAL MANAGEMENT

### Medical

A multidisciplinary team of health care providers may be needed to assist the child with Down syndrome to reach personal maximum potential. During the first year, the focus is on monitoring for GI and cardiac disorders. Between the second and fourth years, medical emphasis is on sleep and behavioral difficulties, thyroid screening, and visual and dental assessment. Frequent infections are a common problem.

### Surgical

Surgery may be required for correction of associated cardiac and GI anomalies.

### Health Promotion

Prenatal diagnosis of Down syndrome is possible through genetic testing, alpha-fetoprotein (AFP) level, or amniotic fluid samples. As a result of increased prenatal diagnosis, approximately 40% of fetuses with Down syndrome in women older than 35 years of age are now electively terminated (James et al., 2002). Therefore, the number of children born with Down syndrome is decreasing. For people born with Down syndrome, life expectancy has increased dramatically in recent decades from 25-years-of-age in 1983 to 7-years-of-age today.

## NURSING MANAGEMENT

Assist caregivers to identify positive features and behaviors of infant. Emphasize that the infant needs play, discipline, and social interactions like every infant. Encourage the caregivers to teach the child socially acceptable behaviors and to express their own fears and concerns.

## NURSING PROCESS

### ASSESSMENT

#### Subjective Data

At birth, it is especially important to elicit the family's health history, the results of amniocentesis (if done), and parental ages. As the infant grows, thoroughly evaluate interaction between the child and caregivers, the caregiver's coping abilities, and the degree to which the child is thriving.

#### Objective Data

During the initial physical examination at birth, assess for the unique features that indicate Down syndrome. As the child grows, assessment of developmental milestones will indicate delays in all areas (language, social, and motor).

### Nursing diagnoses for the infant with Down syndrome include the following:

| NURSING DIAGNOSES | PLANNING/OUTCOMES | NURSING INTERVENTIONS |
|---|---|---|
| *Social Isolation* related to fear of and embarrassment about the child's behavior or appearance | The family will achieve optimal socialization. | Assist in identifying positive features and behaviors in the infant. |
| | | Emphasize that the infant needs play, discipline, and social interaction, as does any infant. |
| | | Encourage the family to teach the child socially acceptable behaviors (e.g., manners and appropriate touch). |
| | | Encourage the family to express feelings and concerns. |
| | | Refer the family to support groups. |
| *Delayed Growth and Development* related to poor sucking abilities and anomalies | The client will maintain a normal growth curve above the fifth percentile. | Explore options for ensuring optimal fluid and calorie intake (e.g., adaptive utensils). |
| | | Encourage self-feeding, when age appropriate. |
| | | Maintain routine. |
| | | Refer to dietitian, as needed. |

**Evaluation**: Evaluate each outcome to determine how it has been met by the client.

## ■ VISUAL IMPAIRMENT

The eye is not fully developed until approximately 10 to 12 years of age. Visual acuity normally increases from a range of 20/50 to 20/80 at birth to a range of 20/20 to 20/30 by age 5 years.

Visual impairments are classified as follows: sighted with eye problems, partially sighted (20/70 to 20/200), and legally blind (20/200 or less). Refractory errors are the most common type of childhood visual disorders.

Strabismus (crossed eye) is caused by lack of coordination of the extraocular muscles. When both eyes are unable to focus simultaneously, the brain suppresses the image from the deviating eye to prevent double vision (diplopia). Amblyopia (blindness from disuse) can develop if strabismus is not treated early. If untreated amblyopia occurs in a child younger than 4 years of age, permanent loss of vision in the deviated eye may result.

Manifestations of visual impairment may include failure to follow an object or to react to bright light, excessive rubbing of the eyes, squinting, tilting of the head, and crossed eyes (after 6 months of age). Visual impairments may be caused by perinatal and postnatal infections; conditions such as sickle-cell disease, juvenile rheumatoid arthritis, glaucoma, cataracts, and retinoblastoma; and injuries.

# MEDICAL–SURGICAL MANAGEMENT

## Medical

Most visual disorders are treated with corrective lenses. Strabismus may require patching of the stronger eye to increase visual stimulation of the weaker eye. The earlier the treatment, the better the chances of normal development and function and adequate vision.

## Surgical

Surgical intervention is required for glaucoma, cataracts, and, sometimes, strabismus.

# NURSING MANAGEMENT

Early detection and referral are crucial in preventing childhood visual impairment. At birth, assess response to visual stimuli, ability to fixate and follow an object to midline, and ability to make eye contact. At 3 months of age, assess the infant for ability to follow moving objects. Crossed eyes after 6 months of age warrants further evaluation. Make referrals to available associations and support groups as needed (see the Resources listed at the end of this chapter).

Provide preoperative and postoperative care when surgical intervention is required. Educate the caregivers about the condition, the prescribed treatment, home care, and follow-up.

# HEARING IMPAIRMENT

At birth, the ear is completely developed. Hearing impairments range from mild to profound and include deaf as well as hard of hearing. Hearing loss is divided into four categories. Conductive (middle-ear hearing loss) is the most common type of hearing impairment and results from interference of transmission of sound to the middle ear. It is usually caused by otitis media. Sensorineural hearing loss (nerve deafness) involves damage to the inner-ear structures and/or auditory nerves. Mixed hearing loss is a combination of conductive and sensorineural loss. It is usually caused by recurrent otitis media. Central hearing loss results from damage to the conduction system between the brainstem and the cerebral cortex.

Infants at risk for hearing loss include those with prenatal, perinatal, and postnatal conditions including a family history of hearing impairments; malformations; low birthweight; asphyxia; infection; CP; Down syndrome; or a history of being administered ototoxic drugs.

Manifestations of hearing impairment in the infant include failure to startle or awaken to a loud sound, to turn the head to sound by 4 months of age, and to babble by 3 months of age. As the child with a hearing impairment matures, language skills are affected, and the child may be perceived as having cognitive as well as behavioral problems.

**CRITICAL THINKING**

**Altered Sensory Functioning**

What can nurses do to decrease the incidence of alterations in sensory function among children?

# MEDICAL–SURGICAL MANAGEMENT

## Medical

Treatment depends on the cause and type of loss. Antibiotics are prescribed for otitis media, which is the most common cause of conduction loss. Sensorineural loss is usually irreversible. Hearing aids or cochlear implants may be recommended.

## Surgical

Insertion of tympanostomy tubes for chronic otitis media is controversial.

# NURSING MANAGEMENT

Detection and prevention are the most important goals for the nurse. Assess all children for hearing acuity at birth, at well-child visits, and whenever there is a complaint specific to the ears. Developmental assessments reveal language delays in infants and children with hearing impairments. When delays are noted, refer the child for further evaluation.

# CHILD ABUSE

Child abuse is any intentional act of physical neglect or physical, emotional, or sexual abuse committed by a person responsible for the care of a child. In 2007, an estimated 794,000 children were victims of maltreatment, and there were an estimated 1,760 child fatalities, with children younger than 1 year accounting for 42.2% of fatalities. Young children are more vulnerable due to their dependency on care givers, small size, and inability to defend themselves. One or both parents are usually responsible for child abuse or neglect fatalities. Fatalities from physical abuse are most often perpetrated by fathers and mothers and commonly result from neglect (USDHHS, 2009).

# PHYSICAL NEGLECT

Physical neglect is failure to provide the adequate hygiene, health care, nutrition, love, nurturing, and supervision required for an infant's normal growth and development. Clinical manifestations of physical neglect in the infant may include inadequate weight gain, dental caries, poor hygiene, and lack of immunizations.

# PHYSICAL ABUSE

Physical punishment that leaves marks, causes injury, or threatens the child's physical or emotional well-being is considered physical abuse. Typical clinical manifestations of physical abuse include bruises on the abdomen, buttocks, genitalia, thighs, and mouth; bruises with distinctive outlines indicative of such things as hangers, belt buckles, hands, teeth, and sticks; bone fractures at various stages of healing; spiral fractures; cerebral edema or hemorrhage; and burns (e.g., from immersion of feet in hot water or from cigarettes). The child may appear sad and forlorn or may actively seek to please.

Predisposing factors to physical abuse include characteristics of the caregiver, child, and environment. Caregivers who abuse their children may have been severely punished as children, have difficulty controlling aggressive impulses, be socially isolated, and have few supportive relationships. Children at greatest risk for abuse are those who are premature, illegitimate, unwanted, brain damaged, hyperactive, physically disabled, or "difficult" (James et al., 2002; Hockenberry et al., 2006). A stressful environment caused by divorce, poverty, unemployment, poor housing, frequent relocation, and drug addiction may contribute to physical abuse; however, abuse occurs at all educational, social, and economic levels.

A more unusual type of abuse is Munchausen syndrome by proxy, also known as pediatric symptom falsification or child abuse. This occurs when a caregiver (usually the mother) causes injury to a child that involves unnecessary and harmful or potentially harmful medical care. Nursing and support staff can frequently help the physician make the right diagnosis by reporting their observations and experiences with the child and caregivers. Videotape surveillance has been recommended to help facilitate capturing a caregiver's misbehavior. Videotaping can help confirm or exclude symptoms reported by the caregiver (Stirling, 2007).

## ■ EMOTIONAL ABUSE

Emotional abuse includes acts or omissions by the caregiver that could cause serious behavioral, cognitive, emotional, or mental disorders. Emotional abuse may involve shaming, ridiculing, embarrassing, or insulting the child and destruction of the child's personal property. Clinical manifestations in the emotionally abused child may include developmental delays, failure to thrive, disruptive behavior, extreme behavior (withdrawal, aggression), unusual fearfulness, obsessions, and suicide attempts.

## ■ SEXUAL ABUSE

Sexual abuse is the exploitation of a child for the sexual gratification of an adult. Common forms of sexual abuse are oral–genital contact, fondling and caressing of the genitals, intercourse (vaginal or anal), rape, sodomy, and prostitution. Possible clinical manifestations in the infant include vaginal discharge; blood-stained diapers; genital redness, pain, itching, or bruising; lax rectal tone; difficulty sitting; and UTIs.

## MEDICAL–SURGICAL MANAGEMENT
### Medical

Diagnosis of abuse is based on a careful history and thorough physical examination. Injuries are treated as needed. All health care providers are legally required to report any suspected child abuse to the local child protective agency.

## NURSING MANAGEMENT

Monitor for inadequate weight gain; lack of immunizations; poor hygiene; bruises; bone fractures at different stages of healing; cerebral edema or hemorrhage; burns; developmental delays; failure to thrive; disruptive behavior; unusual fearfulness; vaginal discharge; blood-stained diaper; genital redness, pain, itching, or bruising; difficulty sitting; and UTIs. Assess child's history and physical examination, parent–infant interactions, child's response to surroundings and strangers, and developmental level.

Report all cases of suspected child abuse to the local child protective agency.

## NURSING PROCESS
### ASSESSMENT
#### Subjective Data

Obtain information about caregiver concerns; a general family history; and a specific child history. Begin with nonthreatening topics to demonstrate concern before asking about suspected abuse. Document verbatim details about the way the injuries occurred and use quotation marks.

#### Objective Data

Physical assessment and documentation must be thorough. Use figure diagrams to document skin injuries. Inconsistencies between what reportedly happened and the extent of injuries constitute a strong indicator of child abuse.

### Nursing diagnoses for the abused child include the following:

| NURSING DIAGNOSES | PLANNING/OUTCOMES | NURSING INTERVENTIONS |
|---|---|---|
| *Risk for Injury* related to family history of abuse/neglect | The client will be free from abuse/neglect. | Use a nonthreatening, nonjudgmental manner when interacting with the caregivers. |
| | | Assess and document the child's history and physical examination results, family history, caregiver–child interactions, the child's response to surroundings and strangers, and the child's developmental level. |
| | | Report all cases of suspected child abuse. |
| | | Assist in removing the child from the unsafe environment. |
| | | Refer the family to social services, as needed. |

*(Continues)*

**Nursing diagnoses for the abused child include the following: (Continued)**

| NURSING DIAGNOSES | PLANNING/OUTCOMES | NURSING INTERVENTIONS |
|---|---|---|
| *Impaired Parenting* related to lack of knowledge | The family will respond to the child's needs appropriately. | Assess the family's strengths, weaknesses, coping mechanisms, and support systems. |
| | | Assess the caregivers' expectations of the child, choice and use of comfort measures, responses to the child, and general knowledge about the child. |
| | | Discuss the parenting that the caregivers received as children. |
| | | Provide information regarding normal growth and development, nutrition, well-child care, and nurturing. |
| | | Role-model when interacting with the child. |
| | | Encourage the caregivers to participate in the child's care. |
| | | Reinforce positive behaviors on the part of the caregivers. |
| | | Assist the family in identifying stressors and options for decreasing stress. |
| | | Refer the parents to a support group such as Parents Anonymous. |

**Evaluation**: Evaluate each outcome to determine how it has been met by the client.

# ENVIRONMENTAL SAFETY

As infants develop and become mobile explorers, environmental safety becomes a major concern for all caregivers. An important role of the nurse is to educate caregivers regarding maintaining a safe environment and administering appropriate aid in the event of an accident. Common environmental safety hazards include poisoning, trauma, suffocation, and drowning.

# POISONING

Poisonous substances can be found everywhere. Commonly ingested substances include cosmetics and other personal care products, medicines, cleaning products, plants, gasoline, toys, lead-based paint, and other miscellaneous foreign substances.

## MEDICAL–SURGICAL MANAGEMENT

### Medical

The poison control center should be called initially and immediately to ascertain whether the child should be treated at home or taken to a treatment center. When the exact substance and amount are unknown, take the child to a treatment center, where complications can be anticipated and life support provided, if needed.

Vomiting is usually initiated immediately to the conscious child, unless the ingested substance is corrosive or highly irritating. Corrosives and irritants can cause further damage to mucous membranes of the esophagus and pharynx if vomited.

When emesis is contraindicated, gastric lavage is used to evacuate the stomach contents. In addition, activated charcoal may be administered to prevent further absorption of the poison.

## Pharmacological

Activated charcoal may be administered orally or through an orogastric tube to absorb the poison and remove it from the body. Activated charcoal may be mixed with a cathartic such as magnesium sulfate (Epsom salts). An antiemetic is sometimes needed.

Magnesium sulfate may be prescribed to promote rapid elimination, thereby decreasing absorption of the poison. Mixing magnesium sulfate with a sweet liquid may enhance its palatability. Results should occur within 2 to 4 hours.

### NURSING MANAGEMENT

Focus on poison prevention as well as on care of the poisoned child. Educate the public about ways to decrease the incidence of poisonings through printed materials such as checklists for poison proofing a home and illustrated first-aid guidelines. Consciousness-raising efforts should be included in each plan of care. Remind caregivers of the importance of keeping the phone number of the poison control center on the phone.

When confronted with a poisoning incident, focus on maintaining vital functions, preventing continued absorption of the poison, preventing complications related to the poisoning and treatment, reducing fear, and educating the caregiver about poison prevention. Once the child's condition is stabilized, exposure to the poison must be terminated. Substances should be removed from the mouth, first manually and then by a sip of water; from the eye with a continuous flush of normal saline; and from the skin by removing contaminated clothing and washing the skin with soap and water.

Once exposure is terminated, identify the substance and consult the poison control center. Procedures to induce vomiting and prevent absorption are initiated as directed by the poison control center.

## CLIENTTEACHING
### Poison Prevention

Advise caregivers of the following poison prevention measures:

- Keep all medicines and household cleaners in original containers with childproof caps and out of reach of children.
- Do not treat medicine like candy *or* candy like medicine.
- Read labels carefully before using medicines and household cleaners.
- Attach the poison control center's phone number to the phone.
- Prevent children from chewing or ingesting plants.
- Be aware of those things at a child's eye level by crawling around the house on hands and knees.
- Regularly wet-mop floors and wet-wipe window components because household dust is a major source of lead (from chipping paint in houses built before 1960).
- Caregivers should wet-mop floors and wet-wipe horizontal surfaces every 2 to 3 weeks.
- Windowsills and wells can contain high levels of leaded dust. They should be kept clean. If feasible, windows should be shut to prevent abrasion of painted surfaces or opened from the top sash.
- Avoid using traditional home remedies that may contain lead.
- Avoid eating candies imported from Mexico because they may be cooked in cookware that contains lead.
- Avoid using containers, cookware, or tableware to store or cook foods or liquids that are not shown to be lead-free.
- Remove recalled toys and toy jewelry immediately from children.
- Toys that have been made in other countries and then imported into the United States (mostly from China) or antique toys and collectibles passed down through generations put children at risk for lead exposure.
- Lead may be found in the paint used on toys or in the plastic used to make toys. Lead is used in plastic toys to stabilize molecules from heat. When the plastic is exposed to substances such as sunlight, air, and detergents, the chemical bond between the lead and plastics breaks down and forms a dust that can then be inhaled or consumed by children.

Source: http://www.cdc.gov/nceh/lead/tips.htm

## CLIENTTEACHING
### Tips for Maintaining a Safe Environment throughout Infancy

At 4 months, infants begin to roll and become very active:

- Keep crib side rails all the way up.
- Do not leave the infant unattended on raised areas such as beds, sofas, changing tables; instead, place on the floor or in a playpen.
- Use walkers away from the stairs.
- Never leave the infant unattended in the tub.
- Place car seat in the center of the back seat and facing backward until the infant weighs 20 pounds or is 12 months old. *Always use a car seat.*

At 6 months, infants begin to crawl, reach, and put things in their mouths:

- Keep the floor swept and be alert for small objects that may be put in the mouth.
- Put gates at the tops and bottoms of stairways.
- Keep bathroom doors closed.
- Dress the infant in clothing that allows freedom of movement.
- Do not leave the infant unattended in highchair.
- Keep cords and plastic bags out of the infant's reach.

At 8 months, infants begin to pull up and walk around furniture:

- Ensure that furniture both inside and outside the house is sturdy enough for the infant to pull self to standing.
- Eliminate containers of water inside and outside the house.
- Avoid dressing the infant in socks without shoes.

At 10 to 12 months, infants may begin to walk:

- Keep exterior doors secure.
- Secure gates around swimming pools.
- Keep appliance doors closed at all times.
- Place the infant weighing more than 20 pounds in a front-facing car seat.

## TRAUMA

Falls and motor vehicle injuries are the most common causes of trauma in infants. Medical–surgical management is dictated by the location and extent of the injury.

### NURSING MANAGEMENT

Preventing trauma or injuries is of utmost importance. Caregivers must stay aware of their infant's abilities as the infant grows and develops and be prepared to provide a safe environment. Every time a nurse encounters a caregiver, provide developmentally appropriate safety information and reminders. Stress car seat safety.

# ■ SUFFOCATION/DROWNING

Suffocation occurs when air exchange is hindered by covering the mouth or nose, applying pressure to the throat and chest, or excluding air (e.g., via refrigerator entrapment).

Drowning can occur in only inches of water. Drowning is a great concern when an infant is in the tub.

# NURSING MANAGEMENT

Educate parents and care providers. Safe cribs have no more than 2 3/8 inch space between the slats, and the crib mattress fits snugly against the slats. The crib is placed out of reach of windows and other furniture that may have cords or strings that could entrap or strangle a child. Other objects that may contribute to suffocation are electrical cords, toys with strings, plastic bags, pieces of balloons, crib mobiles, pieces of hard food, and restraining straps.

Drowning may occur in toilets, buckets of water, tubs, and pools. Remind caregivers that an infant or young child will not roll from the back to the stomach when the child's face is covered with water and that infants are top heavy and do not have the strength to pull themselves out of a bucket if they fall in head first.

## CASE STUDY

J.F. is a 10-month-old female who was brought to the clinic by her grandmother. The grandmother reports that J.F. is irritable, refuses to eat, and does not want to be rocked or cuddled. J.F.'s temperature is 102°F. She had been treated for an upper respiratory infection 10 days ago. A spinal tap indicates that J.F. has meningitis. An IV is started, and antibiotics are administered.

The following questions will guide your development of a nursing care plan for the case study.
1. List subjective and objective data a nurse should obtain about J.F.
2. List three nursing diagnoses and goals for J.F.
3. List three successful outcomes for J.F.
4. How can the spread of this infection be prevented?
5. What must be included in discharge planning if J.F.'s recovery is uneventful?

## SUMMARY

- The most common skin disorders of infancy are diaper rash, eczema, and cradle cap.
- The immaturity of the respiratory system creates hazards for the healthy infant and places the compromised infant at even greater risk of infection.
- Sudden infant death syndrome is the leading cause of death among infants.
- Signs of congenital heart disease in the infant include poor weight gain, poor feeding habits, fatigue, and respiratory infections.
- Iron-deficiency anemia can be prevented largely by teaching caregivers the importance of providing iron-fortified formula to infants until the age of 12 months.
- Possible signs of GI obstruction in the infant include abdominal pain, nausea and vomiting, abdominal distention, and decreased stool output.
- Treatment of colic may involve a change in feeding practices, correction of a stressful environment, and support of the caregivers.

- The most common defects of the GU tract include cryptorchidism, hydrocele, and hypospadias.
- The nursing goals when caring for infants with musculoskeletal impairments focus on preventing both skin breakdown and developmental delays.
- Infants become feverish quickly and must be observed for febrile seizures and protected from injury.
- Routine immunization of infants against *H. Influenzae* type B infection has reduced the incidence of bacterial meningitis.
- Developmental assessment will reveal language and social delays in infants with hearing and visual impairments.
- Inconsistencies between what reportedly happened and the extent of injuries constitute a strong indicator of child abuse.

## REVIEW QUESTIONS

1. The mother of a newborn infant tells the nurse, "He seems to be breathing hard and makes a grunting noise. Is he ok?" The nurse determines that:
   1. the infant must be assessed immediately.

   2. the infant needs oxygen.
   3. the infant is experiencing difficulty transitioning to post-natal life.
   4. the infant is exhibiting normal newborn behavior.

2. An infant diagnosed with ventricular septal defect (VSD) is being discharged to home. The nurse is doing discharge teaching to the mother and explains that when feeding the infant, the mother should:
   1. stimulate the infant to keep his attention.
   2. give large feeds to decrease the amount of time handling the infant.
   3. provide small, frequent, high-caloric feedings.
   4. allow infant to feed lying down.

3. An 8-month-old African-American infant has just been diagnosed with SCA. The nurse determines the parents need further teaching when they state:
   1. "We will keep him well hydrated."
   2. "He will not be immunized."
   3. "We will avoid high altitudes."
   4. "We will avoid extreme temperatures."

4. A nurse is teaching a child safety class at a child day care facility. What is the most important information that the nurse can provide to the child care providers on poisonings?
   1. Strategies to prevent poisonings.
   2. Keeping the child care center clean.
   3. Care of the poisoned child.
   4. Having the phone number to the poison control center readily available.

5. An infant is admitted to the hospital to be tested for Wilms' tumor. Upon assessment, the nurse palpates a mass in the infant's abdomen. The nurse should:
   1. continue palpating the abdomen to accurately document this finding.
   2. auscultate breath sounds and document findings in the chart.
   3. stop palpating immediately and document findings in the chart.
   4. check the infant's blood sugar and document findings in the chart.

6. An appropriate nursing assessment of an infant with spina bifida includes all of the following, except:
   1. head circumference.
   2. checking reflexes.
   3. palpating fontanelles.
   4. abdominal girth.

7. The nurse at a pediatric clinic is teaching the father of a 6-month-old infant diagnosed with atopic dermatitis about home care for the child. The nurse knows the father needs more education when he states:
   1. "I will smoke outside."
   2. "I will keep pets outside."
   3. "I will remove as much dust as possible from his room."
   4. "I will only use perfumed lotions and soaps."

8. A 5-month-old infant girl is being seen at the clinic for gastroesophageal reflux. The nurse teaches the parents strategies to help control and prevent gastroesophageal reflux. Select all of the strategies that apply:
   1. place the infant in a thirty-degree prone position.
   2. provide infant with small, frequent feeds.
   3. thicken formula with cereal.
   4. position in an infant seat to put pressure on the abdomen.
   5. administer orange juice as tolerated.
   6. lay infant on back after feeding.

9. The nurse is providing education regarding use of the Pavlik harness to a family with an infant with developmental dysplasia of the hip (DDH). The nurse has provided accurate information if she tells them:
   1. take off the harness to change diapers.
   2. the harness can be on only 8 to 12 hours a day.
   3. the infant does not have to wear the harness in the car seat.
   4. bathe the infant during the 1 hour the harness is off.

10. The nurse performing a physical assessment notices marks on the client's right leg. What is the most appropriate nursing action?
    1. Tell the mother the marks look like she spanked the infant.
    2. Report this case to the local child protective agency.
    3. Ask the mother how the injury occurred.
    4. Discuss different parenting styles and techniques with the mother.

# REFERENCES/SUGGESTED READINGS

American Academy of Pediatrics, Task Force on Sudden Infant Death Syndrome. (2005). The changing concept of sudden infant death syndrome: Diagnostic coding shifts, controversies regarding the sleeping environment, and new variables to consider in reducing risk. *Pediatrics, 116(5),* 1245–1255.

American Academy of Pediatrics and American Academy of Family Physicians. Subcommittee on Management of Acute Otitis Media. (2004). Diagnosis and management of acute otitis media. *Pediatrics, 113(5),* 1451–1465.

American Academy of Pediatrics. Subcommittee on Hyperbilirubinemia. (2004). Management of hyperbilirubinemia in the newborn infant 35 or more weeks of gestation. *Pediatrics, 114(1),* 297–316.

American Academy of Pediatrics. Committee on Injury, Violence, and Poison Prevention. (2003). Poison treatment in the home. *Pediatrics, 112(5),* 1182–1185.

American Heart Association. (2009). *Congenital cardiovascular defects: statistics.* Retrieved July 10, 2009, from http://216.185.112.5/presenter.jhtml?identifier=4576.

Anderson, R., Kochanek, K., & Murphy, S. (1997). Report of final mortality statistics, 1995. *Monthly Vital Statistics Report 4511* (Suppl. 2). Hyattsville, MD: National Center for Health Statistics.

Applegate, K. (2005). Clinically suspected intussusception in children: Evidence-based review and self-assessment module. *American Journal of Roentgenology, 185,* S175–S183.

Bailey, L., & Berry, R. (2005). Folic acid supplementation and the occurrence of congenital heart defects, orofacial clefts, multiple births, and miscarriage. *American Journal of Clinical Nutrition, 81*(5), 1213–1217.

Ball, J., & Bindler, R. (2007). *Pediatric nursing* (4th ed.). Norwalk, CT: Appleton & Lange.

Barker, E., Sauline, M., & Caristo, A. (2002). Spina bifida. *RN, 65*(12), 33–38.

Bulechek, G., Butcher, H., McCloskey, J., & Dochterman, J. (2007). *Nursing Interventions Classification (NIC)* (5th ed.). St. Louis, MO: Mosby-Elsevier.

Burns, C., Dunn, A., Brady, M., Starr, N., & Blosser, C. (2008). *Pediatric primary care: A handbook for nurse practitioners.* (4th ed.) St. Louis, MO: W.B. Saunders.

Castiglia, P. (1998). Trisomy 21 syndrome: Is there anything new? *Journal of Pediatric Health Care, 12*(1), 35–37.

Centers for Disease Control and Prevention. (2003). Managing acute gastroenteritis among children: Oral rehydration, maintenance, and nutritional therapy. *MMWR 52*(No. RR-16), 1–17.

Clinical Rounds. (2002). SIDS linked to *E. coli. Nursing2002, 32*(7), 34–45.

Cystic Fibrosis Foundation. (2009). *CFTR modulation.* Retrieved from http://www.cff.org/research/DrugDevelopmentPipeline/.

Dowshen, S., Hersheberger, M., & Rutherford, K. (2001). *SIDS: Sudden and silent.* Retrieved August 13, 2009, from http://kidshealth. org/parent/general/sleep/sids.html.

Duncan, B., Ey, J., Holberg, C., Wright, A., Martinez, F., & Taussig, L. M. (1993). Exclusive breast-feeding for at least 4 months protects against otitis media. *Pediatrics 91*(5), 867–872.

Eisenhauer, L., Nichols, L., Spencer, R., & Bergan, F. (1998). *Clinical pharmacology and nursing management* (5th ed.). Philadelphia: Lippincott.

Ellmers, K., & Criddle, L. (2002). Cystic fibrosis. *RN, 65*(9), 61–66.

Estes, M. (2010). *Health assessment & physical examination* (4th ed). Clifton Park, NY: Delmar Cengage Learning.

Finesilver, C. (2002). Down syndrome. *RN, 65*(11), 43–48.

Gartner, L., & Greer, F. (2003). Prevention of rickets and vitamin D deficiency: New guidelines for vitamin D intake. *Pediatrics, 111*(4Pt1), 908.

Godshall, M. (2003). Caring for families of chronically ill kids. *RN, 66*(2), 30–34.

Gorman, K. (1999). Sickle cell disease. *AJN, 99*(3), 38–43.

Hermansen, C., & Lorah, K. (2007). Respiratory distress in the newborn. *American Family Physician, 76*(7), 987–994.

Hockenberry, M., & Wilson, D. (2008). *Wong's nursing care of infants and children* (8th ed.). St. Louis, MO: Mosby.

James, S., Ashwill, J., & Jackson, C. (2007). *Nursing care of children: Principles and practice* (3rd ed.). Philadelphia: W. B. Saunders.

Kaditis, A., & Wald, E. (1998). Viral croup: Current diagnosis and treatment. Pediatric *Infectious Disease Journal, 17*(9), 827–834.

Kamarakrishnan, K., Sparks, R., & Berryhill, W. (2007). Diagnosis and treatment of otitis media. *American Family Physician, 76*(11), 1650–1658.

Kitchens, G. (1995). Relationship of environmental tobacco smoke to otitis media in young children. *Laryngoscope. 105*(5, Part 2), 1–3.

Kline, A. (2003). Pinpointing the cause of pediatric respiratory distress. *Nursing2003, 33*(9), 58–63.

Kuppermann, N., O'Dea, T., Pinchney, L., & Hoecher, C. (2000). Predictors of intussusception in young children. *Archives of Pediatric and Adolescent Medicine, 154*, 250–255.

Marks, M. (1998). *Broadribb's introductory pediatric nursing* (5th ed.). Philadelphia: J. B. Lippincott Williams & Wilkins.

Mayo Clinic. (2009). *Sickle cell anemia.* Retrieved from http://www.mayoclinic.com/health/sickle-cell-anemia/DS00324/DSECTION=lifestyle-and-home-remedies.

Meekins, E. (2002). Would you recognize this pediatric disorder? *RN, 65*(4), 26–30.

Mera, K., & Hackley, B. (2003). Childhood vaccines: How safe are they? *AJN, 103*(2), 79–88.

Miles, M. (2003). Support for parents during a child's hospitalization. *AJN, 103*(2), 62–64.

Moerschel, S. K., Cianciaruso, L. B., & Tracy, L. R. (2008). A practical approach to neonatal jaundice. *American Family Physicians, 77*(9), 1255–1262.

Moorhead, S., Johnson, M., Maas, M., & Swanson, E. (2007). *Nursing Outcomes Classification (NOC)* (4th ed.). St. Louis, MO: Elsevier-Health Sciences Division.

North American Nursing Diagnosis Association International. (2010). *NANDA-I nursing diagnoses: Definitions and classification 2009-2011.* Ames, IA: Wiley-Blackwell.

Orenstein, S., Izadnia, F., & Khan, S. (1999). Gastroesophageal reflux disease in children. *Gastroenterology Clinics of North America, 28*(4), 947–969.

Queenan, J. (2001). *Positional plagiocephaly (flattened head).* Retrieved August 10, 2009, from http://kidshealth.org/parent/general/sleep/positional_plagiocephaly.html.

Roberts, D., Ostapchuk, M., & O'Brien, J. (2004). Infantile colic. *American Family Physician, 70*(4), 735–740.

Sassen, M., Brand, R., & Grote, J. (1997). Risk factors for otitis media with effusion in children 0 to 2 years of age. *American Journal of Otolaryngology 18*(5), 324–330.

Schuman, A. (1997). Disposable diapers? Definitely! *Contemporary Pediatrics, 14*(11), 131–139.

Simmerman, J., & Mauzy, C. (2001). Finally! Babies can get this vaccine. *RN, 64*(7), 28–32.

Spiro, D., Tay, K., Arnold, D., Dziura, J., Baker, M., & Shapiro, E. (2006). Wait-and-see prescription for the treatment of acute otitis media: A randomized controlled trial. *JAMA, 296*(10), 1235–1241.

Spratto, G., & Woods, A. (2009). *2009 PDR nurses' drug handbook.* Clifton Park, NY: Delmar Cengage Learning.

Su, C., Gaskie, S., & Jamieson, B. (2008). What is the best treatment for oral thrush in healthy infants? *The Journal of Family Practice, 57*(7), 484–485.

Swanson, E., Johnson, M., Moorhead, S., & Maas, M. (2007). *Nursing Outcomes Classification (NOC)* (4th ed.). St. Louis, MO: Mosby.

Tinkle, M. (2002). Cystic fibrosis carrier screening. *AWHONN Lifelines, 6*(2), 134–139.

Tully, S., Bar-Haim, Y., & Bradley, R. (1995). Abnormal tympanography after supine bottle feeding. *Journal of Pediatrics, 1995*(126), S105–S111.

Van Riper, M. (2003). A change of plans. *AJN, 103*(6), 71–74.

Wahlgren, D., Hovell, M., Meltzer, S., Hofstetter, C., & Zakarian, J. (1997). Reduction of environmental tobacco smoke exposure in asthmatic children: A 2 year follow-up. *Chest, 111*(1), 81–88.

White, K., Munro, C., & Pickler, R. (1995). Therapeutic implications of recent advances in cystic fibrosis. *MCN, 20*(6), 58–64.

Wittmann-Price, R., & Pope, K. (2002). Universal newborn hearing screening. *AJN, 102*(11), 71–77.

Yetman, R., & Coody, D. (1997). Failure to thrive: A clinical guideline. *Journal of Pediatric Health Care, 11*(3), 134–137.

Zorb, S. (2002). Transplantation offers hope. *RN, 65*(9), 66–68.

## RESOURCES

**American Cleft Palate–Craniofacial Association,** http://www.acpa-cpf.org

**American Lung Association,** http://www.lungusa.org

**American Sickle-Cell Anemia Association,** http://www.ascaa.org

**American SIDS Institute,** http://www.sids.org

**American Society for Deaf Children,** http://www.deafchildren.org

**American Speech-Language-Hearing Association,** http://www.asha.org

**Automotive Safety for Children Program,** http://www.preventinjury.org

**Cystic Fibrosis Foundation,** http://www.cff.org

**Hydrocephalus Association,** http://www.hydroassoc.org

**Kids Health, Nemours Foundation,** http://www.kidshealth.org, www.nemours.org

**La Leche League International,** http://www.llli.org

**National Down Syndrome Society,** http://www.ndss.org

**Sickle Cell Disease Association of America,** http://www.sicklecelldisease.org

**Spina Bifida Association of America,** http://www.sbaa.org

**United Cerebral Palsy National,** http://www.ucpa.org

**Women, Infants and Children (WIC),** http://www.fns.usda.gov/wic

# CHAPTER 8
## Common Problems:
## 1 to 18 Years

## MAKING THE CONNECTION

*Refer to the following chapters to increase your understanding of common pediatric problems:*

*Maternal & Pediatric Nursing*
- *Basics of Pediatric Care*

## LEARNING OBJECTIVES

Upon completion of this chapter, you should be able to:

- Define key terms.
- Discuss the common disorders of the integumentary system in children.
- Differentiate the pathophysiology, common diagnostic tests, treatment, and nursing care for skin conditions in children as compared to adults.
- Differentiate the etiology, medical–surgical management, and nursing care for respiratory conditions in children as compared to adults.
- Describe the causes, assessment, and management of rheumatic fever in children.
- Differentiate the pathophysiology, common diagnostic tests, treatment, and nursing care for digestive conditions in children as compared to adults.
- Differentiate the etiology, medical–surgical management, and nursing care for genitourinary conditions in children as compared to adults.
- Discuss communicable and infectious diseases of childhood, including their causative agents, transmission, incubation periods, contagious periods, prevention, signs and symptoms, treatment, and nursing care.
- Differentiate the etiology, medical–surgical management, and nursing care for orthopedic conditions in children as compared to adults.
- Briefly describe behavioral problems in children, including symptoms, treatment, and nursing care.
- Plan care for a child with any of the common pediatric disorders.

KEY TERMS

acanthosis nigricans          encopresis          Gowers' sign
comedones                     epistaxis           rhinorrhea

# INTRODUCTION

Pediatric nursing focuses on protecting children from illness and injury as well as assisting them to attain optimal levels of functioning, regardless of health status. The pediatric nurse must understand the phases of a child's growth and development (refer to the Life Span Development chapter) and be sensitive to the importance of family interactions. This chapter focuses on common childhood conditions and illnesses affecting all systems of the body; the typical medical and surgical management for these conditions; and nursing management of the child and caregivers.

## RESPIRATORY SYSTEM

Disorders of the respiratory system that occur most often in children include upper-respiratory infections, allergic rhinitis, tonsillitis, asthma, and foreign-body aspiration.

### UPPER-RESPIRATORY INFECTIONS

Common upper-respiratory infections include nasopharyngitis (the common cold), pharyngitis, and influenza.

Nasopharyngitis is usually credited with being the most common childhood respiratory illness. These disorders are generally responsive to supportive therapies, and symptoms typically improve within 3 days. Clinical manifestations, etiology, and management of these common upper-respiratory disorders are presented in Table 8-1.

## NURSING MANAGEMENT

Maintaining fluid intake, providing comfort measures, and preventing spread of infection are the main goals of care for the child with an upper-respiratory infection. The child should not be forced to eat if appetite is decreased. An appropriate diet may include cool, bland fluids and soft foods such as gelatin, soup, mashed potatoes, puddings, hot cereals, and flavored ice pops. Teach caregivers to observe for urinary output and for moist mucous membranes as signs of adequate hydration.

Comfort measures may include warm salt-water gargles (1/4 tsp salt per 8 oz glass of water) and warm or cool compresses applied to the throat. Nasal decongestion may be relieved with normal saline drops before feedings and at bedtime. A cool-mist humidifier at the bedside may also relieve symptoms.

It is important that caregivers know how both to take a child's temperature and to safely administer nonsalicylate antipyretics, such as acetaminophen (Tylenol). Salicylates, such as aspirin, are not used because of the associated risk of Reye's syndrome.

**TABLE 8-1  Distinguishing Characteristics of Common Upper Respiratory Infections**

|  | NASOPHARYNGITIS | PHARYNGITIS | INFLUENZA |
|---|---|---|---|
| **Manifestations** | **Rhinorrhea** (watery nasal discharge), congestion, sneezing, fever, cough, sore throat, muscular aches, and possibly, enlarged lymph nodes | Sore throat; erythema and inflammation of the pharynx and tonsils; fever; enlarged, tender cervical lymph nodes<br><br>Viral: gradual onset, hoarseness, cough, rhinitis, malaise<br><br>Bacterial: abdominal pain, vomiting, headache | Chills, fever, flushed face, myalgia (pain in muscles), cough, rhinitis, headache, sore throat, photophobia, conjunctivitis |
| **Etiology** | Viral | Viral (80%) or bacterial (20%) | Influenza virus |
| **Incidence** | Typically 6 to 9 colds per year, most commonly in the fall and spring | Most common among 4 to 7-year-old children | Highest among school-age children |
| **Management** | Rest, fluids, nonsalicylate antipyretics, oral decongestants, sterile saline nose drops | Rest; fluids; nonsalicylate antipyretics or ibuprofen; warm salt-water gargles; cool, bland liquids; antibiotics for streptococcal infections | Rest, fluids, nonsalicylate Antipyretics |

## CLIENTTEACHING

### Administering Normal Saline Drops

1. Instill two drops.
2. Wait 5 minutes.
3. Instill two more drops.
4. Drops should not be used for more than 3 days.

Teach caregivers and children methods for preventing the spread of infection, such as conscientious hand hygiene, proper disposal of tissues, and covering of the nose and mouth when coughing and sneezing. Also avoid contact with infectious persons. Preventing the spread of infection is especially challenging in school and crowded living environments. Children in day care centers have a higher rate of infection than do children who spend their days in the home.

Untreated streptococcal infections may lead to complications such as rheumatic fever, meningitis, and glomerulonephritis. Emphasize to the caregivers of children with pharyngitis caused by streptococcal infection ("strep throat") the importance of completing the course of prescribed antibiotics.

## ALLERGIC RHINITIS

Allergic rhinitis ("hay fever") is an inflammatory disorder of the nasal mucosa. Most often, it is a seasonal, recurrent response to allergens such as animal dander, house dust, pollens, and molds. Manifestations include rhinorrhea, postnasal drip, sneezing, allergic conjunctivitis, sniffing, itchy nose and palate, dark circles under the eyes, and the "allergic salute" (transverse nasal crease that results from repeatedly pushing nose upward and backward to relieve itching).

## MEDICAL–SURGICAL MANAGEMENT

### Pharmacological

Antihistamines, decongestants, and bronchodilators may be given to relieve symptoms of congestion and difficulty with breathing. Topical intranasal corticosteroids are quite effective in children who do not respond to antihistamines and decongestants. Systemic corticosteroids may be used in extreme cases. Immunotherapy or desensitization to allergens may be initiated if antihistamines and decongestants are not effective in relieving symptoms or are needed chronically. Desensitization is performed for those allergens that produce a positive reaction on skin testing. The allergist sets up a schedule for injections in gradually increasing doses until a maintenance dose is reached. Desensitization is considered to be a safe procedure with considerable benefit for some children. Severe reactions are uncommon. During immunotherapy, children must be observed for signs of anaphylaxis for 30 minutes after each injection.

### Health Promotion

The treatment of choice is to eliminate the allergen from the child's environment. Recommendations for limiting the child's exposure to allergens include avoiding wool and down; using dust-proof covers on bedding; removing carpets, draperies, and blinds from the child's room, if not the whole house; keeping humidity lower than 50%; keeping pets outside; and using air filters.

## NURSING MANAGEMENT

Focus on therapeutic management of the disease. After identification of the allergens, assist the caregivers with allergy proofing the home and administering medications.

Drowsiness, dry mouth, and excitability are side effects of some antihistamines. Combining an antihistamine and decongestant may prevent drowsiness.

## TONSILLITIS

Tonsillitis, a common illness among children, is an inflammation of the tonsils (two masses of lymphoid tissue located at the back of the mouth), resulting from pharyngitis. Tonsils filter and protect the respiratory and alimentary tracts from infection. They normally enlarge progressively between 2 and 10 years of age and reduce during preadolescence. If the tonsils become enlarged from infection, they can interfere with breathing and swallowing and cause partial deafness. Clinical manifestations of tonsillitis include recurrent sore throat; enlarged, bright-red tonsils; mouth breathing; halitosis; nasal speech; fever; difficulty swallowing; and snoring.

## MEDICAL–SURGICAL MANAGEMENT

### Surgical

Tonsillectomy may be warranted in cases of abscesses, upper airway obstruction, and obstructive sleep apnea. Adenoidectomy (removal of lymphoid tissue in the nasal pharynx) is performed in cases of recurrent otitis media with Eustachian tube obstruction or for persistent nasal or airway obstruction. If tonsillectomy can be postponed until 4 or 5 years of age, the apparent need often will have disappeared.

## PROFESSIONALTIP

### Throat Culture

The only reliable means of determining whether pharyngitis is viral or bacterial is with a throat culture. The nurse is most often the person who performs a throat smear for culture, which requires a physician's order. The applicator is swabbed across the tonsils, the posterior edge of the soft palate, and the uvula.

## Pharmacological

Medical treatment includes analgesics for pain, antipyretics for fever, and antibiotics for streptococcal infections.

## NURSING MANAGEMENT

Prepare child for surgery. Use dolls or puppets to assist the child in expressing fears and concerns and acting out the pending experience.

Postoperatively, monitor vital signs, intake and output (I&O), and for signs of blood loss. Maintain child in prone or side-lying position. Encourage intake of cool or cold clear liquids when child is fully awake. Administer analgesic as ordered. Educate child and caregivers to avoid red or brown liquids, using straws, coughing or blowing nose to decrease the risk of spontaneous hemorrhage.

## NURSING PROCESS

### ASSESSMENT

#### Subjective Data

Be sensitive to the child's and caregiver's level of anxiety and offer opportunities for expression of concerns. The use of puppets, dolls, and other materials may be an effective way to allow the child to act out the pending surgical experience and to express concerns and fears.

### Objective Data

Presurgical assessments such as complete blood count (CBC), clotting time, and urinalysis are usually done on an outpatient basis.

Upon admission on the day of surgery, review vital signs and laboratory results for abnormalities, and assess the child for signs of infection (fever, elevated white blood count [WBC], and redness and exudate of the throat). Observe the child's mouth for loose teeth that could be aspirated during anesthesia.

Postoperatively, monitor vital signs and observe for hemorrhage, ability to swallow, and dehydration. The most obvious signs of bleeding from the surgical site are restlessness or anxiety, frequent swallowing, and rapid pulse. Each time vital signs are taken, use a flashlight to observe the pharynx for bleeding.

### ASTHMA

Asthma, a reactive airway disease (RAD), is defined as narrowing or obstruction of the airway triggered by stimuli

**Nursing diagnoses for the child after a tonsillectomy include the following:**

| NURSING DIAGNOSES | PLANNING/OUTCOMES | NURSING INTERVENTIONS |
|---|---|---|
| *Risk for Aspiration* related to unswallowed saliva and postoperative bleeding | The child's airway will remain patent. | Maintain the child in a prone or side-lying position. Monitor vital signs every 15 minutes for 1 hour and hourly for the next 4 hours. Ensure availability of suction equipment. Do not give oral fluids until the child is completely awake. Avoid hot liquids, irritating foods, and use of straws. Instruct the child to avoid coughing and clearing the throat; encourage the child to expectorate secretions into a tissue. |
| *Deficient Risk for Fluid Volume* related to excessive loss through blood loss and decreased oral intake | The child will maintain appropriate fluid intake and demonstrate no signs and symptoms of dehydration | Observe for signs of blood loss, such as frequent swallowing, elevated pulse and respirations, pallor, restlessness and anxiety; report to physician immediately. Maintain intravenous (IV) fluids until the child is taking oral fluids. Encourage intake of cold or cool liquids such as ice pops (no red or brown), noncitric juices, gelatin (no red), and ice chips; introduce milk products only after clear liquids are tolerated. Record hourly I&O, daily weight. |
| *Acute Pain* related to surgical procedure | The child will have pain relief (<3 on a scale of 1 to 10). | rovide nonaspirin analgesic every 4 hours for at least the first 24 hours after surgery. Use age-appropriate pain assessment tools. Encourage the caregivers to stay at the child's bedside to provide reassurance and comfort. |

*(Continues)*

**Nursing diagnoses for the child after a tonsillectomy include the following: (Continued)**

| NURSING DIAGNOSES | PLANNING/OUTCOMES | NURSING INTERVENTIONS |
|---|---|---|
| *Deficient **K**nowledge* (*parents*) related to unfamiliarity with information for discharge care | The caregivers will verbalize an understanding of discharge care. | Instruct the caregivers to:<br><br>• Watch for signs of hemorrhage especially between the fifth and tenth postoperative days.<br>• Watch for signs of infection (persistent earache, temperature over 102°F).<br>• Call physician if bleeding or signs of infection occurs.<br>• Encourage liquids and soft foods as tolerated for 10 days.<br>• Avoid rough, scratchy foods for 3 weeks.<br>• Maintain pain control with nonaspirin analgesics every 4 hours as needed during first week.<br>• Restrict the child's activity to quiet play for 10 days (i.e., no school or vigorous exercise).<br>• Expect the throat to be white in appearance and the mouth odor to be bad for the first week.<br>• Bring child for follow-up visit in 1 to 2 weeks. |

**Evaluation:** Evaluate each outcome to determine how it has been met by the client.

(such as cold air, smoke, viral infection, exercise, stress, drugs, or allergens) and inflammation that leads to mucosal edema and mucus hypersecretion. Asthma is the leading cause of school absenteeism and the most common admitting diagnosis in children's hospitals (Boychuk et al., 2006). Clinical manifestations of asthmatic attacks or episodes include a dry, hacking cough; wheezing; and difficulty breathing. The child may need to sit up to breathe. Attacks may last for hours or days. Thick, tenacious mucus may be expectorated after a coughing episode. In children with repeated acute exacerbations, barrel chest and the use of accessory muscles of respiration are common findings. Chronic asthmatics are usually small according to the standard growth charts. In some cases, episodes no longer occur after puberty, and growth usually catches up in adolescence. A definitive diagnosis of asthma can be made when the airway obstruction (indicated by pulmonary function tests) is reversed with bronchodilators.

## MEDICAL–SURGICAL MANAGEMENT
## Medical

Medical treatment is aimed at preventing airway damage resulting from repeated and severe episodes of asthma. Care

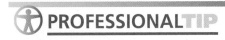

## PROFESSIONALTIP

### Theophylline

The margin of safety is narrow with theophylline. Early adverse effects include tachycardia, irritability, restlessness, insomnia, headache, vomiting, and diarrhea.

is focused on early recognition and treatment of episodes, identification and elimination of allergens, and education of the child and caregivers. Allergy proofing the home along with skin testing followed by desensitization are methods used to control allergens (refer to the section on Allergic Rhinitis).

Educate families about the disease, including ways to prevent attacks; early signs of episodes; drug therapy; appropriate exercise; and chest physiotherapy (CPT), if needed. Early symptoms include increasing cough at night, in the early morning, or in conjunction with activity; respiratory retractions; and wheezing. Using a peak flowmeter is an objective way to measure airway obstruction: families must learn how both to use this device and to record the results.

## Pharmacological

A combination of bronchodilators, short-acting inhaled beta-2 agonists, and anti-inflammatory agents is used to treat asthma. Short-acting bronchodilators, such as beta-2 agonists, are used to treat mild intermittent asthma in children. Short-acting inhaled beta-2 agonists are used with acute symptoms in mild persistent asthma. Long acting bronchodilators, salmeterol xinafoate (Serevent Diskus) and formoterol fumarate (Foradil), are used with moderate and severe persistent asthma. The drugs of choice for long-term mild persistent asthma are inhaled corticosteroids, inhaled antiasthmatics (cromolyn sodium [Crolom] and nedocromil sodium [Tilade]), or oral antiasthmatics (leukotriene modifiers—montelukast sodium [Singulair]) (Spratto & Woods, 2009).

The most commonly prescribed bronchodilator is albuterol (Ventolin). These drugs cause relaxation of bronchial smooth muscle and inhibit the release of mediators from mast cells. Small doses by inhalation are the most effective mode of administration. Bronchodilators may be taken together by inhalation and be given parenterally for additional effect. Repetitive use may mask increasing airway inflammation and hyper-responsiveness. Correct use of the metered-dose inhaler (MDI) is important for maintaining control of asthma symptoms.

Theophylline (Theo-Dur) is the oldest effective bronchodilator. It requires continuous oral or IV administration and is most therapeutic when the serum level measures 10–20 mcg/mL. Educate child and caregivers to monitor for signs of toxicity which include: headache, tachycardia, abdominal pain, and hypotension (Leifer, 2006).

Anti-inflammatory drugs of choice include cromolyn sodium (Crolom) and corticosteroids such as prednisone (Deltasone). Cromolyn is an antiasthmatic, mast cell stabilizer that prevents asthma symptoms by blocking the release of mast cell mediators. Once symptoms start, however, cromolyn is ineffective. Adverse effects associated with cromolyn are airway irritation with mild cough and a bad taste. Corticosteroids effectively reduce mucosal edema and potentiate the effect of bronchodilators. Steroids may be given in inhaled form to reduce the oral dose required and to decrease systemic effects that accompany oral administration. Long-term use of oral steroids is reserved for chronic asthma that has not responded to other drugs. Adverse side effects of long-term oral therapy include Cushing's syndrome, growth suppression, osteoporosis, glaucoma, cataracts, peptic ulcer, hyperglycemia, and decreased resistance to infection (Lenhardt et al., 2006).

## CRITICAL THINKING

### Smoking and Asthma

What teaching would you provide to a caregiver who smokes around a child who has asthma?

## Activity

Children with asthma should not be automatically restricted from physical activity. With adequate treatment, a child with asthma can participate in most physical activities. Sports that do not require sustained exertion, such as gymnastics, baseball, and weight lifting, are well tolerated. Swimming is frequently recommended as an ideal sport because the air is humidified, and breathing increases end expiratory pressure.

## ■ FOREIGN-BODY ASPIRATION

Foreign-body aspiration is the inhalation of any object into the respiratory tract. Commonly aspirated items among children include nuts, grapes, popcorn, hard candy, dried beans, bones, coins, parts of toys, screws, and balloons.

## SAMPLE NURSING CARE PLAN

### The Child with Asthma

M.O., a 5-year-old girl, was admitted to the emergency department (ED) with severe coughing, fever, and difficulty breathing. Crackles and wheezing were evident in all fields upon auscultation. Vital signs were temperature, 102°F; pulse, 160; and respirations, 40. Pulse oximetry was 90%. Her parents had given her Tylenol for what they thought was a "cold." When her condition worsened during the night, they brought her to the ED. M.O. has no history of asthma but has eczema. She has just started kindergarten. Her parents are extremely distraught and are asking many questions. M.O. cries every time anyone enters the room.

**NURSING DIAGNOSIS 1** *Ineffective **A**irway Clearance* related to secretions in the bronchi and exudate in the alveoli as evidenced by difficulty breathing, crackles, and wheezing

**Nursing Outcomes Classification (NOC)**
*Respiratory Status*

**Nursing Interventions Classification (NIC)**
*Airway Suctioning*
*Cough Enhancement*
*Positioning*

| PLANNING/OUTCOMES | NURSING INTERVENTIONS | RATIONALE |
|---|---|---|
| M.O. will have effective airway clearance. | Monitor vital signs, auscultate breath sounds, assess respiratory effort and rate, assess skin color every 15 to 30 minutes, arterial blood gases (ABGs), pulse oximetry, and pulmonary function tests results. | Subtle changes may serve as an early warning of increased airway obstruction. |

*(Continues)*

## SAMPLE NURSING CARE PLAN (Continued)

| PLANNING/OUTCOMES | NURSING INTERVENTIONS | RATIONALE |
|---|---|---|
| | Administer oxygen at the ordered flow rate (if chronic asthmatic, not to exceed 2 L/min). | Decreases hypoxia. Administration of oxygen to a child with chronic carbon dioxide retention may cause respiratory depression. |
| | Position the child upright or for comfort. | Enhances lung expansion. |
| | Ensure availability of suction equipment and tracheostomy tray. | Condition can deteriorate rapidly. |
| | Provide at least 1,600 mL fluids (IV/PO)/24 hours. | Liquefies secretions and replaces insensible fluid losses. |
| | Initiate nothing-by-mouth (NPO) status during periods of severe respiratory distress. | Oral fluid intake during periods of distress can cause aspiration. |
| | Administer ordered medications and assess for therapeutic effect. | Bronchodilators and steroids open airways and decrease edema. |
| | Assess breath sounds before and after CPT. | Theophylline level of >30 can cause serious complication. |
| | Encourage child to cough and deep breathe by blowing bubbles through a wand. | CPT, coughing, and deep breathing help loosen/eliminate secretions. |

## EVALUATION
M.O.'s airway is clear.

**NURSING DIAGNOSIS 2** *Anxiety* related to threat to or change in health status as evidenced by respiratory distress and hospitalization

**Nursing Outcomes Classification (NOC)**
*Coping*
*Anxiety Reduction*

**Nursing Interventions Classification (NIC)**
*Anxiety Reduction*
*Anticipatory Guidance*

| PLANNING/OUTCOMES | NURSING INTERVENTIONS | RATIONALE |
|---|---|---|
| M.O. and her caregivers will demonstrate no signs of anxiety. | Maintain a calm, quiet environment and a reassuring manner. | Decreases oxygen demand and the work of breathing. |
| | Encourage therapeutic play. | Builds rapport and trust. |
| | Keep the caregivers informed of procedures, treatments, and condition of their child. | Builds rapport and trust. Calming the parents can help calm the child. |

## EVALUATION
M.O.'s anxiety level is decreased and her respiration rate is decreased. The parents participate in M.O.'s care.

## SAMPLE NURSING CARE PLAN (Continued)

**NURSING DIAGNOSIS 3** *Deficient **K**nowledge* related to disease process as evidenced by many questions

| Nursing Outcomes Classification (NOC) | Nursing Interventions Classification (NIC) |
|---|---|
| *Knowledge Deficit: Disease Process* | *Teaching: Disease Process* |
| *Knowledge Deficit: Treatment Regimen* | *Teaching: Prescribed Medication* |

| PLANNING/OUTCOMES | NURSING INTERVENTIONS | RATIONALE |
|---|---|---|
| M.O.'s parents will verbalize accurate knowledge about asthma. | Teach parents about the disease, its triggers, and prescribed medications and treatment. | Understanding increases compliance with treatment. |
| | Assess the parents' knowledge about triggers, precipitating factors (such as colds), and allergen control. | Triggers may have been assessed. Knowledge of allergen control may decrease the likelihood of future episodes. |
| | Teach the importance of taking medications as prescribed. | Maintains therapeutic levels. |
| | Teach the importance of exercise and ways to choose appropriate activities based on the child's condition. | Promotes pulmonary and cardiovascular health, enhances self-esteem, and offers peer interaction. |

### EVALUATION

M.O. verbalizes knowledge about disease and treatment in age appropriate terms. M.O.'s caregivers verbalize accurate knowledge about the disease and its treatment.

---

Aspiration may occur at any age but is most common between the ages of 6 months and 4 years. Clinical manifestations may include spasmodic coughing, respiratory distress, or gagging in the absence of fever or other symptoms of illness.

## Medical–Surgical Management

### Medical

Removal of foreign bodies from the respiratory tract is done by direct laryngoscopy or bronchoscopy. After the procedure, the child remains hospitalized for observation of laryngeal edema and respiratory distress. Cool mist is provided and antibiotic therapy ordered if appropriate.

### Health Promotion

It is important that caregivers and child care providers remain watchful as the child gains increased locomotor and manipulative skills and becomes more curious about the environment.

## Nursing Management

After the object has been removed, the main focus of care is prevention. Assess the caregivers' knowledge of safety in relation to the child's developmental level. Encourage parents/caregivers to keep cylindric, spheric, and pliable objects smaller than 1 and 1/4 inches out of children's reach. In addition, supervise children when eating, and cut food into small, irregular pieces.

## CARDIOVASCULAR SYSTEM

A major threat to the child's cardiovascular system is rheumatic fever, which may lead to permanent heart damage and disability.

## RHEUMATIC FEVER

Rheumatic fever is a chronic childhood disease affecting the heart, joints, lungs, and brain. It results from an autoimmune response to untreated group A *beta-hemolytic streptococcus* infections. Clinical manifestations are classified as minor and major. Minor clinical manifestations include fever, listlessness, anorexia, pallor, weight loss, and vague muscle, joint, or abdominal pain. Major clinical manifestations include polyarthritis, chorea (spasmodic twitchings), carditis, erythema marginatum (red skin lesions), and subcutaneous nodules. An elevated antistreptolysin-O (ASO) titer and an anti-DNAse B (both tests indicate a recent streptococcal infection) are common among children with rheumatic fever. The child may have a late complication of chorea known as Sydenham's chorea, perhaps years after the initial rheumatic fever. Chorea is caused inflammatory changes in the neurons of the central nervous system. The child with chorea has purposeless, rapid, involuntary movements of the extremities and trunk of the body (Potts & Mandleco, 2007).

# MEDICAL–SURGICAL MANAGEMENT

## Medical

Diagnosis is made by evaluating presenting signs and symptoms and laboratory test results. A throat culture determines whether the infection is active. Erythrocyte sedimentation rate (ESR), C-reactive protein, and leukocyte count are elevated in the presence of inflammatory processes. An antistreptolysin O-titer (ASO) and anti-DNAse B indicate a previous streptococcal infection. These two tests together confirm the diagnosis of rheumatic fever up to 92% (Potts & Mandleco, 2007). Chest x-ray, electrocardiogram, and echocardiogram may demonstrate evidence of carditis.

The goals of medical management are to treat any existing strep infection, prevent recurrences and heart damage, and alleviate pain and fever. Bed rest is prescribed for the child with carditis until ESR and heart rate are within normal limits.

## Pharmacological

Penicillin, salicylates, and corticosteroids are used to treat rheumatic fever. Long-term administration (as long as 5 years) of penicillin helps prevent the recurrence of rheumatic heart disease. Salicylates relieve pain, reduce inflammation of polyarthritis, and reduce fever. Corticosteroids are used in the presence of carditis. Residual heart disease (congestive heart failure) is treated as needed with digitalis and diuretics. Anticonvulsants may be prescribed to alleviate severe chorea.

## Diet

A low-sodium diet may be prescribed in the presence of congestive heart failure. The intake and output is monitored to prevent dehydration or overhydration.

## Activity

Bed rest is essential to reduce the workload of the heart. The length of bed rest can range from weeks to months depending on the cardiac status. Position the child for comfort and to prevent pressure areas and skin breakdown. A bed cradle may be used to relieve pressure on joints. Ensure safety and protect from falls; keep environment free from bright lights.

## Health Promotion

Continual health supervision for children is the key to prevention of rheumatic fever and resulting heart disease. It is important that children with upper respiratory infections be evaluated for group A *beta-hemolytic streptococcus* and treated with penicillin as prescribed. Prophylactic antibiotics are required prior to any invasive procedure to prevent endocarditis.

# NURSING MANAGEMENT

Maintain child on bed rest. Alternately apply heat and cold to affected joints. Provide distractions such as guided imagery, relaxation, board games, movies, books, or puzzles. Stress importance of evaluating children with upper-respiratory infections and taking penicillin as prescribed even if symptoms disappear.

# NURSING PROCESS

## ASSESSMENT

### Subjective Data

Initially, determine whether any family members or caregivers have had a sore throat or unexplained fever within the past 2 months. Find out when symptoms began; what, if any, treatment was obtained; and if an antibiotic was prescribed, whether it was taken as directed.

### Objective Data

Monitor the child for cardiac complications such as abnormal vital signs, shortness of breath, edema, and precordial pain. Assess joints for tenderness, small lumps, and rapid, purposeless movements. Use age-appropriate tools to assess pain.

| Nursing diagnoses for the child with rheumatic fever include the following: | | |
| --- | --- | --- |
| **NURSING DIAGNOSES** | **PLANNING/OUTCOMES** | **NURSING INTERVENTIONS** |
| *Acute Pain* related to inflamed joints | The child will rate pain ≤3 on a 0 to 10 scale. | Alternate applying heat and cold to affected joints. Reposition the child every 2 hours, handle joints gently. Provide distraction such as guided imagery and relaxation. |
| *Activity Intolerance* related to shortness of breath and pain | The child will tolerate restricted activities. | Limit activities to bed and chair, with bathroom privileges, and meals at the table. Include rest periods alternated with activities such as board games, computer use, movies, puzzles, books, art, and crafts. |

**Nursing diagnoses for the child with rheumatic fever include the following: (Continued)**

| NURSING DIAGNOSES | PLANNING/OUTCOMES | NURSING INTERVENTIONS |
|---|---|---|
| *Risk for Injury* related to weakness and chorea | Child will be injury free. | If the child is experiencing chorea, the mattress may need to be placed on the floor and the child may require assistance going up and down stairs. |
| | | Seizure precautions are taken. |
| | | Teach the importance of evaluating children with upper respiratory infections for streptococcus, and treating with penicillin. |
| *Deficient Knowledge* related to medication administration | The child and caregiver will understand the importance of antibiotic therapy in preventing recurrence of the disease and further heart damage. | Stress the importance of taking penicillin as prescribed even if symptoms disappear. |

**Evaluation:** Evaluate each outcome to determine how it has been met by the client.

# HEMATOLOGIC AND LYMPHATIC SYSTEMS

Leukemia, idiopathic thrombocytopenic purpura, and hemophilia are blood disorders that commonly occur during childhood.

## ■ LEUKEMIA

Leukemia, the most common childhood cancer, is the uncontrolled production of lymphocytes (immature white blood cells). The most common form of leukemia is acute lymphocytic leukemia (ALL). The prognosis has been improving dramatically because of vigorous therapy, but there is concern related to adverse effects of the therapy. Clinical manifestations, the results of neutropenia and decreased red blood cells (RBCs) and platelets, include pallor, weakness, fever, excessive bruising, petechiae, purpura, bone or joint pain, and abdominal pain.

## MEDICAL–SURGICAL MANAGEMENT

### Medical

In addition to the child's history, symptoms, and laboratory studies, bone marrow aspiration is done to confirm the diagnosis of leukemia. The goals of medical intervention are to eradicate the leukemic cells via chemotherapy and to provide supportive care during treatment.

### Surgical

Bone marrow transplant may be recommended after the second remission.

### Pharmacological

A combination of chemotherapy drugs is administered through a subclavian catheter and/or intrathecally to bring about remission. Treatment may last 2 to 3 years. After 30 days of initial treatment, remission can be verified via bone marrow aspiration and lumbar puncture. If remission occurs, the prognosis is good. For the child who suffers a relapse, different drugs are used in an attempt to reinduce a remission. Relapses decrease the probability of survival.

## NURSING MANAGEMENT

Assess the emotional status of the child and the caregivers and identify areas of concern. A plan is made to assist them in working through and resolving their feelings and fears. Explore how the child and caregivers are coping with the illness as well as the treatment.

## ■ IDIOPATHIC THROMBOCYTOPENIC PURPURA

Idiopathic thrombocytopenic purpura (ITP) is a blood disorder associated with a deficit of platelets in the circulatory system. An autoimmune disorder often preceded by a viral infection, ITP may be acute and self-limiting or be chronic and require therapy. The peak age of occurrence is 2 to 4 years. Manifestations include bruising and petechiae.

## MEDICAL–SURGICAL MANAGEMENT

### Medical

Diagnostic evaluation involves gathering a history of viral illness, information about any medications, and a CBC, which will be normal except for a low platelet level. If the history and CBC suggest ITP, bone marrow aspiration may be done to rule out oncological disorders. Most cases are self-limiting, with the platelet count returning to normal within 6 months without therapy. Platelet transfusions may be necessary for the child with chronic ITP if active, uncontrolled bleeding occurs.

# PROFESSIONAL TIP

## Life-Threatening Illness

The following questions can be used in assessing the feelings and fears associated with the diagnosis of life-threatening illness:

- Has the child and/or caregivers been associated with hospitals, nurses, and doctors in the past? If yes, what were the positive and negative aspects of the experience?
- Do the caregivers know anyone diagnosed with a life-threatening illness? If yes, what happened to that person?
- Are there concerns about the child's future? The family or caregiver's future?

## Surgical

When drugs no longer control the thrombocytopenia in a child with chronic ITP, a splenectomy may be indicated. Splenectomy is usually not performed before 5 years of age because of the immaturity of the child's immune system.

## Pharmacological

Steroids and immune globulin are given to block the autoimmune destruction of platelets.

## NURSING MANAGEMENT

Encourage the curtailing of physical activities and sports until condition is resolved. Observe for signs of bleeding. Advise to use soft-bristled toothbrush. Assist parents/caregivers to establish a safe, age-appropriate home environment. Teach the child's caregiver the signs and symptoms of infection.

## NURSING PROCESS

### ASSESSMENT
#### Subjective Data

Caregivers may bring the child to the doctor because of a "red rash" or bruising. The child's activity level may be reported to be normal.

#### Objective Data

Observe for further bleeding (e.g., epistaxis, hematuria, blood in stools) and level of consciousness.

**Nursing diagnoses for the child with ITP include the following:**

| NURSING DIAGNOSES | PLANNING/OUTCOMES | NURSING INTERVENTIONS |
|---|---|---|
| *Risk for Injury* related to low platelet count | The child will be free of injury. | Have the child curtail physical activities and sports until platelets return to normal. |
| | | Encourage the use of a soft-bristled toothbrush to minimize gum bleeding. |
| | | Observe for signs of bleeding. |
| | | Flush the catheter with saline to confirm proper placement of an IV line. |
| *Deficient Knowledge* (Parents) related to disorder and treatment | The caregivers will verbalize an understanding of the disorder and treatment. | Teach the caregivers that ITP should subside within 6 months. |
| | | Teach the caregivers side effects of steroids, such as edema, insomnia, mood changes, poor healing, peptic ulcers, and growth retardation. |
| | | Establish a safe, age-appropriate home environment (e.g., pad table corners, crib rails, and knees and elbows to decrease injury). |
| | | Instruct caregivers to use nonaspirin analgesics and antipyretics. |
| | | Evaluate the child's platelet count weekly. |
| *Risk for Infection* related to chronic use of steroids and/or splenectomy | The child will be free of infection. | Teach the caregivers the signs and symptoms of infection. |
| | | Administer pneumococcus vaccine and/or daily antibiotics, if the child has a splenectomy. |

**Evaluation:** Evaluate each outcome to determine how it has been met by the client.

# ■ HEMOPHILIA

Neonatal bleeding from the umbilical cord or circumcision site may be an early manifestation of severe hemophilia.

Mild hemophilia may not be detected until the toddler becomes mobile, and unusual bruising and bleeding occur from small injuries.

Nursing interventions center on prevention and teaching. Regular physical exercise strengthens muscles and joints and

## CRITICAL THINKING

### Fluid Volume Deficit

What is the priority data to gather when assessing a child for fluid volume deficit? Why?

may decrease the number of bleeding episodes. The infusion of recombinant factor VIII concentrates is the treatment for hemophilia. Recombinant factor concentrates are an effective treatment for hemophilia and prevent the exposure to HIV or hepatitis that previous transfusions caused.

# GASTROINTESTINAL SYSTEM

Gastrointestinal disorders in children interfere with nutrition and fluid and electrolyte balance and have the potential for impairing growth. Common GI disorders of childhood include constipation and parasitic infections.

## ■ CONSTIPATION

Constipation is the infrequent or difficult passage of hard, dry stools. It is most common during the toddler and preschool years because of the child's (and caregivers') efforts at toilet training. School-age children may experience constipation as a result of busy schedules, hesitation to use unfamiliar bathrooms, and limited bathroom privileges. Other potential causes of constipation include lack of fresh fruit and vegetables and grains in the diet, dehydration, lack of exercise, emotional stress, certain drugs, pain from passage of hard stool, excessive milk intake, and a variety of GI tract and systemic disorders and spinal lesions.

Chronic constipation causes an enlarged rectum, which impairs sphincter control, resulting in encopresis (the pas-

### CLIENT TEACHING

#### Guidelines for Preventing Constipation in Children

For toddlers and preschool children:
- Increase cereal, fruit, vegetable, and fluid intake.
- Encourage sitting on the toilet for 5 to 10 minutes after breakfast and after dinner.

For school-age children:
- Allow 1 hour to finish breakfast before leaving for school to allow sufficient time for bathroom use.
- Encourage children to take responsibility for including cereals, fruits, vegetables, and fluids in their diets.
- Encourage children to exercise daily.
- Decrease the anxiety of children by taking time each day to communicate about their day's activities, concerns, and fears.

sage of watery colonic contents around a hard fecal mass). Predisposing factors for encopresis include inadequate or inconsistent toilet training or psychological stress such as that related to starting school or the birth of a sibling. Clinical manifestations of constipation include abdominal pain and cramping without distention; palpable, movable fecal mass and a large amount of stool inside rectum; diarrhea; malaise; anorexia; and headache.

## MEDICAL–SURGICAL MANAGEMENT

### Medical

Abdominal x-rays may reveal a rectum enlarged with stool and gas. The impaction is removed with enemas.

### Pharmacological

Stool softeners or laxatives may be prescribed in an effort to retrain the rectum after the impaction has been removed. Mineral oil may be prescribed to decrease the pain of defecation.

### Diet

Increasing water and fiber intake and limiting milk intake will often decrease constipation and promote defecation.

### Health Promotion

Counseling may be part of the treatment plan, if there is no evidence of physiologic disorders. Establishing and maintaining regular toileting habits, drinking fluids, eating a high-fiber diet, and participating in regular exercise will also help prevent constipation.

## NURSING MANAGEMENT

Focus on teaching caregivers about normal bowel patterns in children and the importance of diet and exercise in maintaining those patterns. Assess the child's diet history and elicit a description of bowel patterns to provide clues to the cause of constipation. Dietary changes may be all that is required to resolve constipation.

Requiring the child to sit on the toilet for 10 minutes approximately 30 minutes after meals encourages regular bowel habits. Caution caregivers about the overuse of laxatives, stool softeners, and enemas. Use of mineral oil may cause soiling from leakage, which should not be mistaken for encopresis.

## ■ INTESTINAL PARASITIC INFECTIONS

Common parasitic infections include giardiasis (a protozoan) and helminths (i.e., pinworms, roundworms, hookworms; see Figures 8-1, 8-2, 8-3, and 8-4). Children are more commonly infected than adults because they frequently put their hands in their mouths. Temperate climates, crowded conditions (i.e., day care centers, schools), untreated water, and poor hygiene practices may contribute to outbreaks of parasitic infections. Appearance, mode of transmission, and clinical manifestations vary, depending on the parasite (Table 8-2).

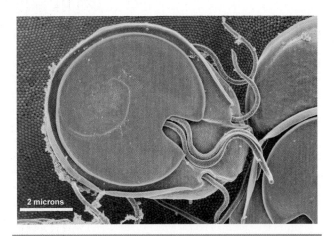

FIGURE 8-1 Scanning electron micrograph (SEM) of a *Giardia muris* trophozoite that had settled atop the mucosal surface of a rat's intestine. The protozoan Giardia causes the diarrheal disease called giardiasis. (*Courtesy of the Centers for Disease Control and Prevention/Photo by Dr. Stan Erlandsen.*)

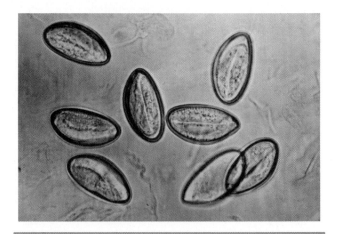

FIGURE 8-2 Human pinworm eggs, captured on cellulose tape. (*Courtesy of the Centers for Disease Control and Prevention.*)

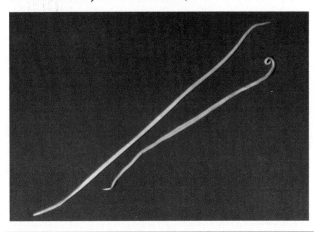
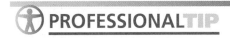

FIGURE 8-3 A 1960 photograph of two roundworms. The larger of the two is the female while the normally smaller male is on the right. Adult worms live in the lumen of the small intestine. Adult roundworms can live for 1 to 2 years and adult female worms can grow over 12 inches in length. (*Courtesy of the Centers for Disease Control and Prevention.*)

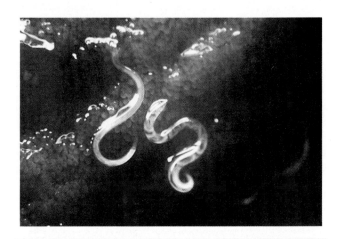

FIGURE 8-4 A photographic enlargement showing hookworms attached to the intestinal mucosa. Barely visible larvae penetrate the skin, are carried to the lungs, go through the respiratory tract to the mouth, are swallowed, and eventually reach the small intestine. This journey takes about a week. (*Courtesy of the Centers for Disease Control and Prevention.*)

## PROFESSIONALTIP

### Quinacrine Hydrochloride (Atabrine HCl)

To disguise the bitter taste of quinacrine tablets, pulverize and mix with jam or honey.

## MEDICAL–SURGICAL MANAGEMENT

### Medical

Identification of a parasitic infection is done with a fecal smear or a microscopic examination. Pinworms may be diagnosed by using cellophane tape to capture eggs from around the anus and then examining them under a microscope.

### Pharmacological

Helminths are treated with oral anthelmintic medications such as pyrantel pamoate (Antiminth) or mebendazole (Vermox). Medication should be repeated 2 to 3 weeks later to eliminate any parasites that may hatch after the initial treatment. All family members and caregivers should also be treated.

Metronidazole (Flagyl) or quinacrine hydrochloride (Atabrine HCl) are effective in treating giardiasis. Alert child care providers to the possibility of a yellow discoloration to the skin for the child on quinacrine hydrochloride (Atabrine HCl).

### Diet

A well-balanced diet with additional protein and iron may be prescribed for the child with hookworms. These nutrients may be depleted from blood loss and malnutrition.

### Health Promotion

Attention to meticulous sanitary practices is essential.

**TABLE 8-2  Common Intestinal Parasites**

| | APPEARANCE | MODE OF TRANSMISSION | CLINICAL MANIFESTATIONS |
|---|---|---|---|
| **Giardiasis** | Microscopic | Ingested cysts<br>Person to person<br>Untreated water<br>Contaminated food<br>Animals<br>Soil<br>Feces | Diarrhea<br>Weight loss<br>Abdominal cramping |
| **Pinworm** | White, threadlike worm | Person to person<br>Ingested or inhaled eggs | Itching around the anus<br>Irritability<br>Distractibility |
| **Roundworm** | Pink worm, 9 to 12 inches in length | Eggs passed from hand to mouth (may migrate to liver and lungs) | Abdominal pain, distention, or obstruction<br>Vomiting<br>Jaundice<br>Pneumonitis |
| **Hookworm** | Microscopic | Skin penetration by contact with contaminated soil (may migrate to lungs) | Dermatitis<br>Anemia<br>Pneumonitis<br>Malnutrition |

COURTESY OF DELMAR CENGAGE LEARNING

## NURSING MANAGEMENT

Assist with collection of specimens, treatment of infections, and prevention of reinfection. Collect stool specimens from diapers, potty chairs, or a toilet covered with clear plastic wrap. Use a tongue blade to place the specimen into the designated and properly labeled container. Provide caregivers with detailed instructions for performing the tape test (see the accompanying Community/Home Health Care box). Provide education regarding the course of treatment and home care.

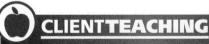

## CLIENT TEACHING

### Preventing Parasitic Infestations

- Care providers should wash hands thoroughly after changing diapers.
- Dispose of soiled diapers in trash receptacles.
- Teach children to wash their hands and fingernails after using the toilet and before eating.
- Wash bedding and undergarments in hot water.
- Regularly use cleaning agents containing bleach in bathrooms.
- Wash all raw fruits and vegetables before eating.
- Cover sandboxes when not in use.
- Avoid swimming pools that allow diapered children.
- Wear shoes outside.

## COMMUNITY/HOME HEALTH CARE

### Instructions for the Tape Test for Pinworms

Perform the test early in the morning, before the child awakens:

1. Wind the tape around the end of a tongue blade, sticky side out.
2. Spread the child's buttocks and press the tape against the anus, rolling the blade from side to side.
3. Place the tongue blade in a glass jar or plastic bag.
4. Take to the lab for microscopic examination. If a glass slide is available, remove the tape from the tongue blade and place it smoothly on the slide, sticky side down.

## ENDOCRINE SYSTEM

A common endocrine disorder in children is type 1, formerly called insulin-dependent, diabetes. The management of diabetes in children presents some unique challenges because of their physical immaturity and dependence on caregivers for care. Stabilizing insulin needs during puberty requires vigilant monitoring of the glucose level and regulating diet, insulin, and exercise. The lifestyle of the entire family or caregivers must change in order to effectively treat the child with diabetes. Family members and caregivers should be familiar with and adhere to the prescribed regimen. Most school-age children are ready and able to learn to give their own injections and should be encouraged to do so.

An increasing number of children, up to 45% of those with diabetes, have type 2 diabetes (American Diabetes Association, 2006). Most of these children are overweight or obese. Testing for type 2 diabetes in children is shown in Table 8-3. They are usually treated initially with nutrition therapy and an exercise program. Eventually, most will require drug therapy. Most pediatric diabetologists use oral agents for children with type 2 diabetes (American Diabetes Association, 2006). For medical–surgical management and nursing management of the child with endocrine disorders, see the endocrine system chapter.

# MUSCULOSKELETAL SYSTEM

Maximizing bone mass in childhood reduces the impact of bone loss related to aging. It is also a critical time for developing lifestyle habits important to maintaining good bone health such as proper nutrition and physical activity (NIH, 2000).

Common musculoskeletal disorders in children include scoliosis, Legg-Calvé-Perthes disease, muscular dystrophy, juvenile arthritis, and fractures.

## SCOLIOSIS

Scoliosis, the most common spinal deformity in children, involves lateral curvature greater than 20 degrees, spinal

### TABLE 8-3 Recommendations for Testing Children for Type 2 Diabetes

*Overweight:* BMI greater than 85th percentile for age and sex, weight for height greater than 85th percentile, or weight greater than 120% of ideal for height

plus

Any two of the following risk factors:
- Family history of type 2 diabetes in first- or second-degree relative
- Being Native American, African American, Hispanic, or Asian/Pacific Islander
- Show signs of insulin resistance or conditions associated with insulin resistance such as **acanthosis nigricans**, a velvety hyperpigmented patch on back of neck, in axilla, or antecubital area; hypertension; dyslipidemia, or polycystic ovarian syndrome (PCOS)

*Age for Testing:* At age 10 years or at onset of puberty, whichever occurs first, and then every 2 years

*Test:* Fasting plasma glucose (FPG) preferred

From: American Diabetes Association. (2006). Type 2 diabetes in children and adolescents. *Diabetes Care, 22*(12), 381. [Online]. Available: www.diabetes.org

## LIFE SPAN CONSIDERATIONS

### Backpacks

A child should be able to stand up straight and maintain good posture when carrying a backpack. Therefore:
- Backpacks should be positioned above the child's buttocks.
- Both straps should be used instead of just one.
- The backpack should not be overloaded so the child has to lean forward when carrying it.

From: Nemours. (2002). School backpacks: How they affect your child's general health. Retrieved December 23, 2003 from www.nemours.org/no/news/releases/2002/020206_ backpack_study.html

rotation, rib asymmetry, and thoracic hypokyphosis (Figure 8-5). It occurs most frequently in prepubescent girls and is usually not caused by any other injury or disease.

Clinical manifestations include visible curve of the spine, posterior rib hump when bending forward, asymmetrical rib cage, and uneven shoulder or pelvic heights. Caregivers may notice that the child's clothes do not fit properly (e.g., uneven hems).

## MEDICAL–SURGICAL MANAGEMENT

### Medical

The goal of medical treatment is to stop the curvature of the spine. Early detection and treatment of scoliosis are essential to successful management. The treatment regimen depends on the degree and progression of the curvature and the reaction of the child and caregivers. Children with mild curvatures

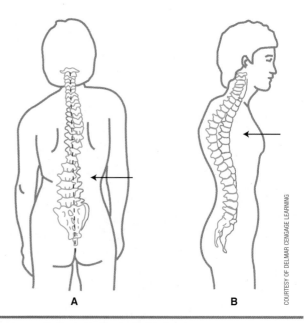

**FIGURE 8-5** *A,* Scoliosis; *B,* Kyphosis

COURTESY OF DELMAR CENGAGE LEARNING

may simply be monitored throughout the growth cycle. Electrical stimulation, bracing, and exercise may be prescribed for children with mild to moderate curvatures.

## Surgical

Surgical intervention may be required for children with curvatures greater than 40 degrees. The goal of surgery is to correct the curvature of the spine with internal fixation and instrumentation.

## NURSING MANAGEMENT

Involve child in the plan of care. Encourage child to perform exercises as prescribed. Provide suggestions to protect bony prominences when wearing a brace.

Postoperatively, assess extremities for color, capillary refill, warmth, sensation, and movement. Log roll the child every 2 hours. Monitor vital signs, for bowel distention, and urinary retention. Assess pain level and provide analgesics as ordered. Teach caregivers about wound care. Discuss restrictions on activity. Emphasize importance of keeping follow-up appointments.

# NURSING PROCESS

## ASSESSMENT

### Subjective Data

Initially, the child may complain of a sore back, improperly fitting clothing, or a slight limp. When being treated with a brace, assess the child for problems related to self-esteem and body image. Ask the child and caregivers to report on the degree of compliance with the prescribed regimen. If the child requires surgery, assess feelings and fears of the child and the family.

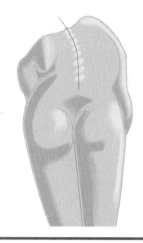

COURTESY OF DELMAR CENGAGE LEARNING

**FIGURE 8-6** Scoliosis screening reveals a rib hump and curved spine.

### Objective Data

Screening for scoliosis is an important role of the nurse. Assess children 10 years of age and older. With clothes removed, observe the back for uneven shoulders and hips, prominent shoulder blade on one side, and curved spine. While bending at the waist and touching the toes, assess the child's back for a rib hump and curved spine (Figure 8-6).

When a brace is in place, continue monitoring the degree of curvature and assess the skin at pressure points for irritation. Progression of the curve may indicate either noncompliance with the prescribed treatment or the need for more aggressive therapy.

Postoperatively, the child is assessed for neurological status, pain, fluid balance, bleeding, and bowel and bladder function. Mobility and nutrition are quickly resumed if there are no complications.

### Nursing diagnoses for the child with scoliosis include the following:

| NURSING DIAGNOSES | PLANNING/OUTCOMES | NURSING INTERVENTIONS |
| --- | --- | --- |
| *Deficient **K**nowledge (parents and child)* related to lack of information about scoliosis, including treatment and surgery | The child and caregiver will verbalize an understanding of and comply with the medical regimen. | Identify the child's and caregiver's knowledge level and areas of concern.<br><br>Inform the child and caregiver that the brace must be worn for prescribed hours per day for recommended length of time.<br><br>Inform the child and caregiver that use of brace may eliminate need for surgery.<br><br>If surgery is necessary, prepare the child and caregiver for the need to log roll the child and the need for the child to cough and have them demonstrate preoperatively. |
| *Disturbed **B**ody Image* related to deformity, bracing, and surgical scar | The child will talk about feelings.<br><br>The child will demonstrate self-confidence. | Involve the child in the plan of care.<br><br>Provide the child with opportunities to ventilate feelings about being different.<br><br>Encourage the child to talk about experiences with friends.<br><br>Help the child select clothing that is stylish yet loose enough to fit over the brace.<br><br>Help the child focus on positive body features (e.g., hair, complexion). |

*(Continues)*

**Nursing diagnoses for the child with scoliosis include the following: (Continued)**

| NURSING DIAGNOSES | PLANNING/OUTCOMES | NURSING INTERVENTIONS |
|---|---|---|
| | | Help the child select activities that will enhance abilities. |
| | | Provide the child with privacy during hospitalization. |
| *Risk for Impaired Skin Integrity* related to wearing of a brace | The child's skin will remain intact. | Have the child wear a knit cotton shirt under the brace. |
| | | Place a protective pad over bony prominences. |
| | | Report reddened areas so that the brace can be adjusted. |
| *Impaired Physical Mobility* related to restricted movement (brace/surgery) | The child will adjust to restricted movement. | Perform exercises as prescribed. |
| | | Instruct the child in how to move with the brace (i.e., climb stairs; get in and out of a vehicle, chair, desk, and bed). |
| *Risk for Injury* related to neurovascular deficit secondary to instrumentation | The child will regain all body functions postoperatively. | Assess all extremities for color, capillary refill, warmth, sensation, and motion. |
| | | Monitor signs of bowel distention and urinary retention. |
| | | Maintain body alignment by logrolling every 2 hours and rolling from a side-lying position to a sitting position. |
| | | Assist with early ambulation postoperatively. |
| *Acute Pain* related to operative procedure | The child will experience pain reduction to an acceptable level. | Assess pain level postoperatively, using pain scale. |
| | | Provide prescribed analgesics around the clock for the first 24 to 48 hours. |
| | | Explore alternate means of relieving pain (e.g., dim lights, music). |
| | | Assess and document the child's response to relief measures. |
| *Deficient Knowledge (parent and child)* related to home care | The child and caregiver will successfully manage postoperative treatment at home. | Teach proper wound care. |
| | | Discuss the importance of a well-balanced diet in maintaining healthy bones. |
| | | Discuss activity restrictions (e.g., lifting no more than 10 pounds) and the length of time they will be in place. |
| | | Have the child demonstrate moving without twisting or bending at the waist. |
| | | Emphasize the importance of keeping follow-up appointments. |

**Evaluation:** Evaluate each outcome to determine how it has been met by the client.

# ■ LEGG-CALVÉ-PERTHES DISEASE

Legg-Calvé-Perthes disease is necrosis of the head of the femur. The disease occurs most commonly in Caucasian boys between the ages of 4 and 8 years. The cause is unknown. Clinical manifestations include hip and knee soreness or stiffness, painful limp, and quadriceps muscle atrophy.

## MEDICAL–SURGICAL MANAGEMENT

### Medical

Diagnosis is made by x-ray. The goal of treatment is to maintain the shape of the femoral head and reduce the risk of permanent stiffness and degenerative arthritis. Methods used to accomplish this goal include traction, bracing, and surgery.

Initially, the child is hospitalized for non–weight-bearing range-of-motion exercises and bed rest. If there is no improvement within 10 days, alternate methods of treatment are usually begun.

Nonsurgical intervention may involve traction followed by the use of a non–weight-bearing abduction brace to position the femoral head in the acetabulum. Exercises maintain muscle integrity during the time that the child is required to wear the brace, for as long as 1 to 3 years.

### Surgical

Surgical intervention is often the treatment of choice because it reduces treatment time and eliminates compliance problems.

The child is usually able to resume normal activities in 3 to 4 months.

## NURSING MANAGEMENT

Maintaining mobility and educating the child and caregivers are the primary nursing goals. Encourage the caregivers and child to adhere to treatment plans and keep follow-up visits. Demonstrate proper application of the abduction brace. Perform skin assessments daily. Encourage the child to maintain muscle integrity via prescribed exercises. Involvement in activities such as horseback riding and swimming may be permitted.

## ■ DUCHENNE MUSCULAR DYSTROPHY

Duchenne muscular dystrophy (DMD) is an x-linked, recessive, hereditary, progressive, degenerative disease of the muscles. The disease occurs almost exclusively among males and is carried by females. Clinical manifestations include delayed motor development, difficulty standing or walking, progressive muscle weakness, increasing abnormalities in gait and posture, lordosis, pelvic waddling, frequent falling, Gowers' sign (walking the hands up legs to move from a sitting to a standing position), and a flat affect and smile. The disease continues into adolescence and young adulthood, when the child usually succumbs to respiratory failure. Children with DMD rarely live beyond 20 years of age. Complications include obesity, contractures, respiratory infections, and cardiac failure. Diagnosis is confirmed by serum enzyme assay, muscle biopsy, and electromyography.

## MEDICAL–SURGICAL MANAGEMENT

### Medical

Initially, therapeutic management is aimed at maintaining ambulation and independence for as long as possible with bracing and physical therapy. Later, therapy is directed at maximizing sitting capabilities, respiratory function, and self-care. Genetic counseling is recommended for caregivers, female siblings, and maternal aunts and their female offspring.

### Surgical

Contractures may be released surgically in order to keep the child as mobile as possible.

## NURSING MANAGEMENT

Monitor children when there is a family history of muscular dystrophy. Encourage physical therapy exercise regimen and use of adaptive devices. Focus on the things the child can do.

## NURSING PROCESS

### ASSESSMENT

#### Subjective Data

When there is a family history of muscular dystrophy, monitor the child carefully. Assess both the family or caregivers' ability to cope with a chronic, debilitating illness and the support systems available.

#### Objective Data

Routinely monitor the child for mobility, self-care abilities, weight gain, and infections.

**Nursing diagnoses for the child with DMD include the following:**

| NURSING DIAGNOSES | PLANNING/OUTCOMES | NURSING INTERVENTIONS |
|---|---|---|
| *Impaired Physical Mobility* related to progressive muscle wasting and contractures | The child will remain physically active. | Reinforce physical therapy exercise regimen. Encourage activity (e.g., school attendance, swimming). Encourage the use of adaptive equipment as needed (e.g., a back brace). |
| *Self-Care Deficit (all)* related to progressive weakness | The child will be able to perform activities of daily living (ADLs) as long as possible. | Instruct the caregivers in ways to adapt the home as needed (e.g., grab bars, overhead sling, raised toilet, wheelchair access). Focus on those things the child can do to prevent frustration. Maintain the child's independence as long as possible (e.g., via an electric wheelchair and portable phone). |
| *Compromised Coping, Family* related to increased demands of care, financial burdens, and needs of other children | The caregivers coping will be effective with the disease process. | Refer the caregivers to resource and support groups. Assist the family or caregivers in anticipating needs and coordinating services. Encourage involvement of extended family and friends. Encourage the family and caregivers to express feelings. |

**Evaluation:** Evaluate each outcome to determine how it has been met by the client.

## JUVENILE ARTHRITIS

Juvenile arthritis (JA) is a systemic, multisystem disorder that affects the body's connective tissue; it is also known as an autoimmune inflammatory disease. There are many different forms of the disease, including juvenile rheumatoid arthritis.

Clinical manifestations include joint swelling accompanied by limited range of motion; pain; tenderness; and inflammation lasting longer than 6 weeks. Complications include blindness and disability. Prognosis is generally good with early detection and treatment.

## MEDICAL–SURGICAL MANAGEMENT

### Medical

The goal of treatment is to maintain mobility and preserve joint function. The therapeutic regimen includes drugs, physical therapy, and/or surgery.

### Surgical

Depending on the severity of the disease, surgery may be necessary to release contractures, correct leg-length discrepancies, and replace joints.

### Pharmacological

Drug therapy includes aspirin, nonsteroidal anti-inflammatory drugs such as ibuprofen (Motrin) and naproxen (Naprosyn), slower-acting antirheumatic drugs such as gold sodium thiomalate (Myochrysine), and penicillamine (Cuprimine). Cytotoxic drugs may be used for severe disease that does not respond to other drugs. Corticosteroids may be used sparingly when the disease is life threatening.

## NURSING MANAGEMENT

Refer to the Immune System chapter.

## FRACTURES

Fractures in children tend to be less complicated and heal more quickly than do those in adults. The bones most commonly fractured in children include the clavicle, femur, tibia, humerus, wrist, and fingers. Fractures in the area of the epiphyseal plate (growth plate) can cause permanent damage and severely impair growth. Greenstick fractures are common

### COMMUNITY/HOME HEALTH CARE

**Juvenile Arthritis**

Home treatment for juvenile rheumatoid arthritis may include the following:
- Exercise, such as swimming and bicycling, to maximize muscle strength and range of motion
- Splints, positioning, and application of heat and cold to provide comfort during painful episodes

among young children because of incomplete ossification. Evidence of old fractures in a young child suggests possible child abuse, whereas fractures in infants may indicate osteogenesis imperfecta (brittle bone disease).

Treatment usually involves realignment and immobilization using traction or closed manipulation and casting.

Refer to the Musculoskeletal System chapter for medical management and the nursing process.

## IMMUNE SYSTEM

Infectious or communicable diseases are not life threatening to most children; however, children with immature or compromised immune systems are at greater risk of developing severe and even fatal complications as the result of communicable diseases.

## COMMUNICABLE DISEASES

A communicable disease is an illness that is directly or indirectly transmitted from one person to another. Infants and young children are more susceptible to infectious diseases because their immune systems are not fully developed until 6 years of age, and their hygiene habits (e.g., covering the mouth when coughing) are lacking. Selected communicable diseases, along with causal agent, transmission mode, communicable period, incubation period, clinical manifestations, potential complications, treatment, and immunity conferment are listed in Table 8-4.

## NURSING MANAGEMENT

Immunization is critical to the health of children. One of the goals of the U.S. government is to immunize 90% of children ages 15 to 35 months by the year 2010 (Healthy People 2010, 2000). Conscientious nurses and health care providers familiarize themselves with immunization schedules and the various frequent revisions to these schedules. The Advisory Committee on Immunization Practices (ACIP) of the U.S. Public Health Service Centers for Disease Control (CDC) and the American Academy of Pediatrics (AAP) Committee on Infectious Diseases are responsible for recommendations regarding vaccinations. Changes in recommendations are published in the *Morbidity and Mortality Weekly Report* for the ACIP and in *Pediatrics* for the AAP.

Recognize barriers to immunizations and educate caregivers about vaccine safety, administration, precautions, and contraindications. Barriers to immunization include long waiting lines, appointment-only systems, inaccessible clinic sites, and inability to speak English. The nurse takes every opportunity to immunize children whenever children enter any health care facility.

Federal law requires health care providers to provide general information about immunizations before administration. This general information includes nature, prevalence, and risks of the disease; type of immunization product to be used; the expected benefits and the risk of side effects of the vaccine; and the need for accurate immunization records. If possible, provide this lengthy information before the immunization appointment so that families have time to read and understand the information and to ask questions. Otherwise, the health care provider must inform parents at the time of administration. Document informed consent of the parent(s).

### TABLE 8-4 Select Common Communicable Diseases

| DISEASE (CAUSAL AGENT) | TRANSMISSION MODE AND COMMUNICABLE PERIOD | INCUBATION PERIOD | CLINICAL MANIFESTATIONS AND POTENTIAL COMPLICATIONS | TREATMENT AND IMMUNITY CONFERMENT |
|---|---|---|---|---|
| Chicken pox (varicella-zoster virus, Figure 8-7) | *Transmission mode:* direct contact, respiratory droplet, airborne particles<br><br>*Communicable period:* 1 day before lesions appear until all lesions crust over | 10–21 days | *Clinical manifestations:* fever, malaise, irritability, and a rash that begins as macules and progresses to fluid-filled papules to crusted lesions.<br><br>*Potential complications:* Reye's syndrome, skin infections, encephalitis | *Treatment:* antihistamines, baths, and lotions for itching<br><br>*Immunity conferment:* natural or with vaccine; may reactivate in adults as herpes zoster |
| Diphtheria (*Corynebacterium diphtheriae*) | *Transmission mode:* direct contact, contact with contaminated articles, or consumption of unpasteurized milk<br><br>*Communicable period:* 2 to 4 weeks in presence of antibiotic treatment, months without treatment | 2–5 days | *Clinical manifestations:* fever, cough, pharyngitis, anorexia, membranous lesion on tonsils, pharynx, or larynx<br><br>*Potential complications:* neuritis, carditis, congestive heart failure, respiratory failure | *Treatment:* Isolation, antitoxin, antibiotics, and analgesics<br><br>*Immunity conferment:* diphtheria, tetanus, and acellular pertussis (DTaP) vaccine; passive immunity conferred by maternal antibodies |
| Erythema infectiosum, or Fifth disease (Parvovirus B19, Figure 8-8) | *Transmission mode:* contact with respiratory secretions and blood<br><br>*Communicable period:* unknown | 4–20 days | *Clinical manifestations:* fiery-red cheeks ("slapped face" appearance); erythematous, maculopapular, lacy rash on trunk then limbs<br><br>*Potential complications:* none | *Treatment: Supportive*<br><br>*Immunity conferment:* no vaccine |
| Hepatitis B, or serum hepatitis (hepatitis B virus [HBV]) | *Transmission mode:* blood, secretions, prenatally, perinatally, sexual contact<br><br>*Communicable period:* throughout clinical course | 50–180 days | *Transmission mode:* mild flulike symptoms, jaundice in adolescents<br><br>*Potential complications:* Liver failure | *Treatment:* supportive care<br><br>*Immunity conferment:* hepatitis B vaccine (Hep B) |

*(Continues)*

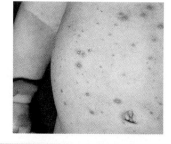

FIGURE 8-7   Varicella (*Courtesy of Robert A. Silverman, M.D., Clinical Associate Professor, Department of Pediatrics, Georgetown University.*)

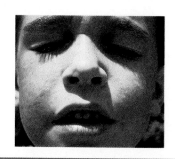

FIGURE 8-8   "Slapped Face" in Erythema Infectiousum (Fifth Disease) (*Courtesy of the Centers for Disease Control and Prevention.*)

**TABLE 8-4 Select Common Communicable Diseases (Continued)**

| DISEASE (CAUSAL AGENT) | TRANSMISSION MODE AND COMMUNICABLE PERIOD | INCUBATION PERIOD | CLINICAL MANIFESTATIONS AND POTENTIAL COMPLICATIONS | TREATMENT AND IMMUNITY CONFERMENT |
|---|---|---|---|---|
| Measles, or rubeola (measles virus, Figure 8-9) | *Transmission mode*: direct or indirect contact with respiratory droplets<br><br>*Communicable period*: 4 days before to 5 days after appearance of rash | 10–21 days | *Clinical manifestations*: fever, runny nose, cough, enlarged lymph nodes, Koplik's spots (small, red spots with blue-white centers on oral mucosa, Figure 8-10), photophobia, maculopapular rash from hairline over entire body<br><br>*Potential complications*: otitis media, pneumonia, encephalitis, airway obstruction | *Treatment*: supportive care<br><br>*Immunity conferment*: measles, mumps, rubella (MMR) vaccine<br><br>*Active*: from infection with causative agent |
| Mononucleosis (Epstein-Barr virus) | *Transmission mode*: direct contact with saliva; blood transfusions; most common in adolescents and young adults<br><br>*Communicable period*: unknown | 30–50 days | *Clinical manifestations*: fever, pharyngitis, fatigue, sore throat, enlarged lymph nodes<br><br>*Potential complications*: splenic rupture, hepatitis, meningitis, encephalitis, Guillain-Barré syndrome | *Treatment*: supportive care, antipyretics, analgesics<br><br>*Immunity conferment*: no vaccine |
| Mumps, or parotitis *(paramyxovirus)* | *Transmission mode*: direct or indirect contact with saliva<br><br>*Communicable period*: 7 days before swelling until 2 to 3 days after swelling subsides | 14–21 days | *Clinical manifestations*: fever, headache, malaise, anorexia, "earache" aggravated by chewing, enlarged parotid gland (Figure 8-11)<br><br>*Potential complications*: orchitis, meningoen-cephalitis, hearing loss | *Treatment*: supportive care, antipyretics, analgesics<br><br>*Immunity conferment*: MMR vaccine, natural; passive: mumps immune globulin |

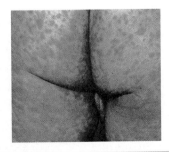

**FIGURE 8-9** Rubeola/Measles (*Courtesy of the Centers for Disease Control and Prevention.*)

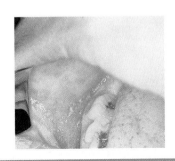

**FIGURE 8-10** Koplik's Spots in Rubeloa (*Courtesy of the Centers for Disease Control and Prevention.*)

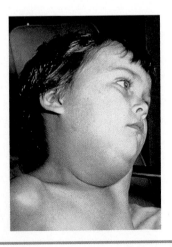

**FIGURE 8-11** Mumps (*Courtesy of the Centers for Disease Control and Prevention.*)

**TABLE 8-4  Select Common Communicable Diseases (Continued)**

| DISEASE (CAUSAL AGENT) | TRANSMISSION MODE AND COMMUNICABLE PERIOD | INCUBATION PERIOD | CLINICAL MANIFESTATIONS AND POTENTIAL COMPLICATIONS | TREATMENT AND IMMUNITY CONFERMENT |
|---|---|---|---|---|
| Pertussis, or whooping cough (*Bordetella pertussis*) | *Transmission mode*: direct contact or respiratory droplets  *Communicable period*: 1 week after exposure until 4 to 6 weeks | 5–21 days | *Clinical manifestations*: upper respiratory symptoms progressing to severe paroxysmal cough with inspiratory whoop  *Potential complications*: pneumonia, otitis media, hemorrhage, convulsions | *Treatment*: antibiotics, supportive care with high humidity  *Immunity conferment*: DTaP vaccine; *active*: from infection with causative agent |
| Poliomyelitis, or infantile paralysis (poliovirus types I, II, III) | *Transmission mode*: fecal–oral, respiratory droplets  *Communicable period*: unknown prior to symptoms, 1 week after symptoms for respiratory contact, up to 6 weeks for fecal contact | 5–14 days | *Clinical manifestations*: fever, headache, abdominal pain, stiff neck, pain and tenderness in lower extremities, paralysis  *Potential complications*: permanent paralysis, respiratory arrest | *Treatment*: supportive, rehabilitative care  *Immunity conferment*: poliovirus vaccine (inactivated) [IPV] or live oral [OPV]; *active*: immunity against a specific strain conferred by disease |
| Roseola, or exanthema subitum (herpesvirus type 6, Figure 8-12) | *Transmission mode*: unknown; appears between 6 months and 2 years of age  *Communicable period*: unknown | Unknown | *Clinical manifestations*: rose-pink, nonpruritic maulopapules on trunk then face, neck, and limbs that fade on pressure  *Potential complications*: febrile seizures | *Treatment*: antipyretics, supportive care  *Immunity conferment*: no vaccine |

(*Continues*)

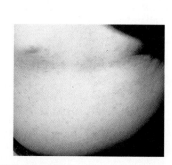

**FIGURE 8-12    Roseola** (*Courtesy of Robert A. Silverman, MD, Clinical Associate Professor, Department of Pediatrics, Georgetown University.*)

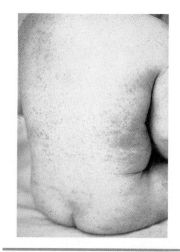

**FIGURE 8-13    Rubella (German Measles/3-Day Measles)** (*Courtesy of the Centers for Disease Control and Prevention.*)

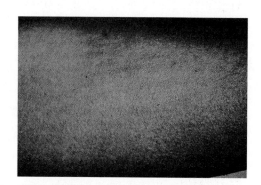

**FIGURE 8-14    Scarlet Fever** (*Courtesy of the Centers for Disease Control and Prevention.*)

**TABLE 8-4 Select Common Communicable Diseases (Continued)**

| DISEASE (CAUSAL AGENT) | TRANSMISSION MODE AND COMMUNICABLE PERIOD | INCUBATION PERIOD | CLINICAL MANIFESTATIONS AND POTENTIAL COMPLICATIONS | TREATMENT AND IMMUNITY CONFERMENT |
|---|---|---|---|---|
| Rubella, or German measles, 3-day measles (Rubella virus, Figure 8-13) | *Transmission mode*: airborne, direct contact with droplets, transplacental<br><br>*Communicable period*: 10 days before symptoms and 15 days after rash appears | 14–21 days | *Clinical manifestations*: fever, headache, malaise, runny nose, anorexia, maculopapular rash progressing from head to extremities<br><br>*Potential complications*: risks for unborn fetus of infected mother; spontaneous abortion, stillbirth, ear, eye, and cardiac anomalies | *Treatment*: supportive care<br><br>*Immunity conferment*: MMR vaccine |
| Scarlet fever, or scarlatina (group A *beta-hemolytic streptococci*, Figure 8-14) | *Transmission mode*: airborne respiratory droplets and contaminated articles<br><br>*Communicable period*: from onset of symptoms until 24 hours after antibiotic therapy is initiated | 1–7 days | *Clinical manifestations*: fever, headache, "strawberry tongue," abdominal pain, sore throat, skin on hands and feet peels in sheets after first week<br><br>*Potential complications*: glomerulonephritis, rheumatic fever | *Treatment*: penicillin, antipyretics, analgesics<br><br>*Immunity conferment*: no immunity |
| Tetanus, or lockjaw (*Clostridium tetani*) | *Transmission mode*: direct contact of skin wound with contaminated soil or implements<br><br>*Communicable period*: not communicable | 3–21 days | *Clinical manifestations*: stiffness of neck and jaw, difficulty breathing<br><br>*Potential complications*: laryngospasm, death | *Treatment*: supportive care<br><br>*Immunity conferment*: DTaP vaccine: passive: from tetanus antitoxin or immune globulin (TIG) |

COURTESY OF DELMAR CENGAGE LEARNING

Be knowledgeable about the safe administration of immunizations. This includes proper storage, reconstitution, sequence, injection site, and technique.

The nurse is responsible for documenting on the child's immunization record the type of vaccine, the date of administration, the manufacturer and lot number, the expiration date, and the administration site. Encourage caregivers to keep and provide immunization records at every health care visit.

# INTEGUMENTARY SYSTEM

Because they are visible and often disfiguring, skin disorders can prove emotionally and psychologically stressful for the child and family/caregivers. It is important to teach families and children strategies to maintain healthy skin. Skin disorders may be caused by infections (bacterial, fungal, viral), infestations (pediculosis, scabies), insects, substances (contact dermatitis), acne, and injuries such as burns.

## :: COMMUNITY/HOME HEALTH CARE

### Preventing Children from Scratching Lesions

To prevent children from scratching lesions:
- Cut the fingernails short.
- Give cool baths.
- Cover the lesions with clothing, when possible.
- At nighttime, cover the hands with socks or gloves.
- During the day, encourage activities that require use of the hands; administer antihistamines or sedatives as needed to control itching.
- Keep the child cool.

## ■ BACTERIAL INFECTIONS

Bacterial infections of the skin are usually caused by staphylococci or streptococci. The two most common skin disorders of childhood resulting from bacterial infections are impetigo and cellulitis.

## IMPETIGO

Impetigo, the most common skin infection of childhood, often begins in an area of broken skin, such as that caused by an insect bite or eczema. The face, mouth, hands, neck, and extremities are the most common sites.

Clinical manifestations include primary lesions (macules that change rapidly to form small, thin-walled vesicles with an erythematous halo), secondary lesions (ruptured vesicles covered by a honey-colored crust over an ulcerated base), pruritus, burning, and lymph node enlargement (Figure 8-15). Lesions usually resolve within 2 weeks. Because impetigo is commonly caused by streptococci, rheumatic fever or glomerulonephritis are possible complications.

### MEDICAL–SURGICAL MANAGEMENT

#### Pharmacological

A topical bactericidal ointment such as polymyxin B sulfate-neomycin (Neosporin) is applied for 5 to 7 days. Children with multiple lesions may require oral antibiotics such as erythromycin (E-Mycin). In extreme and extended situations, parenteral antibiotics may be required.

### NURSING MANAGEMENT

The primary nursing goals are to prevent the spread of infection and promote healing. The child with impetigo is treated at home and should not return to school until 2 days after antibiotics are initiated. Emphasize the importance of taking antibiotics as prescribed.

Encourage caregivers to employ preventive hygiene practices such as sleeping alone, bathing daily with antibacterial soap, using a separate towel, washing hands properly, and using separate eating utensils. Wash the lesions gently three times per day with a warm, soapy washcloth. Remove soaked crusts and

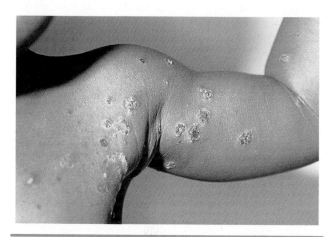

FIGURE 8-15 **Impetigo** (*Courtesy of Robert A. Silverman, MD, Clinical Associate Professor, Department of Pediatrics, Georgetown University.*)

apply topical bactericidal ointment. A small amount of bleeding after crust removal is common. Leave the lesions uncovered. Teach children to keep their fingers away from the lesions.

## CELLULITIS

Cellulitis is a bacterial infection of the skin and subcutaneous tissue. The condition usually affects the face (buccal and periorbital regions) or lower extremities. Children with cellulitis have a history of trauma, impetigo, upper-respiratory infections, sinusitis, otitis media, or tooth abscess. Common causative organisms are staphylococci and streptococci. Clinical manifestations include rapid onset of red or lilac color; tender, hot, edematous skin; and enlarged lymph nodes. Possible complications of cellulitis include septic arthritis, osteomyelitis, meningitis, brain abscess, or blindness.

### MEDICAL–SURGICAL MANAGEMENT

#### Medical

Cellulitis of the extremities is usually treated at home with oral antibiotics and warm compresses. Cellulitis involving the joints or face is extremely serious, requiring hospitalization and IV antibiotics.

#### Surgical

Incision and drainage of the affected area may be necessary if the condition does not improve with treatment.

### NURSING MANAGEMENT

Elevate the affected extremity and immobilize. Apply warm, moist soaks every 4 hours to increase circulation to the affected area, relieve pain, and promote healing. Inform caregivers that failure to administer the entire course of antibiotics as ordered may result in a more serious infection.

## ■ FUNGAL INFECTIONS

Fungal infections are named using the term *tinea* (ringworm) followed by the Latin word for the affected part of the body (Table 8-5).

### NURSING MANAGEMENT

Adequate teaching is essential for successful treatment of tinea. Apply lotion and cream to the entire lesion and extending to approximately 1 inch beyond the lesion. Take oral medication for the full course of treatment, even if symptoms disappear. Proper hygiene is essential.

## ■ VIRAL INFECTIONS

Viral skin infections can produce lesions such as rashes, macules, papules, vesicles, urticaria (hives), and warts. Common communicable diseases of childhood that produce rashes and are preventable through immunizations include rubeola, rubella, and varicella (refer back to Table 8-3). Herpes simplex virus type 1 is a common, contagious skin infection for which there is no cure or prevention.

**TABLE 8-5  Common Fungal Infections**

| INFECTION (SITES) | CLINICAL MANIFESTATIONS | AFFECTED POPULATION | TREATMENT AND PREVENTION |
|---|---|---|---|
| Tinea capitis (scalp) | Erythema, pruritus, scaly scalp with round patches of alopecia | 2- to 10-year-old children | *Treatment*: oral griseofulvin (Fulvicin P/G, Grifulvin V) <br><br> *Prevention*: avoid sharing combs, barber scissors, hats, and towels; avoid direct contact with infected scalp |
| Tinea corporis (trunk, face, extremities) | Ringlike, scaly plaques measuring 1/2 to 1 inch and having pale centers and red margins | Young boys living in hot, humid climates | *Treatment*: antifungal cream applied three times per day until lesions have been gone for 1 week (usually 2 to 4 weeks). <br><br> *Prevention*: treat infected pets |
| Tinea pedis (feet, toes; "athletes foot") | Fissures, red scaly lesions | Adolescents and adults | *Treatment*: daily washing and application of antifungal cream for up to 6 weeks. <br><br> *Prevention*: avoid contaminated floors, sidewalks, and showers; nylon socks; plastic shoes; closed shoes |
| Tinea cruris (inner thighs, inguinal area; "jock itch") | Scaly lesions, erythema, pruritus, possible papules or vesicles | Most commonly, athletes and obese individuals | *Treatment*: oral griseofulvin (Fulvicin P/G, Grifulvin V), sitz baths to soothe <br><br> *Prevention*: wear loose-fitting undergarments to promote dryness |

COURTESY OF DELMAR CENGAGE LEARNING

# HERPES SIMPLEX VIRUS TYPE 1

Herpes simplex virus type 1 (HSV-1) is an often recurrent infection of the mouth ("cold sore," "fever blister"), throat, eyes, or fingers (Figure 8-16). After initial infection, the virus remains dormant within nerve cells and can be reactivated by fever, stress, trauma, sun exposure, menstruation, or immunosuppression. Children suffering from burns, eczema, diaper rash, or immunosuppression are particularly susceptible to HSV-1. Clinical manifestations include clusters of fluid-filled vesicles; ulcerations; swelling; inflammation; pruritus; and severe pain. Lesions usually dry and crust within 7 to 10 days.

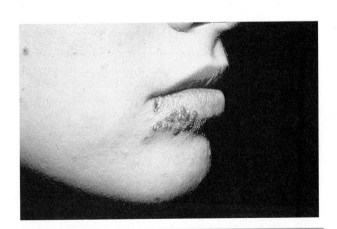

FIGURE 8-16 **Herpes Simplex Virus Type 1** (*Courtesy of Robert A. Silverman, MD, Clinical Associate Professor, Department of Pediatrics, Georgetown University.*)

# MEDICAL–SURGICAL MANAGEMENT

## Medical

Treatment is directed toward relieving symptoms. Usually, children are managed at home by ensuring adequate hydration, pain management, and secondary-infection prevention.

## Pharmacological

Oral acyclovir (Zovirax) is given early in the development of the condition and for recurrent infections. Topical acyclovir cream also is used for recurrent infections. Results are best when applied early in the onset of lesions. Antibiotic ointment may be used to treat secondary infections. Acetaminophen (with or without codeine) and topical and mouth-rinse anesthetics may be prescribed for pain relief.

# NURSING MANAGEMENT

Monitor for dehydration resulting from painful swallowing and for prevention of secondary infection. Offer frozen ice pops, gelatin, noncitrus juices, milk, and flat sodas to help ensure adequate fluid intake despite painful swallowing. Encourage small, frequent feedings of bland, soft foods. Reassure caregivers that fluids are more important than solid food for the first few days.

Teach child to keep hands away from lesions to prevent spreading it to other areas.

Place the hospitalized child in contact isolation or under drainage and secretion precautions. The child is considered contagious until lesions have fallen off or mucous membrane ulcerations have healed.

---

## ::▮:: COMMUNITY/HOME HEALTH CARE

### Caring for the Child with HSV-1

- Wear gloves when suctioning or providing oral care and when handling soiled linens and clothing.
- Practice proper hand hygiene (remembering to wash hands after removing gloves).
- Wash all eating utensils and towels in hot, soapy water.
- Do not eat after the child.
- Prevent the child from putting the fingers in the mouth.
- Use a protective cover such as a sheet when holding and cuddling the child.
- Provide oral fluids that do not irritate the mucous membrane, such as noncitrus juices, flat sodas, milk, and ice pops.
- Provide at least 100 mL (approximately 1/2 cup) /kg/day of fluids for a child weighing less than 20 kg.
- Watch for signs of dehydration, such as dry skin and mucous membranes and decreased urine output (<3 to 4 times per day).
- Administer medications as prescribed.

## ▮ INFESTATIONS

Infestations are one of the major health problems in schools. Common infestations are pediculosis and scabies.

## PEDICULOSIS

Pediculosis (lice) is an infestation that most typically affects the head (capitis), body (corporis), or pubic area (pubis). Pediculosis of the head is the most common infestation seen in children. Lice attach their eggs (nits) to hair shafts close to the scalp. The nits then hatch in approximately 1 week. Clinical manifestations of head lice infestation include "dandruff" (nits) that is not easily removed, severe itching of the scalp, and "bugs" in the hair (usually behind the ears and at the back of the head) (Figure 8-17). Signs and symptoms

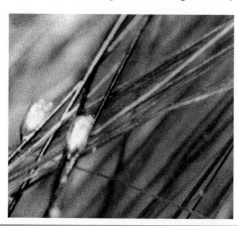

FIGURE 8-17 Nits (*Courtesy of Hogil Pharmaceutical Corporation.*)

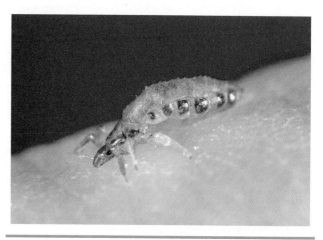

FIGURE 8-18 A female body louse as it was obtaining a blood-meal from a human host, who in this case, happened to be the photographer. Infestation is common, found worldwide, and affects people of all races. Body lice infestations spread rapidly under crowded conditions where hygiene is poor and there is frequent contact among people. (*Courtesy of the Centers for Disease Control and Prevention/provided by Frank Collins, PhD; photo by James Gathany.*)

of body lice infestation include intense pruritus and papular, rose-colored dermatitis in areas under tight-fitting clothing (Figure 8-18). Lice are easily passed from child to child in close-contact situations (e.g., the home, day care centers, and schools) via the sharing of headgear, hair-care products, pillows, blankets, and towels.

## MEDICAL–SURGICAL MANAGEMENT
### Pharmacological

Several anti-lice products are available (Table 8-6).

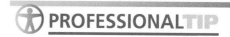

### Checking for Lice

Because lice do not transmit from hair to hands, the use of gloves during head checks is neither necessary nor cost effective.

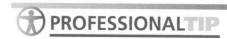

### Manual Removal of Lice

The National Pediculosis Association (NPA) (2009a) advocates early detection and manual removal of nits and lice to prevent the unnecessary use of chemicals. According to the NPA, lindane (Kwell) is the most potentially toxic of all the chemicals available for removing lice and nits. Vacuuming, rather than environmental lice sprays, is a safe and effective way to rid the environment of lice. Lice sprays should not be used in the home or on a child's bedding.

**TABLE 8-6 Anti-Lice Products**

| PRODUCT | TREATMENT | EFFECT |
|---------|-----------|--------|
| permethrin (Nix) | Apply to shampooed hair, leave on for 10 minutes, and rinse out of hair with water; do not re-shampoo for 24 hours | Safely kills lice and nits with one application |
| pyrethrins (TripleX, RID) | Apply to hair as directed; repeat treatment in 1 to 2 weeks, if live nits are present | Safely kills lice and nits; product of choice for those under 2 years of age and for pregnant adolescents |

## NURSING MANAGEMENT

Nursing care for children with pediculosis focuses on screening and education. Encourage caregivers and teachers to incorporate checking for lice into routine daily hygiene. Early detection facilitates immediate removal. There is no need to cut long hair or to shave the child's head, which only draws more attention to the fact that the child is infested.

Teach children that anyone can get lice and that taunting a child who has lice may hurt the child's feelings. Because lice are transmitted from person to person, children should be cautioned about using hair-care products, hats, pillows, blankets, and towels that do not belong to them.

## SCABIES

Scabies results from the impregnated "itch mite" burrowing into the epidermis to lay her eggs. Clinical manifestations include intense pruritus and rash (papules, vesicles, and nodules) found most often on the wrists, finger webs, elbows, axillae, feet, ankles, head, neck, abdomen, waist, groin, and buttocks (Figure 8-19). Secondary infections often occur as a result of scratching the lesions.

## MEDICAL–SURGICAL MANAGEMENT

### Pharmacological

The treatment of choice for scabies is 5% permethrin cream (Elimite, Nix). An oral antihistamine such as diphenhydramine

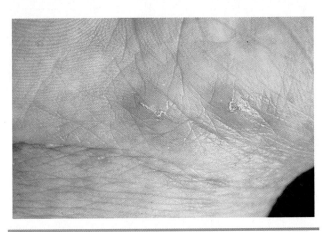

**FIGURE 8-19** Scabies (*Courtesy of Robert A. Silverman, MD, Clinical Associate Professor, Department of Pediatrics, Georgetown University.*)

hydrochloride (Benadryl) or hydroxyzine (Atarax) may be prescribed to relieve pruritus.

## NURSING MANAGEMENT

Nursing management for the child with scabies focuses on promoting healing, preventing secondary infections, and preventing further transmission of the condition. All persons having direct contact with the child, including care providers and those living in the child's house, should be treated. Itching and rash may endure for 2 to 3 weeks.

## ■ BITES/STINGS

Animals (usually dogs), spiders, ticks, and insects (e.g., mosquitoes, fleas) account for the many bites and stings suffered by children. Bites and stings generally cause mild discomfort and are simple to treat; however, in some cases, life-threatening situations result.

## ANIMAL BITES

Animal bites may result from domestic or wild animals but are most commonly caused by a familiar dog. Children younger than 4 years of age are bitten most frequently because of their height and the associated tendency to be near the dog's face. Dog bites usually occur on the face or extremities and can result in crushing and puncture wounds and lacerations.

## COMMUNITY/HOME HEALTH CARE

### Guidelines for Managing Infestations

- Wash bedding, clothing, and stuffed animals in hot water and dry in a hot dryer.
- Vacuum carpets, upholstered seats (in the car and house), mattresses, toys, and nonwashable items. According to the NPA (2009a), there is no need to discard the used vacuum bag.
- The NPA (2009a) does not recommend placing toys or other items in plastic bags.
- The NPA (2009a) recommends manually removing the lice and nits with a special lice removing comb that can be boiled if desired.

## MEDICAL–SURGICAL MANAGEMENT

### Medical

The primary medical concerns for the child who has suffered an animal bite are infections from rabies and tetanus and scarring, especially on the face. Generally, after the wound and surrounding area are thoroughly washed with mild soap and water, a clean dressing is applied.

### 🔬 Pharmacological

If the animal is unvaccinated for rabies, the child will be given a series of immunizations to prevent rabies. Antibiotics may be indicated if the wounds are deep. Tetanus toxoid may be administered, depending on the child's immunization history and the severity of the wound.

## NURSING MANAGEMENT

Focus on prevention and wound care. It is important for children to learn "animal safety rules" in order to prevent bites.

Teach caregivers and children to cleanse wounds properly and observe for signs of infection. Encourage parents to keep their child's immunizations up to date. If rabies immunizations are required, parents must understand the importance of returning for the injections on the appropriate days. Report animal bites to the community animal control agency.

## SPIDER BITES

Bites from black widow and brown recluse spiders demand medical attention. Characteristically, these spiders are nonagressive, avoid light, and bite only in self-defense. Although both spiders inject toxic venom when they bite, the initial bite may go unnoticed. Within a few hours after the bite, however, manifestations surface such as swollen, painful erythema and systemic reactions. Black widow venom is neurotoxic and may cause dizziness, weakness, abdominal pain, paralysis, seizures, and, possibly, death from shock and renal failure. Brown recluse venom is necrotoxic, with the bite progressing to a necrotic ulcer within 1 to 2 weeks. Systemic reactions may include fever, nausea and vomiting, and

joint pain. The recluse bite is not fatal, but the ulcer may take months to heal.

## MEDICAL–SURGICAL MANAGEMENT

### Medical

The child with a black widow spider bite will be hospitalized for supportive care until neurological symptoms subside and renal function is confirmed. The child with a brown recluse bite will require wound care and pain management but will usually not require hospitalization.

### Surgical

Skin grafting may be required for large ulcers resulting from the brown recluse spider bite.

### 🔬 Pharmacological

Antivenin (Lactrodectus mactans) is administered to the child with a black widow spider bite, if the child has no allergy to horse serum. In addition, analgesics, muscle relaxants, and tetanus prophylaxis may be required.

There is no antivenin for the brown recluse spider bite. Antibiotics, corticosteroids, analgesics, and tetanus prophylaxis may be prescribed for the time during which the wound is healing.

## NURSING MANAGEMENT

Focus on wound care, proper administration of medications, and prevention. Teach caregivers and children to be cautious in areas where spiders are likely to live, such as woodpiles and closets.

## TICK BITES

Ticks live in fields and woods. They feed on the blood of mammals (e.g., humans, dogs, livestock, and deer) by embedding their heads into the skin. Tick bites cause pruritic nodules at the site of attachment and, rarely, systemic reactions such as fever, rash, and paralysis. Lyme disease (Figure 8-20) and Rocky Mountain spotted fever are caused by organisms that are transmitted by ticks.

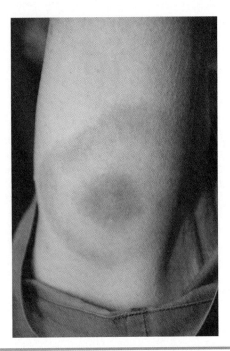

FIGURE 8-20 This "bull's-eye" pattern rash manifested at the site of a tick bite in a client's posterior right upper arm. The client subsequently contracted Lyme disease. Lyme disease patients who are diagnosed early, and receive proper antibiotic treatment, usually recover rapidly and completely. A key component of early diagnosis is recognition of the characteristic Lyme disease bull's-eye rash. (*Courtesy of the Centers for Disease Control and Prevention/photo by James Gathany.*)

## NURSING MANAGEMENT

Preventing tick bites and removing embedded ticks are the primary focus. Remove the tick by grasping the tick's body with blunt, angled forceps or tweezers as close to the skin as possible and pulling straight up in an attempt to remove the embedded head along with the body. Do not twist the tick (American Academy of Family Physicians, 2002). Remove any remaining part of the head or attachment secretions from the tick using a sterile needle, and then thoroughly cleanse hands. Cleanse the attachment site and apply an antiseptic solution.

## INSECT BITES

Insects such as mosquitoes, flies, fleas, and gnats inject foreign proteins when they penetrate the skin to suck blood. Insect bites usually result in itching, erythema, and a small wheal. The severity of the reaction depends on the degree of the child's hypersensitivity.

## MEDICAL–SURGICAL MANAGEMENT
### Medical

Medical management focuses on alleviating itching and preventing infection. Baths and cool compresses may relieve itching and prevent scratching, which can lead to bacterial infections.

### Pharmacological

Antipruritics and antihistamines may be prescribed to control severe itching and facilitate sleep.

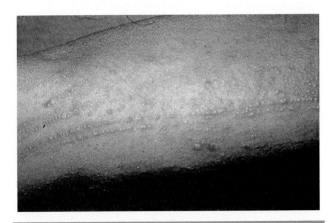

FIGURE 8-21 Contact Dermatitis (*Courtesy of the Centers for Disease Control and Prevention.*)

## NURSING MANAGEMENT

Focus on preventing bites, alleviating itching, and preventing infection. Mattresses, carpets, furniture, and pets may require treatment with insecticides.

## CONTACT DERMATITIS

Contact dermatitis is an inflammatory reaction of the skin to allergens, such as rubber, dyes, nickel, or poison ivy, or to irritants, such as soaps, wool, urine, or stool. Manifestations of allergic contact dermatitis include tiny, itching, weeping blisters over an area of skin (Figure 8-21). Manifestations of irritant contact dermatitis include localized, dry, inflamed, pruritic skin.

## MEDICAL–SURGICAL MANAGEMENT
### Medical

Treatment involves discontinuing exposure to the offending agent, washing the skin thoroughly, and applying cool compresses.

### Pharmacological

Steroid cream (1%) may be applied in a thin layer several times per day after the application of cool compresses. Oral steroids may be prescribed for severe cases.

## NURSING MANAGEMENT

Nursing care is aimed at relieving itching, preventing infection, and identifying and removing offensive substances. In addition to cool compresses, oral antihistamines, antipruritic lotions, and tepid oatmeal baths may relieve itching. Avoid overheating. Teach children to recognize and avoid poison ivy, oak, and sumac.

## ACNE

Acne, one of the most common health problems of adolescence, is a noninfectious, inflammatory disease of the skin involving the sebaceous glands and hair follicles (Figure 8-22). Pathophysiologic factors having the greatest

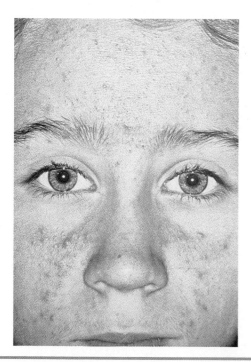

FIGURE 8-22  Acne (*From Acne Vulgaris, by G. Plewig and A. B. Klingman [Eds], 1975, Berlin/Heideberg, Germany; Springer-Verlag. Used with permission.*)

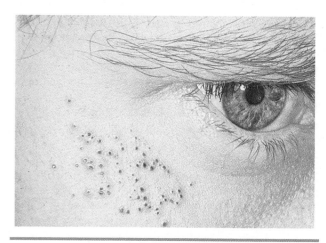

FIGURE 8-23  Open Comedones (*From Acne Vulgaris, by G. Plewig and A. B. Klingman [Eds], 1975, Berlin/Heideberg, Germany; Springer-Verlag. Used with permission.*)

influence on acne development are overproduction of sebum; formation of **comedones**, or whiteheads and blackheads (Figure 8-23); and proliferation of *Propionibacterium acnes* bacteria in the hair follicles.

Manifestations include comedones, papules, pustules, and nodules on the face, neck, back, shoulders, and upper chest. Factors related to the development of acne include elevated hormone levels (especially androgens); predisposition; emotional stress; hot, humid environments; the premenstrual period, in females; and the growth of anaerobic bacteria. The visual lesions of acne, although usually temporary, may be extremely distressing to the adolescent, who is typically very concerned about appearance.

## MEDICAL–SURGICAL MANAGEMENT

### Pharmacological

Treatment is individualized, depending on the severity and types of lesions. The goal is to decrease sebum production and prevent infection with *P. acnes*. Topical agents benzoyl peroxide (Clearasil, Benoxyl) and tretinoin (Retin-A) are available

as cleansers, lotions, creams, sticks, pads, gels, and bars and may be effective for mild cases. Other topical keratolytic agents containing sulfur, resorcinol, or salicylic acid may be prescribed for drying and peeling effects. Topical or oral antibiotics, such as erythromycin and tetracycline preparations, may be administered for infections.

Isotretinoin (Accutane) may be used for nodulocystic acne. Side effects of isotretinoin include dry lips and skin, eye irritation, temporary worsening of acne, **epistaxis** (nosebleed), bleeding and inflammation of the gums, itching, photosensitivity, and joint and muscle pain. In addition, isotretinoin may cause central nervous system, heart, thymus, and craniofacial abnormalities in the fetus.

If isotretinoin is to be prescribed, pregnancy tests are done 2 weeks before initiating, every month during, and 1 month after discontinuing the treatment. All women of childbearing potential are placed on contraception during treatment.

## NURSING MANAGEMENT

A healthy lifestyle, including adequate rest, exercise, and diet, promotes healing of lesions. Be especially sensitive to the adolescent's feelings about the condition, no matter how mild the case may seem.

Educate the adolescent and caregiver about acne and the prescribed treatment. Adolescents are encouraged to take responsibility for implementing the prescribed care.

### ■ BURNS

Burns are the second leading cause of injury deaths among children between 1 and 14 years of age (James, Ashwill, & Droske, 2002). Carelessness of adults, the children's curiosity and increasing mobility, and caretakers' failure to adequately supervise children all contribute to the high incidence of burns among children. In addition, burns are a common form of child abuse. Thermal burns (e.g., from scalding liquids, house fires) are most common, followed by chemical (e.g., from touching or ingesting caustic agents) and electrical (e.g., from wires, curling irons, ovens), respectively.

The major manifestations of burns include severe wounds, pain, fluid and nutritional deficits, respiratory complications, and secondary infections. All systems of the burned child are at risk for complications.

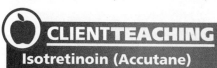

### CLIENT TEACHING

**Isotretinoin (Accutane)**

It is important that adolescent females on isotretinoin who are sexually active use contraceptives 1 month before treatment is started; during treatment; and 1 month after discontinuation of treatment. In addition, children taking isotretinoin should not donate blood during this period.

Smoke inhalation can be fatal. Toxic fumes from burning plastics, polyurethanes, and many fabrics cause cyanide poisoning. Carbon monoxide and cyanide inhalation have the same signs and symptoms: nausea, vomiting, lethargy, confusion, tachycardia, metabolic acidosis, and possibly seizures and coma.

## MEDICAL–SURGICAL MANAGEMENT

### Medical

The severity of the burn injury is assessed on the basis of the percentage of surface burned and the depth of the wound. The Burn Wheel provides an accurate estimate of percentage of body surface area burn in children and by turning the wheel to align the correct values for weight and burns, it provides the amount of fluid resuscitation and continuation needed (Figure 8-24).

The involvement of specific body parts or certain specific burn distributions increase burn severity, regardless of body surface area affected. Burns to the face, hands, feet, perineal area, or anterior chest, and circumferential burns of the thorax or extremity are treated as major because of the potential for functional impairment. Regardless of the amount of tissue destroyed, if smoke inhalation is suspected, there is risk for airway obstruction.

### Pharmacological

Tetanus antitoxin or toxoid should be ordered according to the child's immunization status. Intravenous morphine sulfate is the drug of choice for pain control. Analgesics are

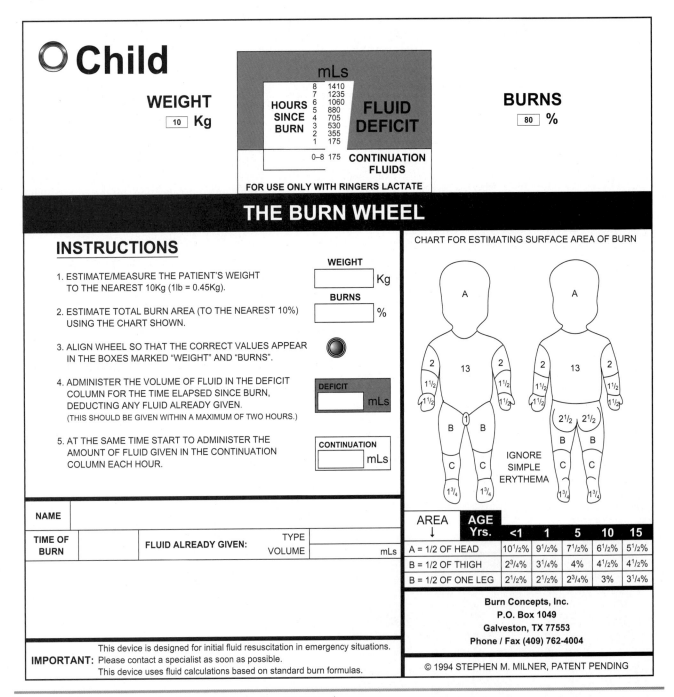

FIGURE 8-24  The Burn Wheel (invented by Stephen M. Milner)

administered 20 to 30 minutes before dressing changes and debridement to provide the most relief possible. Itching may persist for months and may be relieved with medication.

## Health Promotion

Prevention of scarring and contractures is essential for optimal cosmetic and functional recovery. Pressure dressings and suits may need to be worn for more than 1 year to minimize scarring. Physical therapy, initiated at the time of admission and continued until the scars mature, prevents flexion contractures. These treatments add to the child's discomfort.

## NURSING MANAGEMENT

Refer to the Integumentary System chapter for information on nursing management of the child who has been burned.

# URINARY SYSTEM

Acute poststreptococcal glomerulonephritis, nephrotic syndrome, and enuresis are discussed in the following sections.

# ACUTE POSTSTREPTOCOCCAL GLOMERULONEPHRITIS

Glomerulonephritis is an inflammation of the glomeruli of the kidneys. Acute poststreptococcal glomerulonephritis (APSGN) occurs as an immune reaction to streptococcal infection of the throat or skin.

Clinical manifestations of hematuria and periorbital edema usually appear 1 to 3 weeks after a streptococcal infection. Other possible manifestations include decreased urine output, hypertension, fever, and fatigue. The prognosis is excellent.

## MEDICAL–SURGICAL MANAGEMENT
### Medical

The diagnosis of APSGN can be made based on history, presenting symptoms, and laboratory results. There is no treatment for APSGN. Medical management focuses on presenting signs and symptoms and the degree of renal dysfunction. Laboratory values usually return to normal within 6 to 12 weeks.

### Pharmacological

Hypertension may be treated by limiting sodium and water intake or by administering diuretics or antihypertensives.

## NURSING MANAGEMENT

Refer to the Urinary System chapter for information on nursing management of the child with APSGN.

# NEPHROTIC SYNDROME

Nephrotic syndrome refers to kidney disorders characterized by proteinuria, hypoalbuminemia, and edema. The most common childhood nephrotic disorder, minimal change nephrotic syndrome (MCNS), results from minimal alterations of the glomerulus. The cause of the alteration is unknown.

Clinical manifestations include pitting edema (periorbital and dependent), anorexia, fatigue, abdominal pain, increased weight, and normal blood pressure. Potential complications include respiratory compromise and peritonitis. Although the child may experience remissions and exacerbations for months, the prognosis in most cases is good.

## MEDICAL–SURGICAL MANAGEMENT
### Medical

Diagnosis is made based on clinical presentation, age of the child, massive proteinuria (50 mg/kg/day), and hypoalbuminemia (<27g/L).

### Surgical

A kidney biopsy may be done if a lesion other than MCNS is suspected or the child does not respond as expected to pharmacological treatments.

### Pharmacological

The use of corticosteroids such as prednisone (Cortan, Deltasone) induces remission in most cases. Corticosteroid therapy usually produces diuresis within 7 to 14 days. After diuresis occurs, prednisone is continued every other day for 3 days per week. Urine is tested daily for protein until protein has been absent from the urine for up to 7 days. The drug dosage is then gradually decreased and discontinued over a 4-week period. Repeat corticosteroid therapy is administered to children who have relapses after drug therapy is discontinued.

Alkylating agents such as cyclophosphamide (Cytoxan) may be used to reduce symptoms and prevent further relapses in children who do not respond adequately to repeated corticosteroid therapy. The risks and benefits of this therapy must be carefully considered.

When the child is in remission, administration of vaccines for pneumococci and flu should be considered because an exacerbation of nephrotic syndrome can occur following an infection.

### Diet

A general "no-added-salt" diet is recommended. Offer appealing, small, frequent meals to the child, who typically has a poor appetite.

## NURSING MANAGEMENT

Educate the child's caregivers about the disease process. Monitor I&O hourly. Weigh the child daily. Measure abdominal girth and test urine albumin daily. Keep skin clean and dry. Inspect for skin breakdown and turn child every 2 hours. Screen visitors for signs of infection. Follow Standard Precautions carefully.

## NURSING PROCESS

### ASSESSMENT
#### Subjective Data

Question the caregiver about symptom onset, appetite, urine output, irritability, and signs of fatigue.

#### Objective Data

Assess daily weight, abdominal girth, vital signs, and skin for pallor, irritation, breakdown, and edema.

**Nursing diagnoses for the child with MCNS include the following:**

| NURSING DIAGNOSES | PLANNING/OUTCOMES | NURSING INTERVENTIONS |
|---|---|---|
| *Excess **F**luid Volume* related to compromised regulatory mechanism | The child will maintain fluid balance. | Monitor I&O hourly; report urinary output of <2 mL/kg/hr.<br>Weigh daily.<br>Measure abdominal girth daily at the level of the umbilicus.<br>Test urine albumin daily with reagent strips. |
| *Risk for Impaired **S**kin Integrity* related to altered circulation | The child's skin will remain intact. | Inspect the child's skin for breakdown.<br>Turn and reposition the child every 2 hours.<br>Keep the child's skin clean and dry.<br>Use a protective mattress (e.g., eggcrate). |
| *Risk for **I**nfection* related to immunosuppression | The child will remain infection free. | Screen visitors for signs of infection.<br>Practice proper hand hygiene technique.<br>Monitor the child for signs of infection, such as sore throat, cough, fever, abdominal pain.<br>Monitor laboratory values daily. |
| *Deficient **K**nowledge (parent)* related to treatment regimen | The caregiver will follow through with the prescribed treatment. | Educate the caregivers about the disease process.<br>Instruct the caregivers to test urine for albumin, assess for edema and infection, and administer drugs.<br>Instruct the caregiver to allow a return to ADLs once the child is free of edema. |

**Evaluation:** Evaluate each outcome to determine how it has been met by the client.

## ENURESIS

Enuresis is involuntary urination beyond the age when control of urination commonly is acquired. It is not unusual for nocturnal enuresis, or bedwetting, to occur until 8 years of age, because of small bladder capacity and delayed maturation of the neuromuscular system. Most children will outgrow bedwetting without therapeutic intervention.

When enuresis continues to occur beyond the eighth year or recurs in a child who has been dry both day and night for a prolonged period, there may be cause for concern. Possible causes of reoccurring enuresis include urinary tract infections, minor abnormalities of the urinary tract, pinworm infestation, constipation, diabetes, sickle-cell anemia, sexual abuse, stress, and sleep disorders.

## MEDICAL–SURGICAL MANAGEMENT
### Medical

Urinalysis and urine culture are done to rule out infection. Other diagnostic studies are performed to rule out all possible causes. Common treatment approaches for enuresis without a physiologic cause include fluid restriction, bladder stretching exercises, behavioral conditioning (e.g., enuresis alarm), and reward systems.

### Pharmacological

An anticholinergic such as oxybutynin chloride (Ditropan) may reduce uninhibited bladder contractions. Vasopressins such as desmopressin acetate (DDAVP) nasal spray may reduce nighttime urine output. Antidepressants such as imipramine hydrochloride (Tofranil) may be prescribed.

### Other Therapies

If emotional factors are precipitating enuresis, psychosocial support may be an essential part of care. A multidisciplinary team approach is most effective.

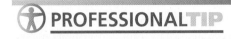

## PROFESSIONALTIP

**Enuresis**

It is most important to provide the caregiver and the child with opportunities to ventilate feelings. The caregiver and the child must be active and willing participants in any plan of care that is implemented. Tell caregivers that reprimanding the child will not improve the outcome.

# PSYCHOSOCIAL DISORDERS

Psychosocial disorders are responses to stressors. Factors influencing an individual's response to stressors include temperament, developmental level, nature and duration of the stressors, past experiences, and coping and adaptive abilities of the family. Possible manifestations in children include depression, anxiety, encopresis, enuresis, passive–aggressive behavior, and learning problems (James, et al., 2002). Some of the psychosocial disorders of childhood include obesity, anorexia nervosa and bulimia nervosa, autism, attention deficit hyperactivity disorder, and suicide.

## ■ OBESITY

Obesity is the excessive accumulation of fat resulting in an increase in body weight to 20% or more above ideal weight. Obesity can be a precursor of cardiovascular disease, hypertension, and diabetes. Factors contributing to obesity include an overconsumption of food; a sedentary lifestyle; a lack of caregiver knowledge regarding nutrition and food preparation; unstructured meals; genetic predisposition; and peer pressure.

## CLIENTTEACHING

### Caring for the Child Who Is Obese

Share the following ideas with caregivers of obese children.

**Nutrition**
- Keep a food diary for 1 week; include time, place, type, and amount of food eaten, and the reasons for eating.
- Set a reasonable weight-loss or weight-maintenance goal.
- Establish and maintain regular mealtimes.
- Serve meals at the table only, preferably with the family.
- Serve meals on a small plate in an effort to decrease quantity of food consumed.
- Encourage the child to eat slowly.
- Keep low-calorie snacks on hand.

**Exercise**
- Get the child involved in regular outside activities.
- Walk instead of ride whenever possible.

**Self-Esteem**
- Weight the child only one time per week.
- Focus on the child's positive assets.
- Provide positive feedback for positive behavior.

**Support**
- Establish a group or buddy system.
- Participate in a support group.

The obese child may overeat to compensate for lack of parenteral love and to relieve stress. As a result of obesity, the child may have low self-esteem, poor body image, difficulty in relationships, and recurring bouts of anxiety and depression.

## MEDICAL–SURGICAL MANAGEMENT

### Medical

Obesity is difficult to treat. Positive outcomes are more likely when the child has a support system, understands the importance of weight reduction, and is actively involved in the plan of care.

### Diet

Meals and snacks should consist of small servings of nutritional foods. Teach the caregiver and child ways to select and prepare foods. Incorporate favorite foods into the menu whenever possible.

### Activity

Incorporate physical exercise into the child's daily routine.

## NURSING MANAGEMENT

Focus on meeting nutritional needs, managing related problems, and promoting self-esteem. Assess weight, exercise, and nutritional intake at predetermined intervals. Provide positive feedback for accomplishments, no matter how small. Discuss and revise goals as needed.

Support groups such as Weight Watchers and Overeaters Anonymous may be helpful. In addition, support groups may be available through schools, summer camps, or children's hospitals. A team approach utilizing a psychiatrist or psychologist, a nutritionist, and a nurse may be appropriate.

## ■ ANOREXIA NERVOSA AND BULIMIA NERVOSA

Anorexia nervosa (AN) and bulimia nervosa (BN) are two of the most common eating disorders among children. AN is self-inflicted starvation; BN is binge-eating followed by purging. These disorders usually begin in middle to late adolescence and can last indefinitely, depending on response to treatment. The incidence is highest among Caucasian girls in the higher socioecomonic classes (Hockenberry et al., 2008). Possible causes of these disorders include sensitivity to social pressure for thinness; distorted body image; and longstanding dysfunctional family patterns.

Clinical manifestations include body weight 15% below that expected for age and height, intense fear of gaining weight, dry skin, brittle nails, downy hair on the back and extremities, amenorrhea, constipation, hypothermia, bradycardia, low blood pressure, fluid and electrolyte imbalances, and anemia. Depression, crying spells, feelings of isolation and loneliness, and suicidal thoughts and feelings are common. Clues to frequent vomiting include dental caries, tooth enamel erosion, and throat irritation. Calluses or abrasions may be noted on the back of the hands, from frequent contact with the teeth while inducing vomiting.

## MEDICAL–SURGICAL MANAGEMENT

### Medical

The goal of medical treatment is to correct malnutrition and resulting complications. A weight gain of 0.1 to 0.2 kg per day is emphasized until the desired weight is attained. Enteral feedings or total parenteral nutrition (TPN) may be necessary to replace lost fluids, protein, and nutrients.

### Pharmacological

Selective serotonin reuptake inhibitors (SSRIs), such as citalopram (Celexa), escitalopram (Lexapro), fluoxetine (Prozac), an sertraline (Zoloft), may decrease binge eating and treat depression (Potts and Mandleco, 2007). SSRIs are also affective with AN.

### Other Therapies

Individual and family therapy are used to address dysfunctional family patterns and assist the adolescent in identifying and dealing with self-esteem and body image issues. Treatment is typically long-term.

## NURSING MANAGEMENT

Refer to the Mental Illness chapter for possible nursing diagnoses for the client with AN or BN and to the Resources listing at the end of this chapter.

## AUTISM

Autism is a complex disorder of brain function involving abnormal emotional, social, and linguistic development. The cause of autism is unknown; however, research suggests it may result from a disturbance in language comprehension, a biochemical problem involving neurotransmitters, or abnormalities in the central nervous system.

Possible clinical manifestations include lack of eye contact, aversion to touch, delayed language development, blank expression, lack of response to verbal stimulation, repetitive behaviors, bizarre body movements, and self-destructive behaviors. Manifestations may vary from mild to severe. The prognosis depends on early detection and the child's response to treatment.

## MEDICAL–SURGICAL MANAGEMENT

### Medical

Diagnosis is based on the presence of specific criteria as listed in *the Diagnostic and Statistical Manual of Mental Disorders,* fourth edition (DSM-IV) (American Psychiatric Association, 1994). In addition, a complete physical and neurological examination is necessary to rule out other disorders such as lead poisoning, phenylketonuria, congenital rubella, and measles encephalitis.

Treatment is provided by a multidisciplinary team and focuses on promoting normal development, social interaction, and learning. Behavior-modification techniques are used to reward desirable behaviors and foster positive coping skills.

---

### CLIENTTEACHING

**Modifying Behavior in the Child Who is Autistic**

- Emphasize the child's positive skills.
- Provide immediate feedback for appropriate behavior.
- Continue social interactions even when the child is unresponsive.
- Provide tactile stimulation such as tickling, holding, cuddling, and shaking hands.
- Teach the child to embrace, kiss, and shake hands.
- Speak in short sentences.
- Use a firm but caring approach.
- Maintain daily routines.

## NURSING MANAGEMENT

Focus on early detection, decreasing environmental stimuli, providing supportive care, maintaining a safe environment, and giving caregivers anticipatory guidance. Monitor growth and development, especially language and social skills. When caring for a child with autism, ascertain the child's routines, rituals, and likes and dislikes. Because autistic children do not do well in unfamiliar environments, it is important that they be surrounded by familiar objects. The child may need assistance with self-care. Keep schedules and care providers as consistent as possible. Close supervision is usually required at all times.

Caregivers need a great deal of support to cope with the challenges of having an autistic child. Assist children to reach their maximum potential through enrollment in special education programs and participation in behavior modification. Some children may achieve independence by adulthood. Inform caregivers about local support groups and refer to the Autism Society of America for current information.

## ATTENTION DEFICIT HYPERACTIVITY DISORDER

Attention-deficit hyperactivity disorder (ADHD) is a developmental disorder characterized by developmentally inappropriate degrees of inattention, overactivity, and impulsivity. The child is usually diagnosed between the ages of 3 and 6 years. Possible clinical manifestations include poor impulse control, distractibility, fidgeting with hands, squirming in seat, excessive talking, and difficulty following instructions.

## MEDICAL–SURGICAL MANAGEMENT

### Medical

Diagnosis may be made based on diagnostic criteria in the *DSM-IV* (American Psychiatric Association, 1994) as well as a complete multidisciplinary evaluation. Treatment focuses on decreasing distractions, modifying behavior (e.g., setting

**CLIENTTEACHING**

**Caring for the Child with ADHD**

- Praise positive behavior and set limits.
- Administer medication as prescribed and with meals.
- Give clear, simple instructions and provide frequent reminders to follow instructions.
- Reduce stimuli in the child's environment (e.g., turning off the TV when the child is trying to do homework).
- Allow for a shortened attention span by providing short teaching sessions and activities that allow for mobility.
- Consult with trained professional for behavior-modification therapy.

limits, ensuring consistency, praising accomplishments), and/or initiating pharmacological therapy.

## Pharmacological

The most commonly prescribed medications include methylphenidate (Ritalin), pemoline (Cylert), and dextroamphetamine (Dexedrine). These drugs stimulate the area of the child's brain that facilitates concentration. Potential side effects include loss of appetite resulting in delayed growth.

## NURSING MANAGEMENT

Focus on improving the child's social interaction and educating the family/caregivers and teachers.

## SUICIDE

Suicide is the third-leading cause of death among adolescents. Boys complete suicide four times more often than do girls, but girls attempt suicide five times more often than do boys. Males tend to use lethal methods such as guns, hanging, and jumping from high elevations, whereas girls more often overdose or cut the wrists. Adolescents who have attempted suicide once are at greatest risk for attempting again. Attempted suicide rarely occurs without warning (Centers for Disease Control and Prevention, 1997a).

Clinical manifestations in the suicidal adolescent may include depression, boredom, restlessness, concentration problems, irritability, lethargy, and intentional misbehavior.

Children at high risk for committing suicide may be experiencing depression, pregnancy, failure in school, drug use, death of a friend or caregiver, problems with a relationship, sexual abuse, chronic illness, or a broken home.

## MEDICAL–SURGICAL MANAGEMENT

### Medical

The child thought to be at high risk for suicide is usually admitted to a psychiatric unit for care. Treatment may include individual, group, and/or family therapy. Negotiating a "No-Suicide" contract is one method that may be used with a suicidal child. In this written and signed contract, the child agrees not to attempt suicide for a negotiated period (e.g., weeks, days, minutes). If at any time the child feels unable to keep the contract, the child agrees to contact help. Children with severe self-abusive behavior may need to be physically or chemically restrained.

### Pharmacological

Drugs that may be used for chemical restraint include diphenhydramine hydrochloride (Benadryl), thioridazine hydrochloride (Mellaril), chlorpromazine (Thorazine), and lorazepam (Ativan). The suicidal child may also require antidepressant and/or antipsychotic medications.

## NURSING MANAGEMENT

Assess risk factors, behaviors, attitude, how lethal is the proposed method of suicide, coping mechanisms, and support system. Be nonjudgmental and show empathy. Remove potentially harmful objects from the environment. Monitor the high-risk child at all times. Administer medications as prescribed. Encourage individual and group therapy for the entire family and keeping all follow-up appointments.

## NURSING PROCESS

### ASSESSMENT

#### Subjective Data

Assess the suicidal child for behaviors, attitudes, risk factors, lethality of the proposed method of suicide, coping mechanisms, and support systems.

#### Objective Data

Observe the child for signs of physical and sexual abuse, self-destructive behaviors, and sudden changes in behavior.

**Nursing diagnoses for the child who is suicidal include the following:**

| NURSING DIAGNOSES | PLANNING/OUTCOMES | NURSING INTERVENTIONS |
|---|---|---|
| *Risk for Self-directed Violence* related to desire to ease emotional pain, solicit attention of others, or avoid responsibility | The child will be less likely to repeat the suicide attempt. | Use a nonjudgmental, empathic approach and a voice and demeanor that are clear, direct, and supportive to discuss feelings and the suicidal event. Remove potentially harmful objects from the environment (e.g., belts, scarves, shoestrings, matches, lighters). |

*(Continues)*

| **Nursing diagnoses for the child who is suicidal include the following: (Continued)** | | |
| --- | --- | --- |
| **NURSING DIAGNOSES** | **PLANNING/OUTCOMES** | **NURSING INTERVENTIONS** |
| | | Monitor the high-risk child at all times, even during bathroom use and sleep. |
| | | Administer prescribed medications. |
| | | Suggest alternate activities for those times when impulsive behavior occurs. |
| | | Restrain the child (as ordered) as an act of care, not punishment. |
| *Interrupted Family Processes* related to relational disturbance or abuse/neglect | The child will feel safe and receive support from others to meet needs. | Encourage individual and group therapy for the entire family to explore personal issues and the need for social support. |
| | | Assist the caregivers to regain the ability to assist the child and manage the home environment. |
| | | Foster caregiver–child interaction. |
| | | Teach the caregivers to monitor the child for sudden changes in behavior. |
| | | Teach the caregivers and child about medication administration. |
| | | Encourage the caregivers to keep follow-up appointments. |

**Evaluation:** Evaluate each outcome to determine how it has been met by the client.

## CASE STUDY

C.P. is a 14-year-old male. He was diagnosed with DMD at 5 years of age. His older brother also had DMD and died 2 years ago at the age of 16. C.P. lives with his parents and 10-year-old sister, L.P. Associated problems include confinement to a wheelchair; contractures of the hips, knees, and ankles; scoliosis requiring a brace; frequent respiratory infections; and obesity. C.P. attends the ninth grade, is a member of the chess club, and enjoys the youth group at his church.

The following questions will guide your development of a nursing care plan for the case study.

1. List the characteristic progression of DMD.
2. Cite three nursing diagnoses and goals for C.P.
3. Identify interventions to help C.P. and his family address the nursing diagnoses identified in question 2.
4. How might genetic counseling benefit this family?
5. Identify resources available to help C.P. and his family cope with DMD.

## SUMMARY

- The most common skin disorders among toddlers and preschoolers are impetigo and dog bites.
- The most common skin disorders among school-age children are pediculosis and scabies.
- The most common skin disorder among adolescents is acne.
- Common respiratory tract infections of childhood include nasopharyngitis, pharyngitis, and influenza.
- Asthma is the leading cause of chronic illness among children.
- Treatment of asthma involves allergen control, drug therapy, controlled exercise, physical therapy, and desensitization.

- Prevention or treatment of group A streptococcal infection in turn prevents rheumatic fever.
- Nursing care of the child with leukemia focuses on preparing the child and family for diagnostic and therapeutic procedures, preventing complications of myelosuppression, managing problems of drug toxicity, and providing emotional support.
- Caregivers of a child with ITP must be able to detect signs of bleeding and know ways to prevent injuries.
- Constipation can be prevented by establishing and maintaining regular toileting habits, drinking fluids, eating a diet high in fiber, and participating in regular exercise.

- Children are more commonly infected with intestinal parasites than are adults because they put their fingers in their mouths more often.
- Obesity can be a precursor to cardiovascular disease, hypertension, and diabetes.
- Acute poststreptococcal glomerulonephritis occurs as an immune reaction to streptococcal infection of the throat or skin.
- Goals for the child with nephrotic syndrome include fluid balance, intact skin, freedom from infection, and compliance with urine testing and drug therapy.
- Goals for children with structural anomalies, such as scoliosis, Legg-Calvé-Perthes disease, and injuries, includes preventing skin breakdown (due to casts and braces) and keeping follow-up appointments.
- Nursing care for the child with DMD focuses on maintaining physical activity, promoting respiratory

function, managing weight, and encouraging age-appropriate social activities.
- Nursing care for the child with juvenile rheumatoid arthritis focuses on preventing injury, controlling pain, enhancing mobility, and encouraging age-appropriate activities.
- Nursing goals for the autistic child may include decreasing environmental stimuli, providing supportive care, maintaining a safe environment, and giving caregivers anticipatory guidance.
- Treatment for the child with ADHD focuses on decreasing distractions, modifying behavior, and initiating drug therapy.
- Suicide is the third leading cause of death among adolescents.
- Child abuse can be classified as physical abuse, physical neglect, emotional abuse, or sexual abuse.

## REVIEW QUESTIONS

1. Determining the causative agent and administering the proper treatment for skin and throat infections may prevent further complications such as:
    1. leukemia.
    2. mononucleosis.
    3. idiopathic thrombocytopenia purpura.
    4. acute post-streptococcal glomerulonephritis.
2. Children with leukemia are at high risk for infection because of:
    1. decreased lymphocytes.
    2. increased red blood cells.
    3. decreased platelets.
    4. decreased neutrophils.
3. Nursing diagnoses for the child with nephrotic syndrome may include:
    1. *Excess **F**luid Volume* related to fluid retention.
    2. ***P**ain* related to operative procedure.
    3. *Impaired Physical **M**obility* related to use of a brace.
    4. *Disturbed **B**ody Image* related to loss of hair.
4. A clinical manifestation of scoliosis is:
    1. lateral curvature of the spine.
    2. necrosis of the femoral head.
    3. quadriceps muscle atrophy.
    4. Gower's sign.
5. Treatment for the child with ADHD includes:
    1. decreasing distractions.
    2. placing in special education class.
    3. prescribing sedatives.
    4. eating a special diet.
6. The pediatric client is experiencing constipation. This condition occurs most frequently in which of the following ages:
    1. toddler and infants.
    2. pre-school and school-aged.

    3. toddler and school-aged.
    4. toddler and pre-school.
7. The nurse educates the caregiver and child regarding juvenile arthritis. Which statement by the caregivers indicates the need for more education?
    1. It is an autoimmune disorder.
    2. There are only two different forms.
    3. Complications can include blindness.
    4. With early treatment, prognosis is good.
8. A client is experiencing pediculosis. The student nurse knows that this is a condition that requires: (Select all that apply.)
    1. standard precautions when screening.
    2. checking for infestation during daily hygiene.
    3. close-contact situations for lice to be passed from person to person.
    4. cutting long hair to prevent further infestation.
    5. the use of lice sprays on a child's bedding.
    6. the use of lindane (Kwell) for lice removal.
9. The pediatric client who is experiencing burns is at risk for which of the following severe complications: (Select all that apply.)
    1. respiratory complications.
    2. fluid and electrolyte imbalances.
    3. cyanide poisoning.
    4. immobility.
    5. functional impairment.
    6. scarring and contractures.
10. The nurse is caring for a pediatric client who is at risk for suicide. Manifestations include all of the following except:
    1. depression and restlessness.
    2. empathy and boredom.
    3. intentional misbehavior and irritability.
    4. difficulty concentrating and lethargy.

# REFERENCES/SUGGESTED READINGS

American Family Physician (AAFP). (2002). Tick removal. Retrieved October 28-2009 from http://www.aafp.org/afp/20020815/643.html

American Psychiatric Association. (2004). *Diagnostic and statistical manual of mental disorders* (6th ed.). Washington, DC: Author.

American Diabetes Association (ADA). (2006). Type 2 diabetes in children and adolescents. *Diabetes Care, 22*(12), 381. Also available at http://www.diabetes.org/ada/Consensus/.

Belson, M., Kingsley, B., & Holmes, A. (2007, January). Risk factors for acute leukemia in children: A review. *Environmental Health Perspectives, 115*(1), 138–145.

Boychuk, R., DeMesa, C., Kiyabu, K., Yamamoto, F., Yamamoto, L., Sanderson, R., et al. (2006). Change in approach and delivery of medical care in children with asthma: Results from a multicenter emergency department educational asthma management program. *Pediatrics, 117*, 145–151.

Bulechek, G., Butcher, H., McCloskey, J., & Dochterman, J., eds. (2008). *Nursing Interventions Classification (NIC)* (5th ed.). St. Louis, MO: Mosby/Elsevier.

Centers for Disease Control and Prevention. (2004a). Status report on the childhood immunization initiative; National, state, and urban area vaccination coverage levels among children aged 19–35 months—United States, 1996. *MMWR, 46*(29), 657–664.

Centers for Disease Control and Prevention. (2004b). Rates of homicide, suicide, and firearm-related death among children—26 industrialized countries. *MMWR, 46*(5), 101–105.

Centers for Disease Control and Prevention. (2006). Update: Vaccine side effects, adverse reactions, contraindications and precautions: Recommendations of the Advisory Committee on Immunization Practices (ACIP). *MMWR, 45*(RR-12), 1–35.

Centers for Disease Control and Prevention. (2008). General recommendations on immunization: Recommendations of the Advisory Committee on Immunization Practices (ACIP), *MMWR, 43*(RR-1), 1–38.

Croom, K., & McCormack, P. (2008, March). Recombinant factor VIIa (Eptacog Alfa): A review of its use in congenital hemophilia with inhibitors, acquired hemophilia, and other congenital bleeding disorders. *BioDrugs, 22*(2), 121.

Eisenhauer, L., Nichols, L., Spencer, R., & Bergan, F. (1998). *Clinical pharmacology & nursing management* (5th ed.). Philadelphia: Lippincott Williams & Wilkins.

Elbein, S., Das, S., Hallman, D., Hanis, C., & Hasstedt, S. (2009, January). Genome-wide linkage and admixture mapping of type 2 diabetes in African American families from the American Diabetes Association GENNID (Genetics of NIDDM) Study Cohort. *Diabetes, 58*(1), 268–267.

Estes, M. (2010). *Health assessment & physical examination* (4th ed.). Clifton Park, NY: Delmar Cengage Learning.

Gradoni, G., & Gradoni, P. (2009, August). Role of an anti-acetonemic diet in reducing the need for tonsillectomy in children with recurrent tonsillitis. *Auris Nasus Larynx, 36*(4), 438–443.

Hayes, L. (2000). Poison emergency? *Nursing2000, 30*(9), 34–39.

Healthy People 2010. (2000). Objectives. Available from http://www.healthypeople.gov/document/html/objectives/14-22.htm.

Herrin, J., & Antoon, A. (2000). Burn injuries. In R. M. Kliegman, S. Jenson, & R. Behrman (Eds.), *Nelson textbook of pediatrics* (16th ed.). Philadelphia: W. B. Saunders.

Hockenberry, M., & Wilson, D. (2008). *Wong's Essentials of Pediatric Care* (8th ed.). St. Louis, MO: Mosby

James, S., Ashwill, J., & Droske, S. (2002). *Nursing care of children: Principles and practice* (2nd ed.). Philadelphia: W. B. Saunders.

Kamienski, M. (2003). Reye syndrome. *AJN, 103*(7), 54–57.

Kliegman, R., Jensen, H., & Behrman, R. (2000). *Nelson's textbook of pediatrics* (16th ed.). Philadelphia: W. B. Saunders.

Kunkel, L., Bachrach, E., Bennett, R., Guyon, J., & Steffen, L. (2006, May). Diagnosis and cell-based therapy for Duchenne muscular dystrophy in humans, mice, and zebrafish. *Journal of Human Genetics, 51*(5), 397–406.

Leifer, G. (2006). *Introduction to Maternity and Pediatric Nursing* (5th ed.). Philadelphia: W.B. Saunders.

Lenhardt, R., Catrambone, C., McDermott, M., Walter, J., Williams, S., & Weiss, K. (2006). Improving pediatric asthma care through surveillance: The Illinois emergency department asthma collaborative. *Pediatrics, 117*, 96–105.

Marks, M. (1998). *Broadribb's introductory pediatric nursing* (5th ed.). Philadelphia: J.B. Lippincott Williams & Wilkins.

Moorhead, S., Johnson, M., Maas, M., & Swanson, E. (2007). *Nursing Outcomes Classification (NOC)* (4th ed.). St. Louis, MO: Mosby.

National Pediculosis Association,® Inc. (2009a) Set the standard. Retrieved October 28, 2009 from http://www.headlice.org/special/doit4 the kids.htm.

National Pediculosis Association,® Inc. (2009b) *The NPA's ten tips for head lice and nit removal*. Retrieved October 28, 2009 from http://www.headlice.org/downloads/tipsremoval.htm.

National Pediculosis Association,® Inc. (2009c) *Treating head lice without toxins*. Retrieved October 28, 2009 from http://www.headlice.org/news/2004/withouttoxins.htm.

Nemours. (2002). School backpacks: How they affect your child's general health. Available from http://www.nemours.org/no/news/releases/2002/020206_backpack_study.html.

North American Nursing Diagnosis Association International. (2010). *NANDA-I nursing diagnoses: Definitions and classification 2009-2011*. Ames, IA: Wiley-Blackwell.

Potts, N., & Mandleco, B. (2007). *Pediatric Nursing: Caring for children and their families* (2nd ed.). Clifton Park, NY: Delmar Cengage Learning.

Ruiz, E. (2001). Type 2 disease in children. *RN, 64*(10), 44–48.

Schultz, T. (2000). Airing differences in pediatric nebulizer therapy. *Nursing2000, 30*(9), 55–57.

Siwula, C. (2003). Managing pediatric emergencies. *Nursing2003, 33*(2), 48–51.

Spratto, G. and Woods, A. (2008). 2009 edition Delmar's nurses drug handbook. Clifton Park, NY: Delmar Cengage Learning.

Thompson, S. (2003). When kids get cancer. *RN, 66*(7), 29–33.

Timby, B., & Harrison, L. (2005). *Fundamental skills and concepts in patient care* (8th ed.). Philadelphia: Lippincott.

VanBoxel, A., & Puhl, P. (2001). Pediatric emergency: Assessing gut pain. *RN, 64*(4), 38–42.

Wong, D., Hockenberry-Eaton, M. (2001). *Wong's essentials of pediatric nursing* (6th ed.). St. Louis, MO: Mosby.

# RESOURCES

**American Academy of Pediatrics (AAP),**
http://www.aap.org

**American Diabetes Association (ADA),**
http://www.diabetes.org

**Autism Society of America (ASA),**
http://www.autism-society.org

**Centers for Disease Control and Prevention,**
http://www.cdc.gov

**Children with Diabetes,** http://www.castleweb.com

**Muscular Dystrophy Association of America,**
http://www.mdausa.org

**National Association of Anorexia Nervosa and Associated Disorders,** http://www.anad.org

**National Association of Pediatric Nurses Associates and Practitioners (NAPNAP),**
http://www.napnap.org

**National Eating Disorders Association,**
http://www.nationaleatingdisorders.org

**National Hemophilia Foundation,**
http://www.hemophilia.org

**The National Pediculosis Association,**
http://www.headlice.org

**National Scoliosis Foundation, Inc.,**
http://www.stepstn.com

**Nemours Foundation,** http://www.nemours.org

**Scoliosis Association, Inc.,**
http://www.scoliosis-assoc.org

# APPENDIX A
## NANDA-I Nursing Diagnoses 2009–2011

**Domain 1**
**Health Promotion**
Ineffective **Health** Maintenance
Ineffective Self **Health** Management
Impaired **Home** Maintenance
Readiness for Enhanced
   **Immunization** Status
Self **Neglect**
Readiness for Enhanced **Nutrition**
Ineffective Family **Therapeutic**
   Regimen Management
Readiness for Enhanced **Self Health**
   Management

**Domain 2**
**Nutrition**
Ineffective Infant **Feeding** Pattern
Imbalanced **Nutrition**: Less Than
   Body Requirements
Imbalanced **Nutrition**: More Than
   Body Requirements
Risk for Imbalanced **Nutrition**: More
   Than Body Requirements
Impaired **Swallowing**
Risk for Unstable Blood **Glucose** Level
Neonatal **Jaundice**
Risk for Impaired **Liver** Function
Risk for **Electrolyte** Imbalance
Readiness for Enhanced **Fluid** Balance

Deficient **Fluid** Volume
Excess **Fluid** Volume
Risk for Deficient **Fluid** Volume
Risk for Imbalanced **Fluid** Volume

**Domain 3**
**Elimination and Exchange**
Functional Urinary **Incontinence**
Overflow Urinary **Incontinence**
Reflex Urinary **Incontinence**
Stress Urinary **Incontinence**
Urge Urinary **Incontinence**
Risk for Urge urinary
   **Incontinence**
Impaired **Urinary** Elimination
Readiness for Enhanced **Urinary**
   Elimination
**Urinary** Retention
**Bowel** Incontinence
**Constipation**
Perceived **Constipation**
Risk for **Constipation**
**Diarrhea**
Dysfunctional Gastrointenstinal
   **Motility**
Risk for Dysfunctional Gastrointestinal
   **Motility**
Impaired **Gas** Exchange

**Domain 4**
**Activity Rest**
**Insomnia**
Disturbed **Sleep** Pattern
**Sleep** Deprivation
Readiness for Enhanced **Sleep**
Risk for **Disuse** Syndrome
Deficient **Diversional** Activity
Sedentary **Lifestyle**
Impaired Bed **Mobility**
Impaired Physical **Mobility**
Impaired Wheelchair **Mobility**
Delayed **Surgical** Recovery
Impaired **Transfer** Ability
Impaired **Walking**
Disturbed **Energy** Field
**Fatigue**
**Activity** Intolerance
Risk for **Activity** Intolerance
Risk for **Bleeding**
Ineffective **Breathing** Pattern
Decreased **Cardiac** Output
Ineffective Peripheral Tissue **Perfusion**
Risk for Decreased Cardiac Tissue
   **Perfusion**
Risk for Ineffective Cerebral Tissue
   **Perfusion**
Risk for Ineffective Gastrointestinal

**Perfusion**

Risk for **Ineffective Renal Perfusion**

Risk for **Shock**

Impaired Spontaneous **Ventilation**

Dysfunctional **Ventilatory** Weaning Response

Readiness for Enhanced **Self-Care**

Bathing **Self-Care** Deficit

Dressing **Self-Care** Deficit

Feeding **Self-Care** Deficit

Toileting **Self-Care** Deficit

**Domain 5**

**Perception/Cognition**

Unilateral **Neglect**

Impaired **Environmental** Interpretation Syndrome

**Wandering**

Disturbed **Sensory** Perception (Specify: Visual, Auditory, Kinesthetic, Gustatory, Tactile, Olfactory)

Acute **Confusion**

Chronic **Confusion**

Risk for Acute **Confusion**

Deficient **Knowledge**

Readiness for Enhanced **Knowledge**

Impaired **Memory**

Readiness for Enhanced **Decision-Making**

Ineffective **Activity** Planning

Impaired Verbal **Communication**

Readiness for Enhanced **Communication**

**Domain 6**

**Self-Perception**

Risk for Compromised Human **Dignity**

**Hopelessness**

Disturbed Personal **Identity**

Risk for **Loneliness**

Readiness for Enhanced **Power**

**Powerlessness**

Risk for **Powerlessness**

Readiness for Enhanced **Self-Concept**

Situational Low **Self-Esteem**

Chronic Low **Self-Esteem**

Risk for Situational Low **Self-Esteem**

Disturbed **Body** Image

**Domain 7**

**Role Relationships**

**Caregiver** Role Strain

Risk for **Caregiver** Role Strain

Impaired **Parenting**

Readiness for Enhanced **Parenting**

Risk for Impaired **Parenting**

Risk for Impaired **Attachment**

Dysfunctional **Family** Processes

Interrupted **Family** Processes

Readiness for Enhanced **Family** Processes

Effective **Breastfeeding**

Ineffective **Breastfeeding**

Interrupted **Breastfeeding**

Parental Role **Conflict**

Readiness for Enhanced **Relationship**

Ineffective **Role** Performance

Impaired **Social** Interaction

**Domain 8**

**Sexuality**

**Sexual** Dysfunction

Ineffective **Sexuality** Pattern

Readiness for Enhanced **Childbearing** Process

Risk for Disturbed **Maternal/Fetal** Dyad

**Domain 9**

**Coping/Stress Tolerance**

**Post-Trauma** Syndrome

Risk for **Post-Trauma** Syndrome

**Rape-Trauma** Syndrome

**Relocation** Stress Syndrome

Risk for **Relocation** Stress Syndrome

**Anxiety**

Death **Anxiety**

Risk-Prone Health **Behavior**

Compromised Family **Coping**

Defensive **Coping**

Disabled Family **Coping**

Ineffective **Coping**

Ineffective Community **Coping**

Readiness for Enhanced **Coping**

Readiness for Enhanced Community **Coping**

Readiness for Enhanced Family **Coping**

Ineffective **Denial**

**Fear**

**Grieving**

Complicated **Grieving**

Risk for Complicated **Grieving**

Impaired Individual **Resilience**

Readiness for Enhanced **Resilience**

Risk for Compromised **Resilience**

Chronic **Sorrow**

**Stress** Overload

**Autonomic** Dysreflexia
Risk for **Autonomic** Dysreflexia
Disorganized **Infant** Behavior
Risk for Disorganized **Infant** Behavior
Readiness for Enhanced Organized **Infant** Behavior
Decreased **Intracranial** Adaptive Capacity

**Domain 10**
**Life Principles**
Readiness for Enhanced **Hope**
Readiness for Enhanced **Spiritual** Well-Being
Decisional **Conflict**
Moral **Distress**
**Noncompliance**
Impaired **Religiosity**
Readiness for Enhanced **Religiosity**
Risk for Impaired **Religiosity**
**Spiritual** Distress
Risk for **Spiritual** Distress

**Domain 11**
**Safety/Protection**
Risk for **Infection**
Ineffective **Airway** Clearance
Risk for **Aspiration**
Risk for Sudden Infant **Death** Syndrome
Impaired **Dentition**
Risk for **Falls**
Risk for **Injury**
Risk for Perioperative-Positioning **Injury**
Impaired **Oral** Mucous Membrane
Risk for **Peripheral** Neurovascular Dysfunction
Ineffective **Protection**
Impaired **Skin** Integrity

Risk for Impaired **Skin** Integrity
Risk for **Suffocation**
Impaired **Tissue** Integrity
Risk for **Trauma**
Risk for Vascular **Trauma**
**Self-Mutilation**
Risk for **Suicide**
Risk for Other-Directed **Violence**
Risk for Self-Directed **Violence**
**Contamination**
Risk for **Contamination**
Risk for **Poisoning**
Latex **Allergy** Response
Risk for Latex **Allergy** Response
Risk for Imbalanced **Body** Temperature
**Hyperthermia**
**Hypothermia**
Ineffective **Thermoregulation**

**Domain 12**
**Comfort**
Readiness for Enhanced **Comfort**
Impaired **Comfort**
**Nausea**
Acute **Pain**
Chronic **Pain**
**Social** Isolation

**Domain 13**
**Growth/Development**
Adult **Failure** to Thrive
Delayed **Growth** and Development
Risk for Disproportionate **Growth**
Risk for Delayed **Development**

# APPENDIX B
# Recommended Immunization Schedules

## Recommended Immunization Schedule for Persons Aged 0 Through 6 Years—United States • 2009
### For those who fall behind or start late, see the catch-up schedule

| Vaccine ▼ Age ► | Birth | 1 month | 2 months | 4 months | 6 months | 12 months | 15 months | 18 months | 19–23 months | 2–3 years | 4–6 years | |
|---|---|---|---|---|---|---|---|---|---|---|---|---|
| Hepatitis B[1] | HepB | HepB | | see footnote 1 | | HepB | | | | | | |
| Rotavirus[2] | | | RV | RV | RV[2] | | | | | | | Range of recommended ages |
| Diphtheria, Tetanus, Pertussis[3] | | | DTaP | DTaP | DTaP | see footnote 3 | DTaP | | | | DTaP | |
| Haemophilus influenzae type b[4] | | | Hib | Hib | Hib[4] | Hib | | | | | | |
| Pneumococcal[5] | | | PCV | PCV | PCV | PCV | | | | | PPSV | Certain high-risk groups |
| Inactivated Poliovirus | | | IPV | IPV | | IPV | | | | | IPV | |
| Influenza[6] | | | | | | Influenza (Yearly) | | | | | | |
| Measles, Mumps, Rubella[7] | | | | | | MMR | | see footnote 7 | | | MMR | |
| Varicella[8] | | | | | | Varicella | | see footnote 8 | | | Varicella | |
| Hepatitis A[9] | | | | | | HepA (2 doses) | | | | HepA Series | | |
| Meningococcal[10] | | | | | | | | | | MCV | | |

This schedule indicates the recommended ages for routine administration of currently licensed vaccines, as of December 1, 2008, for children aged 0 through 6 years. Any dose not administered at the recommended age should be administered at a subsequent visit, when indicated and feasible. Licensed combination vaccines may be used whenever any component of the combination is indicated and other components are not contraindicated and if approved by the Food and Drug Administration for that dose of the series. Providers should consult the relevant Advisory Committee on Immunization Practices statement for detailed recommendations, including high-risk conditions: http://www.cdc.gov/vaccines/pubs/acip-list.htm. Clinically significant adverse events that follow immunization should be reported to the Vaccine Adverse Event Reporting System (VAERS). Guidance about how to obtain and complete a VAERS form is available at http://www.vaers.hhs.gov or by telephone, 800-822-7967.

**1. Hepatitis B vaccine (HepB).** *(Minimum age: birth)*

**At birth:**
- Administer monovalent HepB to all newborns before hospital discharge.
- If mother is hepatitis B surface antigen (HBsAg)-positive, administer HepB and 0.5 mL of hepatitis B immune globulin (HBIG) within 12 hours of birth.
- If mother's HBsAg status is unknown, administer HepB within 12 hours of birth. Determine mother's HBsAg status as soon as possible and, if HBsAg-positive, administer HBIG (no later than age 1 week).

**After the birth dose:**
- The HepB series should be completed with either monovalent HepB or a combination vaccine containing HepB. The second dose should be administered at age 1 or 2 months. The final dose should be administered no earlier than age 24 weeks.
- Infants born to HBsAg-positive mothers should be tested for HBsAg and antibody to HBsAg (anti-HBs) after completion of at least 3 doses of the HepB series, at age 9 through 18 months (generally at the next well-child visit).

**4-month dose:**
- Administration of 4 doses of HepB to infants is permissible when combination vaccines containing HepB are administered after the birth dose.

**2. Rotavirus vaccine (RV).** *(Minimum age: 6 weeks)*
- Administer the first dose at age 6 through 14 weeks (maximum age: 14 weeks 6 days). Vaccination should not be initiated for infants aged 15 weeks or older (i.e., 15 weeks 0 days or older).
- Administer the final dose in the series by age 8 months 0 days.
- If Rotarix® is administered at ages 2 and 4 months, a dose at 6 months is not indicated.

**3. Diphtheria and tetanus toxoids and acellular pertussis vaccine (DTaP).** *(Minimum age: 6 weeks)*
- The fourth dose may be administered as early as age 12 months, provided at least 6 months have elapsed since the third dose.
- Administer the final dose in the series at age 4 through 6 years.

**4. *Haemophilus influenzae* type b conjugate vaccine (Hib).** *(Minimum age: 6 weeks)*
- If PRP-OMP (PedvaxHIB® or Comvax® [HepB-Hib]) is administered at ages 2 and 4 months, a dose at age 6 months is not indicated.
- TriHiBit® (DTaP/Hib) should not be used for doses at ages 2, 4, or 6 months but can be used as the final dose in children aged 12 months or older.

**5. Pneumococcal vaccine.** *(Minimum age: 6 weeks for pneumococcal conjugate vaccine [PCV]; 2 years for pneumococcal polysaccharide vaccine [PPSV])*
- PCV is recommended for all children aged younger than 5 years. Administer 1 dose of PCV to all healthy children aged 24 through 59 months who are not completely vaccinated for their age.
- Administer PPSV to children aged 2 years or older with certain underlying medical conditions (see *MMWR* 2000;49[No. RR-9]), including a cochlear implant.

**6. Influenza vaccine.** *(Minimum age: 6 months for trivalent inactivated influenza vaccine [TIV]; 2 years for live, attenuated influenza vaccine [LAIV])*
- Administer annually to children aged 6 months through 18 years.
- For healthy nonpregnant persons (i.e., those who do not have underlying medical conditions that predispose them to influenza complications) aged 2 through 49 years, either LAIV or TIV may be used.
- Children receiving TIV should receive 0.25 mL if aged 6 through 35 months or 0.5 mL if aged 3 years or older.
- Administer 2 doses (separated by at least 4 weeks) to children aged younger than 9 years who are receiving influenza vaccine for the first time or who were vaccinated for the first time during the previous influenza season but only received 1 dose.

**7. Measles, mumps, and rubella vaccine (MMR).** *(Minimum age: 12 months)*
- Administer the second dose at age 4 through 6 years. However, the second dose may be administered before age 4, provided at least 28 days have elapsed since the first dose.

**8. Varicella vaccine.** *(Minimum age: 12 months)*
- Administer the second dose at age 4 through 6 years. However, the second dose may be administered before age 4, provided at least 3 months have elapsed since the first dose.
- For children aged 12 months through 12 years the minimum interval between doses is 3 months. However, if the second dose was administered at least 28 days after the first dose, it can be accepted as valid.

**9. Hepatitis A vaccine (HepA).** *(Minimum age: 12 months)*
- Administer to all children aged 1 year (i.e., aged 12 through 23 months). Administer 2 doses at least 6 months apart.
- Children not fully vaccinated by age 2 years can be vaccinated at subsequent visits.
- HepA also is recommended for children older than 1 year who live in areas where vaccination programs target older children or who are at increased risk of infection. See *MMWR* 2006;55(No. RR-7).

**10. Meningococcal vaccine.** *(Minimum age: 2 years for meningococcal conjugate vaccine [MCV] and for meningococcal polysaccharide vaccine [MPSV])*
- Administer MCV to children aged 2 through 10 years with terminal complement component deficiency, anatomic or functional asplenia, and certain other high-risk groups. See *MMWR* 2005;54(No. RR-7).
- Persons who received MPSV 3 or more years previously and who remain at increased risk for meningococcal disease should be revaccinated with MCV.

The Recommended Immunization Schedules for Persons Aged 0 Through 18 Years are approved by the Advisory Committee on Immunization Practices (www.cdc.gov/vaccines/recs/acip), the American Academy of Pediatrics (http://www.aap.org), and the American Academy of Family Physicians (http://www.aafp.org).
DEPARTMENT OF HEALTH AND HUMAN SERVICES • CENTERS FOR DISEASE CONTROL AND PREVENTION

# Recommended Immunization Schedule for Persons Aged 7 Through 18 Years—United States • 2009
### For those who fall behind or start late, see the schedule below and the catch-up schedule

| Vaccine ▼        Age ▶ | 7–10 years | 11–12 years | 13–18 years |
|---|---|---|---|
| Tetanus, Diphtheria, Pertussis[1] | see footnote 1 | Tdap | Tdap |
| Human Papillomavirus[2] | see footnote 2 | HPV (3 doses) | HPV Series |
| Meningococcal[3] | MCV | MCV | MCV |
| Influenza[4] | Influenza (Yearly) | | |
| Pneumococcal[5] | PPSV | | |
| Hepatitis A[6] | HepA Series | | |
| Hepatitis B[7] | HepB Series | | |
| Inactivated Poliovirus[8] | IPV Series | | |
| Measles, Mumps, Rubella[9] | MMR Series | | |
| Varicella[10] | Varicella Series | | |

Legend:
- Range of recommended ages
- Catch-up immunization
- Certain high-risk groups

This schedule indicates the recommended ages for routine administration of currently licensed vaccines, as of December 1, 2008, for children aged 7 through 18 years. Any dose not administered at the recommended age should be administered at a subsequent visit, when indicated and feasible. Licensed combination vaccines may be used whenever any component of the combination is indicated and other components are not contraindicated and if approved by the Food and Drug Administration for that dose of the series. Providers should consult the relevant Advisory Committee on Immunization Practices statement for detailed recommendations, including high-risk conditions: http://www.cdc.gov/vaccines/pubs/acip-list.htm. Clinically significant adverse events that follow immunization should be reported to the Vaccine Adverse Event Reporting System (VAERS). Guidance about how to obtain and complete a VAERS form is available at http://www.vaers.hhs.gov or by telephone, 800-822-7967.

1. **Tetanus and diphtheria toxoids and acellular pertussis vaccine (Tdap). (Minimum age: 10 years for BOOSTRIX® and 11 years for ADACEL®)**
   - Administer at age 11 or 12 years for those who have completed the recommended childhood DTP/DTaP vaccination series and have not received a tetanus and diphtheria toxoid (Td) booster dose.
   - Persons aged 13 through 18 years who have not received Tdap should receive a dose.
   - A 5-year interval from the last Td dose is encouraged when Tdap is used as a booster dose; however, a shorter interval may be used if pertussis immunity is needed.

2. **Human papillomavirus vaccine (HPV). (Minimum age: 9 years)**
   - Administer the first dose to females at age 11 or 12 years.
   - Administer the second dose 2 months after the first dose and the third dose 6 months after the first dose (at least 24 weeks after the first dose).
   - Administer the series to females at age 13 through 18 years if not previously vaccinated.

3. **Meningococcal conjugate vaccine (MCV).**
   - Administer at age 11 or 12 years, or at age 13 through 18 years if not previously vaccinated.
   - Administer to previously unvaccinated college freshmen living in a dormitory.
   - MCV is recommended for children aged 2 through 10 years with terminal complement component deficiency, anatomic or functional asplenia, and certain other groups at high risk. See *MMWR* 2005;54(No. RR-7).
   - Persons who received MPSV 5 or more years previously and remain at increased risk for meningococcal disease should be revaccinated with MCV.

4. **Influenza vaccine.**
   - Administer annually to children aged 6 months through 18 years.
   - For healthy nonpregnant persons (i.e., those who do not have underlying medical conditions that predispose them to influenza complications) aged 2 through 49 years, either LAIV or TIV may be used.
   - Administer 2 doses (separated by at least 4 weeks) to children aged younger than 9 years who are receiving influenza vaccine for the first time or who were vaccinated for the first time during the previous influenza season but only received 1 dose.

5. **Pneumococcal polysaccharide vaccine (PPSV).**
   - Administer to children with certain underlying medical conditions (see *MMWR* 1997;46[No. RR-8]), including a cochlear implant. A single revaccination should be administered to children with functional or anatomic asplenia or other immunocompromising condition after 5 years.

6. **Hepatitis A vaccine (HepA).**
   - Administer 2 doses at least 6 months apart.
   - HepA is recommended for children older than 1 year who live in areas where vaccination programs target older children or who are at increased risk of infection. See *MMWR* 2006;55(No. RR-7).

7. **Hepatitis B vaccine (HepB).**
   - Administer the 3-dose series to those not previously vaccinated.
   - A 2-dose series (separated by at least 4 months) of adult formulation Recombivax HB® is licensed for children aged 11 through 15 years.

8. **Inactivated poliovirus vaccine (IPV).**
   - For children who received an all-IPV or all-oral poliovirus (OPV) series, a fourth dose is not necessary if the third dose was administered at age 4 years or older.
   - If both OPV and IPV were administered as part of a series, a total of 4 doses should be administered, regardless of the child's current age.

9. **Measles, mumps, and rubella vaccine (MMR).**
   - If not previously vaccinated, administer 2 doses or the second dose for those who have received only 1 dose, with at least 28 days between doses.

10. **Varicella vaccine.**
   - For persons aged 7 through 18 years without evidence of immunity (see *MMWR* 2007;56[No. RR-4]), administer 2 doses if not previously vaccinated or the second dose if they have received only 1 dose.
   - For persons aged 7 through 12 years, the minimum interval between doses is 3 months. However, if the second dose was administered at least 28 days after the first dose, it can be accepted as valid.
   - For persons aged 13 years and older, the minimum interval between doses is 28 days.

The Recommended Immunization Schedules for Persons Aged 0 Through 18 Years are approved by the Advisory Committee on Immunization Practices (www.cdc.gov/vaccines/recs/acip), the American Academy of Pediatrics (http://www.aap.org), and the American Academy of Family Physicians (http://www.aafp.org).
DEPARTMENT OF HEALTH AND HUMAN SERVICES • CENTERS FOR DISEASE CONTROL AND PREVENTION

# Recommended Adult Immunization Schedule
## UNITED STATES · 2009

Note: These recommendations *must* be read with the footnotes that follow containing number of doses, intervals between doses, and other important information.

## Figure 1. Recommended adult immunization schedule, by vaccine and age group

| VACCINE ▼ / AGE GROUP ▶ | 19–26 years | 27–49 years | 50–59 years | 60–64 years | ≥65 years |
|---|---|---|---|---|---|
| Tetanus, diphtheria, pertussis (Td/Tdap)[1],[*] | Substitute 1-time dose of Tdap for Td booster; then boost with Td every 10 yrs | | | | Td booster every 10 yrs |
| Human papillomavirus (HPV)[2],[*] | 3 doses (females) | | | | |
| Varicella[3],[*] | 2 doses | | | | |
| Zoster[4] | | | | 1 dose | |
| Measles, mumps, rubella (MMR)[5],[*] | 1 or 2 doses | | | 1 dose | |
| Influenza[6],[*] | 1 dose annually | | | | |
| Pneumococcal (polysaccharide)[7,8] | 1 or 2 doses | | | | 1 dose |
| Hepatitis A[9],[*] | 2 doses | | | | |
| Hepatitis B[10],[*] | 3 doses | | | | |
| Meningococcal[11],[*] | 1 or more doses | | | | |

Legend:
- For all persons in this category who meet the age requirements and who lack evidence of immunity (e.g., lack documentation of vaccination or have no evidence of prior infection)
- Recommended if some other risk factor is present (e.g., on the basis of medical, occupational, lifestyle, or other indications)
- No recommendation

*Covered by the Vaccine Injury Compensation Program.

Report all clinically significant postvaccination reactions to the Vaccine Adverse Event Reporting System (VAERS). Reporting forms and instructions on filing a VAERS report are available at www.vaers.hhs.gov or by telephone, 800-822-7967.

Information on how to file a Vaccine Injury Compensation Program claim is available at www.hrsa.gov/vaccinecompensation or by telephone, 800-338-2382. To file a claim for vaccine injury, contact the U.S. Court of Federal Claims, 717 Madison Place, N.W., Washington, D.C. 20005; telephone, 202-357-6400.

Additional information about the vaccines in this schedule, extent of available data, and contraindications for vaccination is also available at www.cdc.gov/vaccines or from the CDC-INFO Contact Center at 800-CDC-INFO (800-232-4636) in English and Spanish, 24 hours a day, 7 days a week.

Use of trade names and commercial sources is for identification only and does not imply endorsement by the U.S. Department of Health and Human Services.

# Figure 2. Vaccines that might be indicated for adults based on medical and other indications

| VACCINE ▼    INDICATION ▶ | Pregnancy | Immuno-compromising conditions (excluding human immunodeficiency virus [HIV])[13] | HIV infection[3,12,13] CD4+ T lympho-cyte count <200 cells/µL | HIV infection[3,12,13] CD4+ T lympho-cyte count ≥200 cells/µL | Diabetes, heart disease, chronic lung disease, chronic alcoholism | Asplenia[12] (including elective splenectomy and terminal complement component deficiencies) | Chronic liver disease | Kidney failure, end-stage renal disease, receipt of hemodialysis | Health-care personnel |
|---|---|---|---|---|---|---|---|---|---|
| Tetanus, diphtheria, pertussis (Td/Tdap)[1,*] | Td | Substitute 1-time dose of Tdap for Td booster; then boost with Td every 10 yrs ||||||||
| Human papillomavirus (HPV)[2,*] | | 3 doses for females through age 26 yrs |||||||| 
| Varicella[3,*] | Contraindicated | | Contraindicated | | 2 doses ||||| 
| Zoster[4] | Contraindicated | | Contraindicated | | | 1 dose |||| 
| Measles, mumps, rubella (MMR)[5,*] | Contraindicated | | Contraindicated | | 1 or 2 doses ||||| 
| Influenza[6,*] | 1 dose TIV annually ||| | 1 or 2 doses | | | | 1 dose TIV or LAIV annually |
| Pneumococcal (polysaccharide)[7,8] | | 1 or 2 doses ||||||||
| Hepatitis A[9,*] | | 2 doses ||||||||
| Hepatitis B[10,*] | | 3 doses ||||||||
| Meningococcal[11,*] | | 1 or more doses ||||||||

*Covered by the Vaccine Injury Compensation Program.

■ For all persons in this category who meet the age requirements and who lack evidence of immunity (e.g., lack documentation of vaccination or have no evidence of prior infection)

■ Recommended if some other risk factor is present (e.g., on the basis of medical, occupational, lifestyle, or other indications)

☐ No recommendation

These schedules indicate the recommended age groups and medical indications for which administration of currently licensed vaccines is commonly indicated for adults ages 19 years and older, as of January 1, 2009. Licensed combination vaccines may be used whenever any components of the combination are indicated and when the vaccine's other components are not contraindicated. For detailed recommendations on all vaccines, including those used primarily for travelers or that are issued during the year, consult the manufacturers' package inserts and the complete statements from the Advisory Committee on Immunization Practices (www.cdc.gov/vaccines/pubs/acip-list.htm).

The recommendations in this schedule were approved by the Centers for Disease Control and Prevention's (CDC) Advisory Committee on Immunization Practices (ACIP), the American Academy of Family Physicians (AAFP), the American College of Obstetricians and Gynecologists (ACOG), and the American College of Physicians (ACP).

DEPARTMENT OF HEALTH AND HUMAN SERVICES
CENTERS FOR DISEASE CONTROL AND PREVENTION

CDC

CS200484-A

# Footnotes

## Recommended Adult Immunization Schedule—UNITED STATES · 2009

**For complete statements by the Advisory Committee on Immunization Practices (ACIP), visit www.cdc.gov/vaccines/pubs/ACIP-list.htm.**

### 1. Tetanus, diphtheria, and acellular pertussis (Td/Tdap) vaccination

Tdap should replace a single dose of Td for adults aged 19 through 64 years who have not received a dose of Tdap previously.

Adults with uncertain or incomplete history of primary vaccination series with tetanus and diphtheria toxoid-containing vaccines should begin or complete a primary vaccination series. A primary series for adults is 3 doses of tetanus and diphtheria toxoid-containing vaccines; administer the first 2 doses at least 4 weeks apart and the third dose 6–12 months after the second. However, Tdap can substitute for any one of the doses of Td in the 3-dose primary series. The booster dose of tetanus and diphtheria toxoid-containing vaccine should be administered to adults who have completed a primary series and if the last vaccination was received 10 or more years previously. Tdap or Td vaccine may be used, as indicated.

If a woman is pregnant and received the last Td vaccination 10 or more years previously, administer Td during the second or third trimester. If the woman received the last Td vaccination less than 10 years previously, administer Tdap during the immediate postpartum period. A dose of Tdap is recommended for postpartum women, close contacts of infants aged less than 12 months, and all health-care personnel with direct patient contact if they have not previously received Tdap. An interval as short as 2 years from the last Td is suggested; shorter intervals can be used. Td may be deferred during pregnancy and Tdap substituted in the immediate postpartum period, or Tdap may be administered instead of Td to a pregnant woman after an informed discussion with the woman.

Consult the ACIP statement for recommendations for administering Td as prophylaxis in wound management.

### 2. Human papillomavirus (HPV) vaccination

HPV vaccination is recommended for all females aged 11 through 26 years (and may begin at 9 years) who have not completed the vaccine series. History of genital warts, abnormal Papanicolaou test, or positive HPV DNA test is not evidence of prior infection with all vaccine HPV types; HPV vaccination is recommended for persons with such histories.

Ideally, vaccine should be administered before potential exposure to HPV through sexual activity; however, females who are sexually active should still be vaccinated consistent with age-based recommendations. Sexually active females who have not been infected with any of the four HPV vaccine types receive the full benefit of the vaccination. Vaccination is less beneficial for females who have already been infected with one or more of the HPV vaccine types.

A complete series consists of 3 doses. The second dose should be administered 2 months after the first dose; the third dose should be administered 6 months after the first dose.

HPV vaccination is not specifically recommended for females with the medical indications described in Figure 2, "Vaccines that might be indicated for adults based on medical and other indications." Because HPV vaccine is not a live-virus vaccine, it may be administered to persons with the medical indications described in Figure 2 for persons with the medical indications described in Figure 2 than in persons who do not have the medical indications described or who are immunocompetent. Health-care personnel are not at increased risk because of occupational exposure, and should be vaccinated consistent with age-based recommendations.

### 3. Varicella vaccination

All adults without evidence of immunity to varicella should receive 2 doses of single-antigen varicella vaccine if not previously vaccinated or the second dose if they have received only one dose unless they have a medical contraindication. Special consideration should be given to those who 1) have close contact with persons at high risk for severe disease (e.g., health-care personnel and family contacts of persons with immunocompromising conditions) or 2) are at high risk for exposure or transmission (e.g., teachers; child care employees; residents and staff members of institutional settings, including correctional institutions; college students; military personnel; adolescents and adults living in households with children; nonpregnant women of childbearing age; and international travelers).

Evidence of immunity to varicella in adults includes any of the following: 1) documentation of 2 doses of varicella vaccine at least 4 weeks apart; 2) U.S.-born before 1980 (although for health-care personnel and pregnant women, birth before 1980 should not be considered evidence of immunity); 3) history of varicella based on diagnosis or verification of varicella by a health-care provider (for a patient reporting a history of or presenting with an atypical case, a mild case, or both, health-care providers should seek either an epidemiologic link with a typical varicella case or to a laboratory-confirmed case or evidence of laboratory confirmation, if it was performed at the time of acute disease); 4) history of herpes zoster based on health-care provider diagnosis or verification of herpes zoster by a health-care provider; or 5) laboratory evidence of immunity or laboratory confirmation of disease.

Pregnant women should be assessed for evidence of varicella immunity. Women who do not have evidence of immunity should receive the first dose of varicella vaccine upon completion or termination of pregnancy and before discharge from the health-care facility. The second dose should be administered 4–8 weeks after the first dose.

### 4. Herpes zoster vaccination

A single dose of zoster vaccine is recommended for adults aged 60 years and older regardless of whether they report a prior episode of herpes zoster. Persons with chronic medical conditions may be vaccinated unless their condition constitutes a contraindication.

### 5. Measles, mumps, rubella (MMR) vaccination

*Measles component:* Adults born before 1957 generally are considered immune to measles. Adults born during or after 1957 should receive 1 or more doses of MMR unless they have a medical contraindication, documentation of 1 or more doses, history of measles based on health-care provider diagnosis, or laboratory evidence of immunity.

A second dose of MMR is recommended for adults who 1) have been recently exposed to measles or are in an outbreak setting; 2) have been vaccinated previously with killed measles vaccine; 3) have been vaccinated with an unknown type of measles vaccine during 1963–1967; 4) are students in postsecondary educational institutions; 5) work in a health-care facility; or 6) plan to travel internationally.

*Mumps component:* Adults born before 1957 generally are considered immune to mumps. Adults born during or after 1957 should receive 1 dose of MMR unless they have a medical contraindication, history of mumps based on health-care provider diagnosis, or laboratory evidence of immunity.

A second dose of MMR is recommended for adults who 1) live in a community experiencing a mumps outbreak and are in an affected age group; 2) are students in postsecondary educational institutions; 3) work in a health-care facility; or 4) plan to travel internationally. For unvaccinated health-care personnel born before 1957 who do not have other evidence of mumps immunity, administering 1 dose on a routine basis should be considered and administering a second dose during an outbreak should be strongly considered.

*Rubella component:* 1 dose of MMR vaccine is recommended for women whose rubella vaccination history is unreliable or who lack laboratory evidence of immunity. For women of childbearing age, regardless of birth year, rubella immunity should be determined and women should be counseled regarding congenital rubella syndrome. Women who do not have evidence of immunity should receive MMR upon completion or termination of pregnancy and before discharge from the health-care facility.

## 6. Influenza vaccination

*Medical indications:* Chronic disorders of the cardiovascular or pulmonary systems, including asthma; chronic metabolic diseases, including diabetes mellitus, renal or hepatic dysfunction, hemoglobinopathies, or immunocompromising conditions (including immunocompromising conditions caused by medications or human immunodeficiency virus [HIV]); any condition that compromises respiratory function or the handling of respiratory secretions or that can increase the risk of aspiration (e.g., cognitive dysfunction, spinal cord injury, or seizure disorder or other neuromuscular disorder); and pregnancy during the influenza season. No data exist on the risk for severe or complicated influenza disease among persons with asplenia; however, influenza is a risk factor for secondary bacterial infections that can cause severe disease among persons with asplenia.

*Occupational indications:* All health-care personnel, including those employed by long-term care and assisted-living facilities, and caregivers of children less than 5 years old.

*Other indications:* Residents of nursing homes and other long-term care and assisted-living facilities; persons likely to transmit influenza to persons at high risk (e.g., in-home household contacts and caregivers of children aged less than 5 years old, persons 65 years old and older and persons of all ages with high-risk condition[s]); and anyone who would like to decrease their risk of getting influenza. Healthy, nonpregnant adults aged less than 50 years without high-risk medical conditions who are not contacts of severely immunocompromised persons in special care units can receive either intranasally administered live, attenuated influenza vaccine (FluMist®) or inactivated vaccine. Other persons should receive the inactivated vaccine.

## 7. Pneumococcal polysaccharide (PPSV) vaccination

*Medical indications:* Chronic lung disease (including asthma); chronic cardiovascular diseases; diabetes mellitus; chronic liver diseases, cirrhosis; chronic alcoholism, chronic renal failure or nephrotic syndrome; functional or anatomic asplenia (e.g., sickle cell disease or splenectomy [if elective splenectomy is planned, vaccinate at least 2 weeks before surgery]); immunocompromising conditions; and cochlear implants and cerebrospinal fluid leaks. Vaccinate as close to HIV diagnosis as possible.

*Other indications:* Residents of nursing homes or long-term care facilities and persons who smoke cigarettes. Routine use of PPSV is not recommended for Alaska Native or American Indian persons younger than 65 years unless they have underlying medical conditions that are PPSV indications. However, public health authorities may consider recommending PPSV for Alaska Natives and American Indians aged 50 through 64 years who are living in areas in which the risk of invasive pneumococcal disease is increased.

## 8. Revaccination with PPSV

One-time revaccination after 5 years for persons with chronic renal failure or nephrotic syndrome; functional or anatomic asplenia (e.g., sickle cell disease or splenectomy); and for persons with immunocompromising conditions. For persons aged 65 years and older, one-time revaccination if they were vaccinated 5 or more years previously and were aged less than 65 years at the time of primary vaccination.

## 9. Hepatitis A vaccination

*Medical indications:* Persons with chronic liver disease and persons who receive clotting factor concentrates.

*Behavioral indications:* Men who have sex with men and persons who use illegal drugs.

*Occupational indications:* Persons working with hepatitis A virus (HAV)-infected primates or with HAV in a research laboratory setting.

*Other indications:* Persons traveling to or working in countries that have high or intermediate endemicity of hepatitis A (a list of countries is available at www.cdc.gov/travel/contentdiseases.aspx) and any person seeking protection from HAV infection.

Single-antigen vaccine formulations should be administered in a 2-dose schedule at either 0 and 6–12 months (Havrix®), or 0 and 6–18 months (Vaqta®). If the combined hepatitis A and hepatitis B vaccine (Twinrix®) is used, administer 3 doses at 0, 1, and 6 months; alternatively, a 4-dose schedule, administered on days 0, 7 and 21 to 30 followed by a booster dose at month 12 may be used.

## 10. Hepatitis B vaccination

*Medical indications:* Persons with end-stage renal disease, including patients receiving hemodialysis; persons with HIV infection; and persons with chronic liver disease.

*Occupational indications:* Health-care personnel and public-safety workers who are exposed to blood or other potentially infectious body fluids.

*Behavioral indications:* Sexually active persons who are not in a long-term, mutually monogamous relationship (e.g., persons with more than 1 sex partner during the previous 6 months); persons seeking evaluation or treatment for a sexually transmitted disease (STD); current or recent injection-drug users; and men who have sex with men.

*Other indications:* Household contacts and sex partners of persons with chronic hepatitis B virus (HBV) infection; clients and staff members of institutions for persons with developmental disabilities; international travelers to countries with high or intermediate prevalence of chronic HBV infection (a list of countries is available at www.cdc.gov/travel/contentdiseases.aspx); and any adult seeking protection from HBV infection.

Hepatitis B vaccination is recommended for all adults in the following settings: STD treatment facilities; HIV testing and treatment facilities; facilities providing drug-abuse treatment and prevention services; health-care settings targeting services to injection-drug users or men who have sex with men; correctional facilities; end-stage renal disease programs and facilities for chronic hemodialysis patients; and institutions and nonresidential daycare facilities for persons with developmental disabilities.

If the combined hepatitis A and hepatitis B vaccine (Twinrix®) is used, administer 3 doses at

0, 1, and 6 months; alternatively, a 4-dose schedule, administered on days 0, 7 and 21 to 30 followed by a booster dose at month 12 may be used.

*Special formulation indications:* For adult patients receiving hemodialysis or with other immunocompromising conditions, 1 dose of 40 μg/mL (Recombivax HB®) administered on a 3-dose schedule or 2 doses of 20 μg/mL (Engerix-B®) administered simultaneously on a 4-dose schedule at 0, 1, 2 and 6 months.

## 11. Meningococcal vaccination

*Medical indications:* Adults with anatomic or functional asplenia, or terminal complement component deficiencies.

*Other indications:* First-year college students living in dormitories; microbiologists who are routinely exposed to isolates of *Neisseria meningitidis*; military recruits; and persons who travel to or live in countries in which meningococcal disease is hyperendemic or epidemic (e.g., the "meningitis belt" of sub-Saharan Africa during the dry season [December–June]), particularly if their contact with local populations will be prolonged. Vaccination is required by the government of Saudi Arabia for all travelers to Mecca during the annual Hajj.

Meningococcal conjugate (MCV) vaccine is preferred for adults with any of the preceding indications who are aged 55 years or younger, although meningococcal polysaccharide vaccine (MPSV) is an acceptable alternative. Revaccination with MCV after 5 years might be indicated for adults previously vaccinated with MPSV who remain at increased risk for infection (e.g., persons residing in areas in which disease is epidemic).

## 12. Selected conditions for which *Haemophilus influenzae* type b (Hib) vaccine may be used

Hib vaccine generally is not recommended for persons aged 5 years and older. No efficacy data are available on which to base a recommendation concerning use of Hib vaccine for older children and adults. However, studies suggest good immunogenicity in persons who have sickle cell disease, leukemia, or HIV infection or who have had a splenectomy; administering 1 dose of vaccine to these persons is not contraindicated.

## 13. Immunocompromising conditions

Inactivated vaccines generally are acceptable (e.g., pneumococcal, meningococcal, and influenza [trivalent inactivated influenza vaccine]), and live vaccines generally are avoided in persons with immune deficiencies or immunocompromising conditions. Information on specific conditions is available at www.cdc.gov/vaccines/pubs/acip-list.htm.

# APPENDIX C
## Abbreviations, Acronyms, and Symbols

| | | | |
|---|---|---|---|
| > | greater than | AIDS | acquired immunodeficiency syndrome |
| < | less than | AJN | *American Journal of Nursing* |
| ʒ | dram | ALFA | Assisted Living Federation of America |
| ℥ | ounce | ALT | alanine aminotransferase |
| ♏ | minum | AMA | against medical advice |
| ā | before | AMA | American Medical Association |
| AAPB | Association of Applied Psychophysiology and Biofeedback | ANA | American Nurses Association |
| | | ANA | antinuclear antibody |
| AARP | American Association of Retired Persons | AoA | Administration on Aging |
| AASM | American Academy of Sleep Medicine | AP | anterior/posterior |
| AAT | animal-assisted therapy | AP | apical pulse |
| AATH | American Association for Therapeutic Humor | APIC | Association for Practitioners in Infection Control and Epidemiology |
| ABC | airway, breathing, circulation | | |
| ABD | abdominal | APRN | advance practice registered nurse |
| ABG | arterial blood gases | APS | Adult Protective Services |
| ABO | blood types | APS | American Pain Society |
| a.c. | before meals | APTT | activated partial thromboplastin time |
| ACIP | Advisory Committee on Immunization Practices | AROM | active range of motion |
| | | AS | left ear |
| ACS | American Cancer Society | ASA | acetylsalicylic acid |
| ACTH | adrenocorticotropic hormone | ASO | antireptolysin-O |
| AD | Alzheimer's disease | AST | aspartate aminotransferase |
| AD | right ear | AT | axillary temperature |
| ad lib | freely, as desired | ATC | around the clock |
| ADA | Americans with Disabilities Act | ATP | adenosine triphosphatase |
| ADH | antidiuretic hormone | AU | both ears |
| ADLs | activities of daily living | $B_1$ | thiamine |
| ADN | associate degree nurse (nursing) | $B_2$ | riboflavin |
| AEB | as evidenced by | $B_6$ | pyridoxine |
| AFP | alpha-fetoprotein | $B_{12}$ | cobolomine |
| AHA | American Hospital Association | BBA | Balanced Budget Act |
| AHCA | American Health Care Association | BE | base excess |
| AHCPR | Agency for Health Care Policy and Research | bid | twice a day |
| AHNA | American Holistic Nurses' Association | BMD | bone mineral density |
| AHRQ | Agency for Healthcare Research and Quality | BMI | body mass index |
| AI | adequate intake | BMR | basal metabolic rate |

| | |
|---|---|
| BP | blood pressure |
| BPH | benign prostatic hypertrophy |
| BPM | beats per minute |
| BSA | body surface area |
| BSE | breast self-examination |
| BSI | body substance isolation |
| BSN | bachelor of science in nursing |
| BUN | blood urea nitrogen |
| c | cup |
| $\bar{c}$ | with |
| C | Celsius |
| Ca | calcium |
| $Ca^{++}$ | calcium ion |
| $CaCl_2$ | calcium chloride |
| C/A | complementary/alternative |
| CAD | coronary artery disease |
| CAI | computer-assisted instruction |
| CAM | complementary/alternative medicine |
| C & S | culture and sensitivity |
| cap | capsule |
| CARF | Commission on Accreditation of Rehabilitation Facilities |
| CAT | computed axial tomography |
| CAT | computerized adaptive testing |
| CBC | complete blood count |
| CBD | common bile duct |
| CBE | charting by exception |
| cc | cubic centimeter |
| CCRC | continuing care retirement community |
| CCU | coronary care unit |
| CDC | Centers for Disease Control and Prevention |
| CEA | carcinoembryonic antigen |
| CEPN-LTC™ | Certification Examination for Practical and Vocational Nurses in Long-Term Care |
| CEU | continuing education unit |
| CHAP | Community Health Accreditation Program |
| CHD | coronary heart disease |
| CHF | congestive heart failure |
| CHIP | Children's Health Insurance Program |
| CHO | carbohydrate (carbon, hydrogen, oxygen) |
| CHON | protein (carbon, hydrogen, oxygen, nitrogen) |
| CK or CPK | creatine kinase or creatine phosphokinase |
| Cl | chlorine, chloride |
| $Cl^-$ | chloride ion |
| CLTC | certified in long-term care |
| cm | centimeter |
| CMS | Centers for Medicare and Medicaid Services |
| CN | cranial nerve |
| CNA | certified nursing assistant |
| CNM | certified nurse midwife |
| CNO | community nursing organization |
| CNS | central nervous system |
| CNS | clinical nurse specialist |
| Co | cobalt |
| $CO_2$ | carbon dioxide |
| $CO_2^-$ | carbon dioxide ion |
| COBRA | Comprehensive Omnibus Budget Reconciliation Act |
| COOH | carboxyl group |
| COPD | chronic obstructive pulmonary disease |
| CPAP | continuous positive airway pressure |
| CPNP | Council of Practical Nursing Programs |
| CPR | cardiopulmonary resuscitation |
| CPR | computerized patient record |
| Cr | chromium |
| CRNA | Certified Registered Nurse Anesthetist |
| CRP | C-reactive protein |
| C&S | culture and sensitivity |
| CSF | cerebrospinal fluid |
| CSM | circulation, sensation, motion |
| CT | computed tomography |
| Cu | copper |
| CVA | cerebrovascular accident |
| CVC | central venous catheter |
| $D_5W$ | dextrose 5% in water |
| D & C | dilatation and curettage |
| DAR | document, action, response |
| dc | discontinue |
| DDB | Disciplinary Data Bank |
| DDS | doctor of dental surgery |
| DEA | Drug Enforcement Agency |
| DHHS | Department of Health and Human Services |
| DIC | disseminated intravascular coagulation |
| DICC | dynamic infusion cavernosometry and cavernosography |
| dL | deciliter |
| DMD | doctor of dental medicine |
| DNA | deoxyribonucleic acid |
| DNR | do not resuscitate |
| DO | doctor of osteopathy |
| DPAHC | durable power of attorney for health care |
| dr | dram, or ʒ |
| DRG | diagnosis-related group |
| DRI | dietary reference intake |
| DSM-IV | *Diagnostic and Statistical Manual of Mental Disorders,* 4th edition |
| DST | dexamethasone suppression test |
| DT | delirium tremens |
| DTaP | diphtheria, tetanus, acellular pertussis |
| DTP | diphtheria, tetanus, pertussis |
| DVT | deep vein thrombosis |
| EAR | estimated average requirement |
| ECF | extended care facility |
| ECF | extracellular fluid |
| ED | emergency department |
| EDTA | ethylenediaminetetraacetic acid |
| EEG | electroencephalograph |
| EGD | esophagogastroduodenoscopy |
| EKG (ECG) | electrocardiogram |
| ELISA | enzyme-linked immunosorbent assay |
| elix | elixir |
| EMG | electromyogram |
| EMLA | eutectic (cream) mixture of local anesthetics |
| EMS | emergency medical services |

| | | | |
|---|---|---|---|
| **EMT** | emergency medical technician | **HFA** | Hospice Foundation of America |
| **EMT-P** | emergency medical technician-paramedic | **Hg** | mercury |
| **EPA** | Environmental Protection Agency | **Hgb** | hemoglobin |
| **EPO** | exclusive provider organization | **Hgbs** | hemoglobins |
| **ER** | emergency room | **HICPAC** | Hospital Infection Control Practices Advisory |
| **ERCP** | endoscopic retrograde | | Committee |
| | cholangiopancreatogram | **HIS** | hospital information system |
| **ERG** | electroretinogram | **HIV** | human immunodeficiency virus |
| **ERT** | estrogen replacement therapy | **HLA** | human leukocyte antigen |
| **ESR** | erythrocyte sedimentation rate | **HMO** | health maintenance organization |
| **ET** | ear (tympanic) temperature | **HPO$_4$** | phosphate |
| **EVAD** | explantable venous access device | **HR** | heart rate |
| **F** | fahrenheit | **HRSA** | Health Resources and Services |
| **FAS** | fetal alcohol syndrome | | Administration |
| **FBS** | fasting blood sugar | **h.s.** | hour of sleep |
| **FCA** | False Claims Act | **I** | iodine |
| **FDA** | Food and Drug Administration | **IADLs** | instrumental activities of daily living |
| **Fe** | iron | **I&O** | intake and output |
| **FeSO$_4$** | iron sulfate | **IASP** | International Association for the Study |
| **fl** | fluid | | of Pain |
| **Fl** | fluorine | **ICF** | intermediate care facility |
| **FOBT** | fecal occult blood test | **ICF** | intracellular fluid |
| **FSH** | follicle-stimulating hormone | **ICN** | International Council of Nurses |
| **ft** | foot or feet | **ICU** | intensive care unit |
| **FVD** | fluid volume deficit | **ID** | identification |
| **g** | gram | **ID** | intradermal |
| **GAO** | General Accounting Office | **IgG** | immunoglobulin G |
| **GAS** | general adaptation syndrome | **IgM** | immunoglobulin M |
| **GCS** | Glasgow Coma Scale | **IHCT** | interdisciplinary health care team |
| **g/dL** | grams per deciliter | **IM** | intramuscular |
| **GED** | general education development | **in** | inch |
| **GER** | gastroesophageal reflux | **INR** | International Normalized Ratio |
| **GFR** | glomerular filtration rate | **I&O** | intake and output |
| **GGT (GGTP)** | gammaglutamy transpeptidase | **IOL** | intraocular lens |
| **GH** | growth hormone | **IOM** | Institute of Medicine |
| **GHB** | glycosylated hemoglobin | **ITT** | insulin tolerance test |
| **GI** | gastrointestinal | **IV** | intravenous |
| **gr** | grain | **IVAD** | implantable vascular access device |
| **gtt** | drop | **IVP** | intravenous push, intravenous pyelogram |
| **GTT** | glucose tolerance test | **IVPB** | intravenous piggyback |
| **gtt/min** | drops per minute | **JCAHO** | Joint Commission on Accreditation of |
| **GU** | genitourinary | | Healthcare Organizations |
| **h** | hour(s) | **K** | potassium |
| **H$^+$** | hydrogen ion | **K$^+$** | potassium ion |
| **H$_2$CO$_3$** | carbonic acid | **kcal** | kilocalorie |
| **H$_2$O** | water | **KCl** | potassium chloride |
| **H&H** | hemoglobin and hematocrit | **kg** | kilogram |
| **HB$_5$AG** | hepatitis B surface antigen | **KS** | ketosteroids |
| **HBV** | hepatitis B virus | **KUB** | kidneys/ureters/bladder |
| **HCFA** | Health Care Financing Administration | **KVO** | keep vein open |
| **hCG** | human chorionic gonadotropin | **L** | liter |
| **HCl** | hydrochloric acid, hydrochloride | **LAS** | local adaptation syndrome |
| **HCO$_3^-$** | bicarbonate ion | **lb** | pound |
| **Hct** | hematocrit | **LDH** | lactic dehydrogenase |
| **HCV** | hepatitis C virus | **LDL** | low density lipoprotein |
| **HDL** | high density lipoprotein | **LE** | lupus erythematosus |
| **HDV** | hepatitis D virus | **LES** | lower esophageal sphincter |
| **Hep B** | hepatitis B | **LFT** | liver function test |

| | |
|---|---|
| LH | luteinizing hormone |
| LLQ | left lower quadrant |
| LMP | last menstrual period |
| L/min | liters per minute |
| LOC | level of consciousness |
| LP | lumbar puncture |
| LP/VN | licensed practical/vocational nurse |
| LPN | licensed practical nurse |
| LUQ | left upper quadrant |
| LVN | licensed vocational nurse |
| m | meter |
| $m^2$ | square meter |
| MAO | monoamine oxidase |
| MAOI | monoamine oxidase inhibitor |
| MAR | medication administration record |
| mcg (or $\mu$g) | microgram |
| MD | doctor of medicine |
| MDI | metered-dose inhaler |
| MDR | multidrug-resistant |
| MDR-TB | multidrug-resistant tuberculosis |
| MDS | minimum data set |
| mEq | milliequivalent |
| mEq/L | milliequivalents per liter |
| mg | milligram |
| mg/dL | milligrams per deciliter |
| Mg | magnesium |
| $Mg^{++}$ | magnesium ion |
| MgCl | magnesium chloride |
| $MgSO_4$ | magnesium sulfate |
| MI | myocardial infarction |
| min | minute |
| mL | milliliter |
| $mm^3$ | cubic millimeter |
| mm Hg | millimeters of mercury |
| mmol/L | millimoles per liter |
| MMR | measles, mumps, rubella |
| Mn | manganese |
| Mo | molybdenum |
| MOM | Milk of Magnesia |
| mOsm/kg | milliosmoles/kilogram |
| MRI | magnetic resonance imaging |
| MRSA | methicillin-resistant *staphylococcus aureus* |
| MS | morphine sulfate |
| MSDS | material safety data sheet |
| MUGA | multi-gated acquisition |
| $N_2$ | nitrogen |
| Na | sodium |
| $Na^+$ | sodium ion |
| $Na_2SO_4$ | sodium sulfate |
| NaCl | sodium chloride |
| NA | not applicable |
| NADSA | National Adult Day Services Associations |
| $NaH_2PO_4$ | sodium dihydrogen phosphate |
| $Na_2HPO_4$ | disodium phosphate |
| NAHC | National Association for Home Care |
| $NaHCO_3$ | sodium bicarbonate |
| $NaHPO_4$ | sodium monohydrogen phosphate |
| NANDA | North American Nursing Diagnosis Association |
| NaOH | sodium hydroxide |
| NAPNE | National Association of Practical Nurse Education |
| NAPNES | National Association for Practical Nurse Education and Services |
| NCCAM | National Center for Complementary and Alternative Medicine |
| NCHS | National Center for Health Statistics |
| NCLEX® | National Council Licensure Examination |
| NCLEX-PN® | National Council Licensure Examination—Practical Nurse |
| NCLEX-RN® | National Council Licensure Examination—Registered Nurse |
| NCLD | National Center for Learning Disabilities |
| NCOA | National Council on Aging |
| NCSBN | National Council of State Boards of Nursing |
| NCVHS | National Committee on Vital and Health Statistics |
| NF | *National Formulary* |
| NFLPN | National Federation of Licensed Practical Nurses, Inc. |
| NG | nasogastric |
| $NH_2$ | amino group |
| NHO | National Hospice Organization |
| NIA | National Institute on Aging |
| NIC | Nursing Interventions Classification |
| NIH | National Institutes of Health |
| NIOSH | National Institute of Occupational Safety and Health |
| NIS | nursing information system |
| NLEA | Nutrition, Labeling, and Education Act |
| NLN | National League for Nursing |
| NLNAC | National League for Nursing Accrediting Commission |
| NMDS | nursing minimum data set |
| NOC | Nursing Outcomes Classification |
| NP | nurse practitioner |
| NPDB | National Practitioner Data Bank |
| NPO | *nil per os,* Latin for "nothing by mouth" |
| NREM | non-rapid eye movement |
| NS | normal saline |
| NSAID | nonsteroidal anti-inflammatory drug |
| NSF | National Sleep Foundation |
| $O_2$ | oxygen |
| OAM | Office of Alternative Medicine |
| O&P | ova and parasite |
| OBRA | Omnibus Budget Reconciliation Act |
| OD | right eye |
| $OH^-$ | hydroxyl |
| OR | operating room |
| ORIF | open reduction/internal fixation |
| OS | left eye |
| OSHA | Occupational Safety and Health Administration |
| OT | occupational therapist |
| OT | oral temperature |

| | |
|---|---|
| OTC | over-the-counter |
| OU | both eyes |
| oz | ounce |
| p̄ | after |
| P | phosphorus |
| P | pulse |
| PA | physician's assistant |
| PA | posterioanterior |
| PaCO$_2$ | partial pressure of carbon dioxide |
| PaO$_2$ | partial pressure of oxygen |
| Pap | Papanicolaou test |
| p.c. | after meals |
| PCA | patient-controlled analgesia |
| PCO$_2$ (PaCO$_2$) | partial pressure of carbon dioxide |
| PCP | primary care provider |
| PCR | polymerase chain reaction |
| PCV | pneumococcal conjugate vaccine |
| PDPH | postdural puncture headache |
| PEG | percutaneous endoscopic gastrostomy |
| PERRLA | pupils equal, round, reactive to light and accommodation |
| PET | positron emission tomography |
| PFT | pulmonary function test |
| pH | potential hydrogen |
| PICC | peripherally inserted central catheter |
| PIE | problem, implementation, evaluation |
| PKU | phenylketonuria |
| PLMS | periodic limb movements in sleep |
| PMI | point of maximum intensity |
| PMR | progressive muscle relaxation |
| PMS | premenstrual syndrome |
| PNI | psychoneuroimmunology |
| PNS | peripheral nervous system |
| po | *per os*, Latin for "by mouth" |
| PO$_2$ (PaO$_2$) | partial pressure of oxygen |
| PO$_4^{--}$ | phosphate ion |
| POMR | problem-oriented medical record |
| POR | problem-oriented record |
| PPBS | post prandial blood sugar |
| PPE | personal protective equipment |
| PPG | post prandial glucose |
| PPO | preferred provider organization |
| PPS | prospective payment system |
| PRA | plama renin activity |
| PRL | prolactin level |
| PRN | *pro re nata*, Latin for "as required" |
| PRO | peer review organization |
| PROM | passive range of motion |
| PSA | prostate specific antigen |
| PSDA | Patient Self-Determination Act |
| PSP | phenolsulfonphtalein |
| pt | pint |
| PT | physical therapist |
| PT | prothrombin time |
| PTH | parathyroid hormone |
| PTSD | post-traumatic stress disorder |
| PTT | partial thromboplastin time |

| | |
|---|---|
| PVD | peripheral vascular disease |
| q | *quaque*, Latin for "every" |
| qd | every day |
| qh | every hour |
| qid | four times a day |
| qod | every other day |
| qs | quantity sufficient |
| q2h | every 2 hours |
| qt | quart |
| R (Resp) | respiration |
| RAIU | radioactive iodine uptake |
| RAST | radio allergosorbent test |
| RBC | red blood count, red blood cell |
| RD | registered dietician |
| RDA | recommended dietary allowance |
| REM | rapid eye movement |
| RF | rheumatoid factor |
| RLQ | right lower quadrant |
| RLS | restless leg syndrome |
| RN | registered nurse |
| RNA | ribonucleic acid |
| RNFA | registered nurse first assistant |
| ROM | range of motion |
| ROS | review of systems |
| RPCH | rural primary care hospital |
| RPh | registered pharmacist |
| RPR | rapid plasma reagin |
| RR | recovery room |
| RSV | respiratory syncytial virus |
| R/T | related to |
| RT | rectal temperature |
| RT | respiratory therapist |
| RTI | respiratory tract infection |
| RUGS | resource utilization group system |
| RUQ | right upper quadrant |
| RWJF | Robert Wood Johnson Foundation |
| s̄ | without |
| S | sulfur |
| SAMe | S-adenosylmethionine |
| SaO$_2$ | oxygen saturation |
| SBC | school-based clinic |
| SC/SQ | subcutaneous |
| SCHIP | State Children's Health Insurance Program |
| Se | selenium |
| SGOT | serum glutamate oxaloacetate transaminase |
| SGPT | serum glutamic pyruvic transaminase |
| SL | sublingual |
| SNF | skilled nursing facility |
| SOAP | subjective data, objective data, assessment, plan |
| SOAPIE | subjective data, objective data, assessment, plan, implementation, evaluation |
| SOAPIER | subjective data, objective data, assessment, plan, implementation, evaluation, revision |
| SPF | sun protection factor |
| s̄s̄ | one half |
| SSA | Social Security Administration |
| STAT | *statim*, Latin for "immediately" |
| STD | sexually transmitted disease |

| | |
|---|---|
| **supp** | suppository |
| **susp** | suspension |
| **SW** | social worker |
| **T** | temperature |
| **T$_3$** | triiodothyronine |
| **T$_4$** | thyroxine |
| **tab** | tablet |
| **TAC** | tetracaine, adrenaline, cocaine |
| **TB** | tuberculosis |
| **Tbsp** | tablespoon |
| **Td** | tetanus/diphtheria |
| **TDD** | telecommunication device for the deaf |
| **TEFRA** | Tax Equity Fiscal Responsibility Act |
| **TENS** | transcutaneous electrical nerve stimulation |
| **TF** | tube feeding |
| **THA** | total hip arthroplasty |
| **TIA** | transient ischemic attack |
| **TIBC** | total iron binding capacity |
| **t.i.d.** | three times a day |
| **TMJ** | temporomandibular joint |
| **t.o.** | telephone order |
| **TPN** | total parenteral nutrition |
| **TPR** | temperature, pulse, respirations |
| **Tr or tinct** | tincture |
| **TRH** | thyrotropin-releasing hormone |
| **TSE** | testicular self examination |
| **TSH** | thyroid-stimulating hormone |
| **tsp** | teaspoon |
| **U** | unit |
| **U/L** | unit per liter |
| **UA** | routine urinalysis |

| | |
|---|---|
| **UAP** | unlicensed assistive personnel |
| **UIS** | Universal Intellectual Standards |
| **UL** | upper intake level |
| **UMLS** | Universal Medical Language System |
| **UNOS** | United Network for Organ Sharing |
| **U-100** | 100 units insulin per cc |
| **UPP** | urethra pressure profile |
| **URQ** | upper right quadrant |
| **USDHHS** | United States Department of Health and Human Services |
| **USP** | *United States Pharmacopeia* |
| **USPHS** | United States Public Health Service |
| **UTI** | urinary tract infection |
| **VA** | Veterans Administration, Veterans Affairs |
| **VAD** | ventricular assist device, vascular access device |
| **VAS** | Visual Analog Scale |
| **VDRL** | venereal disease research laboratory |
| **VLDL** | very low-density lipoprotein |
| **VMA** | vanilymandelic acid |
| **VRE** | vancomycin-resistant enterococci |
| **VS** | vital signs |
| **WASP** | white, Anglo-Saxon, Protestant |
| **WBC** | white blood cell, white blood count |
| **WHO** | World Health Organization |
| **WNL** | within normal limits |
| **WPM** | words per minute |
| **wt** | weight |
| **YWCA** | Young Women's Christian Association |
| **Zn** | Zinc |

# APPENDIX D
# English/Spanish Words and Phrases

Being able to say a few words or phrases in the client's language is one way to show that you care. It lets the client know that you as a nurse are interested in the individual. There are three rules to keep in mind regarding the pronunciation of Spanish words.

- If a word ends in a vowel, or in *n* or *s,* the accent is on the next to the last syllable.
- If the word ends in a consonant other than *n* or *s,* the accent is on the last syllable.
- If the word does not follow these rules, it has a written accent over the vowel of the accented syllable.

Courtesy phrases, names of body parts, and expressions of time and numbers are included in this section for quick reference. The English version will appear first, followed by the Spanish translation and Spanish pronunciation.

## COURTESY PHRASES

| Please | Por favor | Por fah-**vor** |
|---|---|---|
| Thank-you | Grácias | **Grah**-the-as |
| Good morning | Buénos dias | Boo-**ay**-nos **dee**-as |
| Good afternoon | Buénas tardes | Boo-**ay**-nas **tar**-days |
| Good evening | Buénas noches | Boo-**ay**-nas **no**-chays |
| Yes/No | Si/no | See/no |
| Good | Bien | Be-en |
| Bad | Mal | Mahl |
| How many? | ¿Cuántos? | ¿Coo-**ahn**-tos? |
| Where? | ¿Dónde? | ¿**Don**-day? |
| When? | ¿Cuándo? | ¿Coo**ahn**-do? |

## BODY PARTS

| abdomen | el abdomen | el ab-doh-men |
|---|---|---|
| ankle | el tobillo | el to-**beel**-lyo |
| anus | el ano | el **ah**-no |
| anvil (incus) | el yunque | el **yoon**-kay |
| appendix | el apéndice | el ah-**pen**-de-thay |
| aqueous humor | el humor acuoso | el oo-**mor** ah-coo-**o**-so |
| bladder | la vejiga | lah vay-**nee**-gah |
| brain | el cerebro | el thay-**ray**-bro |
| breast | el pecho | el **pay**-cho |
| buttock | la nalga | lah **nahl**-gah |
| calf | la pantorrilla | lah pan-tor-**reel**-lyah |
| cervix | la cerviz | lah ther-**veth** |
| cheek | la mejilla | lah may-**heel**-lyah |

| chin | la barbilla | lah bar-**beel**-lyah |
| choroid | la coroidea | lah co-ro-e-**day**-ah |
| ciliary body | el cuerpo ciliar | el coo-**err**-po the-le-**ar** |
| clitoris | el clítoris | el **clee**-to-ris |
| coccyx | el coxis | el **coc**-sees |
| conjunctiva | la conjuntiva | lah con-hoon-**tee**vah |
| cornea | la córnea | lah **cor**-nay-ah |
| penis | el pene | el **pay**-nay |
| prostate gland | la próstata | lah **pros**-ta-tah |
| pupil | la pupila | lah poo-**pee**-lah |
| rectum | el recto | el **rec**-to |
| retina | la retina | lah ray-**tee**-nah |
| sclera | la esclerótica | lah es-clay-**ro**-te-cah |
| scrotum | el escroto | el es-**cro**-to |
| seminal vesicle | la vesícula seminal | lah vay-**see**-coo-lah say-me-**nahl** |
| shoulder | el hombro | el **om**-bro |
| small intestine | el intestino delgado | el in-tes-**tee**-no del-**gah**-do |
| spinal cord | la médula espinal | lah **may**-doo-lah es-pe-**nahl** |
| spleen | el bazo | el **bah**-tho |
| stirrup (stapes) | el estribo | el es-**tree**-bo |
| stomach | el estómago | el es-**toh**-mah-go |
| temple | la sien | lah se-**ayn** |
| testis | el testículo | el tes-**tee**-coo-lo |
| thigh | el muslo | el **moos**-lo |
| thorax | el tórax | el **to**-rax |
| tongue | la lengua | lah **len**-goo-ah |
| trachea | la tráquea | lah **trah**-kay-ah |
| upper extremities | las extremidades superiores | las ex-tray-me-**dahd**-es soo-pay-re-**or**-es |
| ureter | el uréter | el oo-**ray**-ter |
| uterus | el útero | el **oo**-tay-ro |
| vagina | el vagina | lah vah-**hee**-nah |
| vitreous humor | el humor vítreo | el oo-**mor vee**-tray-o |
| wrist | la muñeca | lah moo-**nyay**-cah |

# EXPRESSIONS OF TIME, CALENDAR, AND NUMBERS

| after meals | después de comer | des-poo-**es** day co-**merr** |
| at bedtime | al acostarse | al ah-cos-**tar**-say |
| before meals | antes de comer | **ahn**-tes day co-**merr** |
| daily | el diario | el de-**ah**-re-o |
| date | la fecha | lah **fay**-chah |
| day | el dia | el **dee**-ah |
| every hour | a cada hora | ah **cah**-dah **o**-rah |
| hour (time) | la hora | lah **o**-rah |
| how often | cada cuánto tiempo | **cah**-dah coo-**ahn**-to te-**em**-po |
| noon | el mediodia | el may-de-o-**dee**-ah |
| now | ahora | ah-**o**-rah |
| once | una vez | **oo**-nah veth |
| today | hoy | **oh**-e |
| tomorrow | mañana | mah-**nyah**-nah |
| tonight | esta noche | **es**-tah **no**-chay |
| week | la semana | lah say-**mah**-nah |
| year | año | **a**-nyo |
| Sunday | el domingo | el do-**meen**-go |
| Monday | el lunes | el **loo**-nes |
| Tuesday | el martes | el **mar**-tes |
| Wednesday | el miércoles | el me-**err**-co-les |
| Thursday | el jueves | el hoo-**ay**ves |
| Friday | el viernes | el ve-**err**-nes |

| Saturday | el sábado | el **sah**-bah-do |
| zero | cero | **thay**-ro |
| one | uno | **oo**-no |
| two | dos | dose |
| three | tres | trays |
| four | cuatro | coo-**ah**-tro |
| five | cinco | **theen**-co |
| six | seis | **say**-ees |
| seven | siete | se-**ay**-tay |
| eight | ocho | **o**-cho |
| nine | nueve | noo-**ay**-vay |
| ten | diez | de-**eth** |

## NURSING CARE SENTENCES AND QUESTIONS

What is your name?
¿Como se llama usted?
¿**Co**-mo say **lyah**-mah oos-**ted?**

I am a student nurse.
Soy estudiente enfermera(o).
Soy es-too-de-**ahn**-tay en-fer-**may**-ra(o).

My name is . . .
Mi nombre es . . .
Mee **nom**-bray es . . .

Do you need a wheelchair?
¿Necesita usted una silla de rueda?
¿Nay-thay-**se**-ta oos-**ted oo**-nah **seel**-lyah day
  roo-**ay**-dah?

How do you feel?
¿Como se siente?
¿**Co**-mo say se-**ayn**-tah?

When is your family coming?
¿Cuándo viene su familia?
¿Coo-**ahn**-do vee-**en**-nah soo fah-**mee**-le-ah?

This is the call light.
Esta es la luz para llamar a la enfermera.
**Es**-tah es lah looth **pah**-ra lyah-**mar** a lah
  en-fer-**may**-ra.

If you need anything, press the button.
Si usted necesita algo, oprima el botón.
See oos-**ted** nay-thay-**se**-ta **ahl**-go o-pre-**ma** el
  bo-**tone.**

Do not turn without calling the nurse.
No se voltee sin llamar a la enfermera.
No say **vol**-tay seen lyah-**mar** a lah en-fer-**may**-ra.

The side rails on your bed are for your protection.
Los rieles del costado están para su protección.
Los re-**el**-es del cos-**tah**-do es-**tahn pah**-ra soo
  pro-tec-the-**on.**

Please do not try to lower or climb over the
  side rail.
Por favor no pretenda bajarlos (barjarlas) o treparse
  sobre ellos.
Por fah-**vor** no pray-**ten**-dah ba-**har**-los o
  tray-**par**-say **so**-bray **ayl**-lyos.

The head nurse is . . .
La jefa de enfermeras es . . .
La **hay**-fay day en-fer-**may**-ras es . . .

Do you need more blankets or another pillow?
¿Necesita usted más frazadas u orta almohada?
¿Nay-thay-**si**-ta oos-**ted** mahs frah-**thad**-dahs oo
  **o**-trah al-mo-**ah**-dah?

You may not smoke in the room.
No se puede fumar en el cuarto.
No say poo-**ay**-day foo-**mar** en el coo-**ar**-to.

Do you want me to turn on (turn off) the lights?
¿Quiere usted que encienda (apague) la luz?
¿Ke-**ay**-ray oos-**ted** day en-the-**en**-dah (a-**pah**-gay)
  lah looth?

Are you thirsty?
¿Tiene usted sed?
¿Tee-**en**-nah oos-**ted** sayd?

Are you allergic to any medication?
¿Es usted alérgico(a) a alguna medicina?
¿Es oos-**ted** ah-**lehr**-hee-co(a) ah ah-**goo**-nah
  nay-de-**thee**-nah?

You may take a bath.
Usted puede bañarse.
Oos-**ted** poo-**ay**-day bah-**nyar**-say.

Do not lock the door, please.
No cierre usted la puerta con llave, por favor.
No the-**err**-ray oos-**ted** lah poo-**err**-tah con **lyah**-vay
  por fah-**vor.**

Call if you feel faint or in need of help.
Llame si usted se siente débil o si necesita ayuda.
**Lyah**-mah see oos-**ted** say se-**ayn**-tah **day**-bil o see
   nay-thay-**se**-ta ah-**yoo**-dah.

Call when you have to go to the toilet.
Llame cuando tenga que ir al inodoro.
**Lyah**-mah coo-**ahn**-do **ten**-gah kay eer al in-o-**do**-ro.

I will give you an enema.
Le pondré una enema.
Lay pon-**dray oo**-nah ay-**nay**-mah.

Turn on your left (right) side.
Voltese a su lado izquierdo (derecho).
Vol-**tay**-say ah soo **lah**-do ith-ke-**er**-do(dah)
   (day-**ray**-cho[cha]).

Here is an appointment card.
Aqui tiene usted una tarjeta con la información escrito.
Ah-**kee** tee-**en**-nah oos-**ted oo**-nah tar-**hay**-tah con lah
   in-for-mah-the-**on** es-**cree**-to.

You are going to be discharged (released) today.
A usted le van a dar de alta hoy.
Ah oos-**ted** lay vahn ah dar day **ahl**-tah **oh**-e.

How did this illness begin?
¿Como empezó esta enfermedad?
¿**Co**-mo em-pa-**tho es**-tah en-fer-may-**dahd**?

Is the pain better after the medicine?
¿Siente usted alivio depués de tomar la medicina?
¿Se-**ayn**-tah oos-**ted** al-**lee**-ve-o des-poo-**es** day to-**mar** lah
   may-de-**thee**-nah?

Where is the pain?
¿Que la duele? (or) Dónde le duele?
¿Kay lah doo-**ay**-le? (or) **Don**-day lay doo-**ay**-le?

Do you have pains in your chest?
¿Tiene usted dolores in el pecho?
¿Tee-**en**-nah oos-**ted** do-**lor**-es en el **pay**-cho?

Are you in pain now?
¿Tiene usted dolores ahora?
¿Tee-**en**-nah oos-**ted** do-**lor**-es ah-**o**-rah?

Is it constant pain or does it come and go?
¿Es un dolor constante o va y vuelve?
¿Es oon do-**lor** cons-**tahn**-tay o vah ee voo-**el**-vah?

Is there anything that makes the pain better?
¿Hay algo que lo alivie?
¿**Ah**-ee **ahl**-go kay lo al-**le**-ve?

Is there anything that makes the pain worse?
¿Hay algo que lo aumente?
¿**Ah**-ee **ahl**-go kay lo ah-oo-**men**-tay?

Where do you feel the pain?
¿Dónde siente usted el dolor?
¿**Don**-day se-**ayn**-tah oos-**ted** el do-**lor**?

Point to where it hurts.
Apunte usted por favor, adonde le duele.
Ah-**poon**-tay oos-**ted** por fah-**vor** ah-**don**-day
   lay doo-**ay**-le.

Show me where it hurts.
Enséñeme usted donde le duele.
En-**say**-nah-may oos-**ted don**-day lay doo-**ay**-le.

Is the pain sharp or dull?
¿Es agudo o sordo el dolor?
¿Es ah-**goo**-do o **sor**-do el do-**lor**?

Do you know where you are?
¿Sabe usted donde esta?
¿Sah-**bay** oos-**ted don**-day es-**tah**?

You are in the hospital.
Usted está en el hospital.
Oos-**ted** es-**tah** en el os-pee-**tahl**.

You will be okay.
Usted va a estar bien.
Oos-**ted** vah a es-**tar** be-en.

Do you have any drug reactions?
¿Tiene usted alguna sensibilidad a productos
   químicos?
¿Te-**en**-nah oos-**ted** al-**goo**-nah sen-se-be-le-**dahd** a
   pro-**dooc**-tos **kee**-me-cos?

Have you seen another doctor or native healer for this
   problem?
¿Ha visto usted a otro médico o curandero tocante a este
   problema?
¿Ah **vees**-to oos-**ted** a o-tro **may**-de-co o coo-ran-**day**-ro
   to-**cahn**-tay a **es**-ah pro-**blay**-mah?

Have you vomited?
¿Ha vomitado usted?
¿Ah vo-me-**tah**-do oos-**ted**?

Do you have any difficulty in breathing?
¿Tiene usted alguna dificultad para respirar?
¿Te-**en**-nah oos-**ted** ah-**goo**-nah de-fe-cool-**tahd pah**-ra
   res-pe-**rar**?

Do you smoke?
¿Fuma usted?
¿Foo-**mar** oos-**ted**?

How many per day?
¿Cuántos al dia?
¿Coo-**ahn**-tos al **dee**-ah?

For how many years?
¿Por cuántos años?
¿por coo-**ahn**-tos **a**-nyos?

Do you awaken in the night because of shortness of
    breath?
¿Se despierta usted por la noche por falta de
    respiración?
¿Say des-pee-**err**-tah oos-**ted** por lah **no**-chay por **fahl**-tah
    day res-pe-rah-the-**on**?

Is any part of your body swollen?
¿Tiene usted alguna parte del cuerpo hinchada?
¿Te-**en**-nah oos-**ted** ah-**goo**-nah **par**-tay del
    coo-**err**-po in-**chah**-da?

How much water do you drink daily?
¿Cuántos vasos de agua bebe usted diariamente?
¿Coo-**ahn**-tos **vah**-sos day **ah**-goo-ah **bay**-be oos-**ted**
    de-ah-re-ah-**men**-tay?

Are you nauseated?
¿Tiene náusea?
¿Te-**en**-nah **nah**-oo-say-ah?

Are you going to vomit?
¿Va a vomitar?
¿Vah a vo-me-**tar**?

When was your last bowel movement?
¿Cuánto tiempo hace que evacúa usted?
¿Coo-**ahn**-to te-**em**-po **ah**-the kay ay-vah-**coo**-ah
    oos-**ted**?

Do you have diarrhea?
¿Tiene usted diarrea?
¿Te-**en**-nah oos-**ted** der-ar-**ray**-ah?

How much do you urinate?
¿Cuánto orina usted?
¿Coo-**ahn**-to o-**re**-nah oos-**ted**?

Did you urinate?
¿Orinó usted?
¿O-re-**no** oos-**ted**?

What color is your urine?
¿De qué color es la orina?
¿Day kay co-**lor** es lah o-**re**-nah?

Call when you have to go to the toilet.
Llame usted cuando tenga que ir al inodoro.
**Lyah**-mah oos-**ted** coo-**ahn**-do **ten**-gah kay eer al
    in-o-**do**-ro.

I need a urine specimen from you.
Necesito una muestra de orina de usted.
Nay-thay-**se**-to **oo**-nah moo-**ays**-trah day o-**re**-nah day
    oos-**ted**.

We will put a tube in your bladder so that you can
    urinate.
Le pondremos un tubo en la vejiga para que puede orinar.
Lay pon-**dray**-mos un **too**-be en lah vay-**hee**-gah **pah**-rah kay
    poo-**ay**-day o-re **nar**.

When was your last menstrual period?
¿Cuándo fue se última menstruación?
¿Coo-**ahn**-do foo-**ay** soo **ool**-te-mah
    mens-troo-ah-the-**on**?

Are you bleeding heavily?
¿Está sangrando mucho?
¿Es-**tah** san-**grahn**-do **moo**-cho?

Take off your clothes, please
Desvístase usted, por favor.
Des-**ves**-tah-say oos-**ted** por-fah-**vor**.

Just relax.
Relaje usted el cuerpo.
Ray-**lah**-he oos-**ted** el coo-**err**-po.

I am going to listen to your chest.
Voy a escucharle el pecho.
Voye a es-coo-**char**-lay el **pay**-cho.

Let me feel your pulse.
Déjeme tomarle el pulso.
**Day**-ha-me to-**bar**-lay el **pool**-so.

I am going to take your temperature.
Voy a tomarle la temperatura.
Voye a to-**mar**-lay lah tem-pay-rah-**too**-rah.

Lie down, please.
Acuéstese, por favor.
Ah-coo-**es**-tah-say por fah-**vor**.

Do you understand?
¿Me comprende usted?
¿May com-**pren**-day oos-**ted**?

That's right.
Así. Bien.
Ah-**see**. **Be**-en.

You are doing very well.
Usted va muy bien.
Oos-**ted** vah **moo**-e **be**-en.

Do not take any medicine from home.
No tome usted ninguna medicina traída de su casa.
No **to**-may oos-**ted** nin-**goon**-ay may-de-**thee**-nah
    trah-**ee**-dah day soo **cah**-sah.

I am going to give you an injection.
Voy a ponerle ana inyección.
Voye a po-**nerr**-lay **oo**-nah in-yec-the-**on**.

Take a sip of water.
Tome usted un traguito de agua.
**To**-may oos-**ted** un trah-**gee**-to day **ah**-goo-ah.

Very good. That was fine.
Muy bien. Excelente.
**Moo**-e **be**-en. **Ex**-thay-**len**-tay.

Don't be nervous.
No se ponga nervioso(a).
No say **pon**-gah ner-ve-**o**-so(ah).

Do you feel dizzy?
¿Se siente vertigo?
¿Say see-**ayn**-tah **verr**-to-go?

Please lie still.
Quédese inmóvil, por favor.
**Kay**-day-say in-**mo**-veel por fah-**vor.**

You must drink lots of liquids.
Usted debe tomar muchos líquidos.
Oos-**ted day**-bay to-**mar moo**-chos **lee**-ke-dos.

## REFERENCES

Kelz, R. K. (1982.) *Conversational Spanish for Medical Personnel.* Clifton Park, NY: Delmar Cengage Learning.
Velazquez de la Cadena, M., Gray, E., & Iribas, J. (1985). *New Revised Velazquez Spanish and English Dictionary.* Clinton, NJ: New Win Publishing, Inc.

# GLOSSARY

## A

**abduction**  Lateral movement away from the body

**ability**  Competence in an activity

**abortion**  Termination of pregnancy before the age of fetal viability, usually 24 weeks

**abruptio placenta**  Premature separation, from the wall of the uterus, of normally implanted placenta

**absorption**  Passage of a drug from the site of administration into the bloodstream; process whereby the end products of digestion pass through the epithelial membranes in the small and large intestines and into the blood or lymph system

**abuse**  Incident involving some type of violation to the client; misuse, excessive, or improper use of a substance, the absence of which does not cause withdrawal symptoms

**acanthosis nigricans**  A velvety hyperpigmented patch on the back of neck, in axilla, or anticubital area found in children with type 2 diabetes

**accreditation**  Process by which a voluntary, nongovernmental agency or organization appraises and grants accredited status to institutions, programs, services, or any combination of these that meet predetermined structure, process, and outcome criteria

**acculturation**  Process of learning beliefs, norms, and behavioral expectations of a group

**acid**  Any substance that in a solution yields hydrogen ions bearing a positive charge

**acidosis**  Condition characterized by an excessive number of hydrogen ions in a solution

**acme**  Peak of a contraction

**acquired immunity**  Formation of antibodies (memory B cells) to protect against future invasions of an already experienced antigen

**acquired immunodeficiency syndrome (AIDS)**  Progressively fatal disease that destroys the immune system and the body's ability to fight infection; caused by the human immunodeficiency virus (HIV)

**acrocyanosis**  Blue coloring of hands and feet

**actively suicidal**  Descriptor of an individual intent upon hurting or killing him- or herself and who is in imminent danger of doing so

**activities of daily living**  Basic care activities that include mobility, bathing, hygiene, grooming, dressing, eating, and toileting

**acupressure**  Technique of releasing blocked energy within an individual when specific points (tsubas) along the meridians are pressed or massaged by the practitioner's fingers, thumbs, and heel of the hands

**acupuncture**  Technique of application of needles and heat to various points on the body to alter the energy flow

**acute pain**  Has a sudden onset, relatively short duration, mild to severe intensity, with a steady decrease in intensity over several days or weeks

**adaptation**  Ongoing process whereby individuals use various responses to adjust to stressors and change; change resulting from assimilation and accommodation

**adaptive energy**  Inner forces that an individual uses to adapt to stress (phrase coined by Selye)

**adaptive measure**  Measure for coping with stress that requires a minimal amount of energy

**addiction**  Overwhelming preoccupation with obtaining and using a drug for its psychic effects; used interchangeably with dependence

**adhesion**  Internal scar tissue from previous surgeries or disease processes

**adjuvant medication**    Drug used to enhance the analgesic efficacy of opioids, treat concurrent symptoms that exacerbate pain, and provide independent analgesia for specific types of pain

**adult day care**    Centers that provide a variety of services in a protective setting for adults who are unable to stay alone but who do not need 24-hour care; the centers are located in a separate unit of a long-term care facility, in a private home, or are freestanding

**adventitious breath sound**    Abnormal sound, including sibilant wheezes (formerly wheezes), sonorous wheezes (formerly rhonchi), fine and course crackles (formerly rales), pleural friction rubs, and stridor

**affect**    Outward expression of mood or emotions

**affective domain**    Area of learning that involves attitudes, beliefs, and emotions

**afferent nerve pathway**    Ascending spinal cord pathway that transmits sensory impulses to the brain

**afferent pain pathway**    Ascending spinal cord

**afterpains**    Discomfort caused by the contracting uterus after the infant's birth

**age appropriate care**    Nursing care that takes into consideration the client's physical, mental, emotional, and spiritual developmental levels

**age of viability**    Gestational age at which a fetus could live outside the uterus, generally considered to be 24 weeks

**agent**    Entity capable of causing disease

**agglutination**    Clumping together of red blood cells

**agglutinin**    Specific kind of antibody whose interaction with antigens is manifested as agglutination

**agglutinogen**    Any antigenic substance that causes agglutination by the production of agglutinin

**agnosia**    Inability to recognize, either by sight or sound, familiar objects such as a hairbrush

**agnostic**    Individual who believes that the existence of God cannot be proved or disproved

**agranulocytosis**    Acute condition causing a severe reduction in the number of granulocytes (basophils, eosinophils, and neutrophils)

**Airborne Precautions**    Measures taken in addition to Standard Precautions and for clients known to have or suspected of having illnesses spread by airborne droplet nuclei

**airborne transmission**    Transfer of an agent to a susceptible host through droplet nuclei or dust particles suspended in the air

**Aldrete Score**    Scoring system for objectively assessing the physical status of clients recovering from anesthesia; serves as a basis for dismissal from the postanesthesia care unit (PACU) and ambulatory surgery; also known as the postanesthetic recovery score

**algor mortis**    Decrease in body temperature after death, resulting in lack of skin elasticity

**alkalosis**    Condition characterized by an excessive loss of hydrogen ions from a solution

**allergen**    Type of antigen commonly found in the environment

**allogeneic**    From a donor of the same species

**alopecia**    Partial or complete baldness or loss of hair

**alternative therapy**    Therapy used instead of conventional or mainstream medical practices

**ambulatory care**    A facility that provides clients diagnostic treatment, medical treatment, preventive care, and rehabilitative care on an outpatient basis

**ambulatory surgery**    Surgical operation performed under general, regional, or local anesthesia, involving less than 24 hours of hospitalization

**amenorrhea**    Absence of menstruation

**amnesia**    Inability to remember things

**amniocentesis**    Withdrawal of amniotic fluid to obtain a sample for specimen examination

**amnion**    Inner fetal membrane originating in the blastocyst

**amniotomy**    Artificial rupture of the membranes

**amphiarthrosis**    Articulation of slightly movable joints such as the vertebrae

**amputation**    Removal of all or part of an extremity

**anabolism**    Constructive process of metabolism whereby new molecules are synthesized and new tissues are formed, as in growth and repair

**analgesia**    Pain relief without producing anesthesia

**analgesic**    Substance that relieves pain

**analyte**    Substance that is measured

**anaphylaxis**    Type I systemic reaction to allergens

**anasarca**    Generalized edema

**anesthesia**    Absence of normal sensation

**anesthesiologist**    Licensed physician educated and skilled in the delivery of anesthesia who also adds to the knowledge of anesthesia through research or other scholarly pursuits

**anesthetist**    Qualified RN, dentist, or medical doctor who administers anesthetics

**aneurysm**    Weakness in the wall of a blood vessel

**anger control assistance**    Nursing intervention aimed at facilitating the expression of anger in an adaptive and nonviolent manner

**angina pectoris**    Chest pain caused by a narrowing of the coronary arteries

**angiocatheter**    Intracatheter with a metal stylet

**angioedema**    Allergic reaction consisting of edema of subcutaneous tissue, mucous membranes, or viscera

**angiogenesis**    Formation of new blood vessels

**angiography**    Visualization of the vascular structures through the use of fluoroscopy with a contrast medium

**angioma**    Benign vascular tumor involving skin and subcutaneous tissue; most are congenital

**anion**    Ion bearing a negative charge

**annulus**   Valvular ring in the heart

**anorexia**   Loss of appetite

**anosognosia**   Lack of awareness of own neurological deficits

**anthrax**   An acute, infectious disease caused by the bacterium Bacillus anthracis, which has an incubation period of 2-60 days; it is an Important potential agent for bioterrorism

**anthropometric measurements**   Measurements of the size, weight, and proportions of the body

**antibody**   Immunoglobulin produced by the body in response to bacteria, viruses, or other antigenic substances; destroys antigens

**anticipatory grief**   Occurrence of grief before an expected loss actually occurs

**anticipatory guidance**   Information, teaching, and guidance given to a client in anticipation of an expected event

**antigen**   Any substance identified by the body as nonself

**antineoplastic**   Agent that inhibits the growth and reproduction of malignant cells

**antioxidant**   Substance that prevents or inhibits oxidation, a chemical process wherein a substance is joined to oxygen

**antipyretic**   Drug used to reduce an abnormally high temperature

**anxiety**   Subjective response that occurs when a person experiences a real or perceived threat to well-being; a diverse feeling of dread or apprehension

**anxiolytic**   Antianxiety medication

**aphasia**   Absence of speech; often the result of a brain lesion

**apheresis**   Removal of unwanted blood components

**appendicitis**   Inflammation of the vermiform appendix

**appropriate for gestational age**   Infant's weight falls between the 90th and 10th percentile for gestational age

**areflexia**   Absence of reflexes

**aromatherapy**   Therapeutic use of concentrated essences or essential oils extracted from plants and flowers

**arousal**   State of wakefulness and alertness

**arterial blood gases**   Measurement of levels of oxygen, carbon dioxide, pH, partial pressure of oxygen ($PO_2$ or $PaO_2$), partial pressure of carbon dioxide ($PCO_2$ or $PaCO_2$), saturation of oxygen ($SaO_2$), and bicarbonate ($HCO_3$) in arterial blood

**arteriography**   Radiographic study of the vascular system following the injection of a radiopaque dye through a catheter

**arteriosclerosis**   Cardiovascular disease wherein plaque forms on the inside of artery walls, reducing the space for blood flow

**arthroplasty**   Replacement of both articular surfaces within a joint capsule

**ascites**   Abnormal accumulation of fluid in the peritoneal cavity

**asepsis**   Absence of pathogenic microorganisms

**aseptic technique**   Collection of principles used to control and/or prevent the transfer of pathogenic microorganisms from sources within (endogenous) and outside (exogenous) the client

**aspiration**   Procedure performed to withdraw fluid that has abnormally collected or to obtain a specimen; also inhalation of secretion or fluids into the pulmonary system

**assent**   Voluntary agreement to participate in a research project or to accept treatment

**assisted living**   A facility that combines housing and services for persons who require assistance with activities of daily living

**asthma**   Condition characterized by intermittent airway obstruction due to antigen antibody reaction

**astigmatism**   Asymmetric focus of light rays on the retina

**ataxia**   Inability to coordinate voluntary muscle action

**atelectasis**   Collapse of a lung or a portion of a lung

**atheist**   Individual who does not believe in God or any other deity

**atherosclerosis**   Cardiovascular disease of fatty deposits on the inner lining, the tunica intima, of vessel walls

**atom**   Smallest unit of an element that still retains the properties of that element and that cannot be altered by any chemical change

**atresia**   Absence or closure of a body orifice

**attachment**   Long-term process that begins during pregnancy and intensifies during the postpartum period, which establishes an enduring bond between parent and child, and develops through reciprocal (parent-to-child and child-to-parent) behaviors

**attitude**   Manner, feeling, or position toward a person or thing

**attribute**   Characteristic that belongs to an individual

**audible wheeze**   Wheeze that can be heard without the aid of a stethoscope

**auditory hallucination**   Perception by an individual that someone is talking when no one in fact is there

**auditory learner**   Person who learns by processing information through hearing

**augmentation of labor**   Stimulation of uterine contractions after spontaneously beginning but having unsatisfactory progress of labor

**aura**   Peculiar sensation preceding a seizure or migraine; may be a taste, smell, sight, sound, dizziness, or just a "funny feeling"

**auscultation**    Physical examination technique that involves listening to sounds in the body that are created by movement of air or fluid

**autoimmune disorder**    Disease wherein the body identifies its own cells as foreign and activates mechanisms to destroy them

**autologous**    From the same organism (person)

**automatism**    Mechanical, repetitive motor behavior performed unconsciously

**autonomic nervous system**    That part of the peripheral nervous system consisting of the sympathetic and parasympathetic nervous systems and controlling unconscious activities

**autonomy**    Self-direction; ethical principle based on the individual's right to choose and the individual's ability to act on that choice

**autopsy**    Examination of a body after death by a pathologist to determine cause of death

**autosomal**    Pertaining to a condition transmitted by a nonsex chromosome

**awareness**    Capacity to perceive sensory impressions through thoughts and actions

**azotemia**    Nitrogenous wastes present in the blood

---

## B

**bacteremia**    Condition of bacteria in the blood

**bactericide**    Bacteria-killing chemicals; found in tears

**ballottement**    Rebounding of the floating fetus when pushed upward through the vagina or abdomen

**bands**    Immature neutrophils

**barium**    Chalky-white contrast medium

**Barrier Precautions**    Use of personal protective equipment, such as masks, gowns, and gloves, to create a barrier between the person and the microorganisms and thus prevent transmission of the microorganism

**basal metabolism**    Energy needed to maintain essential physiologic functions when a person is at complete rest; the lowest level of energy expenditure

**base**    Substance that when dissociated produces ions that will combine with hydrogen ions

**baseline level**    Lab value that serves as a reference point for future value levels

**behavioral tolerance**    Compensatory adjustments of behavior made under the influence of a particular substance

**benign**    Not progressive; favorable for recovery

**bereavement**    Period of grief that follows the death of a loved one

**bioavailability**    Readiness to produce a drug effect

**biofeedback**    Measures physiologic responses that assist individuals to improve their health by using signals from their own bodies

**biologic response modifier**    Agent that destroys malignant cells by stimulating the body's immune system

**biological agent**    Living organism that invades a host, causing disease

**biological clock**    Internal mechanism in a living organism capable of measuring time

**biopsy**    Excision of a small amount of tissue

**bioterrorism**    the purposeful use of a biological preparation for the purposes of harming, killing large numbers of people, and/or instilling fear in large numbers of people

**blanching**    White color of the skin when pressure is applied

**blastic phase**    Intensified phase of leukemia that resembles an acute phase in which there is an increased production of white blood cells

**blastocyst**    Cluster of cells that will develop into the embryo

**bloody show**    Expulsion of cervical secretions, blood-tinged mucus, and the mucus plug that blocked the cervix during pregnancy

**body image**    Individual's perception of physical self, including appearance, function, and ability

**body mass index**    Measurement used to ascertain whether a person's weight is appropriate for height; calculated by dividing the weight in kilograms by the height in meters squared

**body mechanics**    Use of the body to safely and efficiently move or lift objects

**bodymind**    Inseparable connection and operation of thoughts, feelings, and physiologic functions

**bonding**    Rapid process of attachment, parent to infant, that takes place during the sensitive period, the first 30 to 60 minutes after birth

**borborygmi**    High-pitched, loud, rushing sounds produced by the movement of gas in the liquid contents of the intestine

**bradycardia**    Heart rate less than 60 beats per minute in an adult

**bradykinesia**    Slowness of voluntary movement and speech

**bradypnea**    Respiratory rate of 10 or fewer breaths per minute

**Braxton-Hicks contractions**    Irregular, intermittent contractions felt by the pregnant woman toward the end of pregnancy

**breakthrough pain**    Sudden, acute, temporary pain that is usually precipitated by a treatment, a procedure, or unusual activity of the client

**brief dynamic therapy**    Short-term psychotherapy that focuses on resolving core conflicts deriving from personality and living situations

**bronchial sound**   Loud, high-pitched, hollow-sounding breath sound normally heard over the sternum; longer on expiration than inspiration

**bronchiectasis**   Lung disorder characterized by chronic dilation of the bronchi

**bronchitis**   Inflammation of the bronchial tree accompanied by hypersecretion of mucus

**bronchovesicular sound**   Breath sound normally heard in the area of the scapula and near the sternum; medium in pitched blowing sound, with inspiratory and expiratory phases of equal length

**bruxism**   Grinding of teeth during sleep

**buffer**   Substance that attempts to maintain pH range, or hydrogen ion concentration, in the presence of added acids or bases

**burnout**   State of physical and emotional exhaustion occurring when caregivers use up their adaptive energy

**butterfly needle**   Wing-tipped needle

# C

**cachectic**   Being in a state of malnutrition and wasting

**cachexia**   State of malnutrition and protein wasting

**calculus**   Concentration of mineral salts in the body leading to the formation of stone

**calorie**   Amount of heat required to raise the temperature of 1 gram of water 1 degree Celsius

**cancer**   Disease resulting from the uncontrolled growth of cells, which causes malignant cellular tumors

**capitated rate**   Preset fee based on membership rather than services provided; payment system used in managed care

**caput succedaneum**   Edema of the newborn's scalp which is present at birth, may cross suture lines, and is caused by head compression against the cervix

**carcinogen**   Substance that initiates or promotes the development of cancer

**carcinoma**   Cancer occurring in epithelial tissue

**cardiac cycle**   Cycle of an impulse going completely through the conduction system of the heart, and the ventricles contracting

**cardiac output**   Volume of blood pumped per minute by the left ventricle

**cardiac tamponade**   Collection of fluid in the pericardial sac hindering the functioning of the heart

**carrier**   Person who harbors an infectious agent but has no symptoms of disease

**caseation**   Process whereby the center of the primary tubercle formed in the lungs as a result of tuberculosis becomes soft and cheese-like due to decreased perfusion

**catabolism**   Destructive process of metabolism whereby tissues or substances are broken into their component parts

**cataplexy**   Sudden loss of muscle control

**catharsis**   Process of talking out one's feelings; "getting things off the chest" through verbalization

**cation**   Ion bearing a positive charge

**cavitation**   Process whereby a cavity is created in the lung tissue through the liquefaction and rupture of a primary tubercle

**ceiling effect**   Medication dosage beyond which no further analgesia occurs

**cellular immunity**   Type of acquired immunity involving T-cell lymphocytes

**Centers for Disease Control & Prevention (CDC)**   An agency of the federal government that provides for the investigation, identification, prevention, and control of diseases; it plays an important role in preparing for, and disseminating information about, possible terrorist attacks

**central line**   Venous catheter inserted into the superior vena cava through the subclavian or internal or external jugular vein

**central nervous system**   System of the brain and spinal cord

**cephalalgia**   Headache; also known as cephalgia

**cephalhematoma**   Collection of blood between the periosteum and the skull of a newborn; appears several hours to a day after birth, does not cross suture lines, and is caused by the rupturing of the periosteal bridging veins due to friction and pressure during labor and delivery

**cephalopelvic disproportion**   Condition in which the fetal head will not fit through the mother's pelvis

**certification**   Voluntary process that establishes and evaluates standards of care; mandatory for any health care services receiving federal funds

**cerumen**   Earwax

**cervical dilatation**   Enlargement of the cervical opening (os) from 0 to 10 cm (complete dilatation)

**cesarean birth**   Birth of an infant through an incision in the abdomen and uterus

**Chadwick's sign**   Purplish-blue color of the cervix and vagina noted about the eighth week of pregnancy

**chain of custody**   Documentation of the transfer of evidence (of a crime) from one worker to the next in a secure fashion

**chain of infection**   Describes the development of an infectious process

**chalazion**   Cyst of the meibomian glands

**chancre**   Clean, painless, syphilitic primary ulcer appearing 2 to 6 weeks after infection at the site of body contact

**change**   Dynamic process whereby an individual's response to a stressor leads to an alteration in behavior

**change agent**   Person who intentionally creates and implements change

**chemical agent** Substance that interacts with a host, causing disease

**chemical name** Precise description of the drug's chemical formula

**chemical restraint** Medication used to control client behavior

**chemical warfare agents** Poisonous chemicals and gases that are used to harm or kill a large number of persons; examples of chemical agents include nerve agents, blood agents, choking or vomiting agents, and blister or vesicant agents

**Chemical, Biological, Radiological/Nuclear, and Explosive Enhanced Response Force Package** A program of the National Guard that responds rapidly, following a call by the governor, and can be at the scene of a disaster, ready to function in 6 hours; it can also include a surgical suite, if needed

**chemoreceptor** Receptor that monitors the levels of carbon dioxide, oxygen, and pH in the blood

**chemotherapy** Use of drugs to treat illness, especially cancer

**Cheyne-Stokes respirations** Breathing characterized by periods of apnea alternating with periods of dyspnea

**child abuse** Any intentional act of physical, emotional, or sexual abuse or neglect committed by a person responsible for the care of a child

**child life specialist** Health care professional with extensive knowledge of psychology and early childhood development

**chloasma** Darkening of the skin of the forehead and around the eyes during pregnancy; also called the "mask of pregnancy"

**cholecystitis** Inflammation of the gallbladder

**cholelithiasis** Presence of gallstones or calculi in the gallbladder

**cholesterol** Sterol produced by the body and used in the synthesis of steroid hormones

**chorea** Condition characterized by abnormal, involuntary, purposeless movements of all musculature of the body

**chorion** Outer fetal membrane formed from the trophoblast

**chronic acute pain** Discomfort that occurs almost daily over a long period, months or years, and may never stop; also known as progressive pain

**chronic nonmalignant pain** Discomfort that occurs almost daily, has been present for at least 6 months, and ranges from mild to severe in intensity; also known as chronic benign pain

**chronic pain** Discomfort usually defined as long term (lasting 6 months or longer), persistent, nearly constant, or recurrent pain producing significant negative changes in a person's life

**chronobiology** Science of studying biorhythms

**Chvostek's sign** Abnormal spasm of the facial muscles in response to a light tapping of the facial nerve

**chyme** Acidic, semi-fluid paste found in the gastrointestinal tract

**circadian rhythm** Biorhythm that cycles on a daily basis

**circulating nurse** RN responsible and accountable for management of personnel, equipment, supplies, the environment, and communication throughout a surgical procedure

**circumcision** Surgical removal of the prepuce (foreskin), which covers the glans penis

**circumoral cyanosis** Bluish discoloration surrounding the mouth

**cirrhosis** Chronic degenerative changes in the liver cells and thickening of surrounding tissue

**claiming process** Process whereby a family identifies the infant's "likeness to" and the "differences from" family members, and the infant's unique qualities

**clean object** Object on which there are microorganisms that are usually not pathogenic

**cleansing** Removal of soil or organic material from instruments and equipment used in providing client care

**client behavior accident** Mishap resulting from the client's behavior or actions

**clinical** Observing and caring for living clients

**closed reduction** Repair of a fracture done without surgical intervention

**coarse crackle** Moist, low-pitched crackling and gurgling lung sound of long duration

**codependent** Description for persons who live based on what others think of them

**cognition** Intellectual ability to think

**cognitive behavior therapy** Treatment approach aimed at helping a client identify stimuli that cause the client's anxiety, develop plans to respond to those stimuli in a nonanxious manner, and problem-solve when unanticipated anxiety-provoking situations arise

**cognitive domain** Area of learning that involves intellectual understanding

**cognitive reframing** Stress-management technique whereby the individual changes a negative perception of a situation or event to a more positive, less threatening perception

**coitus (copulation)** Sexual act that delivers sperm to the cervix by ejaculation of the erect penis

**cold stress** Excessive heat loss

**colic** Condition of acute abdominal pain

**colonization** Multiplication of microorganisms on or within a host that does not result in cellular injury

**colostomy** Opening created anywhere along the large intestine

**colostrum** Antibody-rich yellow fluid secreted by the breasts during the last trimester of pregnancy and the first 2–3 days after birth; gradually changes to milk

**comedone** Whitehead or blackhead

**command hallucination** Perception by an individual of a voice or voices telling the individual to do something, usually to himself and/or someone else

**communicable agent** Infectious agent transmitted to a client by direct or indirect contact, via vehicle, vector, or airborne route

**communicable disease** Disease caused by a communicable agent

**comorbidity** Simultaneous existence of more than one disease process within an individual

**complementary therapy** Therapy used in conjunction with conventional medical therapies

**complete protein** Protein containing all nine essential amino acids

**complicated grief** Grief associated with traumatic death such as death by accident, violence, or homicide; survivors often have more intense emotions than those associated with normal grief

**compound** Combination of atoms of two or more elements

**compromised host** Person whose normal body defenses are impaired and is therefore susceptible to infection

**computed tomography** Radiological scanning of the body with x-ray beams and radiation detectors to transmit data to a computer that transcribes the data into quantitative measurement and multidimensional images of the internal structures

**conditioning** Teaching a person a behavior until it becomes an automatic response; method of conserving adaptive energy

**conduction** Loss of heat by direct contact with a cooler object

**conductive hearing loss** Condition characterized by the inability of sound waves to reach the inner ear

**confabulation** The making up of information to fill in memory gaps

**congruence** Agreement between two things

**conjunctivitis** Inflammation of the conjunctiva

**consciousness** State of awareness of self, others, and surrounding environment

**constipation** Condition characterized by hard, infrequent stools that are difficult or painful to pass

**Contact Precautions** Measures taken in addition to Standard Precautions for clients known to have or suspected of having illnesses easily spread by direct client contact or by contact with fomites

**contact transmission** Transfer of an agent from an infected person to a host by direct contact with that person, indirect contact with an infected person through a fomite, or close contact with contaminated secretions

**contraception** Measure taken to prevent pregnancy

**contracture** Permanent shortening of a muscle

**contrast medium** Radiopaque substance that facilitates roentgen (x-ray) imaging of the body's internal structures

**convalescent stage** Time period in which acute symptoms of an infection begin to disappear until the client returns to the previous state of health

**convection** Loss of heat by the movement of air

**copulation** Sexual act that delivers sperm to the cervix by ejaculation of the erect penis

**cotyledon** Subdivision of the maternal side of the placenta

**couvade** Development of physical symptoms by the expectant father such as fatigue, depression, headache, backache, and nausea

**crackle** Abnormal breath sound that resembles a popping sound, heard on inhalation and exhalation; not cleared by coughing

**crenation** Condition wherein cells decrease in size, shrivel and wrinkle, and are no longer functional when in a hypertonic solution

**crepitus** Grating or crackling sensation or sound

**cretinism** Congenital lack of thyroid hormones causing defective physical development and mental retardation

**crisis** Acute state of disorganization that occurs when usual coping mechanisms are no longer adequate; stressor that forces an individual to respond and/or adapt in some way

**crisis intervention** Specific technique used to help a person regain equilibrium

**critical thinking** The disciplined intellectual process of applying skillful reasoning, imposing intellectual standards and self-reflective thinking as a guide to a belief or action

**cross-tolerance** Decreased sensitivity to other substances in the same category

**crowning** When the largest diameter of the fetal head is past the vulva

**cryotherapy** Use of cold applications to reduce swelling

**cryptorchidism** Failure of one or both testes to descend

**cultural assimilation** Process whereby members of a minority group are absorbed by the dominant culture, taking on characteristics of the dominant culture

**cultural diversity** Differences among people resulting from ethnic, racial, and cultural variations

**culture** Integrated, dynamic structure of knowledge, attitudes, behaviors, beliefs, ideas, habits, customs, languages, values, symbols, rituals, and ceremonies that are unique to a particular group of people; growing of microorganisms to identify a pathogen

**curative**   To heal or restore health

**curing**   Ridding one of disease

**cutaneous pain**   Discomfort caused by stimulating the cutaneous nerve endings in the skin

**cyanosis**   Bluish discoloration of the skin and mucous membranes observed in lips, nail beds, and earlobes

**cycling**   Alteration in mood between depression and mania

**cystitis**   Inflammation of the urinary bladder

**cystocele**   Downward displacement of the bladder into the anterior vaginal wall

**cytology**   Study of cells

## D

**dawn phenomenon**   Early morning glucose elevation produced by the release of growth hormone

**death rattle**   Noisy respirations in the period preceding death caused by a collection of secretions in the larynx

**debride**   To remove dead or damaged tissue or foreign material from a wound

**decerebration**   Severing of the spinal cord

**decidua**   The endometrium after implantation

**decomposition**   Chemical reaction wherein the bonding between atoms in a molecule is broken and simpler products are formed

**decrement**   Decreasing intensity of a contraction

**defense mechanism**   Unconscious functions protecting the mind from anxiety

**deglutition**   Swallowing of food

**dehiscence**   Complication of wound healing wherein the wound edges separate

**dehydration**   Condition wherein more water is lost from the body than is being replaced

**delirium**   Cognitive changes or acute confusion of rapid onset (less than 6 months)

**delusion**   False belief that misrepresents reality

**dementia**   Organic brain pathology characterized by losses in intellectual functioning and a slow onset (longer than 6 months)

**dental caries**   Cavities

**dependence**   Reliance on a substance to such a degree that abstinence causes functional impairment, physical withdrawal symptoms, and/or psychological craving for the substance; see also addiction

**depersonalization**   Treating an individual as an object rather than as a person

**depolarization**   Contraction of the heart

**depression**   State wherein an individual experiences feelings of extreme sadness, hopelessness, and helplessness

**detoxification**   Elimination of a substance from the body

**development**   Behavioral changes in skills and functional abilities

**dialysate**   Solution used in dialysis, designed to approximate the normal electrolyte structure of plasma and extracellular fluid

**dialysis**   Mechanical means of removing nitrogenous waste from the blood by imitating the function of the nephrons; involves filtration and diffusion of wastes, drugs, and excess electrolytes and/or osmosis of water across a semipermeable membrane into a dialysate solution

**diarthrosis**   Freely movable joint

**didactic**   Systematic presentation of information

**diet therapy**   Treating disease or disorder with special diet

**dietary prescription/order**   Order written by the physician for food, including liquids

**differentiation**   Acquisition of characteristics or functions different from those of the original

**diffusion**   Process whereby a substance moves from an area of higher concentration to an area of lower concentration

**digestion**   Mechanical and chemical processes that convert nutrients into a physically absorbable state

**diplopia**   Double vision

**dirty object**   Object on which there is a high number of microorganisms, some that are potentially pathogenic

**disability**   An individual's lack of ability to complete an activity in the normal manner

**disaster**   A situation or event of greater magnitude than an emergency and that has unforeseen, serious, or immediate threats to public health

**disciplined**   Trained by instruction and exercise

**disenfranchised grief**   Grief not openly acknowledged, socially sanctioned, or publicly shared

**disinfectant**   Chemical solution used to clean inanimate objects

**disinfection**   Elimination of pathogens, with the exception of spores, from inanimate objects

**dislocation**   Injury in which the articular surfaces of a joint are no longer in contact

**disorientation**   State of mental confusion in which awareness of time, place, self, and/or situation is impaired

**disseminated intravascular coagulation** Abnormal stimulation of the clotting mechanism causing small clots throughout the vascular system and widespread bleeding internally, externally, or both

**distraction**   Technique of focusing attention on stimuli other than pain

**distress**   Subjective experience that occurs when stressors evoke an ineffective response

**distribution**   Movement of drugs from the blood into various tissues and body fluids

**diverticula**   Sac-like protrusion of the intestinal wall that results when the mucosa herniates through the bowel wall

**diverticulitis**    Inflammation of one or more diverticula

**diverticulosis**    Condition in which multiple diverticula are present in the colon

**domestic violence**    Aggression and violence involving family members

**dominant culture**    The group whose values prevail within a given society

**Down syndrome**    Congenital chromosomal abnormality; also called trisomy 21

**Droplet Precautions**    Measures taken in addition to Standard Precautions for clients known to have or suspected of having serious illnesses spread by large particle droplets

**drug allergy**    Hypersensitivity to a drug

**drug incompatibility**    Undesired chemical or physical reaction between a drug and a solution, between a drug and the container or tubing, or between two drugs

**drug interaction**    Effect one drug can have on another drug

**drug tolerance**    Reaction that occurs when the body is accustomed to a specific drug that larger doses are needed to produce the desired therapeutic effects

**ductus arteriosus**    Fetal vessel connecting the pulmonay artery to the aorta

**ductus venosus**    Branch of the umbilical vein that enters the inferior vena cava

**duration**    Length of one contraction, from the beginning of the increment to the conclusion of the decrement

**dysarthria**    Difficult and defective speech due to a dysfunction of the muscles used for speech

**dysfunctional grief**    Persistent pattern of intense grief that does not result in reconciliation of feelings

**dysfunctional labor**    Labor with problems of the contractions or of maternal bearing down

**dysmenorrhea**    Painful menstruation

**dyspareunia**    Painful intercourse

**dysphagia**    Difficulty in swallowing

**dysplasia**    Abnormal development

**dyspnea**    Difficulty breathing as observed by labored or forced respirations through the use of accessory muscles in the chest and neck

**dysrhythmia**    Irregularity in the rate, rhythm, or conduction of the electrical system of the heart

**dystocia**    Long, difficult, or abnormal labor caused by any of the four major variables (4 Ps) that affect labor

**dysuria**    Difficult or painful urination

---

## E

**early deceleration**    Reduction in fetal heart rate that begins early in the contraction and virtually mirrors the uterine contraction

**ecchymosis**    Large, irregular hemorrhagic area on the skin; also called a bruise

**eclampsia**    Convulsion occurring in pregnancy-induced hypertension

**ectopic pregnancy**    Pregnancy in which the fertilized ovum is implanted outside the uterine cavity

**edema**    Detectable accumulation of increased interstitial fluid

**effacement**    Thinning of the cervix

**efferent nerve pain pathway**    Descending spinal cord pathway that transmits sensory impulses from the brain

**effluent**    Liquid output from an ileostomy

**electrocardiogram**    Graphic recording of the heart's electrical activity

**electroconvulsive therapy**    Procedure whereby clients are treated with pulses of electrical energy sufficient to cause brief convulsions or seizures

**electroencephalogram**    Graphic recording of the brain's electrical activity

**electrolyte**    Compound that, when dissolved in water or another solvent, dissociates (separates) into ions (electrically charged particles)

**element**    Basic substance of matter

**emancipated minor**    Child who has the legal competency of an adult because of cicumstances involving marriage, divorce, parenting of a child, living independently without parents, or enlistment in the armed services

**embolus**    Mass, such as a blood clot or an air bubble, that circulates in the bloodstream

**embryonic phase**    Development occuring during the first 2 to 8 weeks after fertilization of a human egg

**emergency**    Medical or surgical condition requiring immediate or timely intervention to prevent permanent disability or death

**emergency medical technician (EMT)**    Health care professional trained to provide basic lifesaving measures prior to arrival at the hospital

**emergency nursing**    Care of clients who require emergency interventions

**emotional lability**    Loss of emotional control

**empathy**    Capacity to understand another person's feelings or perception of a situation

**emphysema**    Lung disease wherein air accumulates in the tissues of the lungs

**empowerment**    A process through which an individual is enabled to change situations, and uses resources, skills, and opportunities to do so

**empty calories**    Calories that provide few nutrients

**encephalitis**    Inflammation of the brain

**encoding**    Laying down tracks in areas of the brain to enhance the ability to recall and use information

**encopresis**    Passage of watery colonic contents around a hard fecal mass

**endemic**   Occurring continuously in a particular population and having low mortality

**endocrine**   Group of cells secreting substances directly into the blood or lymph circulation and affecting another part of the body

**endometriosis**   Growth of endometrial tissue on structures outside of the uterus, within the pelvic cavity

**endorphins**   Group of opiate-like substances produced naturally by the brain that raise the pain threshold, produce sedation and euphoria, and promote a sense of well-being

**endoscopy**   Visualization of a body organ or cavity through a scope

**energetic-touch therapy**   Technique of using the hands to direct or redirect the flow of the body's energy fields and enhance balance within those fields

**engagement**   Condition of the widest diameter of the fetal presenting part (head) entering the inlet to the true pelvis

**engorgement**   Distentions and swelling of the breasts in the first few days following delivery

**engrossment**   Parents' intense interest in and preoccupation with the newborn

**enriched**   Descriptor for food in which nutrients that were removed during processing are added back in

**enteral instillation**   Administration of drugs through a gastrointestinal tube

**enteral nutrition**   Feeding method meaning both the ingestion of food orally and the delivery of nutrients through a gastrointestinal tube, but generally meaning the latter

**entrainment**   Infant's ability to move in rhythm to the parent's voice

**enzyme**   Globular protein produced in the body that catalyzes chemical reactions within the cells

**enzyme-linked immunosorbent assay**   Basic screening test currently used to detect antibodies to HIV

**epidemic**   Infecting many people at the same time and in the same geographic area

**epidural analgesia**   Analgesics administered via a catheter that terminates in the epidural space

**episiotomy**   Incision in the perineum to facilitate passage of the baby

**epispadias**   Placement of the urinary meatus on the top of the penis

**epistaxis**   Hemorrhage of the nares or nostrils; also known as nosebleed

**Epstein's pearls**   Small, whitish-yellow epithelial cysts found on the hard palate

**equipment accident**   Accident resulting from the malfunction or improper use of medical equipment

**erythema**   Redness of the skin due to increased blood flow to the area

**erythema toxicum neonatorum**   Pink rash with firm, yellow-white papules or pustules found on the chest, abdomen, back, and/or buttocks of a newborn

**erythematous**   Characterized by redness of the skin

**erythrocytapheresis**   Procedure that removes abnormal red blood cells and replaces them with healthy ones

**erythropoiesis**   Production of red blood cells and their release by the red bone marrow

**eschar**   Dry, dark, leathery scab composed of denatured protein

**ethnicity**   Cultural group's perception of itself or a group identity

**ethnocentrism**   Assumption of cultural superiority and inability to accept another culture's ways

**euglycemia**   Normal blood glucose level

**euphoric**   Characterized by elation out of context to the situation

**eupnea**   Easy respirations with a rate that is age-appropriate

**eustress**   Stress that results in positive outcomes

**evaporation**   Loss of heat when water is changed to a vapor

**evisceration**   Complication of wound healing characterized by a complete separation of wound edges, accompanied by visceral protrusion

**exacerbation**   Increase in the symptoms of a disease

**exclusive provider organization**   Organization wherein care must be delivered by providers in the plan in order for clients to receive any reimbursement

**excretion**   Elimination of drugs or waste products from the body

**Expeditionary Medical Support**   A total package that includes everything necessary to screen, treat, and release clients to other facilities for longer-term care

**exposure**   Contact with an infected person or agent

**extended care facility**   The term refers to any facility that provides care for a long period of time. It has no concrete definition and could refer to either an intermediate or skilled nursing facility

**external respiration**   Exchange of gases between the atmosphere and the lungs

**external version**   Manipulation of the fetus through the mother's abdomen to a presentation facilitating birth

**extracellular fluid**   Fluid outside of the cells; includes interstitial, intravascular, synovial, cerebrospinal, and serous fluids; aqueous and vitreous humor; and endolymph and perilymph

**extravasation**   Escape of fluid into the surrounding tissue

---

## F

**faith**   Confident belief in the truth, value, or trustworthiness of a person, idea, or thing

**false labor**   Contractions that do not cause the cervix to dilate

**family-centered care**  A philosophy of caring recognizing the centrality of the family in the child's life and including the family's contribution and involvement in the plan of care and its delivery (Potts & Mandleco, 2000)

**fasciculation**  Involuntary twitching of muscle fibers

**fat-soluble vitamin**  Vitamin requiring the presence of fats for its absorption from the gastrointestinal tract into the lymphatic system and for cellular metabolism: vitamins A, D, E, and K

**fee for service**  System in which the health care recipient directly pays the provider for services as they are provided

**feedback**  Response from the receiver of a message so that the sender can verify the message

**Ferguson's reflex**  Spontaneous, involutary urge to bear down during labor

**fertilization**  Union of an ovum and a sperm

**fetal attitude**  Relationship of fetal body parts to one another, either flexion or extension

**fetal biophysical profile**  Assessment of five variables: fetal breathing movement, fetal movements of body or limbs, fetal tone (flexion/extension of extremities), amniotic fluid volume, and reactive NST

**fetal lie**  Relationship of the cephalocaudal axis of the fetus to the cephalocaudal axis of the mother, either longitudinal or transverse

**fetal phase**  Intrauterine development from 8 weeks to birth

**fetal position**  Relationship of the identified landmark on the presenting part to the four quadrants of the mother's pelvis

**fetal presentation**  Determined by the fetal lie and the part of the fetus that enters the pelvis first

**fibrinolysis**  Process of breaking fibrin apart

**fight-or-flight response**  State wherein the body becomes physiologically ready to defend itself by either fighting or fleeing from the stressor

**filtration**  Process of fluids and the substances dissolved in them being forced through the cell membrane by hydrostatic pressure

**fine crackle**  Dry, high-pitched crackling and popping lung sounds of short duration

**first assistant**  Physician or RN who assists the surgeon to retract tissue, aids in the removal of blood and fluids at the operative site, and assists with homeostasis and wound closure

**first responders**  Persons who have been identified as the first ones to appear at the scene of a disaster or accident; designated first responders include health care workers, emergency medical personnel, police, and firepersons

**flashback**  Rushing of blood back into intravenous tubing when a negative pressure is created on the tubing; reliving of an original trauma as if the individual were currently experiencing it

**flora**  Microorganisms that occur or have adapted to live in a specific environment, such as intestinal, skin, vaginal, or oral flora

**flow rate**  Volume of fluid to infuse over a set period of time

**fluoroscopy**  Immediate, serial images of the body's structure or function

**fomite**  Object contaminated with an infectious agent

**fontanelle**  Membranous area where sutures meet on the fetal skull

**foramen ovale**  Flap opening in the atrial septum that allows only right-to-left movement of blood

**forceps**  Metal instruments used on the fetal head to provide traction or to provide a method of rotating the fetal head to an occiput-anterior position

**foremilk**  Watery first milk from the breast, high in lactose, like skim milk, and effective in quenching thirst

**formal teaching**  Teaching that takes place at a specific time, in a specific place, and on a specific topic

**fortified**  Descriptor for food in which nutrients not naturally occurring in the food are added to it

**fracture**  Break in the continuity of a bone

**free radical**  Unstable molecule that alters genetic codes and triggers the development of cancer growth in cells

**frequency**  Time for the beginning of one contraction to the beginning of the next contraction

**friction**  Force of two surfaces moving against one another

**fulguration**  Procedure to destroy tissue with long, high-frequency electric sparks

**fundus**  Top of the uterus

**funic souffle**  Sound of the blood pulsating through the umbilical cord; rate the same as the fetal heartbeat

# G

**gastric ulcer**  Erosion in the stomach

**gastritis**  Inflammation of the stomach mucosa

**gate control pain theory**  Theory that proposes that the cognitive, sensory, emotional, and physiologic components of the body can act together to block an individual's perception of pain

**general adaptation syndrome**  Physiologic response that occurs when a person experiences a stressor

**general anesthesia**  Method of producing unconsciousness; amnesia, motionlessness, muscle relaxation, and complete insensibility to pain

**generic name**  Name assigned by the U.S. Adopted Names Council to the manufacturer who first develops a drug

**genogram**  A way to visualize family members, their birth and death dates, or ages and specific health problems

**genuineness**  Sincerity

**germicide**   Chemical that can be applied to both animate and inanimate objects for the purpose of eliminating pathogens

**germinal phase**   Development beginning with conception and lasting approximately 10 to 14 days

**gerontological nursing**   Specialty within nursing that addresses and advocates for the special care needs of older adults

**gerontologist**   Specialist in gerontology in advanced practice nursing, geriatric psychiatry, medicine, and social services

**gerontology**   Study of the effects of normal aging and age-related diseases on human beings

**gingivitis**   Inflammation of the gums

**Glasgow Coma Scale**   Neurological screening test that measures a client's best verbal, motor, and eye response to stimuli

**glucagon**   Hormone secreted by the alpha cells of the pancreas, which stimulate release of glucose by the liver

**gluconeogenesis**   Conversion of amino acids into glucose

**glycogenesis**   Conversion of glucose into glycogen

**glycogenolysis**   Conversion of glycogen into glucose

**glycosuria**   Presence of excessive glucose in the urine

**goiter**   Enlargement of the thyroid gland

**Goodell's sign**   Softening of the cervix noted about the 8th week of pregnancy

**Gower's sign**   Walking the hands up the legs to get from sitting to standing position (as in Duchenne muscular dystrophy)

**granulation tissue**   Delicate connective tissue consisting of fibroblasts, collagen, and capillaries

**graphesthesia**   Ability to identify letters, numbers, or shapes drawn on the skin

**gravida**   Pregnancy, regardless of duration, including present pregnancy

**grief**   Series of intense psychological and physical responses occuring after a loss; these responses are necessary, normal, natural, and adaptive responses to the loss

**growth**   Measurable changes in the physical size of the body and its parts

**gynecomastia**   Abnormal enlargement of one or both breasts in males

## H

**half-life**   Time it takes the body to eliminate half of the blood concentration level of the original dose of medication

**halitosis**   Bad breath

**hallucination**   Sensory perception that occurs in the absence of external stimuli and that is not based on reality

**hallux varus**   Placement of the great toe farther from the other toes

**hand hygiene**   Rubbing together of all surfaces and crevices of the hands using a soap or chemical and water, followed by rinsing in a flowing stream of water

**handicap**   The physical or mental inability to complete a role in one or more major ADL (U.S. Office of Personnel Management, 1987)

**healing**   Process that activates the individual's recovery forces from within; to make whole

**healing touch**   Energy therapy using the hands to clear, energize, and balance the energy field

**health**   According to the World Health Organization, the state of complete physical, mental, and social well-being, not merely the absence of disease or infirmity

**health care delivery system**   Method for providing services to meet the health needs of individuals

**health care surrogate law**   Law enacted by some states that provides a legal means for decision making in the absence of advance directives

**health continuum**   Range of an individual's health, from highest health potential to death

**health history**   Review of the client's functional health patterns prior to the current contact with a health care agency

**health maintenance organization**   Prepaid health plan that provides primary health care services for a preset fee and focuses on cost-effective treatment methods

**hearing**   Act or power of receiving sounds

**heart sound**   Sound heard by auscultating the heart

**Heberden's nodes**   Enlargement and characteristic hypertrophic spurs in the terminal interphalangeal finger joints

**Hegar's sign**   Softening of the uterine isthmus about the 6th week of pregnancy

**HELLP syndrome**   Pregnancy-induced hypertension with liver damage characterized by hemolysis, elevated liver enzymes, and low platelet count

**hemarthrosis**   Bleeding into the joints

**hematemesis**   Vomiting of blood

**hematocrit**   Percentage of red blood cells in a given volume of blood

**hematopoiesis**   Process of blood cell production and development

**hematuria**   Blood in the urine

**hemiparesis**   Weakness of one side of the body

**hemiplegia**   Paralysis of one side of the body

**hemolysis**   Breakdown of red blood cells and the release of hemoglobin

**hemopneumothorax**   Presence of blood and air within the pleural space

**hemorrhagic exudate**   Discharge that has a large component of red blood cells

**hemorrhoid**   Swollen vascular tissue in the rectal area

**hemostasis**   Cessation of bleeding

**hemothorax**   Condition wherein blood accumulates in the pleural space of the lungs

**hepatitis**   Chronic or acute inflammation of the liver

**hesitancy**   Difficulty initiating the urinary stream

**hindmilk**   Follows foremilk, is higher in fat content, leads to weight gain, and is more satisfying

**hirsutism**   Excessive body hair in a masculine distribution

**histamine**   Substance released during allergic reactions

**holistic**   Whole; includes physical, intellectual, sociocultural, psychological, and spiritual aspects as an integrated whole

**Homans' sign**   Test to check for the presence of clots in the leg

**homeostasis**   Balance or equilibrium among the physiologic, psychological, sociocultural, intellectual, and spiritual needs of the body; maintenance of internal environment

**homonymous hemianopia**   Loss of vision in half of the visual field on the same side of both eyes

**hope**   To look forward to with confidence or expectation; a resource clients can use to promote physical, psychological, and spiritual wellness

**hormone**   Substance that initiates or regulates activity of another organ, system, or gland in another part of the body

**hospice**   Humane, compassionate care provided to clients who can no longer benefit from curative treatment and have 6 months or less to live; allows individuals to die with dignity

**host**   Organism that can be affected by an agent

**human immunodeficiency virus (HIV)**   Retrovirus that causes AIDS

**human leukocyte antigen**   Antigen present in human blood

**humoral immunity**   Type of immunity dominated by antibodies

**hydatidiform mole**   Abnormality of the placenta wherein the chorionic villi become fluid filled, grape-like clusters; the trophoblastic tissue proliferates; and there is no viable fetus

**hydramnios (polyhydramnios)**   Excess amount of amniotic fluid

**hydrocele**   Fluid around the testes in the scrotum

**hydrostatic pressure**   Pressure that a fluid exerts against a membrane; also called filtration force

**hygiene**   Study of health and ways of preserving health

**hyperbilirubinemia**   Excess of bilirubin in the blood

**hyperemesis gravidarum**   Excessive vomiting during pregnancy

**hypergylcemia**   Condition wherein the blood glucose level becomes too high as a result of the absence of insulin

**hyperopia**   Farsightedness

**hypersensitivity**   Excessive reaction to a stimulus

**hypersomnia**   Alteration in sleep pattern characterized by excessive sleep, especially in the daytime

**hyperthermia**   Condition in which the core body temperature rises above 106°F

**hypertonic solution**   Solution that has a higher molecular concentration than the cell; also called a hyperosmolar solution

**hypertrophy**   Increase in muscle mass

**hyperuricemia**   Increased uric acid blood level

**hyperventilation**   Breathing characterized by deep, rapid respirations

**hypervigilant**   Condition of constantly scanning the environment for potentially dangerous situations

**hypervolemia**   Increased circulating fluid volume

**hypnosis**   Altered state of consciousness or awareness resembling sleep and during which a person is more receptive to suggestion

**hypoglycemia**   Condition wherein the blood glucose level is exceedingly low

**hypomania**   Mild form of mania without significant impairment

**hypospadias**   Placement of the urinary meatus on the underside of the penis

**hypothermia**   Condition in which the core body temperature drops below 95°F

**hypotonia**   Lax muscle tone

**hypotonic solution**   Solution that has a lower molecular concentration than the cell; also called hypo-osmolar solution

**hypoventilation**   Breathing characterized by shallow respirations

**hypovolemia**   Abnormally low circulatory blood volume

**hypoxemia**   Decreased oxygen level in the blood

## I

**iatrogenic**   Caused by treatment or diagnostic procedures

**ideal self**   The person whom the individual would like to be

**identity**   An individual's conscious description of who he or she is

**idiopathic**   Occurring without a known cause

**idiosyncratic reaction**   Very unpredictable response that may be an overresponse, an underresponse, or an atypical response

**ileal conduit**   Implantation of the ureters into a piece of ileum, which is attached to the abdominal wall as a stoma so urine can be removed from the body

**ileostomy**   Opening created in the small intestine at the ileum

**illness stage**   Time period when the client is manifesting specific signs and symptoms of an infectious agent

**illusion**   Inaccurate perception or misinterpretation of sensory stimuli

**imagery**   Relaxation technique of using the imagination to visualize a pleasant, soothing image

**immune response**   Body's reaction to substances identified as nonself

**immunity**   Body's ability to protect itself from foreign agents or organisms

**immunization**   Process of creating immunity or resistance to infection in an individual

**immunotherapy**   Treatment to suppress or enhance immunologic functioning

**implantable cardioverter-defibrillator (ICD)**   Implantable device that senses a dysrythmia and automatically sends an electrical shock directly to the heart to defibrillate it

**implantable port**   Device made of a radiopaque silicone catheter and a plastic or stainless steel injection port with a self-sealing silicone-rubber septum

**implantation**   Embedding of a fertilized egg into the uterine lining

**impotence**   Inability of an adult male to have an erection firm enough or to maintain it long enough to complete sexual intercourse

**incidence**   Frequency of disease occurrence

**incompetent cervix**   Descriptor for when the cervix begins to dilate, usually during the second trimester

**incomplete protein**   Protein with one or more of the essential amino acids missing

**increment**   Increasing intensity of a contraction

**incubation period**   Time between entry of an infectious agent in the host and the onset of symptoms

**independent nursing intervention**   Nursing action initiated by the nurse and do not require direction or an order from another health care professional

**induction of labor**   Stimulation of uterine contractions before contractions begin spontaneously for the purpose of birthing an infant

**infancy**   Development from the end of the first month to the end of the first year of life

**infection**   Invasion and multiplication of pathogenic microorganims in body tissue that results in cellular injury

**infectious agent**   Microorganism that causes cellular injury

**infertility**   Inability or diminished ability to produce offspring

**infiltration**   Seepage of foreign substances into the interstitial tissue, causing swelling and discomfort at the IV site

**inflammation**   Nonspecific cellular response to tissue injury

**informal teaching**   Teaching that takes place anytime, anyplace, and whenever a learning need is identified

**informed consent**   Legal form signed by a competent client and witnessed by another person that grants permission to the client's physician to perform the procedure described by the physician and that demonstrates the client's understanding of the benefits, risks, and possible complications of the procedure, as well as alternate treatment options

**ingestion**   The taking of food into the digestive tract, generally through the mouth

**initial planning**   Development of a preliminary plan of care by the nurse who performs the admission assessment and gathers the comprehensive admission assessment data

**insensible water loss**   Water loss of which the person is not generally aware

**insomnia**   Difficulty in falling asleep initially or in returning to sleep once awakened

**inspection**   Physical examination technique that involves thorough visual observation

**insulin**   Pancreatic hormone that aids in both the diffusion of glucose into the liver and muscle cells, and the synthesis of glycogen

**intellectual wellness**   Ability to function as an independent person capable of making sound decisions

**intensity**   Strength of the contraction at the acme

**interdependent nursing intervention**   Nursing action that is implemented in a collaborative manner with other health care professionals

**internal respiration**   Exchange of oxygen and carbon dioxide at the cellular level

**interstitial fluid**   Fluid in tissue spaces around each cell

**interval**   Resting period between two contractions

**intoxication**   Reversible effect on the central nervous system soon after the use of a substance

**intracath**   Plastic tube for insertion into a vein

**intracellular fluid**   Fluid within the cells

**intradermal**   Injection into the dermis

**intramuscular**   Injection into the muscle

**intraoperative phase**   Time during the surgical experience that begins when the client is transferred to the operating room table and ends when the client is admitted to the postanesthesia care unit

**intrathecal analgesia**   Administration of analgesics into the subarachnoid space

**intravascular fluid**   Fluid consisting of the plasma in the blood vessels and the lymph in the lymphatic system

**intravenous**   Injection into a vein

**intravenous therapy**   Administration of fluids, electrolytes, nutrients, or medications by the venous route

**intravesical**   Within the urinary bladder

**intussusception**   Telescoping of one part of the intestine into another

**invasive**   Accessing the body tissues, organs, or cavities through some type of instrumentation procedure

**involution**   Return of the reproductive organs, especially the uterus, to their pre-pregnancy size and condition

**ion**   Atom bearing an electrical charge

**ischemia**   Oxygen deprivation, usually due to poor perfusion

**ischemic pain**   Discomfort resulting when the blood supply to an area is restricted or cut off completely

**isolation**   Separation from other persons, especially those with infectious diseases

**isotonic solution**   Solution that has the same molecular concentration as does the cell; also called an isosmolar solution

**isotopes**   Atom of the same element that has a different atomic weight (i.e., different numbers of neutrons in the nucleus)

**iv push (bolus)**   The administration of a large dose of medication in a relatively short time, usually 1–30 minutes

---

### J

**jaundice**   Yellow discoloration of the skin, sclera, mucous membranes, and body fluids that occurs when the liver is unable to fully remove bilirubin from the blood

**Johnsonian intervention**   Confrontational approach to a client with a substance problem that lessens the chance of denial and encourages treatment before the client "hits bottom"

**judgment**   Conclusion based on sound reasoning and supported by evidence

---

### K

**Kardex**   A brief worksheet with basic client care information

**keloid**   Abnormal growth of scar tissue that is elevated, rounded, and firm with irregular, clawlike margins

**keratin**   Tough, fibrous protein produced by cells in the epidermis called keratinocytes

**keratitis**   Inflammation of the cornea

**kernicterus**   Severe neurological damage resulting from a high level of bilirubin (jaundice)

**Kernig's sign**   Diagnostic test for inflammation in the nerve roots; the inability to extend the leg when the thigh is flexed against the abdomen

**ketone**   Acidic by-product of fat metabolism

**ketonuria**   Presence of ketones in the urine

**ketosis**   Condition wherein acids called ketones accumulate in the blood and urine, upsetting the acid–base balance

**kilocalorie**   Equivalent to 1,000 calories

**kinesthetic learner**   Person who learns by processing information through touching, feeling, and doing

**kwashiorkor**   Condition resulting when there is a sudden or recent lack of protein-containing foods

**kyphosis**   Increased roundness of the thoracic spinal curve

---

### L

**lanugo**   Fine hair covering the fetus's body

**large for gestational age**   Infant's weight falls above the 90th percentile for gestational age

**late deceleration**   Reduction in fetal heart rate that begins after the uterus has begun contracting and increases to the baseline level after the uterine contraction has ceased

**learning**   Act or process of acquiring knowledge, skill, or both in a particular subject; process of assimilating knowledge resulting in behavior changes

**learning disability**   Heterogenous group of disorders manifested by significant difficulties in the acquisition and use of listening, speaking, reading, writing, reasoning, or mathematical abilities

**learning plateau**   Peak in the effectiveness of teaching and depth of learning

**learning style**   Individual preference for receiving, processing, and assimilating information about a particular subject

**lecithin**   Major component of surfactant

**Leopold's maneuvers**   Series of specific palpations of the pregnant uterus to determine fetal position and presentation

**let-down reflex**   Neurohormonal reflex that causes milk to be expressed from the alveoli into the lactiferous ducts

**leukocytosis**   Increased number of white blood cells

**leukopenia**   Decreased number of white blood cells

**licensure**   Mandatory system of granting licenses according to specified standards

**life review**   Form of reminiscence wherein a client attempts to come to terms with conflict or to gain meaning from life and die peacefully

**ligation**   Application of a band or tie around a structure

**lightening**   Descent of the fetus into the pelvis, causing the uterus to tip forward, relieving pressure on the diaphragm

**linea nigra**   Dark line on the abdomen from umbilicus to symphysis during the pregnancy

**lipid**   Organic compound that is insoluble in water but soluble in organic solvents such as ether and alcohol; also known as fats

**lipodystrophy**   Atrophy or hypertrophy of subcutaneous fat

**lipoma**   Benign tumor consisting of mature fat cells

**lipoprotein**   Blood lipid bound to protein

**liquefaction necrosis**   Death and subsequent change of tissue to a liquid or semi-liquid state; often descriptive of a primary tubercle

**listening**   Interpreting the sounds heard and attaching meaning to them

**litholapaxy**   Procedure involving crushing of a bladder stone and immediate washing out of the fragments through a catheter

**lithotripsy**   Method of crushing a calculus anyplace in the urinary system with ultrasonic waves

**liver mortis**   Bluish-purple discoloration of the skin that is a by-product of red blood cell destruction; it begins within 20 minutes of death

**living will**   Legal document that allows a person to state preferences about the use of life-sustaining measures should he or she be unable to make his or her wishes known

**local adaptation syndrome**   Physiologic response to a stressor (e.g., trauma, illness) affecting a specific part of the body

**localized infection**   Infection limited to a defined area or single organ

**lochia**   Uterine/vaginal discharge after childbirth; initially bright red, then changing to a pink or pinkish brown, then to a yellowish white

**locomotor**   Pertaining to movement or the ability to move

**long-term care facility**   Health care facility that provides services to individuals who are not acutely ill, have continuing health care needs, and cannot function independently at home

**long-term care managed care**   Care that refers to a spectrum of services provided to individuals who have an ongoing need for health care; traditionally a community-based nursing home licensed for skilled or intermediate care

**long-term goal**   Statement that profiles the desired resolution of the nursing diagnosis over a long period of time, usually weeks or months

**lordosis**   Exaggeration of the curvature of the lumbar spine

**loss**   Any situation, either potential, actual, or perceived, wherein a valued object or person is changed or is not accessible to the individual

**lumbar puncture**   Aspiration of cerebrospinal fluid from the subarachnoid space

**lung stretch receptor**   Receptor that monitors the patterns of breathing and prevents overexpansion of the lungs

**lymphokine**   Chemical substance released by sensitized lymphocytes (T cells) and that assists in antigen destruction

**lymphoma**   Tumor of the lymphatic system

## M

**macrosomia**   Excessive fetal growth characterized by a fetus weighing more than 4,000 g (8.8 lb.)

**magnetic resonance imaging**   Imaging technique that uses radiowaves and a strong magnetic field to make continuous cross-sectional images of the body

**maladaptive measure**   Measure used to avoid conflict or stress

**malignant**   Becoming progessively worse and often resulting in death

**malpractice**   Negligent acts on the part of a professional; relates to the conduct of a person who is acting in a professional capacity

**managed care**   A cost-saving system where a case management, individual, or team control what specialists the client sees, as well as the frequency or duration of that specialty care

**mania**   Extremely elevated mood with accompanying agitated behavior

**marasmus**   Condition resulting from severe malnutrition; afflicts very young children who lack both energy and protein foods as well as vitamins and minerals

**Maslow's hierarchy of needs**   Theory of behavioral motivation based on needs; includes physiologic, safety and security, love and belonging, self-esteem, and self-actualization needs

**mastication**   Chewing food into fine particles and mixing the food with enzymes in saliva

**mastitis**   Inflammation of the breast, generally during breastfeeding

**material principle of justice**   Rationale for determining those times when there can be unequal allocation of scarce resources

**matter**   Anything that occupies space and possesses mass

**maturation**   Process of becoming fully grown and developed; involves physiologic and behavioral aspects

**maturational loss**   Loss that occurs as a person moves from one developmental stage to another

**mechanism of labor**   Series of movements of the fetus as it passes through the pelvis and birth canal

**meconium**   Fecal material stored in the fetal intestines

**meconium ileus**   Impacted feces in the newborn, causing intestinal obstruction

**Medicaid**   Government title program (XIX) that pays for health services for people who are older, poor, or disabled, and for low-income families with dependent children

**medical asepsis**   Practices that reduce the number, growth, and spread of microorganisms

**medical diagnosis**   Clinical judgment by the physician that identifies or determines a specific disease, condition, or pathological state

**medical model**    Traditional approach to health care wherein the focus is on treatment and cure of disease not prevention

**Medicare**    Amendment (Title XVIII) to the Social Security Act that helps finance the health care of persons over 65 years old and younger persons who are permanently disabled to receive Social Security disability benefits

**Medigap insurance**    Insurance plan for persons with Medicare that pays for health care costs not covered by Medicare

**meditation**    An activity that brings the mind and spirit in focus on the present and provokes a sense of peace and relaxation

**melanin**    Pigment that gives skin its color

**melena**    Stool containing partially broken down blood usually black, sticky, and tar-like

**menarche**    Onset of the first menstrual period

**meningitis**    Inflammation of the meninges

**meningocele**    Saclike protrusion along the vertebral column filled with cerebrospinal fluid and meninges

**menopause**    Cessation of menstruation

**menorrhagia**    Excessively heavy menstrual flow

**mental disorder**    Clinically significant behavior or psychological syndrome or pattern that occurs in an individual and is associated with present distress or disability or with a significantly increased risk of suffering, death, pain, disability, or an important loss of freedom (APA, 1994)

**mental illness**    Condition wherein an individual has a distorted view of self, is unable to maintain satisfying personal relationships, and is unable to adapt to the environment

**mentation**    Ability to concentrate, remember, or think abstractly

**metabolic rate**    Rate of energy utilization in the body

**metabolism**    Sum total of all the biological and chemical processes in the body

**metastasis**    Spread of cancer cells to distant areas of the body by way of the lymph system or bloodstream

**metritis**    Inflammation of the uterus including the endometrium and parametrium

**metrorrhagia**    Vaginal bleeding between menstrual periods

**micturition**    Process of expelling urine from the urinary bladder; also called urination or voiding

**middle adulthood**    Development from the ages of 40 years to 65 years

**milia**    Pearly white cysts on the face

**minimum data set**    An assessment tool for assessing a resident's physical, psychological, and psychosocial functioning in a Medicare and Medicaid-certified long-term care facility

**minority group**    Group of people constituting less than a numerical majority of the population and are often labeled and treated differently from others in the society

**miscarriage**    Spontaneous abortion

**misdemeanor**    Offense that is less serious than a felony and may be punished by a fine or by sentence to a local prison for less than 1 year

**misuse**    Use of a legal substance for which it was not intended, or exceeding the recommended dosage of a drug

**mixed agonist-antagonist**    Compound that blocks opioid effects on one receptor type while producing opioid effects on a second receptor type

**mixture**    Substances combined in no specific way

**mnemonic**    Method to aid in association and recall; a memorable sentence created from the first letters of a list of items to be used to recall the items later

**mode of transmission**    Process of the infectious agent moving from the reservoir or source through the portal of exit to the portal of entry of the susceptible "new" host

**modulation**    Central nervous system pathway that selectively inhibits pain transmission by sending signals back down to the dorsal horn of the spinal cord

**molding**    Shaping of the fetal head to adapt to the mother's pelvis during labor

**molecule**    Atoms of the same element that unite with each other

**Mongolian spots**    Large patches of bluish skin on the buttocks of dark-skinned infants

**monounsaturated fatty acid**    Forms a glycerol ester with a double or triple bond; nuts, fowl, and olive oil

**mood**    Subjective report of the way an individual is feeling

**moral maturity**    Ability to decide for oneself what is "right"

**morbidity**    Illness

**mortality**    Death

**morula**    Mass of cells resembling a mulberry

**mourning**    Period during which grief is expressed and integration and resolution of the loss occur

**multigravida**    Condition of being pregnant two or more times

**multipara**    Condition of having delivered twice or more after 24 weeks' gestation

**myelomeningocele**    Saclike protrusion along the vertebral column that is filled with spinal fluid, meninges, nerve roots, and spinal cord

**myocardial infarction**    Necrosis (death) of the myocardium caused by an obstruction in a coronary artery; commonly known as heart attack

**myocarditis**    Inflammation of the myocardium of the heart

**myofascial pain syndrome** Group of muscle disorders characterized by pain, muscle spasm, tenderness, stiffness, and limited motion

**myopia** Nearsightedness

**myringotomy** Surgical incision of the eardrum

**myxedema** Severe hypothyroidism in adults

---

# N

**narcolepsy** Sleep alteration manifested as sudden uncontrollable urges to fall asleep during the daytime

**narrative charting** Chronological account written in paragraphs describes the client's status, the interventions and treatments, and the client's response to treatments

**necrosis** Tissue death as the result of disease or injury

**neglect** Situation wherein a basic need of the client is not being provided

**negligence** General term referring to careless acts on the part of an individual who is not exercising reasonable or prudent judgment

**neonatal stage** First 28 days of life following birth

**neonatal transition** First few hours after birth wherein the newborn makes changes to and stabilizes respiratory and circulatory functions

**neonate** Newborn from birth to 28 days of life

**neoplasm** Any abnormal growth of new tissue

**nephrotoxic** Quality of a substance that causes kidney tissue damage

**nerve agents** Powerful acetylcholinesterase inhibitors that alter cholinergic synaptic transmission at neuroeffector junctions, at skeletal myoneural junctions and autonomic ganglia, and in the central nervous system

**nesting** Surge of energy late in pregnancy when the pregnant woman organizes and cleans the house

**neuralgia** Paroxysmal pain that extends along the course of one or more nerves

**neurogenic shock** Hypotensive situation resulting from the loss of sympathetic control of vital functions from the brain

**neuropeptide** Amino acid produced in the brain and other sites in the body that acts as a chemical communicator

**neurotransmitter** Chemical substance produced by the body that facilitates or inhibits nerve-impulse transmission

**neutral thermal environment** Environment in which the newborn can maintain internal body temperature with minimal oxygen consumption and metabolism

**nevi** Pigmented areas in the skin; commonly known as birthmarks or moles

**nevus flammeus** Large, reddish-purple birthmark usually found on the face or neck and does not blanch with pressure

**nevus vascularis** Birthmark of enlarged superficial blood vessels, elevated and red in color

**nociceptor** Receptive neuron for painful sensations

**nocturia** Awakening at night to void

**nocturnal enuresis** Incontinence that occurs during sleep

**noninvasive** Descriptor for procedure wherein the body is not entered with any type of instrument

**nonmaleficence** Ethical principle based on the obligation to cause no harm to others

**nonshivering thermogenesis** Metabolism of brown fat; process unique to the newborn

**nonverbal communication** Body language or a method of sending a message without words

**nosocomial infection** Infection acquired in the hospital or other health care facility that was not present or incubating at the time of the client's admission

**noxious stimulus** Underlying pathology that causes pain

**nuchal cord** Condition of the umbilical cord being wrapped around the baby's neck

**nuchal rigidity** Pain and rigidity in the neck

**nulligravida** Condition of never having been pregnant

**nullipara** Condition of never having delivered an infant after 24 weeks' gestation

**nursing** The art and science of assisting individuals in learning to care for themselves whenever possible and of caring for them when they are unable to meet their own needs

**nursing audit** Method of evaluating the quality of care provided to clients

**nursing care plan** Written guide of strategies to be implemented to help the client achieve optimal health

**nursing diagnosis** Second step in the nursing process; a clinical judgment about individual, family, or community (aggregate) responses to actual or potential health problems/life processes

**nursing intervention** Action performed by a nurse that helps the client achieve the results specified by the goals and expected outcomes

**nursing interventions classification** Standardized language for nursing interventions

**nursing minimum data set** Elements that should be in clinical records and abstracted for studies on the effectiveness and costs of nursing care

**nursing outcomes classification** Standardized language for nursing outcomes

**nursing practice act** Statute that is enacted by the legislature of a state and that outlines the scope of nursing practice in that state

**nursing process**   Systematic method for providing care to clients, consisting of five steps: assessment, diagnosis, outcome identification and planning, implementation, and evaluation

**nutrition**   All of the processes (ingestion, digestion, absorption, metabolism, and elimination) involved in consuming and using food for energy, maintenance, and growth

**nystagmus**   Constant, involuntary movement of the eye in various directions

---

## O

**obesity**   Weight that is 20% or more above the ideal body weight

**objective data**   Observable and measurable data that are obtained through standard assessment techniques performed during the physical examination and through laboratory and diagnostic tests

**occult blood**   Blood in the stool that can be detected only through a microscope or by chemical means

**occult blood test (guaiac)**   Test for microscopic blood done on stool

**older adulthood**   Development occurring from age 65 years until death

**oligomenorrhea**   Decreased menstrual flow

**oliguria**   Diminished production of urine

**oncology**   Study of tumors

**ongoing assessment**   Type of assessment that includes systematic monitoring of specific problems

**ongoing planning**   Updates the client's plan of care

**onset of action**   Time for the body to respond to a drug after administration

**oophoritis**   Inflammation of the ovary

**open reduction**   Surgical procedure that enables the surgeon to reduce (repair) a fracture under direct visualization

**ophthalmia neonatorum**   Inflammation of a newborn's eyes that results from passing through the birth canal when a gonorrheal or chlamydial infection is present

**opinion**   Subjective belief

**opisthotonos**   Complete arching of the body with only the head and feet on the bed

**opportunistic infection**   Infection in persons with a defective immune system that rarely causes harm in healthy individuals

**oppression**   Condition wherein the rules, values, and ideals of one group are imposed on another group

**orchiectomy**   Removal of a testis

**orientation**   Person's awareness of self in relation to person, place, time, and in some cases, situation

**orthopedics (orthopaedics)**   Branch of medicine that deals with the prevention or correction of the disorders and diseases of the musculoskeletal system

**orthopnea**   Difficulty breathing while lying down

**orthostatic hypotension**   Significant decrease in blood pressure that results when a person moves from a lying or sitting (supine) position to a standing position

**osmolality**   Measurement of the total concentration of dissolved particles (solutes) per kilogram of water

**osmolarity**   Concentration of solutes per liter of cellular fluid

**osmosis**   Movement of a solvent, usually water, through a semipermeable membrane, from a region of higher concentration to a region of lower concentration

**osmotic pressure**   Pressure exerted against the cell membrane by the water inside a cell

**osteoporosis**   Increase in the porosity of bone

**Outcomes and Assessment Information Set**   An outcomes measurable tool developed and implemented to determine the care given and reimbursement required; Outcomes and Assessment Information Set (OASIS) data is reported to the Centers for Medicare and Medicaid Services (CMS)

**overflow incontinence**   Leaking of urine when the bladder becomes very full and distended

**oxidation**   Chemical process of combining with oxygen

**oxidized**   Joined with oxygen

---

## P

**pain**   Unpleasant sensory and emotional experience associated with actual or potential tissue damage or described in terms of such

**pain threshold**   Level of intensity at which pain becomes appreciable or perceptible

**pain tolerance**   Level of intensity or duration of pain that a person is willing to endure

**palliative care**   Care that relieves symptoms, such as pain, but does not alter the course of disease

**pallor**   Abnormal paleness of the skin, seen especially in the face, conjunctiva, nail beds, and oral mucous membranes

**palpation**   Physical examination technique that uses the sense of touch to assess texture, temperature, moisture, organ location and size, vibrations and pulsations, swelling, masses, and tenderness

**pancreatitis**   Acute or chronic inflammation of the pancreas

**Papanicolaou test**   Smear method of examining stained exfoliative cells

**paracentesis**   Aspiration of fluid from the abdominal cavity

**paradoxical reaction**   Opposite effect of that which would normally be expected

**paramedic**   Specialized health care professional trained to provide advanced life support to the client requiring emergency interventions

**paraplegia**    Paralysis of lower extremities

**parasomnia**    Disorders that intrude on sleep in very active ways

**parenteral**    Any route other than the oral-gastrointestinal tract

**parenteral nutrition**    Feeding method whereby nutrients bypass the small intestine and enter the blood directly

**paresthesia**    Abnormal sensation such as burning, prickling, or tingling

**paroxysmal**    Descriptor for a symptom that begins and ends abruptly

**paroxysmal nocturnal dyspnea**    Condition of suddenly awakening, sweating, and having difficulty breathing

**passive euthanasia**    Process of working with the client's dying process

**patency**    Being freely opened

**pathogen**    Microorganism that causes disease

**pathogenicity**    Ability of a microorganism to produce disease

**patient-controlled analgesia**    Device that allows the client to control the delivery of intravenous or subcutaneous pain medication in a safe, effective manner through a programmable pump

**peak plasma level**    Highest blood concentration of a single dose of a drug until the elimination rate equals the rate of absorption

**peer assistance program**    Rehabilitation program that provides an impaired nurse with referrals, professional and peer counseling support groups, and assistance and monitoring back into nursing

**peptic ulcer**    Erosion formed in the esophagus, stomach, or duodenum resulting from acid/pepsin imbalance

**perception**    Ability to experience, recognize, organize, and interpret sensory stimuli

**percussion**    Physical examination technique that uses short, tapping strokes on the surface of the skin to create vibrations of underlying organs

**perfectionism**    Overwhelming expectation of being able to get everything done in a flawless manner

**perfusion**    Blood flow through an organ or body part

**pericardial friction rub**    Short, high-pitched squeak heard as two inflamed pericardial surfaces rub together

**pericardiocentesis**    Removal of fluid from the pericardial sac

**pericarditis**    Inflammation of the membrane sac surrounding the heart

**perineal care**    Cleansing of the external genitalia, perineum, and the surrounding area

**perioperative**    Period of time encompassing the preoperative, intraoperative, and postoperative phases of surgery

**peripheral nervous system**    System of the cranial nerves, spinal nerves, and the autonomic nervous system

**peripheral resistance**    Pressure within a vessel that resists the flow of blood such as plaque buildup or vasoconstriction

**peristalsis**    Rhythmic, coordinated, serial contraction of the smooth muscles of the gastrointestinal tract

**peritonitis**    Inflammation of the peritoneum, the membranous covering of the abdomen

**permeability**    Ability of a membrane to permit substances to pass through it

**petechiae**    Pinpoint hemorrhagic spots on the skin

**phantom limb pain**    Neuropathic pain that occurs after amputation with pain sensations referred to an area in the missing portion of the limb

**pharmacokinetics**    Study of the absorption, distribution, metabolism, and excretion of drugs to determine the relationship between the dose of a drug and the drug's concentration in biological fluids

**phimosis**    Condition wherein the opening in the foreskin is so small that it cannot be pulled back over the glans

**phlebitis**    Inflammation in the wall of a vein without clot formation

**phlebothrombosis**    Formation of a clot because of blood pooling in the vessel, trauma to the vessel's endothelial lining, or a coagulation problem with little or no inflammation in the vessel

**phlebotomist**    Individual who performs venipuncture

**phlebotomy**    Removal of blood from a vein

**phospholipid**    Lipid composed of glycerol, fatty acids, and phosphorus; the structural component of cells

**physical agent**    Factor in the environment capable of causing disease in a host

**physical restraint**    Equipment that reduces the client's movement

**physical wellness**    Healthy body that functions at an optimal level

**physically aggressive**    Descriptor of an individual who threatens or actually harms someone

**physiologic anemia of pregnancy**    Condition of having delivered after 24 weeks' gestation, whether infant is born alive or dead or number of infants born

**phytochemical**    Physiologically active compound present in plants in very small amounts that gives plants flavor, odor, and color

**pica**    Practice of eating substances not considered edible and that have no nutritive value, such as laundry starch, dirt, clay, and freezer frost

**pie charting**    Documentation method using the problem, intervention, evaluation (PIE) format

**piggyback**    Addition of an intravenous solution to infuse concurrently with another infusion

**placenta**   Membranous vascular organ connecting the fetus to the mother, which produces hormones to sustain a pregnancy, supplies the fetus with oxygena and food, and transports waste products out of the fetal system

**placenta previa**   Condition in which the placenta forms over or very near the internal cervical os

**plague**   An infectious disease transmitted by a bite of a flea from a rodent (usually a rat) infected with the bacillus Yersinia pestis; plague is a potential agent of bioterrorism

**planning**   Third step of the nursing process; includes both the establishing of guidelines for the proposed course of nursing action to resolve the nursing diagnoses and developing the client's plan of care

**plateau**   Level at which a drug's blood concentration is maintained

**pleural effusion**   Collection of fluid within the pleural cavity

**pleural friction rub**   Abnormal breath sound that is creaky and grating in nature and is heard on inspiration and expiration

**pleurisy**   Condition arising from inflammation of the pleura, or sac, that encases the lung

**pneumonia**   Inflammation of the bronchioles and alveoli accompanied by consolidation, or solidification of exudate, in the lungs

**pneumothorax**   Condition wherein air or gas accumulates in the pleural space of the lungs, causing the lungs to collapse

**point-of-care charting**   Documentation system that allows health care providers to gain immediate access to client information at the bedside

**poison**   Any substance that when taken into the body interferes with normal physiologic functioning; may be inhaled, injected, ingested, or absorbed by the body

**polydipsia**   Excessive thirst

**polymenorrhea**   Menstrual periods that are abnormally frequent, generally less than every 21 days

**polyp**   Abnormal growth of tissue

**polyphagia**   Increased hunger

**polypharmacy**   Problem of clients taking numerous prescription and over-the-counter medications for the same or various disease processes, with unknown consequences from the resulting combinations of chemical compounds and cumulative side-effects

**polyunsaturated fatty acid**   Forms a glycerol ester with many carbons unbonded to hydrogen atoms; fish, corn, sunflower seeds, soybeans, cotton seeds, and safflower oil

**polyuria**   Increased urination

**Port-a-Cath**   Port that has been implanted under the skin with a catheter inserted into the superior vena cava or right atrium through the subclavian or internal jugular vein

**portal of entry**   Route by which an infectious agent enters the host

**portal of exit**   Route by which an infectious agent leaves the reservoir

**postictal**   After a seizure

**post-mortem care**   Care given immediately after death before the body is moved to the mortuary

**postoperative phase**   Time during the surgical experience that begins at the end of the surgical procedure and ends when the client is discharged, not just from the hospital or institution, but from medical care by the surgeon

**postpartum blues**   Mild transient condition of emotional lability and crying for no apparent reason, which affects up to 80% of women who have just given birth, and lasts about 2 weeks

**postpartum depression**   Condition similar to postpartum blues but is more serious, intense, and persistent

**postpartum hemorrhage**   Blood loss of more than 500 mL after the third stage of labor or 1,000 mL following a cesarean birth

**postpartum psychosis**   Condition more severe than postpartum depression and characterized by delusions and thoughts of self-harm or infant harm

**postprandial**   After eating

**postterm**   Delivery after 42 weeks' gestation

**post-void residual**   Urine that remains in the bladder after urination

**prayer**   A type of communication between an individual and spiritual entities

**preadolescence**   Development from the ages of approximately 10 years to 12 years

**precipitate birth**   Birth occurring suddenly and unexpectantly without a CNM/physician present to assist

**precipitate labor**   Labor lasting less than 3 hours from the onset of contractions to the birth of the infant

**preeclampsia**   Phase of pregnancy-induced hypertension prior to convulsions

**preferred provider organization**   Type of managed care model wherein member choice is limited to providers within the system for full reimbursement and other providers for less reimbursement

**prenatal care**   Care of a woman during pregnancy, before labor

**prenatal stage**   Development beginning with conception and ending with birth

**preoperative phase**   Time during the surgical experience that begins when the client decides to have surgery and ends when the client is transferred to the operating table

**presbycusis**   Sensorineural hearing loss associated with aging

**presbyopia**   Inability of the lens of the eye to change curvature to focus near objects

**preschool stage**   Development from the ages of 3 years to 6 years

**prescriptive authority**   Legal recognition of the ability to prescribe medications

**presenting part**   Part of the fetus in contact with the cervix

**pressured speech**   Rapid, intense style of speech

**preterm**   Delivery after 24 weeks' gestation but before 38 weeks (full term)

**preterm birth**   Birth that takes place before the end of the 37th week of gestation

**preterm labor**   Onset of regular contractions of the uterus that cause cervical changes between 20 and 37 weeks' gestation

**prevention**   Obstructing, thwarting, or hindering a disease or illness

**priapism**   Prolonged erection that does not occur in response to sexual stimulation

**primary care provider**   Health care provider whom a client sees first for health care, typically a family practitioner (physician/nurse), internist, or pediatrician

**primary health care**   Client's point of entry into the health care system; includes assessment, diagnosis, treatment, coordination of care, education, prevention services, and surveillance

**primary hypertension**   High blood pressure, the cause of which is unknown; also known as essential hypertension

**primary prevention**   All practices designed to keep health problems from developing

**primary source**   Major provider of information about a client

**primary tubercle**   Nodule that contains tubercle bacilli and forms within lung tissue

**primigravida**   Condition of being pregnant for the first time

**primipara**   Condition of having delivered once after 24 weeks' gestation

**privacy**   The right to be left alone, to choose care based on personal beliefs, to govern body integrity, and to choose when and how sensitive information is shared (Badzek & Gross, 1999)

**problem-oriented medical record** Documentation method employs a structured, logical format and focuses on the client's problem

**process**   Series of steps or acts that leads to accomplishing some goal or purpose

**procrastination**   Intentionally putting off or delaying something that should be done

**prodromal stage**   Time interval from the onset of nonspecific symptoms until specific symptoms of the infectious process begin to manifest

**professional boundaries**   Limits of the professional relationship that allow for a safe, therapeutic connection between the professional and the client

**progressive muscle relaxation**   Stress-management strategy in which muscles are alternately tensed and relaxed

**projectile vomiting**   Forceful ejection (up to 3 feet) of the contents of the stomach

**prolapsed cord**   Condition in which the umbilical cord lies below the presenting part of the fetus

**prolapsed uterus**   Downward displacement of the uterus into the vagina

**prospective payment**   Predetermined rate paid for each episode of hospitalization based on the client's age and principal diagnosis and the presence or absence of surgery or comorbidity

**protocol**   Series of standing orders or procedures that should be followed under certain specific conditions

**proxemics**   Study of the space between people and its effect on interpersonal behavior

**pruritus**   Severe itching

**pseudocyesis**   False pregnancy

**pseudomenstruation**   Blood-tinged mucus discharge from the vagina of a newborn caused by the withdrawal of maternal hormones

**psychoanalysis**   Therapy focused on uncovering unconscious memories and processes

**psychological wellness**   Enjoyment of creativity, satisfaction of the basic need to love and be loved, understanding of emotions, and ability to maintain control over emotions

**psychomotor domain**   Area of learning that involves performance of motor skills

**psychoneuroimmunology**   Study of the complex relationship among the physical, cognitive, and affective aspects of humans

**psychoprophylaxis**   Mental and physical preparation for childbirth; synonymous with Lamaze

**psychosis**   State wherein an individual has lost the ability to recognize reality

**psychotherapy**   Treatment of mental and emotional disorders through psychological rather than physical methods

**ptosis**   Drooping upper eyelid

**puberty**   Emergence of secondary sex characteristics that signal the beginning of adolescence

**public law**   Law that deals with an individual's relationship to the state

**public self**   What the client thinks others think of him or her

**pudendal block**   Injection of a local anesthetic into the pudendal nerve to provide perineal, external genitalia, and lower vaginal anesthesia

**puerperal (postpartum) infection**    Infection following childbirth occurring between the birth and 6 weeks postpartum

**puerperium**    Term for the first 6 weeks after the birth of an infant

**pulse amplitude**    Measurement of the strength or force exerted by the ejected blood against the arterial wall with each heart contraction

**pulse deficit**    Condition in which the apical pulse rate is greater than the radial pulse rate

**pulse rate**    Indirect measurement of cardiac output obtained by counting the number of peripheral pulse waves over a pulse point

**pulse rhythm**    Regularity of the heartbeat

**purpura**    Reddish-purple patches on the skin indicative of hemorrhage

**purulent exudate**    Discharge resulting from infection; also called pus

**pyelonephritis**    Bacteral infection of the renal pelvis, tubules, and interstitial tissue of one or both kidneys

**pyorrhea**    Periodontal disease

**pyuria**    Pus in the urine

---

# Q

**quadriplegia**    Dysfunction or paralysis of both arms, both legs, and bowel and bladder

**quickening**    Descriptor for when the mother first feels the fetus move, about 16 to 20 weeks' gestation

---

# R

**race**    A group of people with biological similarities

**radiation**    Loss of heat by transfer to cooler near objects, but not through direct contact

**radiation sickness**    An abnormal condition resulting from exposure to ionizing radiation, either purposefully or by accident

**radiography**    Study of x-rays or gamma-ray-exposed film through the action of ionizing radiation

**radiotherapy**    Treatment of cancer with high-energy radiation

**rapport**    Mutual trust established between two people

**readiness for learning**    Evidence of willingness to learn

**real self**    How the individual really thinks about him- or herself

**reasoning**    Use of the elements of thought to solve a problem or settle a question

**reconstructive**    To rebuild or reestablish

**rectocele**    Anterior displacement of the rectum into the posterior vaginal wall

**recurrent acute pain**    Identified by repetitive painful episodes that recur over a prolonged period or throughout a client's lifetime

**referred pain**    Discomfort from the internal organs that is felt in another area of the body

**reframing**    Technique of monitoring negative thoughts and replacing them with positive ones

**regional anesthesia**    Method of temporarily rendering a region of the body insensible to pain

**rehabilitation**    Process or therapy designed to assist individuals to reach their optimal level of physical, mental, and psychosocial functioning

**relapse**    Return to a previous behavior or condition

**relaxation technique**    Method used to decrease anxiety and muscle tension

**religion**    A system of organized beliefs, rituals, and practices with which a person identifies and wishes to be associated

**religious support system**    Group of ministers, priests, nuns, rabbis, shamans, mullahs, or laypersons who are able to meet clients' spiritual needs

**REM movement disorder**    Condition wherein the normal paralysis of REM sleep is absent or incomplete and the sleeper acts out the dream

**remission**    Decrease or absence of symptoms of a disease

**renal colic**    Severe pain in the kidney that radiates to the groin

**repolarization**    Recovery phase of the cardiac muscle

**reportable conditions**    Diseases or injuries that the government requires be reported to the appropriate authority or agency; include suspected abuse and/or neglect, sexually transmitted diseases (STDs), and certain other contagious illnesses that could threaten the health of the general public

**reservoir**    Place where the agent can survive

**resident flora**    Microorganisms that are always present, usually without altering the client's health

**residual urine**    Urine remaining in the bladder after the individual has urinated

**respect**    Acceptance of an individual as is and in a nonjudgmental manner

**respiration**    Process of exchanging oxygen and carbon dioxide

**respite care**    Care and service that provides a break to caregivers and is used for a few hours a week, for an occasional weekend, or for longer periods of time

**rest**    State of mental and physical relaxation and calmness

**restitution**    Rotation of the fetal head back to normal alignment with the shoulders after delivery of the fetal head

**restless leg syndrome**    Condition characterized by uncomfortable sensations of tingling or crawling in the muscles, and twitching, burning, prickling, or deep aching in the foot, calf, or upper leg when at rest

**restraint** Protective device used to limit the physical activity of a client or to immobilize a client or extremity

**resuscitation** Support measures implemented to restore consciousness and life

**reticulocyte** Immature red blood cell

**retroperitoneal** Behind the peritoneum outside the peritoneal cavity

**reverse isolation** Barrier protection designed to prevent infection in clients who are severely compromised and highly susceptible to infection; also known as protective isolation

**reverse tolerance** Phenomenon whereby a smaller amount of substance will elicit the desired psychic effects

**review of systems** Brief account of any recent signs or symptoms related to any body system

**rhinorrhea** Watery nasal discharge

**Ricin** A poison made from the waste products of castor bean processing; a potential agent of bioterrorism because of its ease of dissemination

**rigor mortis** Natural stiffening of muscles after death; begins about 4 hours after death

**risk nursing diagnosis** Nursing diagnosis indicating that a problem does not yet exist but that specific risk factors are present; composed of "Risk for" followed by the diagnostic label and a list of the risk factors

**role** An ascribed or assumed expected behavior in a social position or group

**role performance** Specific behaviors a person exhibits within each role

**rooming-in** Practice of staying with the client 24 hours a day to provide care and comfort

## S

**salpingitis** Inflammation of the fallopian tube

**salt** Product formed when an acid and a base react with each other

**sanguineous** Bloody drainage from a wound or surgical drain

**sarcoma** Cancer occurring in connective tissue

**Sarin** A dangerous man-made nerve agent, first developed as an insecticide that is a potential agent for bioterrorism

**satiety** Feeling of adequate fullness from food

**school-age stage** Development from the ages of 6 years to 10 years

**sclerotherapy** Treatment that involves injecting a chemical into the vein, causing the vein to become sclerosed (hardened) so blood no longer flows through it

**sclerotic** Hardened tissue

**scoliosis** Lateral curvature of the spine

**scrub nurse** RN, LP/VN, or surgical technologist who provides services under the direction of the circulating nurse and who is qualified by training or experience to prepare and maintain the integrity, safety, and efficiency of the sterile field throughout an operation

**sebaceous cyst** Sebaceous gland filled with sebum

**sebum** Oily substance secreted by the sebaceous glands of the skin

**secondary care** Care focused on diagnosis and treatment after the client exhibits symptoms of illness

**secondary hypertension** High blood pressure occurring as a sequel to a pre-existing disease or injury

**secondary prevention** Early detection, screening, diagnosis, and intervention, to reduce the consequences of a health problem

**sedation** Reduction of stress, excitement, or irritability via some central nervous system depression

**self-awareness** Consciously knowing how the self thinks, feels, believes, and behaves at any specific time

**self-care deficit** State wherein an individual is not able to perform one or more activities of daily living

**self-concept** Individual's perception of self; includes self-esteem, body image, and ideal self

**self-efficacy** Belief in one's ability to succeed in attempts to change behavior

**self-esteem** A personal opinion of oneself

**semipermeable membrane** Membrane that allows passage of only certain substances

**sensation** Ability to receive and process stimuli received through the sensory organs

**sensible water loss** Water loss of which the person is aware

**sensitivity** Susceptibility of a pathogen to an antibiotic

**sensorineural hearing loss** Condition in which the inner ear or cochlear portion of cranial nerve VIII is abnormal or diseased

**sensory deficit** Change in the perception of sensory stimuli; can affect any of the senses

**sensory deprivation** State of reduced sensory input from the internal or external environment, manifested by alterations in sensory perception

**sensory overload** State of excessive and sustained multisensory stimulation manifested by behavior change and perceptual distortion

**sensory perception** Ability to receive sensory impressions and, through cortical association, relate the stimuli to past experiences and form an impression of the nature of the stimulus

**seroconversion** Evidence of antibody formation in response to disease or vaccine

**serosanguineous exudate** Discharge that is clear with some blood tinge; seen with surgical incisions

**serous exudate** Discharge composed primarily of serum; is watery in appearance and has a low protein level.

**serum lithium level**   Laboratory test done to determine whether the client's lithium level is within a therapeutic range

**shaman**   Folk healer-priest who uses natural and supernatural forces to help others

**shearing**   Force exerted against the skin by movement or repositioning

**shift report**   Report about each client between shifts

**shock**   Condition of profound hemodynamic and metabolic disturbance characterized by inadequate tissue perfusion and inadequate circulation to the vital organs

**shroud**   Covering for the body after death

**sibilant wheeze**   Abnormal breath sound that is high pitched and musical in nature and is heard on inhalation and exhalation

**sickle**   When red blood cells become crescent-shaped and elongated

**single point of entry**   Common feature of HMOs wherein the client is required to enter the health care system through a point designated by the plan

**single-payer system**   Health care delivery model wherein the government is the only entity to reimburse health care costs

**situational loss**   Loss that takes place in response to external events generally beyond the individual's control

**slander**   Words that are communicated verbally to a third party and that harm or injure the personal or professional reputation of another

**sleep**   State of altered consciousness during which a person has minimal physical activity, changes in levels of consciousness, and a slowing of physiologic processes

**sleep apnea**   A period during sleep of not breathing; often associated with heavy snoring

**sleep cycle**   Sequence of sleep beginning with the four stages of NREM sleep, a return to stage 3 and then stage 2 (first phase), followed by the first REM sleep (second phase)

**sleep deprivation**   Prolonged inadequate quality and quantity of sleep

**small for gestational age**   Infant's weight falls below the 10th percentile for gestational age

**smallpox (variola)**   A highly contagious and frequently fatal viral disease, which is a potential agent for a bioterroristic attack; there are two varieties, known as variola major and variola minor

**Snellen Chart**   Chart containing various-sized letters with standardized numbers at the end of each line of letters

**sociocultural wellness**   Ability to appreciate the needs of others and to care about one's environment and the inhabitants of it

**somatic nervous system**   Nerves that connect the central nervous system to the skin and skeletal muscles and control conscious activities

**somatic pain**   Nonlocalized discomfort originating in tendons, ligaments, and nerves

**somnambulism**   Sleepwalking

**Somogyi phenomenon**   In response to hypoglycemia, the release of glucose-elevating hormones (epinephrine, cortisol, glucose), which produces a hyperglycemic state

**sonorous wheeze**   Abnormal breath sound that is low pitched and snoring in nature and is louder on expiration

**spermatogenesis**   Production of sperm

**spina bifida occulta**   Failure of the vertebral arch to close

**spinal shock**   Cessation of motor, sensory, autonomic, and reflex impulses below the level of injury; characterized by flaccid paralysis of all skeletal muscles, loss of spinal reflexes, loss of sensation, and absence of autonomic function below the level of injury

**spiritual care**   Recognition of and assistance toward meeting spiritual needs

**spiritual distress**   A client in this situation may have a troubled, fragmented, or possibly disintegrating spirit

**spiritual needs**   Individual's desire to find purpose and meaning in life, pain, and death

**spiritual wellness**   Inner strength and peace

**spirituality**   The core of a person's being, a higher experience or transcendence of oneself

**spore**   Bacteria in a resistant stage that can withstand unfavorable environments

**sprain**   Injury to ligaments surrounding a joint caused by a sudden twist, wrench, or fall

**stable**   Alert with vital signs within the client's normal range

**staff development**   Delivery of instruction to assist nurses achieve the goals of the employer

**standard**   Level or degree of quality

**Standard Precautions**   Preventive practices to be used in the care of all clients in hospitals regardless of their diagnosis or presumed infection status

**standards of practice**   Guidelines established to direct nursing care

**startle response**   Overreaction to minor sounds or noises

**stasis dermatitis**   Inflammation of the skin due to decreased circulation

**station**   Relationship of the fetal presenting part to the ischial spines

**status asthmaticus**   Persistent, intractable asthma attack

**status epilepticus**   Acute, prolonged episode of seizure activity that lasts at least 30 minutes and may or may not involve loss of consciousness

**statutory law**   Law enacted by legislative bodies

**steatorrhea**   Fatty stool

**stent** Tiny metal tube with holes in it that prevents a vessel from collapsing and keeps the atherosclerotic plaque pressed against the vessel wall; any material used to hold tissue in place or provide support

**stereognosis** Ability to recognize an object by feel

**stereotyping** Belief that all people within the same ethnic, racial, or cultural group act the same way, sharing the same beliefs and attitudes

**sterile** Without microorganisms

**sterile conscience** Individual's personal sense of honesty and integrity with regard to adherence to the principles of aseptic technique, including prompt admission and correction of any errors and omissions

**sterile field** Area surrounding the client and the surgical site that is free from all microorganisms; created by draping of the work area and the client with sterile drape

**sterilization** Destroying all microorganisms, including spores

**stock supply** Medications dispensed and labeled in large quantities for storage in the medication room or nursing unit

**stoma** Surgical opening between a cavity and the surface of the body

**stomatitis** Inflammation of the oral mucosa

**strabismus** Inability of the eyes to focus in the same direction

**strain** Injury to a muscle or tendon due to overuse or overstretching

**stress** Nonspecific response to any demand made on the body (Selye, 1974)

**stress incontinence** Leakage of urine when a person does anything that strains the abdomen, such as coughing, laughing, jogging, dancing, sneezing, lifting, making a quick movement, or even walking

**stress test** Measure of a client's cardiovascular response to exercise

**stressor** Any situation, event, or agent that produces stress

**striae gravidarum** Reddish streaks frequently found on the abdomen, thighs, buttocks, and breasts; also called "stretch marks"

**stridor** High-pitched, harsh sound heard on inspiration when the trachea or larynx is obstructed

**stroke volume** Volume of blood pumped by the ventricle with each contraction

**stye** Pustular inflammation of an eyelash follicle or sebaceous gland on the eyelid margin

**subacute care** Short-term, aggressive care for clients who are out of the acute stage of illness but who still require skilled nursing, monitoring, and ongoing treatment

**subcutaneous** Injection into the subcutaneous tissue

**subinvolution** Incomplete return of the uterus to its prepregnant size and consistency

**subluxation** Partial separation of an articular surface

**substance** A drug, legal or illegal, that may cause physical or mental impairment

**suicidal ideations** Thoughts of hurting or killing oneself

**supine hypotensive syndrome** Lowering of blood pressure in a pregnant woman when lying supine due to compression of the vena cava by the enlarged, heavy uterus

**surfactant** Phospholipids that are present in the lungs and lower surface tension to prevent collapse of the airways

**surgery** Treatment of injury, disease, or deformity through invasive operative methods

**suture** Thin, fibrous, membrane-covered space between skull bones

**synarthrosis** Immovable joint

**syndactyly** Fusion of two or more fingers or toes

**synergism** Result of two or more agents working together to achieve a greater effect than either could produce alone

**synthesiasis** Hearing colors and seeing sounds

**synthesis** Chemical reaction when two or more atoms, called reactants, bond and form a more complex molecular product; putting data together in a new way

## T

**tachycardia** Heart rate in excess of 100 beats per minute in an adult

**tachypnea** Respiratory rate greater than 24 beats per minute

**talipes equinovarus** A congenital deformity in which the foot and ankle are twisted inward and cannot be moved to a midline position; also known as clubfoot

**teaching** Active process wherein one individual shares information with another as a means to facilitate learning and thereby promote behavioral changes

**teaching strategy** Technique to promote learning

**teaching–learning process** Planned interaction that promotes a behavioral change that is not a result of maturation or coincidence

**telangiectasic nevi** Birthmarks of dilated capillaries that blanch with pressure; also called stork-bites

**telangiestasia** Permanent dilation of groups of superficial capillaries and venules; commonly known as "spider veins"

**telehealth** An electronic information services that offer increased client and family participation; for example, nurse and client use interactive videos, telephone cardiac rate monitoring with EKG readout, digital subscriber lines, and Internet transmission of data

**telemedicine**   An element of telehealth permitting physicians to provide care through a telecommunication system

**teleology**   Ethical theory that states that the value of a situation is determined by its consequences

**tenesmus**   Spasmodic contradiction of the anal or bladder sphincter, causing pain and a persistent urge to empty the bowel or bladder

**teratogen**   Agent such as radiation, drugs, viruses, and other microorganisms capable of causing abnormal fetal development

**teratogenic**   Causing abnormal development of the embryo

**teratogenic substance**   Substance that crosses the placenta and impairs normal growth and development

**term**   Descriptor for a pregnancy between 38 and 42 weeks' gestation

**terrorism**   Instilling fear in large groups of persons by using any product, weapon, or the threat of using a harmful act or substance to kill or injure people

**tertiary care**   Care focused on restoring the client to the state of health that existed before the development of an illness; if unattainable, then care is directed to attaining the optimal level of health possible

**tertiary prevention**   Treatment of an illness or disease after symptoms have appeared, so as to prevent further progression

**tetany**   Sharp flexion of the wrist and ankle joints, involving muscle twitching or cramps

**therapeutic communication**   Communication that is purposeful and goal directed, creating a beneficial outcome for the client

**therapeutic massage**   Application of hand pressure and motion to improve the recipient's well-being

**therapeutic procedure accident**   Accident that occurs during the delivery of medical or nursing interventions

**therapeutic touch**   Technique of assessing alterations in a person's energy fields and using the hands to direct energy to achieve a balanced state

**thermogenesis**   Production of heat

**thermoregulation**   Maintenance of body temperature

**thoracentesis**   Aspiration of fluid from the pleural cavity

**thrombocytopenia**   Decrease in the number of platelets in the blood

**thrombophlebitis**   Formation of a clot due to an inflammation in the wall of the vessel

**thrombosis**   Formation of a clot due to an inflammation in the wall of the vessel

**thrombus**   Formed clot that remains at the site where it formed

**time management**   System to help meet goals through problem solving

**tinnitus**   Ringing sound in the ear

**tocolysis**   Process of stopping labor with medications

**tocolytic agent**   Medication that inhibits uterine contractions

**toddler stage**   Development begins at approximately 12 to 18 months of age, when a child begins to walk, and ends at approximately 3 years of age

**tolerance**   Decreased sensitivity to subsequent doses of the same substance; an increased dose of the substance is needed to produce the same desired effect

**tophi**   Subcutaneous nodules of sodium urate crystals

**tort**   Civil wrong committed by a person against another person or property

**tort law**   Enforcement of duties and rights among individuals and independent of contractual agreements

**touch**   Means of perceiving or experiencing through tactile sensation

**toxic effect**   Reaction that occurs when the body cannot metabolize a drug and the drug accumulates in the blood

**trade (brand) name**   Name assigned to a drug by the pharmaceutical company; always capitalized

**transcendence**   A state of being or existence above and beyond the limits of material experience

**transcutaneous electrical nerve stimulation**   Process of applying a low-voltage electrical current to the skin through cutaneous electrodes

**transducer**   Instrument that converts electrical energy to sound waves

**transduction**   Noxious stimulus that triggers electrical activity in the endings of afferent nerve fibers (nociceptors)

**transmission**   Process whereby the pain impulse travels from the receiving nociceptors to the spinal cord

**Transmission-based Precautions**   Practices designed for clients documented as, or suspected of, being infected with highly transmissible or epidemiologically important pathogens for which additional precautions beyond Standard Precautions are required to interrupt transmission in hospitals

**trauma**   Wound or injury

**traumatic imagery**   Imagining the feelings of horror felt by the victim or reliving the horror of the incident

**triage**   Classification of clients to determine priority of need and proper place of treatment

**triglyceride**   Lipid compound consisting of three fatty acids and a glycerol molecule

**trocar**  Sharply pointed surgical instrument contained in a cannula

**Trousseau's sign**  Carpal spasm caused by inflating a blood pressure cuff above the client's systolic pressure and leaving it in place for 3 minutes

**trust**  Ability to rely on an individual's character and ability

**tumor marker**  Substance found in the serum that indicates the possible presence of malignancy

**turgor**  Normal resiliency of the skin

**type and cross-match**  Laboratory test that identifies the client's blood type (e.g., A or B) and determines the compatibility of the blood between potential donor and recipient

## U

**ultrasound**  Use of high-frequency sound waves to visualize deep body structures; also called an echogram or sonogram

**umbilical cord**  Structure that connects the fetus to the placenta

**uncomplicated grief**  Grief reaction normally following a significant loss

**unilateral neglect**  Failure to recognize or care for one side of the body

**unit dose form**  System of packaging and labeling each dose of medication by the pharmacy, usually for a 24-hour period

**urethrocele**  Downward displacement of the urethra into the vagina

**urethrostomy**  Formation of a permanent fistula opening into the urethra

**urge incontinence**  Inability to suppress the sudden urge or need to urinate

**urgent care center**  A facility designed for the effective and efficient treatment of acute illnesses and injuries; clients do not require an appointment, do not see the same provider consistently, and are usually seen in the order of arrival or the order of acuity

**urobilinogen**  Colorless derivative of bilirubin formed by the normal bacterial action of intestinal flora on bilirubin

**urticaria**  Allergic reaction causing raised pruritic, red, nontender wheals on the skin; also called hives

**uterine retraction**  Unique ability of the muscle fibers of the uterus to remain shortened to a small degree after each contraction

**uterine souffle**  Sound of blood pulsating through the uterus and placenta

**utility**  Ethical principle that states that an act must result in the greatest positive benefit for the greatest number of people involved

## V

**value system**  Individual's collection of inner beliefs that guides the way the person acts and helps determine the choices the person makes

**values**  Influences on the development of beliefs and attitudes rather than behaviors; a principle, standard, or quality considered worthwhile or desirable

**values clarification**  Process of analyzing one's own values to better understand those things that are truly important

**variable deceleration**  Reduction in fetal heart rate that has no relationship to contractions of the uterus

**vasectomy**  Surgical resection of the vas deferens

**venipuncture**  Puncturing of a vein with a needle to aspirate blood

**ventilation**  Movement of gases into and out of the lungs

**veracity**  Ethical principle based on truthfulness (neither lying nor deceiving others)

**verbal communication**  Using words, either spoken or written, to send a message

**verbally aggressive**  Descriptor of an individual who says things in a loud and/or intimidating manner

**vernix caseosa**  White, creamy substance covering a fetus's body

**vertigo**  Dizziness

**vesicant**  Agent that may produce blisters and tissue necrosis

**vesicular sound**  Soft, breezy, low-pitched sound heard longer on inspiration than expiration resulting from air moving through the smaller airways over the lung periphery, with the exception of the scapular area

**villi**  Finger-like projections that line the small intestine

**viral load test**  Test that measures copies of HIV RNA

**visceral pain**  Discomfort felt in the internal organs

**visual hallucination**  Perception by an individual that something is present when nothing in fact is

**visual learner**  Person who learns by processing information through seeing

**vitamin**  Organic compounds essential to life and health

**vitiligo**  Depigmentation of the skin caused by destruction of melanocytes; appears as milk-white patches on the skin

**void**  Process of urine elimination

**volvulus**  Twisting of a bowel on itself

## W

**water-soluble vitamin**  Vitamin that must be ingested daily in normal quantities because it is not stored in the body: vitamins C and B-complex

**wellness** State of optimal health wherein an individual maximizes human potential, moves toward integration of human functioning, has greater self-awareness and self-satisfaction, and takes responsibility for health

**Western blot test** Confirmatory test used to detect HIV infection

**Wharton's jelly** Thick substance surrounding and protecting the vessels of the umbilical cord

**whistleblowing** Calling public attention to unethical, illegal, or incompetent actions of others

**windowing** Cutting a hole in a plaster cast to relieve pressure on the skin or a bony area and to permit visualization of the underlying body part

**witch's milk** A whitish fluid secreted by a newborn's nipples

**withdrawal** Symptoms produced when a substance on which an individual has dependence is no longer used by that individual

**word salad** Nonsensical combination of words that is meaningless to others

**wound** Disruption in the integrity of body tissue

## Y

**yin and yang** Opposing forces that yield health when in balance

**young adulthood** Development from the ages of 21 years through approximately 40 years

## Z

**zoonotic disease** A disease of animals that is directly transmissible to humans from the primary animal host

**zygote** Fertilized ovum

# INDEX

Page numbers followed by "f" denote figures, "t" denote tables, and "b" denote boxes.